T0215165

Monoclonal Antibodies, Cytokines, and Arthritis

INFLAMMATORY DISEASE AND THERAPY

Series Editor

Daniel E. Furst
*University of Medicine and Dentistry
of New Jersey
Robert Wood Johnson Medical School
New Brunswick, New Jersey
and Pharmaceuticals Division
CIBA-GEIGY Corporation
Summit, New Jersey*

Monoclonal Antibodies, Cytokines, and Arthritis

Mediators of Inflammation and Therapy

edited by
Thomas F. Kresina

Miriam Hospital
Brown University
International Health Institute
Providence, Rhode Island

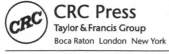
CRC Press
Taylor & Francis Group
Boca Raton London New York

CRC Press is an imprint of the
Taylor & Francis Group, an **informa** business

CRC Press
Taylor & Francis Group
6000 Broken Sound Parkway NW, Suite 300
Boca Raton, FL 33487-2742

First issued in paperback 2019

© 1991 by Taylor & Francis Group, LLC
CRC Press is an imprint of Taylor & Francis Group, an Informa business

No claim to original U.S. Government works

ISBN-13: 978-0-8247-8116-3 (hbk)
ISBN-13: 978-0-367-40298-3 (pbk)

Library of Congress Cataloging--in--Publication Data

Monoclonal antibodies, cytokines, and arthritis: mediators of
    inflammation and therapy/edited by Thomas F. Kresina.
        p.   cm.
    Includes bibliographical references and index.
    ISBN 0-8247-8116-3 (alk. paper)
        1. Arthritis-- --Immunotherapy. 2. Monoclonal antibodies--
    --Therapeutic use-- --Testing. 3. Cytokines-- --Physiological effect.
    4. Arthritis-- --Immunological aspects. 5. Arthritis-- --Animal models.
    I. Kresina, Thomas F.
        [DNLM: 1. Antibodies, Monoclonal-- --therapeutic use. 2. Arthritis,
    Rheumatoid-- --therapy. 3. Cytokines-- --physiology. 4. Immunotherapy.
    WE 346 M751]
    RC933.M66   1991
    616.7'22061-- --dc20
    DNLM/DLC
    for Library of Congress   91–6715
                                                                    CIP

Visit the Taylor & Francis Web site at
http://www.taylorandfrancis.com

and the CRC Press Web site at
http://www.crcpress.com

Dedicated with Love to My Daughters

RACHEL ANN, JENNIFER LYNN
and REBECCA MARIE

Series Introduction

As knowledge of inflammation and immunology has flourished over the last decade, understanding of the pathogenesis and therapy of inflammatory and immunologically mediated diseases has also progressed. This has been particularly true in the rheumatic diseases, including infectious rheumatic diseases, those rheumatic diseases associated with gastrointestinal inflammation, immunologically mediated diseases, various forms of vasculitis, metabolic diseases with rheumatic manifestations, and so forth.

Marcel Dekker, Inc., which specializes in high-quality monographs in a variety of focused medical disciplines, has supplied up-to-date, detailed, and practical information for both the practicing physician and research scientist. The Inflammatory Disease and Therapy Series addresses a number of carefully chosen topics of interest to practicing physicians, rheumatologists, and research scientists. These topics include a wide range of therapeutic options, basic research as it applies to human disease, and diagnostic tools that may arise from the burgeoning knowledge about inflammation and immunology.

Daniel E. Furst

Preface

In recent years musculoskeletal research has generated new technologies for the potential amelioration of inflammation and the resultant pathology in musculoskeletal diseases. Three significant advances in biomedical research have influenced the rapid development of new avenues of musculoskeletal disease research. The first is technological innovations that allow for stable antibody-secreting hybridomas which generate both murine and human monoclonal antibodies. Second, modern recombinant DNA technology allows for the identification and further characterization of these monoclonal antibodies as well as the delineation of cellular receptors in autoimmunity. The third advance is the discovery and elucidation of the mechanisms by which the cells communicate both specifically and nonspecifically, that is, through cytokines or serological determinants such as idiotype–anti-idiotype interactions. The present textbook represents a sampling of the new and novel approaches to the amelioration of musculoskeletal disease pathology generated by these avenues of research.

This book emphasizes two aspects: prevention and therapy. Where applicable, these new technologies are focused on their application to human autoimmune diseases. But this volume mainly discusses and details the use of experimentally preventive or therapeutic methodologies in animal models of rheumatic diseases. It is hoped that this emphasis will further stimulate therapeutic and preventive investigations in musculoskeletal diseases, as well as new concepts for the development of experimental therapies with application to human populations. Thus, the initial chapters focus on human autoimmune diseases, emphasizing potential horizons and useful application of monoclonal antibodies in the rheumatic diseases. Also, the generation of human monoclonal antibodies and the ability to recover specific autoantibodies as clonal hybridoma-derived antibodies is summarized.

Subsequent chapters deal conceptually with biological therapies for rheumatoid arthritis—the cellular and molecular interactions in the induction of inflammation—with specific emphasis on the language of cellular interactions and delineation of cytokines in rheumatic diseases. Additional contributions show that inhibitors to specific cytokines could have a role in the prevention or therapy of rheumatic diseases, through either the direct inhibition of cartilage pathology or the regulation of specific enzymatic activities that degrade cartilage. Alternatively, cytokine antagonists could act as immunomodulators of arthritis pathology through their regulation of additional cytokine mediators that bind components of the extracellular matrix.

The role of T cells in experimental arthritis is investigated through two differing systems, examining heat-shock proteins, T-cell-derived antigen binding proteins, as well as the concept of antigen mimicry. Immunotherapy in the rheumatic diseases is emphasized by the use of anti-T-cell antibodies or anti-HMC or cytokine receptor antibodies and their effect on the regulation of experimentally induced arthritis pathology.

Also discussed is the role of B cells and antibodies in collagen-induced arthritis and in experimental spondylarthritis and immune synovitis. In the latter two models, emphasis is on the role of antiproteoglycan antibodies. Subsequent chapters deal with the breakdown products of proteoglycans of the extracellular matrix as a potential noninvasive marker of rheumatic diseases. Other contributions focus on the idiotypy of antibodies in arthritis and related diseases. Idiotype-anti-idiotype serology of rheumatoid factor and anti-DNA antibodies and the role of the idioype–anti-idiotype network conclude the selected topics on potential new or future therapeutic and preventive methodologies for the musculoskeletal diseases.

The information that follows would make Aesculapius and Hygieia, the Greek gods of therapy and prevention, smile. It is hoped that this compilation will serve as a stepping-stone to future therapeutic intervention and will be coupled with present therapy to form additional combination therapy protocols, thereby expanding the arsenal of weapons available to combat the rheumatic diseases.

Thomas F. Kresina

Contents

Contents

Contributors

Nabih I. Abdou, M.D., Ph.D. St. Luke's Hospital of Kansas City, Kansas City, Missouri

Mary Ann Accavitti, Ph.D. University of Alabama at Birmingham, Birmingham, Alabama

Howard Amital-Teplizki, M.D. Sheba Medical Center and Tel-Aviv University Medical School, Tel-Hashomer, Israel

Subhashis Banerjee, M.D. McGill University and Shriners Hospital for Crippled Children, Montreal, Quebec, Canada

Claude C. A. Bernard, Ph.D. Brain-Behaviour Research Institute, LaTrobe University, Bundoora, Victoria, Australia

Claire J. P. Boog, Ph.D. Faculty of Veterinary Medicine, University of Utrecht, Utrecht, The Netherlands

Edit Buzás, M.D. University of Medicine, Debrecen, Hungary

Giles V. Campion, M.D., M.R.C.P. Rush-Presbyterian-St. Luke's Medical Center, Chicago, Illinois

Dennis A. Carson, M.D.* Scripps Clinic and Research Foundation, La Jolla, California

Nancy L. Carteron, M.D. Veterans Administration Medical Center and the University of California, San Francisco, California

Pojen P. Chen, Ph.D.* Scripps Clinic and Research Foundation, La Jolla, California

Eric Dayer, M.D. Institut Central des Hôpitaux Valaisans, Sion, Switzerland

Gene DiPasquale, Ph.D. Pharmaceuticals Division, CIBA-GEIGY, Summit, New Jersey

Edward G. Engleman, M.D. Stanford University Medical Center, Stanford University School of Medicine, Stanford, California

Steven K. H. Foung, M.D. Stanford University Medical Center, Stanford University School of Medicine, Stanford, California

Susan Alpert Galel, M.D. Stanford University Medical Center, Stanford University School of Medicine, Stanford, California

Tibor T. Glant, M.D., Ph.D., D.Sc. Rush-Presbyterian-St. Luke's Medical Center, Chicago, Illinois, and the University of Medicine, Debrecen, Hungary

Christian Herzog, M.D. University of Basel, Basel, Switzerland

Gloria C. Higgins, Ph.D., M.D. College of Medicine, University of Tennessee, Memphis, Tennessee

Els J. M. Hogervorst Faculty of Veterinary Medicine, University of Utrecht, Utrecht, The Netherlands

Rikard Holmdahl, M.D., Ph.D. Uppsala University, Uppsala, Sweden

William J. Koopman, M.D. University of Alabama at Birmingham, Birmingham Veterans' Administration Hospital, Birmingham, Alabama

Thomas F. Kresina, Ph.D. Miriam Hospital and Brown University International Health Institute, Providence, Rhode Island

Klaus E. Kuettner, Ph.D. Rush-Presbyterian-St. Luke's Medical Center, Chicago, Illinois

Edward V. Lally, M.D. Brown University School of Medicine, Roger Williams General Hospital, Providence, Rhode Island

---

Present affiliation: University of California, San Diego, La Jolla, California.

Mary Ellen Lenz, M.S. Rush-Presbyterian-St. Luke's Medical Center, Chicago, Illinois

Ian R. Mackay, M.D. Centre for Molecular Biology and Medicine, Monash University, Clayton, Victoria, Australia

Brian A. Maldonado, Ph.D. Rush-Presbyterian-St. Luke's Medical Center, Chicago, Illinois

Katalin Mikecz, M.D., Ph.D. Rush-Presbyterian-St. Luke's Medical Center, Chicago, Illinois, and the University of Medicine, Debrecen, Hungary

Wolfgang Müller, M.D. University of Basel, Basel, Switzerland

Werner J. Pichler, M.D. Institute of Clinical Immunology, Inselspital, Berne, Switzerland

A. Robin Poole, Ph.D., D.Sc. Shriners Hospital for Crippled Children and McGill University, Montreal, Quebec, Canada

Arnold E. Postlethwaite, M.D. University of Tennessee, and Veterans' Administration Medical Center, Memphis, Tennessee

Merrill J. Rowley, Ph.D. Centre for Molecular Biology and Medicine, Monash University, Clayton, Victoria, Australia

Thomas J. Schnitzer, M.D., Ph.D. Rush-Presbyterian-St. Luke's Medical Center, Chicago, Illinois

Yehuda Shoenfeld, M.D. Sheba Medical Center and Tel-Aviv University Medical School, Tel-Hashomer, Israel

Ralph E. Schrohenloher, Ph.D. University of Alabama of Birmingham, Birmingham, Alabama

Donna J. Spannaus-Martin, Ph.D. Miriam Hospital and Brown University International Health Institute, Providence, Rhode Island

Vibeke Strand, M.D. XOMA Corporation, Berkeley, and University of California San Francisco School of Medicine, San Francisco, California

Ronsuke Suenaga, M.D. Research Laboratory, St. Luke's Hospital of Kansas City, Kansas City, Missouri

M. Barry E. Sweet, M.D., Ph.D. University of the Witwatersrand, Johannesburg, South Africa

Eugene J.-M. A. Thonar, Ph.D. Rush-Presbyterian-St. Luke's Medical Center, Chicago, Illinois

David E. Trentham, M.D.   Harvard Medical School and Beth Israel Hospital, Boston, Massachusetts

Mieke C. J. van Bruggen   University Hospital St. Radboud, Nijmegen, The Netherlands

Levinus B. A. van de Putte, Ph.D.   University Hospital St. Radboud, Nijmegen, The Netherlands

Wim B. van den Berg, Ph.D.   University Hospital St. Radboud, Nijmegen, The Netherlands

Maries F. van den Broek, Ph.D.   University Hospital St. Radboud, Nijmegen, The Netherlands

Ruurd van der Zee, Ph.D.   National Institute of Public Health and Environmental Protection, Bilthoven, The Netherlands

Willem van Eden, M.D., Ph.D.   Faculty of Veterinary Medicine, University of Utrecht, Utrecht, The Netherlands

Jan D. A. van Embden, Ph.D.   National Institute of Public Health and Environmental Protection, Bilthoven, The Netherlands

Peter L. E. M. van Lent   University Hospital St. Radboud, Nijmegen, The Netherlands

Sharon M. Wahl, Ph.D.   National Institute of Dental Research, National Institutes of Health, Bethesda, Maryland

Christoph Walker*   Institute of Clinical Immunology, Inselspital, Berne, Switzerland

Marca H. M. Wauben   Faculty of Veterinary Medicine, University of Utrecht, Utrecht, The Netherlands

James M. Williams, Ph.D.   Rush-Presbyterian-St. Luke's Medical Center, Chicago, Illinois

Paul H. Wooley, Ph.D.   Wayne State University Medical School, Detroit, Michigan

David Wofsy, M.D.   Veterans Administration Medical Center and the University of California, San Francisco, California

---

Present affiliation: Swiss Institute of Allergy and Asthma Research, Davos, Switzerland.

1

Monoclonal Antibodies: New Horizons in the Treatment of Human Autoimmune Disease

William J. Koopman

University of Alabama at Birmingham, Birmingham Veterans' Administration Hospital, Birmingham, Alabama

I. INTRODUCTION

The remarkable impact of monoclonal antibody (MAb) technology on biomedical research is amply documented within this volume. Moreover, continued refinements in MAb technology coupled with sustained progress in elucidation of the events underlying immune responses at the molecular level virtually ensure that subsequent editions of such volumes will be welcome.

Although high expectations exist regarding the efficacy of MAb therapy in human autoimmune diseases, it is clear that practical difficulties require solutions before these hopes are fulfilled. Host responses to therapeutic MAb and modulation of target antigens exemplify such difficulties. These problems not withstanding, a particularly appealing feature of MAbs in the therapy of autoimmune disease relates to their potential disease specificity. Antibodies directed at antigens expressed on broad lymphoid cell subsets (e.g., CD4, CD8, and CD3) or their products [e.g., interleukin-2 (IL-2), and interferon-γ] in themselves may have a role, but strategies employing such antibodies are also likely to suppress desirable immune responses with attendant adverse consequences. Unfortunately, significant gaps exist regarding the pathogenesis of many autoimmune diseases, which limits the options available for specific MAb therapy at this time. The target antigens for such diseases as rheumatoid arthritis (RA), ankylosing spondylitis (AS), and polymyositis (PM) remain unknown. Lack of such information retards efforts to identify variable region elements of the T (and B) cell repertoire essential to the induction and perpetuation of such diseases. Lessons learned from the study of reasonably well defined animal models of autoimmune disease, such as experimental allergic encephalomyelitis (EAE) in mice and rats, teach that the "filling in" of these knowledge gaps related to human autoimmune processes will enhance the likelihood of developing successful approaches to MAb therapy in human disease.

In this chapter, attention is directed toward a consideration of strategies for specific MAb therapy in human autoimmune disease.

II. IMMUNE RECOGNITION: FUNDAMENTAL CONCEPTS

The central role of helper T (T_H) cells in regulating both cellular and humoral immune responses is clear (1). Experience with anti-CD4 MAb therapy in several animal models of autoimmune disease, including collagen arthritis (2), murine systemic lupus erythematosus (SLE) (3), murine myasthenia gravis (4), EAE in mice (5) and rats (6), and murine diabetes (7), strongly indicates the efficacy of this approach and, by inference, the critical role of T_H cells in the induction and/or perpetuation of these diseases. Understanding of the minimal activation requirements for T_H cells therefore provides a framework for designing more specific interventions in these diseases.

Antigen-induced activation of T cells involves a complementary interaction between the binding site of the T cell receptor (TCR) and a complex on the surface of the antigen presenting cell (APC) consisting of an antigen fragment associated with an appropriate major histocompatibility complex (MHC) molecule (Fig. 1). Three polymorphic structures therefore determine the specificity of this interaction—the MHC antigen binding cleft, the bound antigen peptide, and the TCR binding site (generated by the variable regions of the TCR β and α chains— or, alternatively, the TCR γ and δ chains). In the case of CD8$^+$ cytotoxic T cells (Tc) the recognized antigen fragment is associated with an MHC class I molecule, whereas CD4$^+$ T_H cells recognize a complex consisting of an antigen fragment bound to an MHC class II molecule. It is presumed that Tc are of critical importance in the pathogenesis of class I MHC gene-associated diseases, like AS, and T_H likely play a central role in diseases associated with MHC class II genes, such as RA.

Successful crystallization of a prototypic human class I MHC molecule has provided direct visualization of the antigen binding cleft in this molecule (8). A similar structural model for the antigen binding groove of class II MHC molecules has been proposed (9), and it is only a matter of time until crystallographic studies permit elucidation of the architecture of the binding cleft of these molecules. Precise identification and determination of the primary structure of the MHC molecule variable regions associated with specific diseases will provide critical

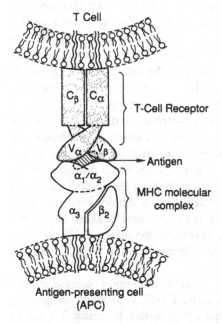

T Cell

T-Cell Receptor

Antigen

MHC molecular complex

Antigen-presenting cell
(APC)

Figure 1 Schematic representation of structures involved in antigen recognition by T cells. The T cell receptor (TCR) consists of two disulfide-bonded polypeptide chains designated α and β. Each TCR polypeptide possesses a variable region (V α or V β) and a constant region (C_α or C_β). The two V regions interact to form a binding site complementary to a complex composed of an antigen fragment occupying the antigen binding cleft of a self MHC molecules. In this diagram a MHC class I molecule is depicted consisting of an α heavy chain (with three domains designated α_1, α_2, and α_3) and β_2-migroglobulin. [From Kumar, V., Kono, D. H., Urban, J. L., and Hood, L. (1989). The T-cell receptor repertoire and autoimmune diseases. In: Annual Review of Immunology. Paul, W. E., Fathman, C. G., and Metzger, H., eds., Annual Reviews, Palo Alto, CA, p. 658. Reproduced with permission from the *Annual Review of Immunology*, Vol. 7. © 1989 by Annual Reviews, Inc.]

information suitable for ultimate modeling of the three-dimensional structure of the antigen binding sites relevant to disease pathogenesis. In this regard, considerable progress has been made in the elucidation of DRβ1 and DQβ1 variable region amino acid sequences associated with susceptibility to rheumatoid arthritis and insulin-dependent diabetes, respectively (10,11).

It should be stressed that information concerning the structure of MHC antigen binding clefts associated with disease susceptibility is also likely to provide important clues concerning the responsible antigen. At the very least, such information may permit the design of blocking peptides that preclude MHC binding by the offending antigen. Experimental evidence that different peptides can compete for MHC binding and T cell activation support the feasibility of this approach (12). Recently, Adorini and colleagues demonstrated that administration of a murine lysozyme peptide can block T cell priming in mice by a foreign lysozyme peptide, apparently by occupying binding sites on the relevant MHC molecule (I-A^k) (13). A complicating factor with regard to this strategy relates to the complexity of the immune response to the responsible target antigen(s). The possibility that multiple epitopes of the parent antigen may contribute to disease pathogenesis would obviously complicate strategies directed toward blockade of antigen-specific T cell activation. In the case of EAE, some strain variability exists regarding the dominant peptide on the inducing antigen (myelin basic protein , MBP) recognized by effector T cells responsible for mediating the disease. In strains PL and BIO.PL the major response to MBP involves amino acids (aa) 1–49 (14–16), whereas in the SJL strain an MBP peptide consisting of aa 89–101, which contains at least three overlapping epitopes, is immunodominant (17,18). Whether these variations are strictly related to MHC differences in the respective strains is not yet clear.

The remaining target for specific intervention in autoimmune disease encompasses the varible region of TCR structures on T cells capable of recognizing the MHC molecule-antigen peptide complex responsible for induction and/or perpetuation of the disease. Similarly, targeting of variable region structures on Ig molecules (idiotypes) directed against the disease-related antigen may be useful in diseases in which humoral immunity contributes to disease pathogenesis (e.g., myasthenia and SLE).

Evidence for a restricted variable region gene contribution to disease pathogenesis in some animal models provides encouragement for this approach. Indeed, in the PL mouse a highly restricted pattern of V region use is exhibited by T cells capable of mediating EAE; approximately 80% use $V_\beta 8.2$ and 100% a member of the $V_\alpha 4$ gene family (14–16,19). Restricted Ig idiotypes associated with pathologic autoantibody responses have been observed in murine models of lupus, particularly anti-DNA responses (20–22). In the human the identification of critical TCR variable region gene products in autoimune disease is hampered by lack of information in most cases concerning the responsible antigen(s). Interpretation of reports indicating restricted TCR V region gene expression at sites of tissue injury in RA (23,24) is therefore difficult in the absence of direct identification of the T cells responsible for causing the disease.

III. STRATEGIES FOR SPECIFIC MONOCLONAL ANTIBODY THERAPY OF HUMAN AUTOIMMUNE DISEASE

An optimal therapeutic agent for an autoimmune disease would abrogate a process(es) essential to the perpetuation of the disease without interrupting homeostatic immune functions. Evidence suggesting a central role for T cells in the pathogenesis of immune-mediated diseases is convincing and argues for the development of therapeutic modalities directed at T cell recognition events unique to each particular disease. Obviously such an approach must be regarded as a simplistic generalization, and indeed, a prominent role for B cells, perhaps independent of T cells, has been suggested for some autoimmune diseases. Nonetheless, the concept of tailoring interventions to the immune recognition events underlying a particular disease (be they T and/or B cell related) offers hope for avoiding unwanted suppression of otherwise beneficial immune system processes.

Other chapters in this volume convincingly document the exquisite specificity attainable with MAb technology in a variety of disciplines. Clearly it is this quality that renders so appealing the application of MAb technology to disease therapy. The possibility of designing MAbs capable of specifically blocking T (or B) cell recognition events critical in the pathogenesis of an autoimmune disease seems feasible; indeed, initial experiences with MAb therapy in animal models of autoimmune disease is particularly promising in this regard (see later). In considering the current model of recognition events underlying antigen-induced activation of T cells, two sites emerge as candidates for targets of MAb therapy: the antigen fragment-MHC molecule complex and the binding site of the complementary T cell receptor.

A. Antigen-MHC Complex

Monoclonal antibodies directed against MHC molecules have been effectively employed in the treatment of several animal models of autoimmune disease, include EAE (25), autoimmune thyroiditis (26), myasthenia gravis (27), and collagen-induced arthritis (28). In each case the MAb has been directed against the MHC class II allele associated with susceptibility to the disease and, therefore, likely recognizes an epitope related to the allele-specific hypervariable region sequence(s) located in the amino-terminal α_1 and β_1 domains of the molecule (there is essentially no experience with animal models of class I MHC-related autoimmune diseases). By inference it is presumed these MAbs bind to an epitope situated in or near the antigen binding cleft of the targeted MHC molecule and thereby interfere with antigen recognition by pathogenic T cells. Unfortunately, direct evidence supporting this mechanism of action for anti-MHC MAbs in animal models of autoimmune disease is lacking.

The aforementioned advances in identification of disease-associated MHC alleles in the human coupled with information concerning the variable region primary structures of these alleles should facilitate efforts to construct high-affinity MAbs directed against the antigen binding cleft of these molecules. These "antigen surrogates" would be anticipated to compete effectively with the antigen peptides responsible for inducing and/or perpetuating the disease. An obstacle likely to be encountered in the use of such antibodies is the induction of host antibodies directed against the MAb with resultant neutralization and potentially adverse clinical sequelae (29,30). Efforts to construct chimeric MAbs consisting of murine immunoglobulin variable regions grafted onto human constant and framework regions offers a promising approach to minimizing immunogenic "foreign" determinants present on the administered MAb (31,32). Alternatively, the successful construction of synthetic peptides derived from heavy- and light-chain complementary-determining regions that retain the antigen-binding properties of the parent MAb (33,34) is another promising approach to reducing host responses. Administration of anti-CD4 MAb in animal models has been associated with tolerance induction for simultaneously administered antigens (35,36) and therefore might be useful in circumventing host responses to anti-MHC MAb (or derived peptides).

An attractive feature of therapeutic strategies directed toward developing disease-specific anti-MHC MAbs relates to the fact that identification of the responsible antigen(s) is not essential. Nonetheless, evidence that dominant responses to disease-inciting antigens may involve several epitopes (e.g., EAE) raises the distinct possibility that multiple MHC alleles may need to be targeted for a particular disease.

B. T Cell Receptor Variable Region Determinants

Selective targeting of T cells bearing variable region structures complementary to the inciting antigen-MHC complex represents an alternative approach to disease-specific MAb therapy. As alluded to previously, EAE in some murine strains (PL) and the Lewis rat is associated with highly restricted expression of V_β and V_α gene products on encephalitogenic T cells. Administration of MAb directed against these TCR structures abrogates the development of EAE in both mice and rats (15,37).

It remains to be determined whether other autoimmune diseases are associated with highly restricted patterns of TCR V region use by pathogenetic T cells. In this regard mapping studies in the collagen-induced arthritis model in mice have implicated genomic TCR genes in the V_β 6 family as contributing to disease susceptibility (38).

In the absence of more detailed information concerning antigen(s) responsible for perpetuating a particular disease and the attendant TCR variable region genes associated with recognition of that antigen, it might be argued that strategies directed toward targeting disease-related TCR variable region structures are distant possibilities. Advances in modeling of disease-related MHC antigen binding clefts, however, may provide insights concerning aspects of the three-dimensional structure of complementary TCR V region structures and perhaps facilitate the development of MAbs directed against these V region conformations. Monoclonal anti-idiotype antibodies directed against MAbs reactive with disease-related MHC alleles would be of particular interest in this regard, since it is anticipated that binding sites of some of these anti-MHC antibodies might resemble those of TCR structures complementary to the MHC-antigen fragment complex. Thus, anti-ids might be useful probes for these complementary TCR structures.

A similar approach involves targeting Ig variable region structures associated with antibodies that play a pathologic role in a particular disease. In the case of murine SLE models, some success has been reported following the administration of anti-idiotypic MAbs directed against dominant anti-DNA antibody idiotypes expressed in the disease (39,40). The emergence of nonidiotypic bearing anti-DNA antibodies following such treatment, however, reflects the plasticity of the B cell repertoire, which represents a formidable obstacle likely to be encountered with this approach.

IV. SUMMARY

The emergence of considerable information concerning the stuctures involved in antigen recognition by T cells provides a useful framework for designing disease-specific therapeutic interventions. Administration of MAbs targeted against disease-related MHC alleles or TCR V region determinants has proven useful in ameliorating several autoimmune diseases in animal models, probably by virtue of interrupting T cell recognition events critical to the pathogenesis of these diseases. Progress in the identification of disease-related MHC alleles in human autoimmune disease should facilitate the development of potentially efficacious MAbs directed against these molecules. Gaps exist in our knowledge concerning the antigen(s) responsible for perpetuating human autoimmune diseases and the TCR V region structures employed in the recognition of these antigens; nonetheless, continued progress in the elucidation of disease-related TCR V region structures coupled with increasingly detailed knowledge of the configuration of disease-related MHC antigen binding clefts should facilitate construction of MAbs directed against these structures. The future availability of MAbs that bind disease-specific T cell recognition structures should ultimately provide a useful adjunct in the therapy of autoimmune diseases.

ACKNOWLEDGMENTS

Funding for this research supported in part by grants AR-03555 and AI-18745 and the Veterans Administration Research Program.

Appreciation is expressed to Mrs. Boula Constantine and Sandra Reid for their skillful preparation of this manuscript.

REFERENCES

1. Weiss, A. (1989). T lymphocytes. In: Textbook of Rheumatology. Kelley, W.N., Harris, E.D., Ruddy, S., and Sledge, C.B., eds. W.B. Saunders, Philadelphia, p. 148.
2. Ranges, G.E., Sriram, S., and Cooper, S.M. (1985). Prevention of type II collagen-induced arthritis by in vivo treatment with anti-L3T4. J. Exp. Med. 162:1105.
3. Wofsy, D., and Seaman, W.E. (1985). Successful treatment of autoimmunity in NZB/NZW F$_1$ mice with monoclonal antibody to L3T4. J. Exp. Med. 161:378.
4. Christadoss, P., and Dauphinée, M. (1986). Immunotherapy for myasthenia gravis: A murine model. J. Immunol. 136:2437.
5. Waldor, M.K., Sriram, S., Hardy, R., Herzenberg, L.A., Lanier, L., Tim, M., and Steinman, L. (1985). Reversal of experimental allergic encephalomyelitis with monoclonal antibody to a T-cell subset marker. Science 227:415.
6. Brostoff, S.W., and Mason, D.W. (1984). Experimental allergic encephalomyelitis: Successful treatment in vivo with a monoclonal antibody that recognizes T helper cells. J. Immunol. 133:1938.
7. Wang, Y., Hao, L., Gill, R.C., and Lafferty, K.J. (1987). Autoimmune disease in the NOD mouse is L3T4 T-lymphocyte dependent. Diabetes 36:535.
8. Bjorkman, P.J., Saper, M.A., Samraoui, B., Bennett, W.S., Strominger, J.L., and Wiley, D.C. (1988). Structure of the human class I histocompatibility antigen, HLA-A2. Nature 329:506.
9. Brown, J.H., Jardetzky, T., Saper, M.A., Samraoui, B., Bjorkman, P.J., and Wiley, D.C. (1988). A hypothetical model of the foreign antigen binding site of class II histocompatibility molecules. Nature 332:845.
10. Todd, J.A., Bell, J.J., and McDevitt, H.O. (1987). HLA-DQβ gene contributes to susceptibility and resistance to insulin-dependent diabetes mellitus. Nature 329:599.
11. Winchester, R.J., and Gregersen, P.K. (1988). The molecular basis of susceptibility to rheumatoid arthritis: The conformational equivalence hypothesis. Springer Semin. Immunopathol. 10:119.
12. Guillet, J.-G., Lai, M.Z., Brinte, T.J., Buus, S., Sette, A., Grey, H.M., Smith, J.A., and Gefter, M.L. (1987). Immunological self non-self discrimination. Science 235:865.
13. Adorini, L., Muller, S., Cardinaux, F., Lehmann, P.V., Falcioni, F., and Nagy, Z.A. (1988). In vivo competition between self peptides and foreign antigens in T-cell activation. Nature 334:623.
14. Acha-Orbea, H., Mitchell, D.J., Timmermann, L., Wraith, D.C., Tausch, G.S., Waldor, M.K., Zamvil, S.S., McDevitt, H.O., and Steinman, L. (1988). Limited heterogeneity of T cell receptors from lymphocytes mediating autoimmune encephalomyelitis allows specific immune intervention. Cell 54:263.
15. Urban, J.L., Kumar, V., Kono, D.H., Gomez, C., Horvath, S.J., Clayton, J., Ando, D.G., Sercarz, E.E., and Hood, L. (1988). Restricted use of T cell receptor V geners in autoimmune encephalomyelitis raises possibilities for antibody therapy. Cell 54:577.
16. Burns, F.R., Li, X., Shen, N., Offner, H., Chou, Y.K., Vandenbark, A., and Heber-Katz, E. (1989). Both rat and mouse T cell receptors specific for the encelphalitogenic determinants of myelin basic protein use similar Vα and Vβ chain genes. J. Exp. Med. 169:27.

17. Kono, D.H., Urban, J.L., Horvath, S.J., Ando, D.G., Saavedra, R.A., and Hood, L. (1988). Two minor determinants of myelin basic protein induce experimental allergic encephalomyelitis in SJL/J mice. J. Exp. Med. 168:213.

18. Sakai, K., Sinha, A.A., Mitchell, D.J., Zamvil, S.S., Rothbard, J.B., McDevitt, H.O., and Steinman, L. (1988). Involvement of distinct murine T-cell receptors in the autoimmune encephalitogenic response to nested epitopes of myelin basic protein. Proc. Natl. Acad. Sci. USA 85:8608.

19. Zamvil, S.S., Mitchell, D.J., Lee, N.E., Moore, A.C., Waldor, M.K., Sakai, K., Rothbard, J.B., McDevitt, H.O., Steinman, L., and Acha-Orbea, H. (1988). Predominant expression of a T cell receptor Vβ8 gene subfamily in autoimmune encephalomyelitis. J. Exp. Med. 167:1586.

20. Rauch, J., Murphy, E., Roths, J.B., Stollar, B.D., and Schwartz, R.S. (1982). A high frequency idiotypic marker of anti-DNA antibodies in MRL-1pr/1pr mice. J. Immunol. 129:236.

21. Hahn, B.H., and Ebling, F.H. (1987). Idiotypic restriction in murine lupus. High frequency of three public idiotypes on serum IgG in nephritic NZBxNZW F$_1$ mice. J. Immunol. 138:2110.

22. Gavalchin, J., Seder, R.A., and Datta, S.K. (1987). The NZBxSWR model of lupus nephritis. 1. Cross-reactive idiotypes of monoclonal anti-DNA antibodies in relation to antigenic specificity, charge, and allotype. Identification of interconnected idiotype families inherited from the normal SWR and autoimmune NZB parents. J. Immunol. 138:128.

23. Savill, C.M., Delves, P.J., Kioussis, K., Walker, P., Lydyard, P.M., Colaco, B., Shipley, M., and Roitt, I.M. (1987). A minority of patients with rheumatoid arthritis show a dominant rearrangement of T-cell receptor β chain genes in synovial lymphocytes. Scand. J. Immunol. 25:629.

24. Stamenkovic, I., Stegagno, M., Wright, K.A., Krane, S.M., Amento, E.P., Colvin, R.B., Duquesnoy, R.J., and Kurnick, J.T. (1988). Clonal dominance among T-lymphocyte infiltrates in arthritis. Proc. Natl. Acad. Sci. USA 85:1179.

25. Steinman, L., Rosenbaum, J.T., Sriram, S., and McDevitt, H.O. (1981). In vivo effects of antibodies to immune response gene products: Prevention of experimental allergic encephalomyelitis. Proc. Natl. Acad. Sci. USA 78:7111.

26. Vladutiu, A.O., and Steinman, L. (1987). Inhibition of experimental autoimmune thyroiditis in mice by anti-I-A antibodies. Cell. Immunol. 109:169.

27. Waldor, M.K., Sriram, S., McDevitt, H.O., and Steinman, L. (1983). In vivo therapy with monoclonal anti-I-A antibody suppresses immune responses to acetylcholine receptor. Proc. Natl. Acad. Sci. USA 80:2713.

28. Wooley, P.H., Luthra, H.S., Lafuse, W.P., Huse, A., Stuart, J.M., and David, C.S. (1985). Type II collagen-induced arthritis in mice. III. Suppression of arthritis by using monoclonal and polyclonal anti-Ia antisera. J. Immunol. 134:2366.

29. Jonker, M., Neuhaus, P., Zurcher, C., Fucello, A., and Goldstein, G. (1985). OKT4 and OKT4A antibody treatment as immunosuppression for kidney transplantation in rhesus monkeys. Transplantation 39:247.

30. Wofsy, D., Ledbetter, J.A., Hendler, P.L., and Searman, W.E. (1985). Treatment of murine lupus with a monoclonal anti-cell antibody. J. Immunol. 134:852.

31. Morrison, S.I., Johnson, M.J., Herzenberg, L.A., and Oi, V.T. (1984). Chimaeric human antibody molecules: Mouse antigen binding domains with human constant region domains. Proc. Natl. Acad. Sci. USA 81:6857.

32. Verhoeyen, M., Milstein, C., and Winter, G. (1988). Reshaping human antibodies: Grafting an antilysozyme activity. Science 239:1534.

33. Williams, W.V., Moss, D.A., Kieber-Emmens, T., Cohen, J.A., Myers, J.N., Weinber, D.B., and Greene, M.I. (1989). Development of biologically active peptides based on antibody structure. Proc. Natl. Acad. Sci. USA 86:5537.

34. Taub, R., Gould, R.J., Garsky, V.M., Ciccarone, T.M., Hoxie, J., Friedman, P.A., and Shattil, S.J., (1989). A monoclonal antibody against the platelet fibrinogen receptor contains a sequence that mimics a receptor recognition domain in fibrinogen J. Biol. Chem. 246:259.

35. Benjamin, R.J., and Waldmann, H. (1986). Induction of tolerance by monoclonal antibody therapy. Nature 320:449.

36. Gutstein, N.L., Seaman, W.E., Scott, J.H., and Wofsy, D. (1986). Induction of immune tolerance by administration of monoclonal antibody to L3T4. J. Immunol. 137:1127.

37. Owhashi, M., and Heber-Katz, E. (1988). Protection from experimental allergic encephalomyelitis conferred by a monoclonal antibody directed against a shared idiotype on T cell receptors specific for myelin basic protein. J. Exp. Med. 168:2153.

38. Banerjee, S.J., Haqqu, T.M., Luthra, H.S., Stuart, J.M., and David, C.S. (1988). Possible role of $V\beta$ T cell receptor genes in susceptibility to collagen-induced arthritis in mice. J. Exp. Med. 167:832.

39. Hahn, B.F., and Ebling, F.M. (1984). Suppression of murine lupus nephritis by administration of an anti-idiotypic antibody to DNA. J. Immunol. 132:187.

40. Teitelbaum, D., Rauch, J., Stollar, B.D., and Schwartz, R.S. (1984). In vivo effects of antibodies against a high frequency idiotype of anti-DNA antibodies. J. Immunol. 132:1282.

2

Therapeutic Application of Monoclonal Antibodies in the Rheumatic Diseases

Edward V. Lally
*Brown University School of Medicine, Roger Williams General Hospital,
Providence, Rhode Island*

I. INTRODUCTION

Successful, long-term pharmacologic management of rheumatic diseases has been
an elusive goal for physicians caring for individuals with these chronic disorders.
Arguably, there has been no single major development in the field of rheumatologic
therapeutics since the introduction of compound E in 1948 and its treatment of
patients with rheumatoid arthritis (1). Over the past four decades, however, the
quality of life in patients with rheumatic disease has been enhanced significantly
as a result of many factors, including improved methods for earlier diagnosis,
advances in the pharmacologic treatment of complications of rheumatic disease,
recognition of the importance of optimizing functional outcomes, and acceptable
management strategies for end-organ failure under some circumstances. In certain diseases, survival has also been prolonged. Nonetheless, there is mounting
frustration among rheumatologists over the fundamental inability to alter or modify
the natural course of most rheumatic disorders. This sentiment has been expressed
most vocally in the area of rheumatoid arthritis (2–5). Long-term studies evaluating
"second-line" or disease-modifying agents in this disorder have demonstrated
relatively little improvement in outcome and a high degree of patient and physician dissatisfaction with currently available antirheumatic drugs. The development of safe and effective therapies capable of predictably modulating

rheumatic disease expression for extendened periods is one of the most pressing issues in contemporary rheumatology.

Pharmacologic antirheumatic therapy has been developed traditionally through empiric channels. The beneficial effect of gold salts in rheumatoid arthritis was noted initially when this agent was administered as antimicrobial therapy because of its use in tuberculosis and the belief that rheumatoid arthritis was caused by an infectious agent (6). More recently, methotrexate has been employed successfully for the treatment of both rheumatoid and psoriatic arthritis (7–9), although the rationale for its use as well as its specific mechanism of action is not well understood (10). Drug treatment for arthritis remains largely empiric and produces symptomatic clinical improvement by reducing inflammation or by "suppressing" the immune system at multiple levels. Anti-inflammatory agents and cytotoxic or immunosuppressive drugs have dominated antirheumatic drug therapy for many years.

The great majority, if not all, of the rheumatic diseases are characterized by mild or profound abnormalities of immunologic function. Significant advances in molecular biology and immunogenetics have led to the identification of disease susceptibility genes that directly or indirectly promote clinical disease expression. Our understanding of inflammatory mediators as well as of the integrative circuits required for facile communication between immunocompetent cells has clarified pathophysiologic mechanisms in many rheumatic diseases. For the full impact of these discoveries to be realized, this accumulated knowledge must be applied innovatively to develop more specific means for modulating the immune system in a restricted yet specific and beneficial fashion.

As an accompaniment to recently acquired insight into immune dysregulation, several new therapeutic modalities for the treatment of rheumatic disease have been proposed on theoretical grounds, have been implemented in a few areas, and have been reviewed recently (11–15). Clinical trials of these therapies in humans are scarce, but they appear to offer potential for rheumatic disease modification. The present chapter reviews comprehensively the rationale for the use of monoclonal antibodies to treat a variety of rheumatic diseases and the preliminary results from a few small clinical trials that have been reported. Although the use of such antibodies as specific immunopharmacologic agents requires extensive study, this application holds considerable promise for antirheumatic therapy in the future.

II. MONOCLONAL ANTIBODIES AS THERAPEUTIC AGENTS

The era of monoclonal antibody (MAb) therapy began in 1975 when Köhler and Milstein generated MAbs from a B cell hybridoma (16). The next decade witnessed the mass production of large quantities of rodent MAbs for diagnostic and therapeutic use (17,18). Among other purposes, MAbs have been used to identify and characterize subpopulations of immunocompetent cells based on the specific reactivity of these reagents with cell surface receptors and activation antigens. The distribution of these cells in the circulation and in tissues under both normal and pathologic conditions has been analyzed using MAb technology. In rheumatology, MAbs directed against cell surface receptors, immune response gene products, circulating informational molecules, and components of connective tissue degradation have provided substantial insight into the pathogenesis of several rheumatic diseases, particularly rheumatoid arthritis and systemic lupus erythematosus. Since the advent of MAb technology, it has been particularly attractive to consider these compounds as therapeutic agents. Using MAbs, it is theoretically possible to modulate the immune network by acting to enhance or inhibit specific pathways in a highly predictable fashion to improve or correct immunologic abnormalities. It would also be possible to employ MAbs as carrier proteins for transporting chemotherapeutic agents to targeted cells or tissues. MAbs have been employed therapeutically in experimental systems to test efficacy in diseases with suitable animal models. For routine use in human disease, however, it will be necessary to develop and perfect human MAbs since immune reactions to "foreign"MAbs will hamper the regular administration of such proteins raised in other species.

The use of MAbs as therapeutic agents has been studied most extensively in the area of cancer treatment. In theory, MAbs against specific surface receptors on malignant cells home to, and bind uniformly to, these antigens. This interaction activates complement-mediated cytolysis or the antibody-antigen complex itself attracts cytotoxic lymphocytes. Tumor cells are killed. It is also possible to conjugate MAbs to a variety of cytotoxic agents that might exert their beneficial effect only on specific malignant cells and leave normal cell populations intact. In 1980, the first report of MAbs as anticancer agents in humans was published (19). Initial treatment efforts with MAbs in malignant disease employed murine sources, but more recently human MAbs have been developed for this purpose (20). This form of cancer immunotherapy has great potential, but it is still in its early stages and several pitfalls have already developed during its implementation (20).

The other clinical setting in which MAb therapy has matured is in organ transplantation. Anti-CD3 MAbs (MAbs directed against T cells) have been used in renal transplantation with beneficial results (21,22). These murine MAbs have been shown not only to suppress T cell function but also to enhance T cell activation and lymphokine release (23-25). Presumably because of this latter effect, significant toxicity has been reported in preliminary studies (24-27).

Major adverse reactions from MAb therapy in the areas of oncology and organ transplantation underscore the difficulty of administering murine proteins to humans. Predictably, patients may develop both acute systemic reactions from cytokine release and immune responses against these mouse proteins that would limit their use for long-term treatment. It is clear that MAbs as practical therapeutic agents will have to be generated from human sources. Techniques for the development of human lymphocyte hybridomas and high-titer monospecific antibodies have been refined (28–31) but not perfected (32). It is apparent that generating and utilizing human MAbs as therapeutic agents may be more complex than anticipated, and the need for more vigorous study in this area has been stressed (32).

The therapeutic use of MAbs in cancer and organ transplantation, as well as in animal models of autoimmune disease, has provided background for the potential utility of both murine and human MAbs in the management of patients with rheumatic disorders. The remainder of this chapter reviews the currently available evidence and future directions for the role of MAbs as antirheumatic agents in specific diseases.

III. RHEUMATOID ARTHRITIS

Rheumatoid arthritis (RA) is the prototypic inflammatory joint disease characterized by immunogenetic susceptibility, by profound abnormalities of humoral and cell-mediated immunity, by immunologically driven chronic synovitis, and by variable clinical expression, including the potential for joint destruction and for significant extra-articular manifestations (33,34). It is likely that adult RA can be understood on the basis of class II major histocompatibility complex (MHC) gene product expression and its selective influence on the immune system (33,35–37). Within the past decade, insights regarding the etiopathogenesis of RA have emerged from the arena of molecular biology at an accelerated pace. It is vital that developments regarding the genetic and immunologic aspects of RA be applied directly to the treatment of patients with this disease. Conventional therapies for RA have been palliative only in the short term, have been poorly studied methodologically, and have been associated with significant toxicity. Prevailing knowledge of the etiopathogenesis of RA, although imprecise, nonetheless provides a basis for the implementation of unique treatment strategies directed at specific, rather than global, abnormalities of immune function and regulation in this disorder. It should be possible to apply this knowledge to develop new pharmacologic agents that could potentially replace existing remedies.

The use of traditional "disease-modifying" antirheumatic drugs (DMARDs) or second-line agents has been based almost totally on empiricism, and the exact mechanism of action of most agents in this category remains obscure. The therapeutic benefit of these compounds as well as their proposed mechanisms of action have been reviewed (38,39). In patients with severe or refractory RA, there has been recent consideration given to combination chemotherapy with "cocktails" of traditional DMARDs and cytotoxic agents (40,41). Short-term improvement in some clinical parameters has been observed in certain patients in this category, but substantial long-term benefit has not been demonstrated and major toxicity with this form of treatment is predictable. Other forms of investigational therapy in RA have also been considered (42).

It is apparent that currently available DMARDs and broad-spectrum immunosuppressive agents do not provide the practicing physician with a suitable spectrum of therapeutic options in the long-term management of RA. Indeed, there has been renewed scrutiny recently of the concept of disease modification or remission in RA (2–5). In addition, there is increased recognition that RA is associated not only with significant morbidity but also with increased mortality (43). This latter observation imparts renewed urgency to the development of more specific and potent antirheumatic drugs. There is speculation and optimism that newer pharmacologic and nonpharmacologic interventions in RA, based on a clearer understanding of immune dysfunction in this disease, might potentially provide for successful patient management over many years (13–15).

Future immunomodulatory therapy in RA will be focused, in part, on the use of MAbs directed at specific targets in the pathogenetic schema of this disorder. Potentially, MAbs can be directed against cell surface receptors to stimulate or inhibit cell function, against soluble factors to block or enhance their effect, or against idiotypes of antibodies to regulate this important network. There are many theoretical points of intervention in RA, but the most attractive component targeted to date has been the T lymphocyte. The primary role of the CD4$^+$ T helper cell in the rheumatoid process (33,44–46), the accumulated knowledge of T cell activation in RA (47–49), and the anecdotal clinical experience with anti-T cell antibodies in animal models (50,51) and in human disease (52–54) have led to the use of MAb against T cells in RA.

In many therapeutic trials, clinical improvement in RA has been associated with preferential reduction or depletion of T cell subsets by a variety of methods. This observation has been demonstrated using gold (55), D-penicillamine (56,57), antimalarial compounds (57), thoracic duct drainage (58), lymphapheresis (59), lymphoplasmapheresis (60), and total lymphoid irradiation (61,62). More recently, cyclosporin A, a specific inhibitor of T helper cell activation (via inhibition of interleukin-2 production), has produced clinical improvement in RA (63–65).

In animal models, it has been possible to abrogate specific immune responses by pretreatment with anti-T cell antibodies. Wofsy and colleagues (66–68) prevented the development of nephritis in NZB × NZW mice by treating them with MAbs against L3T4, the murine analog of the CD4 T helper cell receptor in humans. Models of inflammatory arthritis have also been manipulated with MAbs reagents. Type II collagen-induced arthritis in mice (50) and adjuvant arthritis in rats (51) have been inhibited by pretreatment with anti-L3T4 and anti-CD4 MAbs, respectively.

There have been a few pilot studies analyzing the use of murine MAbs directed against T cell surface receptors in small numbers of patients with RA (Table 1). Herzog and colleagues (52) treated four patients with RA and one patient with

Table 1 Monoclonal Antibody Therapy in Patients with Rheumatic Disease[a]

Source of MAb	Directed against	Diagnosis	No. patients	Comments	Reference
Mouse	CD4	RA	4	All improved, 3–5 months; no side effects	Herzog et al. (52)
		PsA	1		
NS	CD5	R	16	8 initially responded, 3 with prolonged benefit; decrease in CD5+ cells; frequent allergic reactions	Caperton et al. (53)
Mouse	CD7	RA	4	2 transiently improved; no side effects; all developed antimouse Ig antibodies	Kirkham et al. (54)
Rat	IL-2R	RA	3	2 excellent responses for 3 months; no significant side effects	Kyle et al. (78)

[a]RA, rheumatoid arthritis; PsA, psoriatic arthritis; IL-2R, interleukin-2 receptor; NS, not stated.

psoriatic arthritis with intravenous monoclonal anti-CD4 MAbs for 7 days. There were no side effects, and all patients showed clinical improvement. Interestingly, three of the patients showed sustained clinical improvement after 5 months. A group of 16 patients with severe chronic RA were treated with MAbs against the pan-T cell antigen CD5 coupled to ricin A chain (XomaZyme H65) by Caperton and colleagues (53). Dose-dependent decreases in circulating CD5$^+$ lymphocytes were demonstrated in all patients, and 8 of 16 noted initial clinical improvement. Prolonged benefit at 5–7 months was noted in 3 patients. However, antibodies against the murine MAbs developed in treated patients and precluded repeated dosing.

Since it is expected that MAbs directed against pan-T-cell surface determinants react with all populations of T cells, including those subserving normal immune function, more specific MAb therapy might be directed at activated T cells and their surface receptors. Murine anti-CD7 MABs were used by Kirkham and colleagues to treat four patients with RA, and transient improvement occurred in two (54). MAbs against this particular T cell surface antigen were used because CD7 has been associated with T cell activation and many T cells bearing this antigen have been noted in the rheumatoid synovium (47). In this study, however, antimouse IgG antibodies developed in all patients by day 10 or 11 and resulted in minor allergic reactions.

Interleukin-2 (IL-2) is produced by mitogen-stimulated CD4$^+$ and CD8$^+$ T cells, and decreased concentrations of IL-2 and diminished IL-2 responsiveness have been described in RA (69–71). Recently, these abnormalities have been ascribed to an inhibitory factor produced in the synovial membrane (72,73). During active RA, IL-2 receptors (IL-2R) on circulating lymphocytes are decreased (74) and increased concentrations of soluble IL-2Rs have been noted in the serum and synovial fluid of RA and appear to correlate with disease activity (75,76). MAbs against IL-2Rs have been used in mice to suppress collagen-induced arthritis (77). Kyle and colleagues (78) treated three patients with refractory RA with a rat MAb against the IL-2R on activated T cells. Two patients showed a sustained beneficial response for 3 months and did not develop significant side effects. It would also appear feasible to direct MAbs against class II MHC antigens on the surface of activated T cells or antigen-presenting cells (APC) to abolish or abrogate antigen-driven immune events in RA (79). Pretreatment with monoclonal anti-Ia antibodies has been shown to inhibit murine collagen-induced arthritis (80), but this form of treatment has not been evaluated in human clinical trials.

Downregulation of rheumatoid factor (RF) production by B cells in RA might be accomplished using anti-idiotypic antibodies against cross-reactive idiotypes in RA (81). In vitro suppression by anti-idiotypic antibodies of RF from B lymphocytes in RA has been demonstrated (82) and could represent a means of influencing humoral immune dysregulation in this disorder. It is also theoretically possible to develop MAbs against B cells and their products, against various stimulatory and inhibitory cytokines, or against complement receptors in RA to effect clinical improvement. However, extending these concepts to the bedside will require additional years of investigation.

Finally, the same questions from the clinical arena that currently are pertinent regarding DMARDs will be applicable when evaluating MAb therapy in RA. Which patients will be candidates for these agents? At what stage in RA should they be introduced? Will they be cycled or given on a regular basis? Will concomitant therapy with other rheumatic drugs (e.g., nonsteroidal anti-inflammatory drugs) be feasible? Will they affect radiologic progression and be truly disease modifying? What will be their short- and long-term toxicity profiles? The current standards for detailed, methodologically sound clinical trials employed in the evaluation of antirheumatic agents in RA will need to be applied to MAb therapy to answer many of these questions.

IV. SYSTEMIC LUPUS ERYTHEMATOSUS

Systemic lupus erythematosus (SLE) in its fully expressed form serves as the classic human model for autoimmune disease. Animal models, particularly murine lupus, have provided significant insight into the nature of autoantibody production and its control by immunoregulatory cells (83). An array of autoantibodies are found in the serum of patients with SLE and may be directed at organ- or tissue-specific antigens, at cells or cell surface receptors, at cytoplasmic or nuclear constituents, or at circulating proteins, polypeptides, glycoproteins, nucleic acids, and nucleoproteins (84,85). Tissue injury and clinical disease expression in SLE may result directly from cytotoxic autoantibodies (e.g., hemolytic anemia or thrombocytopenia) or, more characteristically, from the deposition of cytotoxic antibody-autoantigen immune complexes in blood vessels and tissues (e.g., vasculitis, glomerulonephritis, serositis, and synovitis). The most specific autoantibodies in SLE are those directed against double-stranded DNA.

The clinical manifestations of SLE are protean and range from asymptomatic, "serologically active" SLE to fully expressed multisystemic disease associated with critical organ damage and significant mortality (86,87). Management strategies in SLE are developed based on the severity of clinical involvement (88). Most patients with SLE are controlled effectively with general supportive measures, anti-inflammatory medication, and symptomatic treatment for specific organ involvement. Severe compromise of major organs or cell lines in SLE usually requires therapy with corticosteroids and/or other generalized immunosuppressive agents, such as azathioprine or cyclophosphamide. The ability of these drugs or other therapeutic interventions to modify or retard the course of SLE or reduce mortality from this disorder has never been proved (89). Over the past four decades an increase in survival in SLE has been noted (87), but this improvement likely results from earlier diagnosis, better pharmacologic management of cardiovascular and infectious complications, and acceptable therapeutic alternatives for end-stage renal disease.

A better understanding of immunopathogenetic mechanisms in SLE should enable physicians to expect the development of more specific pharmacologic interventions designed to reverse or improve immune system abnormalities in this disorder. The use of MAbs as chemotherapeutic agents targeted to specific immune sites in SLE could lead potentially to better disease management and improved quality of life for lupus patients. To date, immunomanipulative therapy with MAbs in SLE has concentrated on three areas: T cell subpopulations and their surface receptors, soluble immune mediators, and idiotypic determinants on autoantibodies.

Investigations in murine lupus have demonstrated that autoimmune responses can be retarded by the use of MAbs directed against T cells. Wofsy, with Seaman, successfully treated murine lupus in NZB × NZW F_1 mice with rat anti-T cell antibodies (66–68). In these studies, MAbs were directed against the L3T4 surface molecule on T helper-inducer cells. This form of treatment significantly reduced circulating L3T4$^+$ T cells, diminished autoantibody concentrations, retarded renal disease, and prolonged life in these animals without eliciting antirat Ig reactions. These investigators subsequently treated the same strain of murine lupus with F(ab')$_2$ fragments of anti-L3T4 MAb and demonstrated similar inhibition of autoimmunity without T helper cell depletion (90). This experiment is highly significant since specific immunosuppression in this situation is quickly reversed with cessation of MAb therapy. Anti-L3T4 MAbs may exert a beneficial effect by blocking the interaction of T helper cells with antigenic determinants on antigen presenting cells (APCs) presented in the context of class II MHC molecules. Alternatively, or additionally, these MAbs could block T cell activation or activation-related events after binding to the surface antigens. These experiments using anti-T helper cell antibodies provide a rationale for the development of human MAbs directed against CD4$^+$ T helper cells. More careful study is required, however, to determine the differential effects of these MAbs on subsets of CD4$^+$ cells and on cells in various stages of activation.

MAb therapy in SLE might be directed more specifically at activated T cells and targeted to activation molecules, including Il-2Rs or class II MHC gene products. As in RA both decreased IL-2 production (91,92) and responsiveness (91,93) have been demonstrated in SLE. Recently, increased concentrations of soluble IL-2Rs were found in SLE and appear to correlate with disease activity (94,95). Anti-IL-2R MAbs have been demonstrated to suppress murine lupus nephritis (96). However, in mice, MAb therapy against IL-2Rs produces an inhibition of T suppressor-cytotoxic T cell responses, not of T helper cell responses (97), and also has been associated with increased levels of soluble IL-2R (98). Since cytotoxic T cell responses in SLE may already be impaired and since increased disease activity in human SLE may be associated with increased concentrations of soluble IL-2R (94,95), anti-IL-2R therapy in humans should be approached cautiously. Furthermore, in a recent report, therapy with cyclosporin A, a potent inhibitor of IL-2 production, was associated with an exacerbation of neurologic disease in SLE (99).

MAb therapy directed at class II MHC surface antigens on activated T cells has been considered in autoimmune diseases (79,100). Anti-I-A MAbs have been used to prevent experimental allergic encephalitis in mice (101) and to treat murine lupus nephritis (102). By suppressing haplotype-specific humoral immunity, this form of treatment could block antigen-specific responses that are under the control of immune response genes without interfering with normal immune function (103).

Another focus of MAbs in SLE is on their use as anti-idiotypic antibodies. Anti-idiotypic antibodies to anti-DNA have been shown to produce decreased levels of autoantibodies and disease suppression in murine lupus nephritis (104,105). Conjugation of anti-idiotypic MAbs with cytotoxic drugs could also eliminate B cell clones producing particular autoantibodies (106). However, not all autoantibodies are pathogenic and idiotypic restitution has been demonstrated in anti-DNA antibodies found in glomerular lesions of patients with SLE (107). Antiidiotypic antibodies to immunoglobulins not involved in the pathogenic sequence in SLE may be ineffective or may even augment the production of autoantibodies (108). Nonetheless, downregulation of autoantibody production by MAb therapy under some circumstances may have important clinical implications in SLE (109).

MAb therapy holds considerable promise for specific immunologic management of patients with SLE. MAbs against T cell subpopulations, against activation surface antigens, and against idiotypic determinants on autoantibodies have been investigated in experimental systems and have potential for human application. However, the intricate network of competing circuitry in SLE mandates that extreme caution be used when targeting therapy at isolated components studied in vitro. Refined manipulation of immune system components in experimental animals must be followed by controlled studies in patients with SLE to test therapeutic hypotheses. The era of routine MAb therapy in SLE appears to be several years away.

V. OTHER RHEUMATIC DISEASES

Newer immunomanipulative therapy, including MAbs, for the rheumatic diseases has been studied most extensively in RA and SLE. Both disorders represent rather common clinical syndromes with potential for significant progressive articular destruction and/or life-threatening multisystemic complications. Sophisticated techniques for studying immune dysfunction have been applied extensively in RA and SLE, and both diseases have suitable, albeit imperfect, animal models with which to study pathogenetic mechanisms and explore avenues for potential immunotherapy. Not surprisingly, antirheumatic therapy with MAbs has been evaluated almost exclusively in the context of these two conditions. However, abnormal regulatory circuits between immunocompetent cells are consistently noted in almost all rheumatic diseases. Although the sense of urgency to develop new treatment strategies for RA and SLE does not apply to most other rheumatic disorders, insight regarding immunopathology might be applied to develop more direct and specific therapy in such diseases. The application of MAb technology to treat rheumatic diseases other than RA and SLE is theoretical at present, but it is worth considering how these agents might be utilized for more specific immunomodulation.

A. Osteoarthritis

Osteoarthritis (OA), the most common type of chronic arthritis, is characterized by articular cartilage degradation, particularly of the major matrix macromolecule, proteoglycan, and by reactive new bone formation in the subchondral plate and at the joint margins (110,111). A clearer understanding of chondrocyte metabolism and the structure and function of cartilage collagens and proteoglycans has established that articular cartilage is truly a dynamic biologic tissue in both health and disease. Chondrocyte function and matrix synthesis are controlled tightly by mechanical, hormonal, and autocrine factors (111). The critical mismatch in OA is the inability of chondrocytes to increase their synthesis of new matrix at or above the rate of enzymatic degradation. The concept of OA as a "wear-and-tear," degenerative arthritis has been replaced by a model of cartilage pathology resulting from various metabolic and immunologic abnormalities. For example, soluble factors, particularly interleukin-1 (IL-1), released from the synovium in both primary and secondary OA, are important in mediating cartilage degradation (112–114). Lymphocytic infiltrates in the synovial membrane in OA are found commonly (115,116), and chondrocytes from osteoarthritic cartilage can be activated and induced to express Ia antigens by γ-interferon (117,118).

Clinically, OA results in pain and dysfunction in affected joints. Management strategies for symptomatic patients with OA include optimizing biomechanical advantages (especially in the spine and weight-bearing joints), providing physical therapy measures, administering pharmacologic agents to relieve pain and reduce inflammation, and considering an array of options for surgical intervention under appropriate circumstances (119). Treatment in OA is empiric, and there is little convincing evidence that available therapy is "disease modifying." Future directions for the treatment of OA include the development of agents refined to enhance chondrocyte synthetic capacity in a controlled fashion and/or inhibit mediators responsible for matrix depletion.

In the setting of cartilage biology and OA, MAbs have been employed most often as immunodiagnostic agents. MAbs directed against proteoglycans and their subunits and against type II collagen have been employed as measures of cartilage-specific breakdown products in OA (120–124). Their value as specific markers for early OA has been debated recently (125,126). The role of MAbs as therapeutic agents has not been explored in experimental models or in human OA. However, as an appreciation of the immunologic control of cartilage homeostasis and breakdown emerges, it should be possible to direct MAb therapy at particular targets in this area. T cells, particularly T helper-inducer cells, have been identified in the synovial membrane of patients with primary OA (116,127). The role of these cells in mediating cartilage damage in OA is uncertain, but their modulation by MAb therapy may be feasible. It has also been demonstrated that the cytokines IL-1, tumor necrosis factor α and interferon-γ may all potentially induce cartilage breakdown and inhibit proteoglycan synthesis in OA (112,114,128,129). Future MAb therapy directed at these cytokines or their cell surface receptors may provide a means for modulating disease expression in OA.

B. HLA-B27-Associated Arthropathies

The HLA-B27-associated arthropathies (seronegative spondyloarthropathies) comprise ankylosing spondylitis (AS), Reiter's syndrome (RS) and reactive arthritis (ReA), psoriatic arthritis (PsA), and the arthropathy of inflammatory bowel disease (AIBD). There is a highly significant association of these disorders with the class I MHC allele, HLA-B27. Approximately 96% of patients with the prototype disease, AS, are B27 positive (130) and significant proportions (60–80%) of patients with RS, ReA, PsA, and AIBD also carry this allele, depending in part on the presence or absence of spondylitis (131). The exact relationship between the B27 allele and the immunopathology of these disorders is uncertain (132,133). One hypothesis concerning the role of B27 in these diseases relates to "molecular mimicry" and implicates sequences on the hypervariable region of the B27 molecule that are homologous with antigenic determinants associated with certain infectious agents, particularly enteric pathogens (134,135). The molecular mimicry model, however, has been re-examined recently in AS (135,136) as well as in other diseases in this category (137).

Abnormalities of cell-mediated immunity have been studied in the B27-associated arthropathies. Populations of circulating T helper-inducer and T suppressor-cytotoxic cells in AS and ReA have been found to be normal (132,138,139). CD4$^+$ helper/inducer T cells are increased in the synovial fluid of patients with RS (140), whereas both CD4$^+$ and CD8$^+$ cells have been found to occur in equal proportions in the synovium of patients with AS (141). The recent descriptions of RS (142) and PsA (143) developing in patients with the acquired immunodeficiency syndrome (AIDS) raise questions regarding the primary role of the CD4$^+$ T cell in B27-related disorders. Since CD8$^+$ suppressor-cytotoxic T cells recognize foreign antigen in the context of class I surface molecules, the interaction between putative microbial antiens, CD8+ and CD4+ T cells, and HLA-B27 (or a closely linked allele) might be partly responsible for the induction of clinical disease in these disorders.

The seronegative spondyloarthropathies, as a group, are managed in remarkably similar fashion. Since the proportion of patients with progressive joint destruction and serious extraarticular manifestations in these disorders is lower than in RA, attention is focused on supportive care, physical therapy modalities, including exercise, and pharmacologic management with nonsteroidal anti-inflammatory drugs. The necessity for developing novel treatments for the few patients in this category with "refractory" disease is seldom debated among rheumatologists (144,145). Immunosuppressive therapy has been used successfully in small numbers of patients with RS (145,146) and PsA (9,147) with unremitting disease. Recently, cyclosporine has been shown to be of benefit in patients with psoriasis (148), and this may relate to its effect on CD4+ T cell function. There is currently no evidence that any single antirheumatic drug or specific intervention has the potential to modify the course of these diseases.

The strength of the association beween B27 and the seronegative spondyloarthropathies is so great that it is tempting to consider immunomanipulative therapy against the B27 molecule itself or against various T cell responses to this surface antigen. MAb therapy could potentially be useful in this regard, although such treatment has not been attempted to date. Until recently, the lack of a suitable animal model for B27-associated arthropathies has precluded the development and testing of therapeutic MAbs in this setting. However, the ability to transmit B27 genetic information in the transgenic mouse (149) may allow for future study in a controlled experimental system.

C. Systemic Sclerosis

Systemic sclerosis (SSc, scleroderma) is an acquired disorder of connective tissue with characteristic abnormalities of the microvascular circulation and fibrosis of affected organs and tissues (150). Dysregulation of connective tissue synthesis at the level of gene transcription has now been recognized as a significant defect in SSc (151,152). Although circulating autoantibodies are found in a great majority of patients with SSc, a more central pathogenetic role in this disorder has been attributed to abnormalities of cell-mediated immunity (150,152,153). Decreased numbers of circulating T lymphocytes have been found in SSc (154), as well as a reduced population of CD8+ suppressor cells (155). A critical role for natural killer cells have been proposed based on the reduced peripheral blood activity of these cells in early diffuse SSc (156). T cell activation has also been demonstrated in the peripheral blood (157) and in the dermal lesions (158) of SSc. Enhanced IL-2 production, particularly by CD4+ cells, correlates with early disease activity in this disorder (159,160) and supports a role for activated T cells in the pathogenesis of SSc.

At the present time, specific disease-modifying therapy for SSc is unavailable and current treatment regimens are empiric (150,161). As interconnecting immune circuits are unraveled in the pathogenetic scheme of SSc, it will be theoretically possible to direct intervention at specific abnormalities along these pathways. MAbs may be developed to interfere with critical cellular function or to block overactivity of various growth factors. Potential targets for MAb therapy would be T cells and/or their activation antigens, mast cells and their secreted products, fibroblasts, and cytokines or their receptors. Since there are no clinical studies to date using these agents in SSc, their potential beneficial effect is speculative. Information gained from the use of MAb therapy in other diseases, particularly RA and SLE, may stimulate investigations into their therapeutic application in SSc.

D. Inflammatory Muscle Disease

A central role for T cells in the pathogenesis of dermatomyositis/polymyositis (DM/PM) has been established (162). Traditional treatment for DM/PM has employed high-dose corticosteroids as first-line therapy (162). In patients refractory to these agents, or in whom toxicity develops, azathioprine, cyclophosphamide and methotrexate have all been used successfully (163–165). Recently, the success of "specific" immunomodulatory therapy in DM/PM with cyclosporin A (166,167) and total lymphoid irradiation (168,169) raises the possibility that anti T cell therapy with MAbs can be effective in patients with inflammatory muscle disease. At the present time, however, there are no clinical trials using MAb therapy to treat DM/PM. Data collected from therapeutic studies of MAbs in RA and SLE may provide a rationale for their use in PM/DM.

VI. CONCLUSIONS

Recent technological developments in the generation of MAbs have expanded their potentional role as therapeutic agents in the rheumatic diseases. In experimental systems, MAbs most often have targeted CD4$^+$ T cells, activation antigens (including class II MHC molecules and IL-2 receptors), and idiotypic determinants on autoantibodies. Beneficial prophylactic or therapeutic results have been demonstrated in animal models of inflammatory arthritis and autoimmunity. Small numbers of patients with rheumatic disease have been treated with MAbs, but their therapeutic application in humans require considerable additional study. Normal immune function and the immune dysregulation characteristically observed in the rheumatic diseases comprise complex multicomponent systems. Intervention along these pathways, even when carried out with monospecific MAbs that can be targeted, may produce unexpected amplification or inhibition of immune function. Furthermore, with the development of human MAbs, it will be important to package these agents pharmacologically and to analyze their pharmacokinetics, including biologic distribution, therapeutic plasma levels, elimination pathways, and drug-drug interactions. In this regard, it appears that the routine use of biologically active and pharmacologically available MAbs is several years away.

Although the era of immunologically targeted, high-technology drug therapy has begun, the associated optimism must be tempered. Careful clinical evaluation of new antirheumatic therapies, including MAbs, is as essential as the critical experiments that led to their development. MAbs deserve much more comprehensive study before they can be touted as panaceas for the rheumatic diseases.

REFERENCES

1. Hench, P.S., Kendall, V.C., Slocumb, C.H., and Polley, H.F. (1949). The effect of a hormone of the adrenal cortex (17-hydroxy-11-dehydrocorticosterone: compound E) and of pituitary adrenocorticotropic hormone on rheumatoid arthritis. Proc. Mayo Clin. 24:181–197.
2. Iannuzzi, L., Dawson, N., Zein, N., Kushner, I. (1983). Does drug therapy slow radiographic deterioration in rheumatoid arthritis? N. Engl. J. Med.; 309:1023–1028.
3. Scott, D. L., Symmons, D.P.M., Coulton, B.L., and Popert, A.J. (1987). Long-term outcome of treating rheumatoid arthritis: Results after 20 years. Lancet 1:1108–1111.
4. Gabriel, S.E., and Luthra, H.S. (1988). Rheumatoid arthritis: Can the long-term outcome be altered? Mayo Clin. Proc. 63:58–68.
5. Kushner, I. (1989). Does aggressive therapy of rheumatoid arthritis affect outcome (editorial)? J. Rheumatol. 16:1–4.
6. Forestier, J. (1935). Rheumatoid arthritis and its treatment by gold salts. The results of six years' experience. J. Lab. Clin. Med. 20:827–840.
7. Weinblatt, M.E., Coblyn, J.S., Fox, D. A., Fraser, P. A., Holdsworth, D.E., Glass, D.N., and Trentham, D.E. (1985). Efficacy of low-dose methotrexate in rheumatoid arthritis. N. Engl. J. Med. 312:818–822.
8. Kremer, J.M., and Lee, J.K. (1988). A long-term prospective study of the use of methotrexate in rheumatoid arthritis. Update ater a mean of fifty-three months. Arthritis Rheum. 31:577–584.
9. Wilkens, R.F. (1989). The use of methotrexate in the treatment of psoriatic arthritis. In: Methotrexate Therapy in Rheumatic Disease. Wilke, W.S., ed. Marcel Dekker, New York, pp. 287–294.
10. Bertino, J.R., and Dicker, A.P. (1989). On the mechanism of methotrexate action in rheumatoid arthritis. In: Methotrexate Therapy in Rheumatic Disease. Wilke, W.S., ed. Marcel Dekker, New York, pp. 129–144.
11. Dibner, M.D., and Ackerman, N.R., (1986). Biotechnology and new therapies for arthritis (editorial). J. Rheumatol. 13:997–999.

12. Ben-Yehuda, O., Tomer, Y., and Shoenfeld, Y. (1988). Advances in therapy of autoimmune diseases. Semin. Arthritis Rheum. 17:206–220.
13. Pincus, S.H. (1989). Immunoregulation and experimental therapies. In: Arthritis and Allied Conditions, McCarty, D.J., ed. Lea & Febiger, Philadelphia, pp. 622–645.
14. Klippel, J.H., Strober, S., and Wofsy, D. (1989). New therapies for the rheumatic diseases. Bull. Rheum. Dis. 38:1–8.
15. Trentham, D.E. (1989). Rheumatologic therapy for the 1990s. Evolution or revolution? Rheum. Dis. Clin. North Am. 15:407–412.
16. Köhler, G., and Milstein, C. (1975). Continuous cultures of fused cells secreting antibody of predefined specificity. Nature 256:495–497.
17. Diamond, B.A., Yelton, D.E., and Scharff, M.D. (1981). Monoclonal antibodies. A new technology for producing serologic reagents. N. Engl. J. Med. 304:1344–1349.
18. DePinho, R.A., Feldman, L.B., and Scharff, M.D. (1986). Tailor-made monoclonal antibodies. Ann. Intern. Med. 104:225–233.
19. Nadler, L.M., Stashenko, P., Hardy, R., Kaplan, W.D., Button, L.N., Kufe, D.W., Antman, S.H., and Schlossman, S.F., (1980). Serotherapy of a patient with a monoclonal antibody directed against a human lymphoma-associated antigen. Cancer Res. 40:3147–3154.
20. Dillman, R.O. (1989). Monoclonal antibodies for treating cancer. Ann. Intern. Med. 111:592–603.
21. Ortho Multicenter Transplant Study Group (1985). A randomized clinical trial of OKT3 monoclonal antibody for acute rejection of cadaveric renal transplant. N. Engl. J. Med. 313:337–342.
22. Ackerman, J.R., Lefor, W.M., Kahana, L., Weinstein, S., and Shires, D.L. (1988). Prophylatic use of OKT3 in renal transplantation: Part of a prospective randomized multicenter trial. Transplant. Proc. 20:242–244.
23. Hirsch, R., Gress, R.E., Pluznik, D.H., Eckhaus, and Bluestone, J.A. (1989). Effects of in vivo administration of anti-CD3 monoclonal antibody of T cell function in mice. II. In vivo activation of T cells. J. Immunol. 142:1737–1743.
24. Hirsch, R., Gress, R. E., and Bluestone, J.A. (1989). Anti-CD3 antibody for autoimmune disease, a cautionary note (letter). Lancet 1:1390.
25. Chatenoud, L., Ferran, C., and Bach, J.F. (1989). In-vivo anti-CD3 treatment of autoimmune patients (letter). Lancet 2:164.
26. Abramowicz, D., Schandene, L., Goldman, M., Crusiaux, A., Vereerstraeten, P., DePauw, L., Wybran, J., Kinnaert, P., Dupont, E., and Toussaint, C. (1989). Release of tumor necrosis factor, interleukin-2 and gamma-interferon in serum after injection of OKT3 monoclonal antibody in kidney transplant recepients. Transplantation 47:606–608.
27. Schatenoud, L., Ferran, C., Reuter, A., Legendre, C., Gevaert, Y., Kreis, H., Franchimont, P., and Bach, J. (1989). Systemic reaction to the anti-T-cell monoclonal antibody OKT3 in relation to serum levels of tumor necrosis factor and interferon-α (letter). N. Engl. J. Med. 320:1420–1421.
28. Olsson, L., and Kaplan, H.S. (1980). Human-human hybridomas producing monoclonal antibodies of predefined antigenic specificity. Immunology 77:5429–5431.

29. Carson, D.A., and Freimark, B. D. (1986). Human lymphocyte hybridomas and monoclonal antibodies. Adv. Immunol. 38:275–311.

30. Posner, M.R., Elboim, H., and Santos, D. (1987). The construction and use of a human-mouse myeloma analogue suitable for the routine production of hybridomas secreting human monoclonal antibodies. Hybridoma 6:611–625.

31. James, K., and Bell, G.T. (1987). Human monoclonal antibody production. Current status and future prospects. J. Immunol. Methods 100:5–21.

32. James, K., (1989). Human monoclonal antibody technology—Are its achievements, challenges, and potential appreciated? (editorial). Scand. J. Immunol. 29:257–264.

33. Zvaifler, N.J. (1989). Etiology and pathogenesis of rheumatoid arthritis. In: Arthritis and Allied Conditions, 11th ed. D.J. McCarty, ed. Lea & Febiger, Philadelphia, pp. 659–673.

34. Harris, E.D. (1989). The clinical features of rheumatoid arthritis. In: Textbook of Rheumatology, 3rd ed., Kelly, W.N., Harris, E.D., Jr., Ruddy, S., and Sledge, C.B. eds. W.B. Saunders, Philadelphia, pp. 943–981.

35. Gregersen, P.K., Silver, J., and Winchester, R. J. (1987). The shared epitope hypothesis. An approach to understanding the molecular genetics of susceptibility to rheumatoid arthritis. Arthritis Rheum. 30:1205–1213.

36. Nepom, G.T. (1988). Structural and genetic features of human leukocytic antigen class II elements associated with rheumatoid arthritis. Am. J. Med. (1989). 85(Suppl. 6A):12–13.

37. Moral, T.A., and Fathman, C.G. (1989). Immunogenetics of rheumatoid arthritis (editorial). J. Rheumatol. 16:421–423.

38. Bunch, T.W., and O'Duffy, J.D. (1980). Disease-modifying drugs for progressive rheumatoid arthritis. Mayo Clin. Proc. 55:161–179.

39. Tsokos, C.G., (1987). Immunomodulatory treatment in patients with rheumatic diseases: Mechanisms of action. Semin. Arthritis Rheum. 17:24–38.

40. McCarty, D.J., and Carrera, G.F. (1982). Intractable rheumatoid arthritis. Treatment with combined cyclophosphamide, azathioprine, and hydroxychloroquine. JAMA 248:1718–1723.

41. Walters, M.T., and Cawley, M.I.D. (1988). Combined suppressive drug treatment in severe refractory rheumatoid disease: An analysis of the relative effects of parenteral methylprednisolone, cyclophosphmide and sodium aurothiomalate. Ann. Rheum. Dis. 47:924–929.

42. Yunus, M.B. (1988). Investigational therapy in rheumatoid arthritis: A critical review. Semin. Arthritis Rheum. 17:163–184.

43. Pincus, T., and Callahan, L.F. (1986). Taking mortality in rheumatoid arthritis seriously—predictive markers, socioeconomic status and comorbidity (editorial). J. Rheumatol. 13:841–845.

44. Janossy, G., Panayi, G., Duke, O., Bofill, M., Poulter, L.W., and Goldstein, G. (1981). Rheumatoid arthritis: A disease of T-lymphocyte/macrophage immunoregulation. Lancet 2:839–842.

45. Morimoto, C., Romain, P.L., Fox, D.A., Anderson, P., DiMaggio, M., Levine, H., and Schlossman, S.F. (1988). Abnormalities in CD4+ T-lymphocyte subsets in inflammatory rheumatic diseases. Am. J. Med. 84:817–825.

46. Lasky, H.P., Bauer, K., and Pope, R.M. (1988). Increased helper inducer and decreased suppressor inducer phenotypes in the rheumatoid joint. Arthritis Rheum. 31:52–58.

47. Poulter, L.W., Duke, O., Panayi, G.S., Hobb, S., Raftery, M.J., and Janossy, G. (1985). Activated T-lymphocytes of the synovial membrane in rheumatoid arthritis and other arthropathies. Scand. J. Immunol. 22:683–690.

48. Keystone, E.C., Poplonski, L., Miller, R.G., Gorcyzynski, R., and Gladman, D. (1986). In vivo activation of lymphocytes in rheumatoid arthritis. J. Rheumatol. 13:694–699.

49. Cush, J.J., and Lipsky, P.E. (1988). Phenotypic analysis of synovial tissue and peripheral blood lymphocytes isolated from patients with rheumatoid arthritis. Arthritis Rheum. 31:1230–1238.

50. Ranges, G.E., Sriram, S., and Cooper, S.M. (1985). Prevention of type II collagen-induced arthritis by in vivo treatment with anti-L3T4. J. Expl. Med. 162:1105–1110.

51. Billingham, M.E.J., Griffin, E., and Hicks, C. (1988). Induction of tolerance to arthritis induction with anti-CD4 monoclonal antibodies (abstract). Br. J. Rheumatol. 27(Suppl. 2):34.

52. Herzog, C., Walker, C., Pichler, W., Aeschlimann, A., Wassmer, P. Stockinger, H., Knapp, W., Rieber, P., and Mueller, W. (1987). Monoclonal anti-CD4 in arthritis. Lancet 2:1461–1462.

53. Caperton, E., Byers, V., Shephard, J., Ackerman, S., and Scannon, P.J. (1989). Treatment of refractory rheumatoid arthritis (RA) with anti-lymphocyte immunotoxin (abstract). Arthritis Rheum. 32(Suppl.):S130.

54. Kirkham, B., Chikanza, I., Pitzalis, C., Kingsley, G.H., Grahame, R., Gibson, T., and Panayi, G.S. (1988). Response to monoclonal CD7 antibody in rheumatoid arthritis. Lancet 1:589.

55. Griswold, D.W., Lee, J.C., Poste, G., and Hanna, N. (1985). Modulation of macrophage-lymphocyte interactions by the antiarthritic gold compound, auranofin. J. Rheumatol. 12:490–497.

56. Lipsky, P.E. (1984). Immunosuppression by D-penicillamine in vitro. Inhibition of human T lymphocyte proliferation by copper or ceruloplasmin-dependent generation of hydrogen peroxide and protection by monocytes. J. Clin. Invest. 73:53–65.

57. Karlsson-Parra, A., Svenson, K., Hallgren, R., Klareskog, L., and Forsum, U. (1986). Peripheral blood T-lymphocyte subsets in active rheumatoid arthritis—effects of different therapies on previously untreated patients. J. Rheumatol. 13:263–268.

58. Ueo, T., Tanaka, S., Tominaga, Y., Ogawa, H., and Sakurami, T. (1979). The effect of thoracic duct drainage on lymphocyte dynamics and clinical symptoms in patients with rheumatoid arthritis. Arthritis Rheum. 22:1405–1412.

59. Karsh, J., Klippel, J.H., Plotz, P.H., Decker, J.L., Wright, D.G., and Flye, M.W. (1981). Lymphapheresis in rheumatoid arthritis. A randomized trial. Arthritis Rheum. 24:867–873.

60. Verdickt, W., Dequeker, J., Ceuppens, J.L., Stevens, E., Gautama, K., and Vermylen, C. (1983). Effect of lymphoplasmapheresis on clinical indices and T cell subsets in rheumatoid arthritis. A double-blind controlled study. Arthritis Rheum. 26:1419–1426.

61. Kotzin, B.L., Strober, S., Engleman, E.G., Calin, A., Hoppe, R.T., Kansas, G.S., Terrell, C.P., and Kaplan, H.S. (1981). Treatment of intractable rheumatoid arthritis with total lymphoid irradiation. N. Engl. J. Med. 305:969–976.

62. Gaston, J.S.H., Strober, S., Solovera, J.J., Gandour, D., Lane, N., Schurman, D., Hoppe, T., Chin, R.C., Eugui, E.M., Vaughn, J.H., and Allison, A.C. (1988). Dissection of the mechanisms of immune injury in rheumatoid arthritis, using total lymphoid irradiation. Arthritis Rheum. 31:21–30.

63. Weinblatt, M.E., Coblyn, J.S., Fraser, P.A., Anderson, R.J., Spragg, J., Trentham, D.E., and Austen, K.F. (1987). Cyclosporin A treatment of refractory rheumatoid arthritis. Arthritis Rheum. 30:11–17.

64. Dougados, M., Awada, H. and Amor, B. (1988). Cyclosporin in rheumatoid arthritis: A double bind placebo controlled study in 52 patients. Ann Rheum. Dis. 47:127–133.

65. Yocum, D.E., Klippel, J.H., Wilder, R.L., Gerber, N.L., Austin, H.A., Wahl, S.M., Lesko, L. Minor, J. R., Preuss, H.G., Yarboro, C., Berkehile, C., and Dougherty, S. (1988). Cyclosporin A in severe treatment-refractory rheumatoid arthritis. A randomized study. Ann. Intern. Med. 109:863–869.

66. Wofsy, D., and Seaman, W.E. (1985). Successful treatment of autoimmunity in NZB/NZW F1 mice with monoclonal antibody to L3T4. J. Exp. Med. 161:378–391.

67. Wofsy, D. (1986). Administration of monoclonal anti-T-cell antibodies retards murine lupus in BXSB mice. J. Immunol. 136:4554–4560.

68. Wofsy, D., and Seaman, W.E. (1987). Reversal of advanced murine lupus in NZB/NZW F1 mice by treatment with monoclonal antibody to L3T4. J. Immunol. 138:3247–3253.

69. Tan, P., Shore, A., Leary, P., and Keystone, E.C. (1984). Interleukin abnormalities in recently active rheumatoid arthritis. J. Immunol. 11:593–596.

70. Combe, B., Pope, R.M., Fischbach, M., Darnell, B., Baron, S., and Talal, N. (1985). Interleukin-2 in rheumatoid arthritis: Production of and response to interleukin-2 in rheumatoid synovial fluid, synovial tissue and peripheral blood. Clin. Exp. Immunol. 59:520–528.

71. McKenna, R.M., Ofosu-Appiah, W., Warrington, R.J., and Wilkins, J.A. (1986). Interleukin 2 production and responsiveness in active and inactive rheumatoid arthritis. J. Rheumatol 13:28–32.

72. Kashiwado, T., Miossec, P., Oppenheimer-Marks, N., and Ziff, M. (1987). Inhibitor of interleukin-2 synthesis and response in rheumatoid synovial fluid. Arthritis Rheum. 30:1339–1346.

73. Smith, M.D., Haynes, D.R., and Roberts-Thomson, P.J. (1989). Interleukin-2 and interleukin 2 inhibitors in human serum and synovial fluid. I. Characterization of the inhibitor and its mechanism of action. J. Rheumatol. 16:149–157.

74. Emery, P., Wood, N., Gentry, K., Stockman, A., Kackay, I.R., and Bernard O. (1988). High-affinity interleukin-2 receptors on blood lymphocytes are decreased during active rheumatoid arthritis. Arthritis Rheum. 31:1176–1181.

75. Symons, J.A., Wood, N.C., DiGiovine, F.S., and Duff, G.W. (1988). Soluble IL-2 receptor in rheumatoid arthritis. Correlation with disease activity, IL-1 and IL-2 inhibition. J. Immunol. 141:2612–2618.

76. Campen, D.H., Horwitz, D.A., Quismorio, F.P., Ehresmann, G.R., and Martin,
     W.J. (1988). Serum levels of interleukin-2 receptor and activity of rheumatic diseases
     characterized by immune system activation. Arthritis Rheum. 31:1358–1364.
77. Banerjee, S., Wei, B.Y., Hillman, K., Kuthra, H.S., and David, C.S. (1988). Im-
     munosuppression of collagen-induced arthritis in mice with an anti-IL-2 receptor an-
     tibody. J. Immunol. 141:1150–1154.
78. Kyle, V., Coughlan, R.J., Tighe, H., Waldmann, H., and Hazelman, B.L. (1989).
     Beneficial effect of monoclonal antibody to interleukin 2 receptor on activated T cells
     in rheumatoid arthritis. Ann. Rheum. Dis. 48:428–429.
79. Sany, J. (1988). Treatment of rheumatoid arthritis by antibodies directed against class
     II MHC antigens. Scand. J. Rheumatol. (Suppl.) 76:289–295.
80. Cooper, S.M., Sriram, S., and Ranges, G.E. (1988). Suppression of murine collagen-
     induced arthritis with monoclonal anti-Ia antibodies and augmentation with IFN-γ.
     J. Immunol. 141:1958–1962.
81. Carson, D.A., Chen, P.P., Kipps, T.J., Radoux, V., Jirik, F.R., Goldfien, R.D.,
     Fox, R.I., Silverman, G.J., and Fong, S. (1987). Idiotypic and genetic studies of
     human rheumatoid factors. Arthritis Rheum. 30:1321–1325.
82. Takeuchi, T., Hosono, O.P., Koide, J., Homma, M., and Abe, T. (1985). Suppres-
     sion of rheumatoid factor synthesis by antiidiotypic antibody in rheumatoid arthritis
     patients with cross-reactive idiotypes. Arthritis Rheum. 28:873–880.
83. Steinberg, A.D., Raveche, E.S., Laskin, C.A., Smith, H.R., Santoro, T., Miller,
     M.L., and Plotz, P.H. (1984). Systemic lupus erythematosus: Insights from animal
     models. Ann. Intern. Med. 100:714–727.
84. Mackay, I.R. (1987). Autoimmunity in relation to lupus erythematosus. In: Dubois'
     Lupus Erythematosus, 3rd ed. Wallace, D.J., and Dubois, E.L., eds. Lea & Febiger,
     Philadelphia, pp. 44–52.
85. Woods, V.L., and Zvaifler, N.J. (1989). Pathogenesis of systemic lupus
     erythematosus. In: Textbook of Rheumatology, 3rd ed. Kelly, W.N., Harris, E.D.,
     Jr., Ruddy, S., and Sledge, D.B., eds. W.B. Saunders, Philadelphia, pp. 1077–1100.
86. Dubois, D.L., and Wallace, D.J. Clinical and laboratory manifestations of systemic
     lupus erythematosus. In: Dubois' Lupus Erythematosus, 3rd ed., Wallace, D.J., and
     Dubois, E.L., eds. Lea & Febiger, Philadelphia, pp. 317–449.
87. Bresnihan, B. (1989). Outcome and survival in systemic lupus erythematosus. Ann.
     Rheum. Dis. 48:443–445.
88. Rothfield, N.F. (1989). Systemic lupus erythematosus: Clinical aspects and treat-
     ment. In: Arthritis and Allied Conditions, 11th ed. McCarty, D.J. (ed.), Lea &
     Febiger, Philadelphia, pp. 1022–1048.
89. Lieberman, J.D., and Schatten, S. (1988). Treatment: Disease-modifying therapies.
     Clin. Rheum. Dis. 14:223–243.
90. Carteron, N.L., Schimenti, C.L., and Wofsy, D. (1989). Treatment of murine lupus
     with F(ab')2 fragments of monoclonal antibody to L3T4. Suppression of autoim-
     munity does not depend on T helper cell depletion. J. Immunol. 142:1470–1475.
91. Alcocer-Varela, J., and Alarcon-Segovia, D. (1982). Decreased production of and
     response to interleukin-2 by cultured lymphocytes of patients with systemic lupus
     erythematosus. J. Clin. Invest. 69:1388–1392.

92. Linker-Israeli, M., Bakke, A.C., Kitridou, R.C., Gendler, S., Gillis, S., and Horwitz, D.A. (1983). Defective production of interleukin 1 and interleukin 2 in patients with systemic lupus erythematosus (SLE). J. Immunol. 130:2651–2655.
93. Lakhanpal, S., and Handwerger, B.S. (1987). Interleukin 2 receptors and responsiveness to recombinant human interleukin 2 in patients with systemic lupus erythematosus. Mayo Clin. Proc. 62:3–7.
94. Wolf, R.E., and Brelsford, W.G. (1988). Soluble interleukin-2 receptors in systemic lupus erythematosus. Arthritis Rheum. 31:729–735.
95. Tokano, Y., Murashima, A., Takasaki, Y., Hashimoto, H., Okumura, K., and Hirose, S. (1989). Relation between soluble interleukin 2 receptor and clinical findings in patients with systemic lupus erythematosus. Ann. Rheum. Dis. 48:803–809.
96. Kelley, V.E., Gaulton, G.N., Hattori, M., Ikegami, H., Eisenbarth, G., and Strom, T.V. (1988). Anti-interleukin 2 receptor antibody suppresses murine diabetic insulitis and lupus nephritis. J. Immunol. 140:59–61.
97. Leist, T.P., Kohler, M., Eppler, M., and Zinkernagel, R.M. (1989). Effects of treatment with IL-2 receptor specific monoclonal antibody in mice. Inhibition of cytotoxic T cell responses but not of T help. J. Immunol. 143:628–632.
98. Volk, H.D., Josimovic-Alasevic, O., Ross, M., and Diamantstein, T. (1989). The therapeutic efficacy of an anti-IL-2 receptor monoclonal antibody correlates with an increase in serum soluble IL-2 receptor levels. Clin. Exp. Immunol. 76:121–125.
99. Makeover, D., Freundlich, B., and Zurier, R.B. (1988). Relapse of systemic lupus erythematosus in a patient receiving cylosporine A. J. Rheumatol. 15:117–119.
100. Todd, J.A., Acha-Orbea, H., Bell, J.I., Chao, N., Fronek, Z., Jacob, C.O., McDermott, M., Sinha, A.A., Timmerman, L., Steinman, L., and McDevitt, H.O. (1988). A molecular basis for MHC class II-associated autoimmunity. Science 240:1003–1009.
101. Steinman, L., Rosenbaum, J. T., Sriram, S., and McDevitt, H.O. (1981). In vivo effects of antibodies to immune response gene products: Prevention of experimental allergic encephalitis. Proc. Natl. Acad. Sci. USA 78:7111–7114.
102. Adelman, N.E., Watling, D.L., and McDevitt, H.O. (1983). Treatment of (NZB × NZW) F1 disease with anti-I-A monoclonal antibodies. J. Exp. Med. 154:1350–1355.
103. Rosenbaum, J.T., Adelman, N.E., and McDevitt, H.O. (1981). In vivo effects of antibodies to immune response gene products. I. Haplotype-specific suppression of humoral immune responses with a monoclonal anti-I-A. J. Exp. Med. 154:1694–1702.
104. Hahn, B.H., and Ebling, F.M. (1983). Suppression of NZB/NZW murine nephritis by administration of syngeneic monoclonal antibody to DNA. Possible role of anti-idiotypic antibodies. J. Clin. Invest. 71:1728–1736.
105. Hahn, B.H., and Ebling, F.M. (1984). Suppression of murine lupus nephritis by administration of an anti-idiotypic antibody to anti-DNA. J. Immunol. 132:187–191.
106. Sasaki, T., Muryoi, T., Takai, O., Tamate, E., Ono, Y., Koide, Y, Ishida, N., and Yoshinga, K. (1986). Selective elimination of anti-DNA antibody-producing cells by antiidiotypic antibody conjugated with neocarzinostatin. J. Clin. Invest. 77:1382–1386.

107. Kalunian, K.C., Panosian-Sahakian, N., Ebling, F.M., Cohen, A.H., Louie, J.S., Kaine, J., and Hahn, B.H. (1989). Idiotypic characteristics of immunoglobulins associated with systemic lupus erythematosus. Studies of antibodies in glomeruli of humans. Arthritis Rheum. 32:513–522.

108. Teitelbaum, D., Rauch, J., Stollar, D.B., and Schwartz, R.S. (1984). In vivo effects of antibodies against a high frequency idiotype of anti-DNA antibodies in MRL mice. J. Immunol. 132:1282–1285.

109. Wats, R.A., and Isenberg, D.A. (1988). Idiotypes and anti-idiotypes: What are they trying to tell us? Ann. Rheum. Dis. 47:705–707.

110. Mankin, H.J., and Brandt, K.D. (1989). Pathogenesis of osteoarthritis. In: Textbook of Rheumatology, 3rd ed. Kelly, W.N. Harris, E.D., Jr., Ruddy, S., and Sledge, D.B. eds. W.B. Saunders, Philadelphia, pp 1469–1479.

111. Hamerman, D. (1989). The biology of osteoarthritis. N. Engl. J. Med. 320:1322–1330.

112. Dingle, J.T., Page Thomas, D.P., King, B., and Bard, D.R. (1987). In vivo studies of articular tissue damage mediated by catabolin/interleukin 1. Ann. Rheum. Dis. 46:527–533.

113. Appel, A.M., Hopson, C.N., and Herman, J.H. (1988). Modulation of cartilage proteoglycan synthesis by osteoarthritic synovium. J. Rheumatol. 15:1515–1524.

114. Morales, T.I., and Hascall, V.C. (1989). Factors involved in the regulation of proteoglycan metabolism in articular cartilage. Arthritis Rheum. 32:1197–1201.

115. Goldenberg, D.L., Egan, M.S., and Cohen, A.S. (1982). Inflammatory synovitis in degenerative joint disease. J. Rheumatol. 9:204–209.

116. Revell, P.A., Mayston, V., Lalor, P., and Mapp, P. (1988). The synovial membrane in osteoarthritis: A histological study including the characterization of the cellular infiltrate present in inflammatory osteoarthritis using monoclonal antibodies. Ann. Rheum. Dis. 47:300–307.

117. Burmester, G.R., Menche, D., Merryman, P., Klein, M., and Winchester, R. (1983). Application of monoclonal antibodies to the characterization of cells eluted from human articular cartilage. Expression of Ia antigens from certain diseases and identification of an 85-kD cell surface molecule accumulated in the pericellular matrix. Arthritis Rheum. 26:1187–1195.

118. Jahn, B., Burmester, G.R., Schmid, H., Weseloh, G., Rohwer, P., and Kalden, J.R. (1987). Changes in cell surface antigen expression on human articular chondrocytes induced by gamma-interferon. Induction of Ia antigens. Arthritis Rheum. 30:64–74.

119. Brandt, K.D. (1989). Management of osteoarthritis. In: Textbook of Rheumatology, 3rd, ed. Kelly, W.N., Harris, E.D., Jr., Ruddy, S., and Sledge, C.B., eds. W.B. Saunders, Philadelphia, pp. 1501–1512.

120. Kresina, T.F., Malemud, C.J., and Moskowitz, R.W. (19867). Analyis of osteoarthritic cartilage using monoclonal antibodies reactive with rabbit proteogylcan. Arthritis Rheum. 29:863–871.

121. Thonar, E.J.A., Lenz, M.E., Klintworth, G.K., Caterson, B., Pachman, L.M., Glickman, P., Katz, R., Huff, J., and Kuettner, K.E. (1985). Quantification of

keratan sulfate in blood as a marker of cartilage catabolism. Arthritis Rheum. 28:1367–1376.

122. Witter, J., Roughley, P.J., Webber, C., Roberts, N., Keystone, E., and Poole, A.R. (1987). The immunologic detection and characterization of cartilage proteoglycan degradation products in synovial fluids of patients with arthritis. Arthritis Rheum. 30:519–529.

123. Posner, M.R., Barrach, H.J., Elboim, H.S., Nivens, K., Santos, D.J., Chichester, C.O., and Lally, E.V. (1989). The generation of hybridomas secreting human monoclonal antibodies reactive with type II collagen. Hybridoma. 8:187–197.

124. Moreland, L.W., Stewart, T., Gay, R.E., Huang, G.Q., McGee, N., and Gay, S. (1989). Immunohistologic demonstration of type II collagen in synovial fluid phagocytes of osteoarthritis and rheumatoid arthritis patients. Arthritis Rheum. 32:1458–1464.

125. Hascall, V.C., and Glant, T.T. (1987). Proteoglycan epitopes as potential markers of normal and pathologic cartilage metabolism. Arthritis Rheum. 30:586–588.

126. Brandt, K.D. (1989). A pessimistic view of serologic markers for diagnosis and management of osteoarthritis. Biochemical, immunologic and clinicopathologic barriers. J. Rheumatol. (Suppl. 18) 16:39–42.

127. Reidbord, H.E., and Osial, T.A. (1987). Synovial lymphocyte subsets in rheumatoid arthritis and degenerative joint disease. J. Rheumatol 14:1089–1094.

128. Saklatvala, J. (1986). Tumour necrosis factor α stimulates resorption and inhibits synthesis of proteogylcan in cartilage. Nature 322:547–549.

129. Goldring, M.B., Sandell, L.A., Stephenson, M.L., Amento, E.P., and Krane, S.M. (1985). Immune interferon suppresses levels of procollagen mRNA and type II collagen synthesis in human chondrocytes (abstract). Arthritis Rheum. 28(Suppl.):542.

130. Kahn, M.A. (1984). Ankylosing spondylitis. In: Spondyloarthropathies. Calin, A. (ed.) Grune & Stratton, Orlando, FL, pp. 69–117.

131. Arnett, F.C. (1984). HLA and the spondyloarthropathies. In: Spondyloarthropathies. Calin, A. (ed.) Grune & Stratton, Orlando, FL, pp. 297–321.

132. McGuigan, L.E., Geczy, A.F., and Edmonds, J.P. (1985). The immunopathology of ankylosing spondylitis—a review. Semin. Arthritis Rheum. 15:81–105.

133. Calin, A. (1989). Ankylosing spondylitis. In: Textbook of Rheumatology, 3rd ed. Kelly, W.N., Harris, E.D., Jr., Ruddy, S., and Sledge, C.B., eds. W.B. Saunders, Philadelphia, pp. 1021–1027.

134. Oldstone, M.B.A. (1987). Molecular mimicry and autoimmune disease. Cell 50:819–820.

135. Yu, D.T.Y., Choo, S.Y., and Schaack, T. (1989). Molecular mimicry in HLA—B27-related arthritis. Ann. Intern. Med. 111:581–591.

136. Geczy A.F., Prendergast, J.K., Sullivan, J.S., Upfold, L.I., McGuigan, L.E., Bashir, H.V., Prendergast, M., and Edmonds, J.P., (1987). HLA-B27, molecular mimicry, and ankylosing spondylitis: Popular misconceptions. Ann. Rheum. Dis. 46:171–172.

137. Inman, D., Chiu, B., Johnston, M.E.A., and Falk, J. (1986). Molecule mimicry in Reiter's syndrome: Cytotoxicity and ELISA studies of HLA-microbial relationships. Immunology 58:501–506.

138. Vinje, O., Dobloug, J.H., Forre, O., Moller, P., and Mellbye, O.J. (1982). Immunoregulatory T cells in the peripheral blood of patients with Bechterew's syndrome. Ann. Rheum. Dis. 41:41–46.

139. Veys, E.M., Verbruggen, G., Hermanns, P., Mielants, H., Van Bruewaene, P., DeBrabanter, G., DeLandsheere, D., and Immesoete, C. (1983). Peripheral blood T lymphocytes sub-populations in HLA-B27 related rheumatic diseases: Ankylosing spondylitis and reactive synovitis. J. Rheumatol. 10:140–143.

140. Nordstrom, D., Konttinen, Y.T., Bergroth, V., and Leirisalo-Reto, M. (1985). Synovial fluid cells in Reiter's syndrome. Ann. Rheum. Dis. 44:852–856.

141. Kidd, B.L., Moore, K., Walters, M.T., Smith, J.L., and Cawley, M.I.D. (1989). Immunohistological features of synovitis in ankylosing spondylitis: A comparison with rheumatoid arthritis. Ann. Rheum. Dis. 48:92–98.

142. Winchester, R., Berstein, D.H., Fischer, H.D., Enlow, R., and Solomon, G. (1987). The co-occurrence of Reiter's syndrome and acquired immunodeficiency. Ann. Intern. Med. 106:19–26.

143. Espinoza, L.R., Berman, A., Vasey, F.B., Cahalin, C., Nelson, R., and Germain, B.F. (1988). Psoriatic arthritis and acquired immunodeficiency syndrome. Arthritis Rheum. 31:1034–1040.

144. Rosenthal, M. (1979). Is there a place for corticosteroids or immune modulation in treating Reiter's syndrome or ankylosing spondylitis? Ann. Rheum. Dis. 38(Suppl.):100–101.

145. Lally, E.V., and Ho, G. (1985). A review of methotrexate therapy in Reiter syndrome. Semin. Arthritis Rheum. 15:139–145.

146. Calin, A. (1986). A placebo controlled, crossover study of azathioprine in Reiter's syndrome. Ann. Rheum. Dis. 45:653–655.

147. Vasey, F.B., and Espinoza, L.R. (1984). Psoriatic arthropathy In: Spondyloarthropathies. Calin. A. ed. Grune & Stratton, Orlando, FL, pp. 151–185.

148. Ellis, C.N., Gorsulowski, D.C., Hamilton, T.A., Billings, J.K., Brown, M.D., Headington, J.T., Cooper, K.D., Baadsgaard, O., Duell, E.A., Annesley, T.M., Turcotte, J.G., and Voorhees, J.J. (1986). Cyclosporine improves psoriasis in a double-blind study. JAMA 256:3110–3116.

149. Taurog, J.D., Lowen, L., Forman, J., and Hammer, R.E. (1988). HLA-B27 in inbred and non-inbred transgenic mice. Cell surface expression and recognition as an alloantigen in the absence of human β_2-microglobulin. J. Immunol. 141:4020–4023.

150. Seibold, J.R. (1989). Scleroderma. In: Textbook of Rheumatology, 3rd ed. Kelly, W.N., Harris, E.D., Jr., Ruddy, S., and Sledge, C.B., eds. W.B. Saunders, Philadelphia, pp. 1215–1234.

151. Ohta, A., and Uitto, J. (1987). Procollagen gene expression by scleroderma fibroblasts in culture. Inhibition of collagen production and reduction of proα1 (I) and proα1 (III) collagen messenger RNA steady-state levels by retinoids. Arthritis Rheum. 30:404–411.

152. LeRoy, E.C., Smith, E.A., Kahaleh, M.B., Trojanowska, M., and Silver, R.M. (1989). A strategy for determining the pathogensis of systemic sclerosis. Is transforming growth factor β the answer? Arthritis Rheum. 32:817–825.

153. Kahaleh, M.B., and LeRoy, E.C. (1989). The immune basis for human fibrotic disease especially scleroderma (systemic sclerosis). Clin. Asp. Autoimmun. 3:19–28.
154. Inoshita, T., Whiteside, T.L., Rodnan, G.P., and Taylor, F.H. (1981). Abnormalities of T lymphocyte subsets in patients with systemic sclerosis (PSS, scleroderma). J. Lab. Clin. Med. 97:264–277.
155. Whiteside, T.L., Kumagai, Y., Roumm, A.D., Almendinger, R., and Rodnan G.P. (1983). Suppressor cell function and T lymphocyte sub-populations in peripheral blood of patients with progressive systemic sclerosis. Arthritis Rheum. 26:841–847.
156. Miller, E.B., Hiserodt, J.C., Hunt, L.E., Steen, V.D., and Medsger, T.A. (1988). Reduced natural killer cell activity in patients with systemic sclerosis. Correlation with clinical disease type. Arthritis Rheum. 31:1515–1522.
157. Kahan, A., Gerfaux, J., Kahan, A., Joret, A.M., Menkes, C.J., and Amor, B. (1989). Increased proto-oncogene expression in peripheral blood T lymphocytes from patients with systemic sclerosis. Arthritis Rheum. 32:430–436.
158. Roumm, A.D., Whiteside, T.L., Metsger, T.A., and Rodnan, G.P. (1984). Lymphocytes in the skin of patients with progressive systemic sclerosis. Quantification, subtyping, and clinical correlations. Arthritis Rheum. 27:645–653.
159. Umehara, H., Kumagai, S., Ishida, H., Suginoshita, T., Maeda, M., and Imura, H. (1988). Enhanced production of interleukin-2 in patients with progressive systemic sclerosis. Hyperactivity of CD4-positive T cells? Arthritis Rheum. 31:401–407.
160. Kahaleh, M.B., and LeRoy, E.C. (1989). Interleukin-2 in scleroderma: Correlation of serum level with extent of skin involvement and disease duration. Ann. Intern. Med. 110:446–450
161. Wollheim, F.A., and Akesson, A. (1989). Treatment of systemic sclerosis in 1988. Semin. Arthritis Rheum. 18:181–188.
162. Plotz, P.H., Dalakas, M., Leff, R.L., Love, L.A., Miller, F.W., and Cronin, M.E. (1989). Current concepts in the idiopathic inflammatory myopathies: Polymyositis, dermatomyositis, and related disorders. Ann. Intern. Med. 111:143–157.
163. Bunch, T.W. (1981). Prednisone and azathioprine for polymyositis: Long-term followup. Arthritis Rheum. 24:45–48.
164. Bombardieri, S., Hughes, G.R.V., Neri, R., Del Bravo, P., and Del Bono, L. (1989). Cyclophosphamide in severe polymyositis (letter). Lancet 1:1138–1139.
165. Lally, E. V. (1989). The use of methotrexate in the treatment of Reiter's syndrome, polymyositis/dermatomyositis, and other connective tissue diseases. In: Methotrexate Therapy in Rheumatic Disease, Wilke, W.S., ed. Marcel Dekker, New York, pp. 295–312.
166. Zabel, T., Leimenstoll, G., and Gross, W.L. (1984). Cyclosporin for acute dermatomyositis (letter). Lancet 1:343.
167. Heckmatt, J., Hasson, N., Saunders C., Thompson, N., Peters, A.M., Cambridge, G., Rose, M., Hyde, S.A., and Dubowitz, V. (1989) Cyclosporin in juvenile dermatomyositis. Lancet 1:1063–1066.
168. Engel, W.K., Lichter, A.S., and Galdi, A.P. (1981). Polymyositis: Remarkable response to total body irradiation (letter). Lancet 1:658.
169. Morgan, S.H., Bernstein, R.M., Coppen, J., Halnan, K.E., and Hughes, G.R.V. (1985). Total body irradiation and the course of polymyositis. Arthritis Rheum. 28:831–834.

3

Treatment of Patients with Rheumatoid Arthritis with Anti-CD4 Monoclonal Antibodies

Christian Herzog and Wolfgang Müller
University of Basel, Basel, Switzerland

Christoph Walker* and Werner J. Pichler
Institute of Clinical Immunology, Inselspital, Berne, Switzerland

I. INTRODUCTION

Rheumatoid arthritis (RA) is a disease of unknown etiology with substantial evidence that T lymphocytes, specifically CD4$^+$ cells, play an important role in the pathogenesis of the rheumatoid inflammatory process: (1) Immunohistology of synovial membranes showed that CD4 cells are several times more numerous than those bearing the CD8 antigens and that the CD4 cells are in close apposition to major histocompatibility complex (MHC) class II bearing accessory cells (1,2). (2) RA is genetically linked to HLA class II structures, specifically HLA DR3 and 4, which are membrane structures for presenting antigenic fragments to CD4$^+$ cells (3). (3) The clinical improvement of RA after total lymphoid irradiation (TLI) can be attributed to a quantitative and functional impairment of CD 4 cells (4,5).

Since the immunosuppressive therapy of RA is unsatisfactory, new treatments are at present under study. These include therapies with interferon-γ (IFN-γ), cyclosporin A, and monoclonal antibodies (MAbs) (6). In humans, MAb have already been used to reverse renal allograft rejection and to treat cancer and multiple sclerosis (7–9). In mice they have been used to prevent and/or reverse autoimmune diseases, including systemic lupus erythematosus, multiple sclerosis, and rheumatoid arthritislike diseases (10–13). However, both in humans and in mice

---

Present Affiliation: Swiss Institute of Allergy and Asthma Research, Davos, Switzerland.

the use of MAbs has generally been complicated by the development of a host immune response to therapy (7–13). An exception to this rule occurs if one treats mice with rat MAbs to L3T4, the mouse homolog for the human CD4 antigen. Treatment of mice with rat MABs to L3T4 not only fails to elicit a humoral and cellular immunity, it also retards autoimmunity and allows induction of tolerance to some antigens (14–16). These observations made CD4 MAb a promising candidate for an effective treatment of rheumatoid arthritis.

In the present study we summarize our experience with anti-CD4 MAb treatment in eight patients with arthritis (17,18). The results presented provide some insight to the distribution of T cell subsets during such a treatment and suggest an involvement of CD4 cells in the pathogenesis of rheumatoid arthritis, as a beneficial effect of CD4 MAb treatment was seen on the clinical course of RA. In addition, our studies regarding the mechanism of the immunosuppressive effect of anti-CD4 MAb treatment are also reviewed (18).

II. MATERIALS AND METHODS

A. Patients

A group of seven patients with clinically severe RA who fullfilled the American Rheumatism Association criteria (19) for definite or classic RA and one patient with clinically active psoriatic arthritis (patient 2) were evaluated (Table 1). Excluded from the study were patients with a serious concomitant medical illness.

At the entry and follow-up visits various laboratory parameters were evaluated (Table 2). A complete list of previous basic therapy is given in Table 3. Patient 1 had been previously treated with TLI (1984). Before the start of therapy, cytotoxic drugs, antimetabolites, gold, and D-penicillamine were discontinued for at least 8 weeks. Prednisone was given continuously in a dose of 5 mg/day before, during, and after antibody therapy in patients 1–7 but was stopped before MAb therapy in patient 8.

B. Characteristics of Monoclonal Anti-CD4 Antibodies Chosen for Study

Both antibodies VIT4 and MT151 have been characterized biochemically and immunologically (20) and were prepared for in vivo use according to the recommendations published in collaboration with the Gesellschaft für Immunologie (21). Studies by Sattentau et al. (22) suggested that both MAbs detect a similar epitope on the CD4 antigen as they similarly inhibited human immunodeficiency virus (HIV)-induced syncytium formation and showed the same cross-competition pattern between monoclonal antibodies to CD4 (see Ref. 22 and own observations). These in vitro nonmodulating antibodies of the mouse IgG_{2a} isotype induced

Table 1 Patient Characteristics

Age	
Mean	51
Range	36–70
Sex	
Female	4
Male	4
Disease	
Rheumatoid arthritis	7
Psoriatic arthritis	1
Disease duration, years	
Mean	8.6
Range	4–13
Anatomic stage	
II	3
III	5
Functional class	
II	2
III	6
Rheumatoid factor titer, 1:600	6
Prednisone, 5 mg/day	7

complement-dependent cytotoxicity in the presence of rabbit but not of human complement.

C. Administration of Anti-CD4 Antibodies

Before therapy, the patients received 5 mg of the antihistamine clemastin IV (Tavegyl) daily. At 7 a.m. the MAb was administered intravenously over 15 minutes (diluted in 20 ml 0.9% NaCl) at a dosage of 10 mg daily for 7 days. Prednisone at a dose of 5 mg daily (PO) was maintained (except in patient 8), and patients were allowed to take a small dose of an NSAID. A total of six patients were hospitalized during treatment, but fully mobilized. Patients 3 and 7 were treated on an out patient basis.

D. Clinical Assessment

The clinical disease variables determined at each visit consisted of (1) Ritchie index, (2) duration of morning stiffness, (3) evaluation of pain by visual analog scale, and (4) mean grip strength for both hands.

Overall responses to treatment were judged using the following arbitrary designations: (1) therapeutic remission, defined by the preliminary criteria of the

Table 2 Treatment Plan and Clinical and Laboratory Investigations[a]

	Before treatment	Day											
		1	2	3	4	5	6	7	8	14	21	
Clinical investigations													
Morning stiffness	x	x	x	x	x	x	x	x	x	x	x	Weekly
Pain assessment												
Ritchie articular index												
Laboratory investigations													
ESR, HB, thrombocytes, RC WBC and differential, serum creatinine, urine status, SGOT, SGPT, AP	x	x		x		x		x	x	x	x	Weekly
Ic, complement factors C3, C4	x	x	x						x	x		Every 4 weeks
Rheumatoid factors, CRP	x								x	x		Every 4 weeks
AB to EBV, HSV-1	x	x										
Skin multitest	x				x							Day 56
T, B cells and subsets and functional analysis (lymphocyte stimulation, antibody coating, antigen modulation, MLC)[b]	x	x	x				x	x				
Serum levels of CD4			x	x	x	x	x	x				
Antimouse response			x	x	x	x	x	x	x		x	Weekly

[a]Monoclonal anti-CD4 antibodies, 10 mg/day.
[b]At 7 (before injection), 9, and 11 a.m. and 5 p.m.

Table 3 Previous Basic Therapy[a]

	Patient							
	1	2	3	4	5	6	7	8
	IL-1 release inhibitor, TLI	Salazosulfapyridine, IL-1 release inhibitor, retinoid			Podophyllin, salazosulfapyridine, azoridine	Podophyllin	Retinoid, salazosulfapyridine	Podophyllin
Gold salts	+	+	+	+	+	+	+	+
D-penicillamine	+	-	+	+	+	+	-	-
Antimalarial drugs	+	+	+	+	+	-	-	+
Azathioprine	+	+	+	+	-	-	-	+
Methotrexate	-	+	-	-	+	-	-	-
Cyclosporin A	+	+	-	-	-	-	-	-

[a] All patients were continuously on prednisolone 5 mg/day, which was stopped only in patient 8 before and during therapy.

American Rheumatism Association (23); (2) marked improvement of the Ritchie articular index or of pain assessment, defined as a decrease of 50% or more at week 12 or 16 compared with the value at entry; (3) moderate improvement; defined as a decrease of 30–50% on an index; (4) no change, designated when an index remained within 30% of its original value; and (5) worsening, designated by an increase of 30% or more in an index.

E. Analysis of Lymphocyte Subsets

Monoclonal antibodies for cell identification and stimulation were obtained from Behringwerke [Marburg, FRG; BMA030-F(ab')$_2$], Coulter Clone (Hialeh, FL; 2H4 and 4B4), Becton Dickinson (Mountain View, CA; Leu-4, Leu-3a, Leu-2a, Leu-16, anti-HLA-DR, anti-IL-2 receptor, and Leu-7), Ortho Diagnostic System (Raritan, NJ; OKT3) and Biotest (Frankfurt on Main, FRG; Clonab T4). Leu-3a and Clonab T4 react with an epitope of CD4 that is distinct from the MTI5I binding site and is not cross-blocked by MT151 (our observation) (18).

Specific binding of MAb was analyzed according to standard methods, recommended by Becton Dickinson Monoclonal Center (Mountain View, CA) using a cytofluorograph (model 50H, Ortho Instruments).

F. Cell Preparations and Lymphocyte Cultures

Peripheral blood mononuclear cells were isolated from heparin-stabilized blood by Ficoll-Ronpacon 440 density gradient centrifugation (Pharmacia Fine Chemicals, Uppsala, Sweden). Cell density was adjusted to 1×10^6 cells per ml and proliferative response to mitogens, antigens, and alloantigens evaluated using standard procedures (17,18).

Selective T cell stimulation was achieved by combined cross-linking of a nonmitogenic anti-CD3 antibody fragment [BMO30-F(ab')$_2$] with subset-specific anti-T cell antibodies (24,25). Cell cultures were performed on goat antimouse IgG-coated culture plates.

To determine activated T cell subsets, cells were stained with FITC-labeled anti-CD4 or anti-CD8 antibodies and the degree of activation was evaluated by phycoerythrin-labeled anti-IL-2 receptor antibodies.

G. Measurement of Circulating Anti-CD4 MAb Serum Levels and Antimouse Antibodies

Serum levels of VIT4 and MT151 were measured with an enzyme-linked immunosorbent assay (ELISA). Detection of antimouse antibodies was achieved with a competition ELISA (17).

H. Statistical Analysis

The statistical significance of the changes in clinical and laboratory parameters was determined by means of the improved Wilcoxon test.

III. RESULTS

A. Changes in Clinical Parameters Following Anti-CD4 MAb Treatment

None of the eight patients developed severe side effects to the monoclonal antibody treatment. Only patient 4 had low-grade fever for 1 day. As shown in Fig. 1, significant improvement in the clinical variables of morning stiffness (mean 59%), pain assessment (74%), and Ritchie articular index (70%) occurred in all eight patients within 1 week after initiation of therapy. Follow-up examination of these clinical parameters after 16 weeks showed stabilization of the underlying disease in some patients. The amelioration lasted in patient 2 for 5½ months, in patient 3 for 8 months, and in patients 5, 6, and 8 for >12 months. Clinical improvement in patient 1 lasted only for 3 weeks; nevertheless, a dramatic improvement of a vasculitis in the right thumb could be noted. Patient 4 felt better for only about 8 weeks. Patient 7 showed in general only marginal improvement of clinical symptoms. No difference in efficacy between VIT4 and MT151 treatment was observed (patients 1–3 were treated with VIT 4 and patients 4–8 with MT151).

Patients 1–7 received 5 mg prednisone per day, whereas patient 8 was treated only with MT151 antibody alone. Since patient 8 showed the same clinical improvement, the observed changes in clinical parameters are most likely due to a specific effect of the CD4 treatment. The good clinical response was not accompanied by significant changes in such laboratory parameters as erythrocyte sedimentation rate (ESR), CRP, rheumatoid factors, creatinine, or immune complexes, either during therapy or in the follow-up period.

B. Changes in Lymphocyte Subsets After In Vivo Anti-CD4 Antibody Treatment

Relative numbers of CD3, CD4, CD8 and "injected antibody" (MT151) positive cells were determined 1 day before and 2, 4, and 24 h after treatment with 10 mg VIT4 or MT151. As shown in Fig. 2, CD4 antibody treatment of patients with rheumatoid arthritis induced a selective elimination of CD3- and CD4-positive cells. In contrast, a relative increase in CD8-positive cells was found. Injected antibody-positive cells were detectable for 11 h after treatment. Maximal fluoroescence intensity, which correlates with the amount of bound antibody per

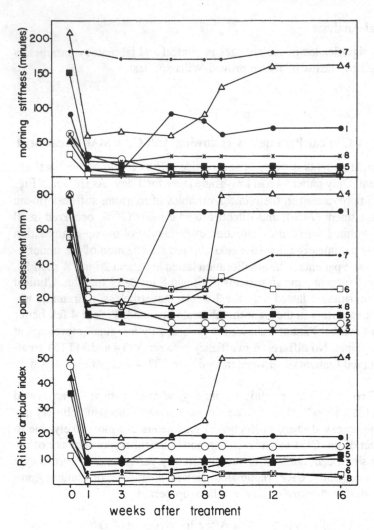

Figure 1 Changes in duration of morning stiffness, pain assessment, and Ritchie articular index after anti-CD4 MAb treatment. Follow-up examination of the clinical parameters of eight patients treated with the anti-CD4 MAb VIT4 (patients 1–3) or MT151 (patients 4–8) over 16 weeks after initiation of therapy. The improvement after 1 week was highly significant for all three parameters (stiffness, $p < 0.01$; pain, $p < 0.001$; Ritchie, $p < 0.001$). Patient 2 had psoriatic arthritis. [From Herzog et al. (17).]

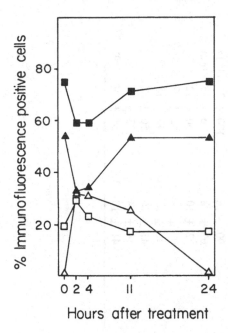

Figure 2 Changes in lymphocyte subsets after in vivo anti-CD4 antibody treatment. Relative numbers of CD3 (■), CD4 (▲), CD8 (□), and injected antibody-positive cells (△) were determined before and 2, 4, 11, and 24 h after injection of 10 mg VIT4. Results are mean values of the three VIT4 injections (percentage immunofluorescence-positive cells). Note the short decrease in CD3$^+$ and CD4$^+$ cells and that ~30% of the circulating cells were coated with VIT4.

cell, was found 2 h after antibody infusion. At that time point, the mouse antibody concentration in serum was still higher than 1 μg/ml. The change in cell distribution was transient and returned to normal levels within 24 h.

The decrease in anti-CD4–positive cells was not due to antigenic modulation since the percentage of CD3-positive cells also decreased and the percentage of cells stained by CD8 increased. Moreover, the CD4-positive cells were still stainable by the anti-CD4 antibody Leu-3a, which binds to a different CD4 epitope than does MT151.

As shown in Table 4, administration of prednisone alone induced a diminution of all lymphocytes subsets (CD4, CD8, B, natural killer, NK, CD45R lymphocytes). Injection of anti-CD4 MAb further reduced CD3 and CD4 cells without affecting the other lymphocyte subsets.

Interestingly, administration of CD4 MAb predominantly eliminated only one of the two main subsets of CD4-positive cells, as CD4$^+$ CDw29$^+$ cells were

Table 4 Changes in Leukocyte and Lymphocyte Subsets after αCD4 MAb Treatment

	Cells mm^{-3} before treatment			% Control 2 h after treatment			
	Day −1	Day 1	Day 5	Day −1		Day 1	Day 5
Leukocytes	6630[a]	6450[b]	7580[b]	113 ± 13[a]		108 ± 10[b] (100)[c]	104 ± 11[b] (87)[c]
Neutrophils	3880	4360	4290	140 ± 16		140 ± 14 (109)	141 ± 1 (87)
Monocytes	350	360	390	97 ± 15	$p < 0.005$[d]	53 ± 17 (69)	73 ± 17 (73)
Lymphocytes	2220	1530	2650	63 ± 4	$p < 0.05$	44 ± 4 (73)	54 ± 8 (67)
CD3 (Leu-4)	1770	1150	1980	61 ± 4		36 ± 6 (67)	48 ± 10 (73)
CD4 (Leu-3a)	1260	830	1510	58 ± 5	$p < 0.05$	28 ± 7 (30)	40 ± 8 (49)
CD8 (Leu-2a)	490	270	410	78 ± 9		67 ± 4 (112)	66 ± 10 (109)
B cell s(Leu-16)	110	170	360	72 ± 9	$p < 0.05$	69 ± 10	75 ± 15 (86)
NK cells (Leu-7)	220	150	170	87 ± 17		90 ± 16	100 ± 23 (111)
HLA-DR	230	190	450	73 ± 5		60 ± 8	76 ± 13 (80)
IL-2 receptor	40	60	150	80 ± 20		42 ± 10	50 ± 12
CD45R (2H4)	640	640	1100	66 ± 9		61 ± 2	62 ± 9
CDw29 (4B4)	ND	870	1520	ND		36 ± 3	48 ± 13
CD45R/CD4	190	340	590	48 ± 2		41 ± 16	56 ± 17
CDw29/CD4	ND	490	950	ND		14 ± 4	33 ± 12
T4/T8 ratio	3.03	3.46	4.00	75 ± 8		41 ± 10 (39)	51 ± 9 (49)

[a] Only 3 patients.
[b] Mean value + SD of 7 patients.
[c] One patient without prednisone.
[d] Only significantly different values between day −1 and day 1 are given.

more decreased than the CD4$^+$ CD45R$^+$ cells (Table 4). Quite striking was also the effect of CD4 MAb treatment on the distribution of monocytes, which was not altered by 5 mg prednisone but decreased by <30% with CD4 treatment.

C. Effect of Anti-CD4 MAb Treatment on Functional Parameters of T Cells

The delayed-type hypersensitivity reaction to a battery of recall antigens (Multitest Mérieux) disappeared in four patients during anti-CD4 MAb treatment (17,26). These patients again showed positive reactions 8 weeks after completion of therapy.

The consequence of the altered cell distribution and in vivo coating of CD4 cells on functional parameters in vitro is described in detail in Figs. 3 through 5. A reduced proliferative response to mitogens, antigens, or alloantigens was observed 2 and 4 h after antibody treatment but was normalized within 24 h (like the T cell subset distribution, Fig. 3).

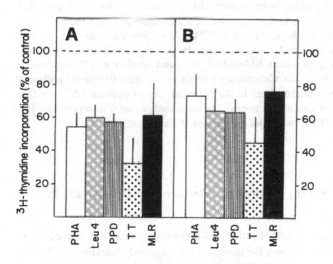

Figure 3 Proliferative response to mitogens, antigens, and alloantigens after in vivo anti-CD4 antibody treatment. Mononuclear cells were stimulated with PHA (1:2000), the anti-CD3 antibody Leu-4 (20 ng/ml), tuberculin PPD (20 µg/ml), tetanus toxoid (2 LFU/ml), or alloantigens (MLR) before or 2 h (A) or 4 h (B) after the injection of 10 mg MT151 (day 1). Results are expressed as the percentage of [³H]thymidine incorporation of cultures before antibody treatment (mean of four experiments ± SD). (From Walker et al. (18).]

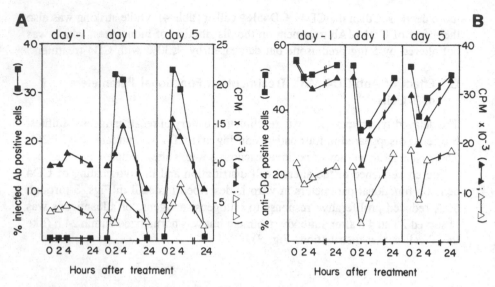

Figure 4   Selective T cell subset proliferation induced by dual-antibody stimulation. (A) Mononuclear cells before and 2, 4, and 24 h after injection of MT151 at days 1 and 5 were stimulated by cross-linking the anti-CD4 antibody (coated in vivo) with BMA030-F(ab')$_2$ (10 ng/ml added in vitro) with (▲) or without (△) the addition of rIL-2 (250 U/ml) for 2 days. [^{3}H] thymidine incorporation was compared with the amount of injected antibody-positive cells (■) as stained by FITC-labeled goat antimouse Ig. (B) Total CD4-positive cells (■) stained by Leu-3a were correlated with the proliferative response obtained with CD4$^+$ cells to which BMA030-F(ab')$_2$ and another anti-CD4 antibody (Clonab T4) were added (10 ng/ml). Cultures were performed by cross-linking the antibodies on goat antimouse coated culture plates in the presence (▲) or absence (△) of rIL-2. Results are mean values of four experiments. The same analysis were also performed on day −1, on which no MT151 was injected. [From Walker et al. (18).]

D.   Selective T Cell Subset Proliferation Induced by Dual-Antibody Stimulation

To address the question of whether anti-CD4 antibody-coated cells were refractory to further stimulation, we used the model of dual-antibody stimulation (24,25). The anti-CD3 antibody fragment BMA030-F(ab')$_2$ is per se nonmitogenic. Cross-linking it with a T cell subset-specific antibody induces selective T cell stimulation (dual-antibody stimulation; Refs. 24 and 25). Using this method, it should be possible to selectively activate T cells coated in vivo by cross-linking the in vivo cell-bound antibody (MT151) with in vitro added BMA030-F (ab')$_2$.

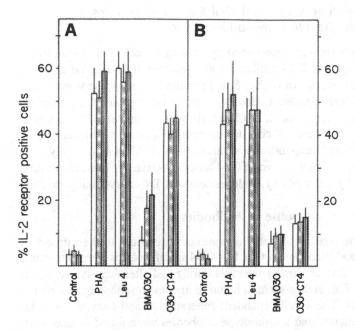

Figure 5 Double-immunofluorescence analysis of mitogen-activated T cell subset after in vivo MT151 treatment. Mononuclear cells before (□) and 2 h (▩) and 4 h (Ⅲ) after the first injection of 10 mg MT151 were stimulated with PHA (1:2000), Leu-4 (20 ng/ml), BMA030-F(ab′)$_2$ (10 ng/ml) or BMA030-F (ab′)$_2$ plus Clonab T4 (10 ng/ml). After 2 days T cell subsets were determined by staining the cells by FITC-labeled anti-CD4 (A) or anti-CD8 (B) antibodies, and activation was evaluated by phycoerythrin-labeled anti-IL-2 receptor antibodies. Results are expressed as a percentage of IL-2 receptor-positive cells within either CD4 or CD8 subsets (mean values of four experiments ± SD). (From Walker et al. (18).]

As shown in Fig. 4, the patients' mononuclear cells were stimulated before and 2 and 4 h after anti-CD4 antibody injection. The stimulation was achieved by cross-linking the in vivo coated antibody (MT151) with BMA030-F(ab′)$_2$. The proliferation was compared with the number of injected antibody-positive (MT151/FITC goat antimouse Ig) cells. A close correlation between the number of CD4-positive cells and maximal CD4 stimulation can be observed. Before MT151 injection, BMA030-F(ab′)$_2$ + IL-2 was only poorly mitogenic. After the start of MT151 injection, the percentage of cells reactive with FITC goat antimouse antibodies and the proliferative response to in vitro added BMA030-F(ab′)$_2$ increased.

E. Characterization of Activated T Cell Subsets After Mitogen Stimulation by Double Immunofluorescence

Activated T cell subsets were determined by staining the cells either with FITC-labeled anti-CD4 or anti-CD8 antibodies and phycoerythrin-labeled anti-IL-2 receptor antibodies. As shown in Fig. 5, the proliferative response was reduced 2 and 4 h after antibody treatment. However, this reduced proliferative response was not due to a selective blockade of CD4 cells by the bound anti-CD4 antibody as the proportion of activated T cell subsets remained constant. Moreover, the in vivo coating allowed dual-antibody stimulation of the CD4 subset only. This observation emphasizes that in vivo MT151 antibody-coated cells were not functionally impaired by the antibody, independent of CD4 cross-linking or not.

F. Development of Antimouse Ig Antibodies

To test whether the patients mounted an antimouse response to the infused antibodies, IgG antibody titers against the two CD4 specific MAbs were determined in serum samples taken at various intervals during and after therapy. As shown in Table 5, in six of the eight patients a humoral immune response against murine IgG_{2a} was detected. The T-cell-dependent generation of anti-isotype antibodies occurred in all patients, and anti-idiotype antibodies were found in one of the eight patients.

In two patients blocking antibodies were detected. Most antimouse antibodies were detectable shortly after treatment. Only one patient had a high-titer antimouse Ig response.

IV. DISCUSSION

Although a disease like RA has a variable course, the data from this open study suggest that treatment with monoclonal anti-CD4 antibodies has an effect on circulating T cells and may possibly influence the course of recalcitrant rheumatoid arthritis. The clinical parameters were improved after 7 days of therapy in all patients (in patient 7 only marginally), and follow-up examinations revealed a persistent improvement for up to > 12 months.

None of the eight patients developed a severe adverse reaction to the MAb. Unlike the patients treated with TLI, our population was not found to develop severe viral or bacterial infections. A known recurrent herpes zoster (patient 4) was also not reactivated.

It is likely that the beneficial effect of the anti-CD4 antibody treatment is due to its immunosuppressive efficacy, which was also nicely demonstrated in the transient loss of skin test reactivity (17,26).

The cell analysis data show that infusion of 10 mg anti-CD4 antibody induced a transient and not complete elimination of CD4-positive cells from the peripheral

Table 5 Human Antibody Response to the Murine Anti-CD4 Antibody

	Antimouse Ig[a] (U)			Blocking
			Blocking	anti-Id
Patient	During	After	antimouse Ig	antibodies
1	—	200, week 4	(+) week 4	—
2	—	200, week 1	+, week 12	—
3	—	100, week 2	—	—
4	—	< 100	—	—
5	100, day 4	200, week 4	—	—
6	—	200, week 3	—	(+) week 4
7	—	400, week 1	—	—
		800, week 2		
8	—	< 100		

[a]Values of 100 U (= 100 ng) and above are positive.

blood. Mainly the CD4 CDw29[+] T cell subset was diminished, which is interesting, as this subset is overrepresented in synovial fluid of patients with RA (6). The residual CD4 cells were coated by the infused antibody without modulation of the CD4 antigen. Besides T cells, monocytes were also diminished by anti-CD4 treatment. In one patient the synovial fluid cells could be also analyzed after MAb treatment and were found to be CD4-antibody coated (data not shown).

There are several mechanism by which MAbs to CD 4 might exert an immunosuppressive effect and thus alleviate the symptoms of RA. These include blocking of CD4 MHC (class II) interaction, transmission of a negative signal to CD4 cells, and depletion of CD4 cells (27,28). Also, coaggregation of CD4 with a TCR CD3 complex, which occurs when CD4[+] cells are stimulated (29), may be inhibited.

The functional studies speak against the transmission of a negative signal to CD4 cells by MT151 treatment as (1) mitogen stimulation revealed that the proportion of mitogen-activated CD4[+] cells did not differ before and after MT151 treatment; and (2) the in vivo coating of CD4 cells with MT151 did not block the CD4 cell reactivity, since cross-linking the MT151 injected in vivo with BMA030-F(ab')$_2$ added in vitro resulted in enhanced proliferation. In the absence of a demonstrable negative signal transmitted by the anti-CD4 antibodies to CD4 cells, we propose that the diminished proliferative response and probably also the clinical improvement following anti-CD4 antibody therapy is due to an altered cell distribution and/or to an interference of the anti-CD4 antibodies with CD4-accessory cell interaction or TCR-CD4 coaggregation.

The finding that noncirculating cells were coated by the infused MAbs, that free circulating MAb was found in the presence of maximal binding to CD4 cells, and that delayed hyperreactivity reactions in the skin were suppressed indicate that the 10 mg MAb injected daily was sufficient to cover circulating and probably also tissue CD4$^+$ cells for some hours. The short duration of this coating suggests, however, that the therapeutic efficacy may be increased by an additional injection after 10–12 h. Studies are underway to use 20 mg anti-CD4 antibodies per day (30). Moreover, anti-CD4 antibodies may differ in their capacity to remove CD4 cells from the circulation, as another anti-CD4 antibody was found to persistently diminish CD4 cells from the circulation (Burmester and Emmrich, Erlangen, FRG, personal communication).

In contrast to the mouse system, the two anti-CD4 antibodies used were immunogenic in human, as most patients developed an antimouse response. The antimouse response in our patients was, however, quite weak as only in one patient were high antibody titers observed. Indeed, retreatment with the same anti-CD4 antibody was repeatedly performed in a follow-up study and was tolerated without problems (30). Since treatment with the same CD4 antibodies in renal transplant patients generally induced a higher immune response it is likely that the underlying rheumatic disease may be a cofactor for the poor antibody response.

In conclusion, this pilot study of the two anti-CD4 antibodies MT151 and VIT4 shows that the treatment was well tolerated. With the dosage of 10 mg/day over 7 days, an immediate clinical improvement was observed. The treatment reduced T cell-mediated functions in vivo and in vitro, but these changes were only transient and are not sufficient explanation for the long-lasting improvement of clinical parameters in some patients.

V. SUMMARY

A group of eight patients with severe arthritis were treated for 7 days with daily 10 mg anti-CD4 antibody (VIT4 or MT151). No side effects were observed. A partial or complete remission of rheumatoid arthritis was induced in seven patients, which lasted between 3 weeks and > 12 months. Laboratory parameters were not changed. However, the treatment induced a drastic fall in circulating T cells, mainly of the CD4$^+$ CDw29$^+$ subset, which lasted for 8–10 h. After 24 h, before the next treatment, the lymphocyte values were normalized again. Six of eight patients developed a weak antimouse Ig response. Five of eight patients had a transient skin anergy during treatment. Functional analysis of in vivo antibody-coated CD4+ cells revealed an intact proliferative response, suggesting that mainly the altered cell distribution contributes to the impaired immune response. We conclude that mouse anti-CD4 monoclonal antibody treatment is well tolerated and that the cellular immunologic changes observed are short-lasting.

the low incidence of side effects may justify further clinical studies to evaluate the clinical efficacy of such treatment.

ACKNOWLEDGMENTS

This work was supported by grants 3.612.087 and 3.705.087 of Swiss National Foundation. We thank Mrs. M. Bader for excellent secretarial assistance, and Academic Press, London, for permission of reproduction of figures and tables from our original work, which appeared in J. Autoimmun. (17,18).

REFERENCES

1. Harris, E.D., Jr. (1986). Pathogenesis of rheumatoid arthritis. In: Textbook of Rheumatology. Kelly, W.N., Harris, E.D., Ruddy, S., and Sledge, C.B., eds. W.B. Saunders, Philadelphia, p. 886.
2. Duke, O., Panayi, G.S., Janossy, G., and Poulter, L.W. (1982). An immunohistological analysis of lymphocyte subpopulations and their microenvironment in the synovial membranes of patients with rheumatoid arthritis using monoclonal antibodies. Clin. Exp. Immunol. 49:22.
3. Stastny, P. (1978). Association of the B-cell alloantigen DRw4 with rheumatoid arthritis. N. Engl. J. Med. 298:869.
4. Trentham, D.E., Belli, J.A., Anderson, R.J., Buchley, J.A., Goetzl, E.S., David, J.R., and Austen, K.F. (1981). Clinical and immunologic effects of fractionated total lymphoid irradiation in refractory rheumatoid arthritis. N. Engl. J. Med. 305:976.
5. Kotzin, B., Strober, S., Engleman, E.F., Calin, A., Hoppe, R., Kansan, I.S., Terrell, C.P., and Kaplan, H.S. (1981). Treatment of intractable rheumatoid arthritis with total lymphoid irradiation. N. Engl. J. Med. 305:969.
6. Herzog, C., Walker, C., and Pichler, W.J. (1989). New therapeutic approaches in rheumatoid arthritis. Concept Immunopathol. 7:79.
7. Ortho Multicenter Transplant Study Group (1985). A randomized clinical trial of OKT3 monoclolnal antibody for acute rejection of cadaveric renal transplants. N. Engl. J. Med. 313:337.
8. Dillmann, R. O. (1986). Monoclonal antibody: Intravenous therapy in lymphoproliferative disorders. In: Monoclonal Antibodies. Diagnostic and Therapeutic Use in Tumor and Transplantation. Chatterjee, S.N. ed., PSG Publishing Company, Littleton, MA, p. 21.
9. Hafler, D.A., Ritz, J., Schlossmann, St. A., and Wainer, H.L. (1988). Anti CD4 and anti CD2 monoclonal antibody infusions in subjects with multiple sclerosis. J. Immunol. 141:131.
10. Wofsy, D., Ledbetter, J.A., Hendler, P.L., and Seaman, W.E. (1985). Treatment of murine lupus with monoclonal anti-T cell antibody. J. Immunol. 134:852.
11. Waldor, M.K., Sriram, S., Hardy, R., Herzenberg, L.A., Herzenber, L.A., Lanier, L., Lim, M, and Steinman, L. (1985). Reversal of experimental allergic encephalomyelitis with monoclonal antibody to a T cell subset marker. Science 227:415.

12. Ranges, G.E., Sriram, S., and Cooper, S.M. (1985). Prevention of type II collagen-induced arthritis by in vivo treatment with anti-L3T4. J. Exp. Med. 162:1105.

13. Sedgwick, J.D., and Mason, D.W. (1986). The mechanism of inhibition of experimental allergic encephalomyelitis in the rat by monoclonal antibody against CD4. J. Neuroimmunol. 13:217.

14. Benjamin, R.J., and Waldmann, H. (1986). Induction of tolerance by monoclonal antibody therapy. Nature 320:449.

15. Gutstein, N.L., Seaman, W.E., Scott, J.H., and Wofsy, D. (1986). Induction of immune tolerance by administration of monoclonal antibody to L3T4. J. Immunol. 137:1127.

16. Carteron, N.L., Wofsy, D., and Seaman, W.E. (1988). Induction of immune tolerance during administration of monoclonal antibody to L3T4 does not depend on depletion of L3T4+ cells. J. Immunol. 140:713.

17. Herzog, C., Walker, C., Müller, W., Rieber, P., Reiter, C., Riethmüller, G., Wassmer, P., Stockinger, H., Madic, O., and Pichler, W.J. (1989). Anti-CD4 antibody treatment of patients with rheumatoid arthritis. I. Effect on clinical course and circulating T cells. J. Autoimmun. 2:627.

18. Walker, C., Herzog, C., Rieber, P., Riethmüller, G., Müller, W., and Pichler, W.J. (1989). Anti-CD4 antibody treatment of patients with rheumatoid arthritis. II. Effect of in vivo treatment on in vitro proliferative response of CD4 cells. J. Autoimmun. 2:643.

19. Ropes, M.W., Bennet, G.A., Cobb, S., Jacox, R., and Jessar, R.A., (1958). 1958 Revision of diagnostic criteria for rheumatoid arthritis. Bull. Rheum. Dis. 9:175.

20. Reinherz, E.L., Haynes, B.F., Nadler, L.M., and Bernstein, I.D., eds. (1986). Leucocyte Typing II, Vol. 1 Springer-Verlag, Berlin.

21. Emmrich, F. (1987). Empfehlungen für die Herstellung und Prüfung in vivo applizierbarer monoklonaler Antikörper. Dtsch. Med. Wochenschr. 112:194.

22. Sattentau, Q.J., Dalgleish, A.G., Weiss, R.A., and Beverley, P.C.L. (1986). Epitopes of the CD 4 antigen and HIV infection. Science 243:1120.

23. Pinals, R.S., Masi, A.T., Larsen, R.A., and the Subcommittee for Criteria of Remission in Rheumatoid Arthritis of the American Rheumatism Association Diagnostic and therapeutic criteria committee (1981). Preliminary criteria for clinical remission in rheumatoid arthritis. Arthritis Rheum 24:1308.

24. Walker, C., Bettens, F., and Pichler, W.J. (1987). Activation of T cells by cross-linking an anti-CD3 antibody with a second anti-T cells antibody: Mechanism and subset-specific activation. Eur. J. Immunol. 17:873.

25. Walker, C., Bettens, F., and Pichler, W.J. (1987). T cell activation by cross-linking anti-CD3 antibodies with second anti-T cell antibodies: Dual antibody cross-linking mimics physical monocyte interaction. Eur. J. Immunol. 17:1611.

26. Herzog, C., Walker, C., Pichler, W.J., et al. (1987). Monoclonal anti-CD4 in arthritis (letter). Lancet 2:1461.

27. Wassmer, P., Chan, C., Lögdberg, L., and Shevach, E.M., (1985). Role of the L3T4-antigen in T cell activation. II. Inhibition of T cell activation by monoclonal anti-13T4 antibodies in the absence of accessory cells. J. Immunol 135:2237.

28. Bank, I., and Chess, L. (1985). Perturbation of the T4 molecule transmits a negative signal to T cells. J. Exp. Med. 162:1294.
29. Saizawa, K., Rojo, J., and Janeway, C.A., Jr. (1987). Evidence for a physical association of CD4 and the CD3: $\alpha:\beta$ T-cell receptor. Nature 328:260.
30. Reiter, C., Krieger, K., Schattenkirchner, M., Riethmüller, G., and Rieber, E.P. (1989). Treatment of patients with rheumatoid arthritis (RA) with anti CD4 monoclonal antibodies. Abstract 125-40. 7th Int. Congress of Immunol. Berlin.

4

Human Monoclonal Autoantibodies

Susan Alpert Galel, Edgar G. Engleman, and Steven K. H. Foung
Stanford University Medical Center, Stanford University School of Medicine,
Stanford, California

I. INTRODUCTION

Although multiple autoreactive antibodies have been found in the sera of patients with autoimmune diseases, the role of autoantibodies in the pathogenesis of these disorders has been difficult to determine. By "capturing" individual autoantibodies in vitro in high concentration, monoclonal antibody technology permits a precise analysis of the binding specificity and functional effects of individual autoantibodies.

Many laboratories have successfully utilized human monoclonal antibody technology to isolate autoreactive antibodies from patients with autoimmune disorders. These include anti-red cell antibodies from patients with autoimmune hemolytic anemia (1), antiplatelet antibodies from patients with idiopathic thrombocytopenic purpura (2), collagen-reactive antibodies from patients with arthritis and polychondritis (3), rheumatoid factor from patients with rheumatoid arthritis and cryoglobulinemia (4), and multiple organ reactive antibodies from patients with diabetes mellitus and other autoimmune endocrine disorders (5). Multiple investigators have successfully isolated DNA-reactive autoantibodies from patients with autoimmune disease (6,7).

These monoclonal autoantibodies have contributed to our understanding of autoimmune disease on several levels. First, with high-titer preparations of isolated autoantibodies, one can precisely define the target antigens to which the antibodies

57

bind. From this, in turn, one can determine the potential functional effects of each antibody and thereby evaluate its contribution to the pathogenesis of disease. Further evaluation of the clinical significance of particular autoantibodies can be derived by surveying patient sera and tissues for the presence of specific antibodies through the use of anti-idiotypes generated against the monoclonals. Surveys using anti-idiotypes have revealed a striking prevalence of expression of particular idiotypes in certain patient populations as well as on multiple autoantibodies of diverse specificity (8). Furthermore, analysis of monoclonal autoantibodies at a molecular level has revealed common genetic origins of many autoantibodies (4). The significance of these characteristics common to multiple autoantibodies is discussed in later chapters of this book.

In this chapter we describe the techniques currently available for the production of human monoclonal antibodies. We demonstrate how these techniques can be successfully utilized to analyze the B cell repertoire in human autoimmune disease.

II. PRODUCTION OF HUMAN MONOCLONAL ANTIBODIES

A. B Cell Activation

Human monoclonal antibody production involves the isolation and immortalization of a single antibody-producing human B cell. It appears that to immortalize antibody production in vitro, the B cell must be activated toward immunoglobulin secretion at the time of immortalization. In both the murine and human systems, optimal activation is achieved through in vivo immunization, resulting from either natural infection or active immunization. In the human system, an increased number of activated, antigen-specific B cells may be found in the circulating blood approximately 1 week after in vivo challenge (9). In the absence of in vivo immunization, it may still be possible to isolate B cells specific for a defined antigen if they are represented within the B cell repertoire. However, to generate specific antibody production from these cells in vitro, it is necessary to activate them toward antibody production, which can be accomplished in vitro with the use of polyclonal stimulators.

B. Polyclonal Stimulation

The two most commonly used polyclonal activators of human B cells are pokeweed mitogen (PWM) and the Epstein-Barr virus (EBV). For PWM activation, B cells are cultured in the presence of T cells and pokeweed mitogen. B cells are harvested after 2–5 days, before terminal differentiation, and immortalized through fusion with an established myeloma or lymphoblastoid cell line.

Although some laboratories have had good success with the pokeweed mitogen stimulation-fusion technique (6), it has been more popular to use EBV stimulation as the primary step for in vitro B cell activation. EBV readily infects human B cells after binding to their complement receptors and induces both proliferation and antibody secretion. Unlike PWM stimulation, which drives B cells to terminal differentiation, the immunoglobulin-secreting cells resulting from EBV infection continue to proliferate indefinitely. A certain percentage of EBV-infected B cells become "transformed" and can be grown and maintained in vitro as long-term cell lines.

Therefore, EBV activation and transformation alone has been used as a means of producing human monoclonal antibodies (10). Human B cells are infected with EBV, and culture supernatants are tested for the desired antibody after 2–3 weeks of culture. Cell cultures that contain the desired antibody are cloned repeatedly at limiting dilution, and clone supernatants are assayed for the secretion of the desired immunoglobulin. In this way it may be possible to isolate a monoclonal lymphoblastoid cell line that secretes a specific human antibody. This technique, although successful in some instances, is not, however, a reliable means of generating a long-term source of antibody (see later). It is more advantageous to use EBV to stimulate B cells to secrete immunoglobulin and proliferate and to follow this with fusion to produce a hybridoma cell line that can then be cloned and maintained in long-term tissue culture.

C. B Cell Selection

Because B cells of a given specificity are represented in very low frequencies (estimated $1/10^5$–$1/10^4$ B cells) (11,12), it is desirable to enrich the B cell preparation for the cells of the desired specificity before attempting hybridoma formation. The specific enrichment of B cells can be accomplished through a variety of methods. Most enrichment techniques take advantage of the fact that resting B cells bear their specific antibody on their surface and therefore can be positively selected by physically binding them into contact with their specific antigen. For soluble antigens, this can be accomplished by rosetting the B cell preparation with antigen-coated red cells (13). For cell surface antigens, antigen-specific enrichment has been reportedly accomplished by "panning" B cells on plates coated with the target cells (14). By enriching for the relatively rare antigen-specific B cell and then expanding the enriched population through EBV infection, it has been possible to isolate specific antibody-secreting cells from very small starting numbers of resting B cells (15).

D. In Vitro Immunization

Although the combination of B cell selection and polyclonal activation could theoretically be used to generate in vitro any antibody represented in the B cell repertoire, in practice human monoclonal antibody technology has been most successful thus far in isolating antibodies following specific in vivo stimulation. It appears that specific antigen stimulation is the most effective means of activating and expanding the desired B cell population. Because one is obviously constrained in the ability to immunize human subjects to specific antigens, much effort has been placed on developing techniques to accomplish primary immunization of human cells in vitro.

The requirements for successful primary in vitro immunization have not yet been clearly defined, although a number of investigators have achieved encouraging results (16). In general, there is agreement that several elements must be present in vitro in addition to the B cells:

1. Antigen, often coupled to a protein carrier.
2. Polyclonal stimulators (e.g., pokeweed mitogen or lipopolysaccharide).
3. Source of interleukin-2 and B cell growth and differentiation factors (e.g., culture supernatants from phytohemagglutinin-activated mononuclear cell cultures).
4. T cells and "accessory cells": Some investigators have reported that it is necessary to remove CD8$^+$ suppressor precursors that bear histamine receptors or to inactivate them with cimetidine before culture, although other investigators have found no such requirement (reviewed in Ref. 16). Others have found that removal of a lysosome-rich fraction of peripheral blood mononuclear cells (including monocytes and natural killer cells) results in marked enhancement of B cell activation (17).

For in vitro activation, the mixtures are cultured for 4–7 days and the activated B cells are harvested and immortalized through fusion.

In the hands of some investigators, in vitro immunization systems show remarkable promise for expanding the applicability of human monoclonal antibody technology. However, a reproducibly successful protocol remains to be defined.

E. B Cell Immortalization: EBV Infection Versus Hybridoma Formation

After the antigen-specific B cell has been activated either in vivo or in vitro, it must be cloned and rendered immortal in such a way as to maintain stable antibody production in long-term tissue culture. As noted earlier, EBV infection, which is often used as a polyclonal B cell activator, can result in the "transformation," that is, immortalization, of the infected B cells. Therefore, some investigators have used EBV infection alone as means of generating antigen-specific B cell lines. Unfortunately, this technique has serious limitations. First, EBV-infected B cells are relatively difficult to clone, and specific antibody production is often lost during the attempts to isolate the B cell of desired specificity. Second, even cloned EBV-infected cell lines tend to lose antibody production over time. Whether this is due to cessation of antibody production or to overgrowth of nonsecreting clones is not clear, but this occurrence limits the availability of the desired antibody.

Therefore, most investigators have found it more reliable to immortalize antigen-specific B cells through physical fusion with long-term cell lines, that is, through the formation of "hybridoma" cells. The ideal fusing partner for hybridomas appears to be a stable cell line that does not secrete immunoglobulin but has the machinery for antibody production (such as a myeloma or lymphoblastoid cell line), that can be readily separated from hybrid cells after fusion (i.e., selectable), and that generates stable, easily clonable antibody-secreting hybrids with activated human B cells. A wide variety of fusing partners have been reported of both murine and human origin (18). The major differences between fusing partners relate to their efficiency of fusion, the level of antibody secretion in the resulting hybrids, and the stability of the hybrids in long-term tissue culture.

We have previously described the development of a selectable (HGPRT deficient, ouabain sensitive) human-mouse heteromyeloma cell line, SBC-H20 (19). This cell line has an excellent fusing efficiency and generates stable hybridomas that secrete 1–20 μg/ml of antibody in long-term tissue culture, which is similar to the levels of antibody production achievable with murine hybridomas.

The hybridoma formation is accomplished through physical fusion of the activated B cell with the fusing partner cell line. Most often, this has been achieved by mixing the cells in the presence of polyethylene glycol (PEG) (18). However, a technology has recently been developed for achieving fusion of cells through electrical breakdown of their membranes (20). In our hands, this "electrofusion" has shown distinct advantages over PEG in that it appears to result in a greater efficiency of fusion and can be used to fuse extremely small numbers of activated B cells (21). Therefore, we currently use electrofusion exclusively for all hybridoma formation. The approach of EBV activation with subsequent fusion by PEG or electrofusion has been effective in the production of human monoclonal antibodies to a variety of antigens (Table 1).

Following fusion, hybridoma cells are allowed to grow, and after 2–3 weeks, culture supernatants are tested for the presence of antibody of desired specificity. Colonies secreting the desired antibody are cloned by limiting dilution, and clone supernatants are again assayed for specific immunoglobulin. After repeated cloning, the cells secreting the desired antibody are grown in bulk culture, from which immunoglobulin can be collected in unlimited quantities and concentrated or purified for further use.

We will demonstrate how these techniques can be manipulated to isolate autoreactive monoclonal antibodies from the B cells of patients with autoimmune disease. Our experience illustrates that the ability to "capture" autoantibodies in vitro can result not only in an improved understanding of autoimmune disease, but also in the generation of reagents that identify previously unrecognized human tissue antigens of functional importance.

Table 1   Human Monoclonal Antibodies Derived from Human-Mouse Heteromyelomas

Fusogen	Antigen	Ig Class	Reference
PEG	Type A red blood cells	IgM	22
	$Rh_0(D)$	IgG, IgM	23
	rh^G	IgG	24
	T cell	IgM	25
	VZV	IgG	26
	EBV	IgM	19
	Mycobacterium leprae	IgM	19
	HIV	IgG	27
	HLA class II	IgM	28a
Electrofusion	HCMV	IgG	21
	VZV	IgG	28b
	HLA class I	IgM	28c

III. PRODUCTION OF HUMAN MONOCLONAL ANTI-T CELL ANTIBODIES

A variety of immunoregulatory abnormalities have been identified in patients with the autoimmune diseases systemic lupus erythematosus (SLE) and juvenile rheumatoid arthritis (JRA) (29–33). It has been suggested that some of the cellular dysfunction may be due to depletion of immunoregulatory subsets of lymphocytes by cytotoxic anti-T cell autoantibodies. Cytotoxic autoantibodies reactive with T lymphocytes have been described in the sera of patients with these disorders (33–41). However, the precise specificity of these autoantibodies has been difficult to determine because of low titers and multiple specificities of antibody in human serum. We have utilized human monoclonal antibody technology to isolate from patients with autoimmune disease monoclonal antibodies reactive with human T cell surface molecules.

We first screened the sera of patients with autoimmune disease for the presence of antibodies to T cell surface molecules by incubating patient sera with T cells from normal blood donors. Antibody binding to T cells was detected with FITC-conjugated goat antihuman immunoglobulin and analysis on a cytofluorograph. By this method, 16 of 40 patients with SLE and 9 of 23 patients with JRA were found to have T cell binding antibodies in their sera. Binding patterns vary greatly, with some patients showing strong reactivity with almost all T cells and other patients showing reactivity with less than 50% of cells (Fig. 1). Initially, patients with strongly reactive antibodies were selected for attempts to isolate human monoclonal anti-T cell antibodies.

B lymphocytes were isolated from the peripheral blood of these patients and

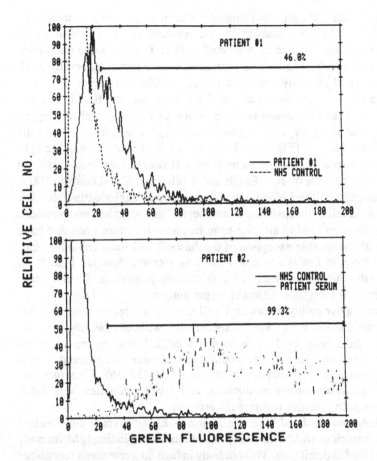

Figure 1 Staining patterns of normal and SLE sera on T cells. E rosette (+) lymphocytes (10⁶) from a healthy donor were incubated at 4 °C with 100 μl normal human serum or SLE patient serum, as indicated, stained with FITC-conjugated goat antihuman Ig, and analyzed on an Ortho System 50H cell sorter.

then either fused directly or activated with Epstein-Barr virus and then fused with the SBC-H20 cell line. Hybrid supernatants were screened for the presence of human immunoglobulin by enzyme-linked immunosorbent assay (ELISA). It was observed that fusions of freshly drawn B cells yielded many hybrids (fusion frequency approximately 5 per 10⁵ B cells) but only a low level of antibody secretion in the hybrids. However, if patient B cells were first stimulated in vitro with Epstein-Barr virus before fusion, there was an even greater fusing efficiency and much improved level of immunoglobulin secretion, with 50–80% of hybrids secreting greater than 500 ng/ml of immunoglobulin. Hybrid supernatants containing immunoglobulin were assayed for the presence of anti-T cell antibody by indirect immunofluorescence as described earlier. T cell-reactive antibodies were concentrated by ultrafiltration to saturating concentration (generally 5–10 μg/ml). Concentrated antibody was used for all specificity analyses.

By this method we were able to successfully isolate from the B cells of a patient with SLE a human monoclonal antibody with clear reactivity with T lymphocytes (Fig. 2B). Subsequently, a second antibody was generated from spleen cells of another patient with SLE (Fig. 2C). These two antibodies are both of the IgM class and show similar staining patterns on T cells. However, they show distinctly different reactivity patterns on non-T cells and T cell lines. SLE-I binds to 100% of lymphocytes and to all red blood cells (spontaneously agglutinating all adult and cord red blood cells). It also binds to monocytes, granulocytes, and platelets. In fact, it was found to bind to all long-term human cell culture lines that have been tested, with the notable exception of the Jurkat T cell line. The other antibody, SLE-II, binds to few if any non-T lymphocytes and does not bind at all to red blood cells. Therefore, despite similar staining patterns on T cells, these antibodies appear to recognize different target antigens.

After confirming our ability to isolate T cell-reactive antibodies from patients with autoimmune disease, we decided to see whether we could identify any antibodies that recognize only a subset of human T cells. It was reported that the sera of some patients with juvenile rheumatoid arthritis were preferentially cytotoxic for functionally distinct subpopulations of T cells (33–36). Therefore, we next attempted to isolate human monoclonal anti-T cell antibodies from the B cells of patients with juvenile rheumatoid arthritis.

Antibody JRA-I was isolated from the fusion of EBV-activated cells from a patient with polyarticular JRA. Characteristics of this T cell binding IgM antibody have been described in detail (25). This antibody in high concentrations recognizes approximately 80% of normal T cells. It shows striking preferential cytotoxicity to functionally distinct T cell subsets, preferentially killing Leu-8$^+$ cells within the CD4$^+$ T cell subset, and sparing Leu-8$^-$ cells. Functionally, this would result in preservation of T cell help for immunoglobulin synthesis, carried out by Leu-8$^-$, CD4$^+$ cells, but loss of T cell suppressor activity due to depletion of the suppressor-inducer subset (Leu-8$^+$, CD4$^+$ cells). Thus, the specificity of this JRA-I monoclonal antibody shows a remarkable similarity to the JRA sera characterized by Morimoto et al. (35,42), which functionally also caused a preferential depletion of suppressor-inducer activity from the CD4$^+$ population.

Within the CD8$^+$ T cell subset, JRA-I antibody preferentially spares natural killer cells (25). Thus, JRA-I appears to define a previously unrecognized T cell surface molecule expressed differentially on functionally distinct T cell subsets. The binding pattern of JRA-I does not correlate with the reactivities of any of a large panel of defined murine monoclonal antibodies.

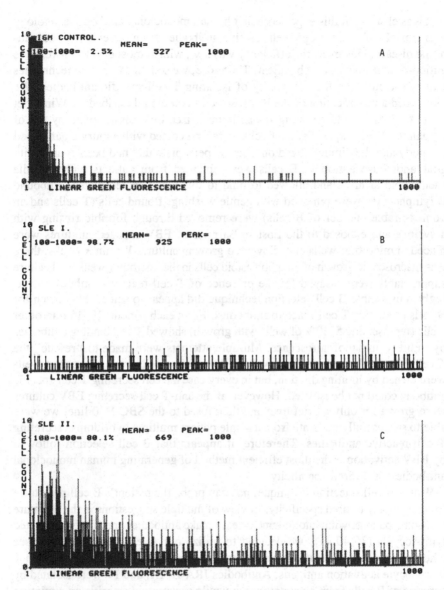

Figure 2 Staining patterns of two human monoclonal antibodies reacting with human T cells. Hybridoma supernatants (100 μl) were incubated with 10^6 E rosette (+) lymphocytes at 4 °C followed by staining with FITC-conjugated goat antihuman IgM and analysis on an Ortho Cytofluorograf System 50H. (A) T cell binding pattern of a control supernatant that contained an equal concentration of a human IgM monoclonal antibody directed against type A red blood cells. (B and C) T cell binding patterns of the SLE I and II hybridoma supernatants (see text).

It was clear from this experience that human monoclonal antibody technology was capable of generating T cell reactive antibodies from patients with autoimmune disease. However, the efficiency was low, with at most one T cell-reactive antibody isolated from each patient. Therefore, we sought to develop techniques that would improve the probability of isolating T cell-specific antibodies. We developed a modification of the B cell selection method described by Winger et al. (14). First, the target antigen was immobilized on a plastic plate by use of a "panning" technique. Target T cells were first coated with a murine pan-T cell antibody and then immobilized on a sterile petri plate that had been coated with goat antimouse antibody. B cells were obtained from patients with juvenile rheumatoid arthritis and allowed to bind to the T cell-coated plates. Unbound B lymphocytes were removed with gentle washing. Bound cells (T cells and an unmeasurable number of B cells) were removed through forcible rinsing with a syringe and exposed to the Epstein-Barr virus. EBV-exposed mixtures were placed in microtiter wells and allowed to grow in culture. Within 3 weeks, there was macroscopic growth of lymphoblastoid cells in the microtiter wells, and culture supernatants were assayed for the presence of T cell-reactive antibody. Strikingly, this simple B cell selection technique did appear to selectively enrich for B cells producing T cell-reactive antibodies. From each patient, 10–15 microtiter wells (representing 5–10% of wells with growth) showed T cell binding antibodies by indirect immunofluorescence. Multiple attempts were made to "rescue" the T cell-specific clones from these wells. EBV-infected cells from the positive wells were cloned by limiting dilution, but in every case the cell secreting T cell-specific antibody could not be isolated. However, if the anti-T cell-secreting EBV cultures were grown for only a brief time and then fused to the SBC-H20 line, we were able to successfully generate from a single patient multiple hybridomas secreting T cell-reactive antibodies. Therefore, it appears that B cell selection followed by EBV activation is the most efficient method of generating human monoclonal antibodies of desired specificity.

With a B cell selection technique, one can probe the patient's B cell repertoire for cells of any desired specificity. In view of multiple suggestions in the literature that some patients with autoimmune disease make antibodies specific for activated lymphocytes (36,40,41), we decided to utilize our selection technique to see whether we could generate human monoclonal antibodies that defined human T lymphocyte activation antigens. Antibodies JRA-II, III, and IV were isolated by panning of B cells from a patient with juvenile rheumatoid arthritis on a mixture of resting and activated T lymphocytes. EBV culture supernatants were screened by indirect immunofluorescence for reactivity with both resting and PHA-activated T cells, and positive wells were pooled and fused. Three T cell-reactive hybrids, JRA-II, III, and IV, were isolated from a single patient by this method. Antibody JRA-IV shows very strong binding to all resting T cells. However, JRA-II and III show preferential staining of activated cells. JRA-III binds weakly to resting

T cells but strongly to most T cells after PHA activation. It appears that this recognizes an antigen that may be expressed on all T cells but that has enhanced expression with activation. However, JRA-II, from the same patient, binds brightly to a small percentage (10–25%) of resting T cells and extremely brightly to all T cells after PHA activation (see Fig. 3). This latter pattern is unlike that of any other reported T cell "activation antigens," such as HLA class II, interleukin-2 (IL-2) receptor, and transferrin receptor, which are not expressed to this extent by resting cells. This antibody binds brightly to all cycling cell lines (both T cell and non-T cell) tested thus far but does not bind to mature (noncycling) red blood cells.

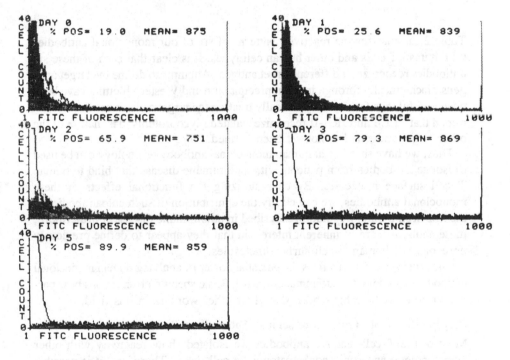

Figure 3 Binding pattern of JRA-II antibody on resting and activated T lymphocytes. E rosette (+) lymphocytes (10^6), freshly isolated or exposed to PHA (μg/ml) for 1–5 days, were incubated in 100 μl concentrated JRA-II for 45 minutes at 4 °C. Cells were then washed, stained with FITC-conjugated goat antihuman IgM, and analyzed on an Ortho Cytofluorograf System 50H. Shaded area represents the fluorescence pattern obtained with the JRA-II antibody. The solid line represents the binding pattern of an equal concentration of a control human IgM monoclonal antibody directed against the group A red blood cell antigen.

Table 2   Reactivity of Human Monoclonal Anti-T Cell Antibodies with Other Cell Types[a]

		T lymphocytes	RBC	Platelets	Monocytes	Cell lines Endothelial	T cell
SLE	I	4+	2+	2+	1+	4+	Neg Jurkat
	II	3+	—	—	1+	—	Variable
JRA	I	2+	—	—	—	—	Variable
	II	1+[b]	—	2+	1+	4+	4+ all
	III	2+	—	—	1+	2+	Variable
	IV	4+	—	—	—	—	Variable

[a]Reactivity with RBC was assessed by hemagglutination. Reactivity with other cells and cell lines was assessed by indirect immunofluorescence and analysis on an Ortho System 50H Cytofluorograf.
[b]4+ on all activated cells and cell lines.

Table 2 summarizes the reactivity patterns of six of our monoclonal antibodies with human T cells and other human cell types. It is clear that each of these six antibodies recognizes a different target antigen. Attempts to define the target antigens biochemically through immunoprecipitation and Western blotting have been unsuccessful thus far. By enzymatically treating the target cells, it has been determined that SLE-I and JRA-II recognize sialated glycoproteins. The nature of the other target antigens has not yet been defined.

Thus, we have shown that human monoclonal antibody technology can be used to isolate antibodies from patients with autoimmune disease that bind to human T cell surface molecules. By characterizing the functional effects of these monoclonal antibodies, we can clarify the contribution of such autoantibodies to the impaired immunoregulation described in autoimmune disease. Furthermore, these antibodies are of inherent interest in that they appear to define previously unrecognized human T cell surface molecules.

Our experience demonstrates the potential power of applying human monoclonal antibody technology to autoimmune disease. Some specific observations bear particular note, as they have been shared by other workers in this field.

Polyspecificity of Human Monoclonal Autoantibodies

Most of the T cell-reactive antibodies we isolated show reactivity with other hematopoietic and some nonhematopoietic cell types. Therefore, it is possible that antilymphocyte autoantibodies may cause wide-ranging functional effects. Similarly, Shoenfeld et al. have found that the DNA-reactive monoclonal antibodies that they have isolated also show a remarkable degree of polyspecificity. That is, individual DNA-reactive monoclonal antibodies bind to a wide variety of targets, including native DNA, single-stranded DNA, synthetic polynucleotides, cardiolipin, lymphocytes, platelets, cytoskeletal proteins, and some mycobacterial antigens (6,43–46). However, there is significant variability from antibody to antibody in the precise pattern of cross-reactivity. The remarkable cross-reactivity of human monoclonal autoantibodies raises interesting questions regarding the original stimulus for such antibodies and raises the possibility that a single autoantibody could be involved in a wide range of clinical effects.

Requirement for In Vitro Activation

It is the general experience that it is extremely difficult to isolate human monoclonal antibodies from circulating lymphocytes of patients with autoimmune disease without performing in vitro activation of the cells. This is somewhat difficult to understand in view of the fact that the patients are usually selected for the presence of autoantibody in their serum at the time that their B cells are obtained. It is likely, however, that most of the serum antibody was generated by B lymphocytes in the lymphoid organs, rather than by circulating cells. Therefore, to isolate autoantibodies from circulating cells, it appears necessary to activate the cells with polyclonal stimulators in vitro before fusion. This has been the general experience in our laboratory as well as others in this field (1–3,5,6). Shoenfeld et al. have used pokeweed mitogen to activate the B cells of their patients (6), although most other laboratories have utilized the Epstein-Barr virus technique.

Demonstration of Clinical Relevance

Because most of the monoclonal autoantibodies have been generated with the aid of in vitro polyclonal stimulation, it must be demonstrated that the antibodies generated in vitro have relevance to the autoantibodies detected in vivo. Clinical relevance may be demonstrated through a variety of techniques. First, as we have done, one can compare the binding specificity or functional effects of the monoclonal antibodies to those of patient sera. Second, one can look for competitive effects of the monoclonal antibody versus patient sera. Finally, one can generate an anti-idiotype antibody directed against the monoclonal and use this to demonstrate expression of the monoclonal idiotype in patient sera. Shoenfeld et al. used this third approach to identify an idiotype common to many monoclonal anti-DNA antibodies and have demonstrated the expression of this idiotype in a large percentage of patients with SLE both in their serum and at the site of tissue damage (8).

Immunoglobulin Class

All the T cell-reactive monoclonal antibodies we have generated have been of the IgM class. This has also been a common experience of other investigators generating human monoclonal autoantibodies in vitro (1–3,5,6). The preponderance of IgM monoclonal antibodies generated in vitro may simply reflect the prevalence of B cells in circulation that are "programmed" for IgM secretion.

It is possible that monoclonal autoantibodies of the IgG class may be isolated more frequently when B cells are obtained instead from sites of involved tissue (3). Alternatively, it has been suggested that the restriction to the IgM class as well as the apparently limited genetic diversity of autoantibodies may signify that certain autoantibodies arise from a specific subset of B lymphocytes designated CD5$^+$ (47). In this regard, recent studies in our laboratory of the origin of anti-DNA antibodies in SLE patients indicate that both CD5$^+$ and CD5$^-$ B cells can produce IgM and IgG anti-DNA antibodies. However, the mechanism of induction of antibody secretion by these two populations appears to differ (48). It will be of interest to analyze the specificity and genetic diversity of monoclonal autoantibodies derived from each of these B cell subsets.

IV. SUMMARY

Human monoclonal antibody technology, through its ability to isolate large quantities of individual antibodies, provides the ideal tool to define the specificity of individual autoantibodies and to determine their functional and clinical significance. These antibodies are not only helpful in understanding the significance of autoantibodies in autoimmune disease but are of inherent interest in that they appear to define previously unrecognized human tissue antigens.

Using a combination of B cell selection and in vitro activation, human monoclonal antibody technology enables one to isolate virtually any antibody represented within the human B cell repertoire. For reagent production, recombinant DNA techniques recently described may represent a more efficient way to generate and select for immunoglobulins of a desired specificity (49). These techniques, based on random recombination of heavy- and light-chain genes, may generate an even greater diversity of antibodies than are represented by the repertoire of intact B cells. However, to evaluate antibodies involved in human disease, the monoclonal antibody technique used should be one that reflects the immunoglobulins encoded by B cells in vivo. Therefore, the techniques described in this chapter represent the ideal approach to an evaluation of the role of antibodies in the pathogenesis or resolution of human disease.

ACKNOWLEDGMENTS

The work described here was supported by grants from the state of California and the National Institutes of Health (AM 32075 and AI 11313). Dr. Alpert Galel was a fellow of the Arthritis Foundation. The authors thank Michelle Hempy for her excellent technical assistance.

REFERENCES

1. Andrzejewski, C., Young, P.J., Goldman, J., Spitalnik, S.L., and Silberstein, L.E. (1989). Production of human warm-reacting red cell monoclonal autoantibodies by Epstein-Barr virus transformation. Transfusion 29:196-200.
2. Nugent, D.J. (1989). Human monoclonal autoantibodies to characterize platelet antigens in immune-mediated thrombocytopenia. Blut 59:52-58.
3. Posner, M.R., Barrach, H.J., Elboim, H.S., Nivens, K. Santos, D.J., Chichester, C.O., and Lally, E.V. (1989). The generation of hybridomas secreting human monoclonal antibodies reactive with type II collagen. Hybridoma 8:187-197.
4. Fong, S., Chen, P.P., Gilbertson, T.A., Weber, J.R., Fox, R.I., and Carson, D.A. (1986). Expression of three cross-reactive idiotypes on rheumatoid factor autoantibodies from patients with autoimmune diseases and seropositive adults. J. Immunol. 137:122-128.
5. Satoh, J., Prabhakar, B.S., Haspel, M.V., Ginsberg-Fellner, F., and Notkins, A.L. (1983). Human monoclonal autoantibodies that react with multiple endocrine organs. N. Engl. J. Med. 309:217-220.
6. Shoenfeld, Y., Hsu-Lin, S.C., Gabriels, J.E., Silberstein, L.E., Furie, B.C., Furie, B., Stollar, B.D., and Schwartz, R.S. (1982). Production of autoantibodies by human-human hybridomas. J. Clin. Invest. 70:205-208.
7. Rauch, J., Massicotte, H., and Tannenbaum, H. (1985). Hybridoma anti-DNA autoantibodies from patients with rheumatoid arthritis and systemic lupus erythematosus demonstrate similar nucleic acid binding characteristics. J. Immunol. 134:180-186.
8. Shoenfeld, Y., and Isenberg, D. (1987). DNA antibody idiotypes: A review of their genetic, clinical, and immunopathologic features, Semin. Arthritis Rheum. 16:245-252.
9. Burnett, K.G., Leung, J.P., and Martinis, J. (1985). Human monoclonal antibodies to defined antigens. In: Human Hybridomas and Monoclonal Antibodies. Engleman, E.G., Foung, S.K.H., Larrick, J., and Raubitschek, A., eds. Plenum Press, New York, pp. 113-133.
10. Crawford, D.H. (1985). Production of human monoclonal antibodies using Epstein-Barr virus. In: Human Hybridomas and Monoclonal Antibodies. Engleman, E.G., Foung, S.K.H., Larrick, J., and Raubitschek, A., eds. Plenum Press, New York, pp. 37-53.
11. Stevens, R.H., Macy, E., Morrow, C., and Saxon, A. (1979). Characterization of a circulating subpopulation of spontaneous antitetanus toxoid antibody producing B cells following in vivo booster immunization. J. Immunol. 122:2498-2504.
12. Golding, B., Inghirami, G., Peters, E., Hoffman, T., Balow, J.E., and Tsokos, G.C. (1987). In vitro generated human monoclonal trinitrophenyl-specific B cell lines. Evidence that human and murine anti-trinitrophenyl monoclonal antibodies cross-react with Escherichia coli β-galactosidase. J. Immunol. 139:4061-4066.
13. Steinitz, M., Koskimies, S., Klein, G., and Makela, O. (1979). Establishment of specific antibody producing human lines by antigen preselection and Epstein-Barr (EBV) transformation. Clin. Lab. Immunol. 2:1-7.
14. Winger, L., Winger, C., Shastry, P., Russell, A., and Longenecker, M. (1983). Efficient generation in vitro, from human peripheral blood cells, of monoclonal

Epstein-Barr virus transformants producing specific antibody to a variety of antigens
without prior deliberate immunization. Proc. Natl. Acad. Sci. USA 80:4484–4488.

15. Steinitz, M., Tamir, S., and Goldfarb, A. (1984). Human anti-pneumococci antibody
produced by an Epstein-Barr virus (EBV)-immortalized cell line. J. Immunol.
132:877–882.

16. Borrebaeck, C.A.K. (1988). Human mAbs produced by primary in-vitro immunization. Immunol. Today 9:355–359.

17. Borrebaeck, C.A.K. (1988). Human monoclonal antibodies produced from primary
in vitro immunized leucine methyl ester-treated peripheral blood lymphocytes. In:
In Vitro Immunization in Hybridoma Technology. Borrebaeck, C.A.K., ed. Elsevier
Science, Amsterdam, pp. 209–229.

18. Engleman, E.G., Foung, S.K.H., Larrick, J., and Raubitschek, A., eds. (1985).
Human Hybridomas and Monoclonal Antibodies. Plenum Press, New York.

19. Foung, S.K.H., Perkins, S., Arvin, A., Lifson, J., Mohagheghpour, N., Fishwild,
D., Grumet, F.C., and Engleman, E.G. (1985). Production of human monoclonal
antibodies using a human-mouse fusion partner. In: Human Hybridomas and
Monoclonal Antibodies. Engleman, E.G., Foung, S.K.H., Larrick, J., and
Raubitschek, A., eds. Plenum Press, New York, pp. 135–148.

20. Zimmermann, U. (1987). Electrofusion of cells. In: Methods of Hybridoma Formation. Bartal, A.H., and Hirshaut, Y., eds. Humana Press, Clifton, NJ, p. 97.

21. Foung, S.K.H., and Perkins, S. (1989). Electric field-induced cell fusion and human
monoclonal antibodies. J. Immunol. Methods 116:117–122.

22. Foung, S.K.H., Perkins, S., Raubitschek, A., Larrick, J., Lizak, G., Fishwild, D.,
Engleman, E.G., and Grumet, F.C. (1984). Rescue of human monoclonal antibody
production from an EBV-transformed B cell line by fusion to a human-mouse
hybridoma. J. Immunol. Methods 70:83–90.

23. Foung, S.K.H., Blunt, J.A., Wu, P.S., Ahearn, P., Winn, L.C., Engleman, E.G.,
and Grumet, F.C. (1987). Human monoclonal antibodies to $Rh_O(D)$. Vox Sang.
53:44–47.

24. Foung, S.K.H., Blunt, J., Perkins, S., Winn, L., and Grumet, F.C. (1986). A human
monoclonal antibody to rh^G. Vox Sang. 50:160–163.

25. Alpert, S.D., Turek, P.J., Foung, S.K.H., and Engleman, E.G. (1987). Human
monoclonal anti-T cell antibody from a patient with juvenile rheumatoid arthritis.
J. Immunol. 138:104–108.

26. Foung, S.K.H., Perkins, S., Koropchak, C., Fishwild, D., Wittek, A., Engleman,
E.G., Grumet, F.C., and Arvin, A. (1985). Human monoclonal antibodies neutralizing
Varicella-Zoster virus. J. Infect. Dis. 152:280–285.

27. Banapour, B., Rosenthal, K., Rabin, L., Sharma, V., Young, L., Fernandez, J.,
Engleman, E., McGrath, M., Reyes, G, and Lifson, J. (1987). Characterization and
epitope mapping of a human monoclonal antibody reactive with the envelope glycoprotein of human immunodeficiency virus. J. Immunol. 139:4027–4033.

28a. Foung, S.K.H. Manuscript in preparation.

28b. Foung, S.K.H., Bradshaw, P.A., and Emanuel,D. (1990). Uses of human mono-
clonal antibodies to human cytomegalovirus and Varicella-Zoster virus. In:
Therapeutic Monoclonal Antibodies. Borrebaeck, C. and Larrick, J. Eds. Stockton
Press, New York. In press.

28c. Wallace, E.F., Foung, S.K.H., Bradbury, K., Pask, S.L., and Grumet, F.C. (1990). Generation of a human hybridoma producing a pure anti-HLA-A2 monoclonal antibody. Human Immunol. 28:65–69.

29. Sakane, T., Steinberg, A.D., and Green, I. (1978). Studies of immune functions of patients with systemic lupus erythematosus. I. Dysfunction of suppressor T-cell activity related to impaired generation of, rather than response to, suppressor cells. Arthritis Rheum. 21:657–664.

30. Fauci, A.S., Steinberg, A.D., Haynes, B.F., and Whalen, G. (1978). Immunoregulatory aberrations in systemic lupus erythematosus. J. Immunol. 121:1473–1479.

31. Sakane, T., Steinberg, A.D., and Green, I. (1978). Failure of autologous mixed lymphocyte reactions between T and non-T cells in patients with systemic lupus erythematosus. Proc. Natl. Acad. Sci. USA 75:3464–3468.

32. Tsokos, G.C., and Balow, J.E. (1981). Cytotoxic responses to alloantigens in systemic lupus erythematosus. J. Clin. Immunol. 1:208–216.

33. Strelkauskas, A.J., Callery, R. T., McDowell, J., Borel, Y., and Schlossman, S.F. (1978). Direct evidence for loss of human suppressor cells during active autoimmune disease. Proc. Natl. Acad. Sci. USA 75:5150–5154.

34. Morimoto, C., Reinherz, E.L., Borel, Y., Mantzouranis, E., Steinberg, A.D., and Schlossman, S.F. (1981). Autoantibody to an immunoregulatory inducer population in patients with juvenile rheumatoid arthritis. J. Clin. Invest. 67:753–761.

35. Morimoto, C., Reinherz, E.L., Borel, Y., and Schlossman, S.F. (1983). Direct demonstration of the human suppressor inducer subset by anti-T cell antibodies. J. Immunol. 130:157–161.

36. Barron, K.S., Lewis, D.E., Brewer, E.J., Marcus, D.M., and Shearer, W.T. (1984). Cytotoxic anti-T cell antibodies in children with juvenile rheumatoid arthritis. Arthritis Rheum. 27:1272–1280.

37. Morimoto, C., Reinherz, E.L., Abe, T., Homma, M., and Schlossman, S.F. (1980). Characteristics of anti-T antibodies in systemic lupus erythematosus: Evidence for selective reactivity with normal suppressor cells defined by monoclonal antibodies. Clin. Immunol. Immunopathol. 16:474–484.

38. Sakane, T., Steinberg, A.D., Reeves, J.P., and Green, I. (1979). Studies of immune functions of patients with systemic lupus erythematosus. Complement-dependent immunoglobulin M anti-thymus-derived cell antibodies preferentially inactivate suppressor cells. J. Clin. Invest. 63:954–965.

39. Morimoto, C., Reinherz, E.L., Schlossman, S.F., Schur, P.H., Mills, J.A., and Steinberg, A.D. (1980). Alterations in immunoregulatory T cell subsets in active systemic lupus erythematosus. J. Clin. Invest. 66:1171–1174.

40. Litvin, D.A., Cohen, P.L., and Winfield, J.B. (1983). Characterization of warm reactive IgG anti-lymphocyte antibodies in systemic lupus erythematosus. Relative specificity for mitogen-activated T cells and their soluble products. J. Immunol. 130:181–186.

41. Yamada, A., and Winfield, J.B. (1984). Inhibition of soluble antigen-induced T cell proliferation by warm-reactive antibodies to activated T cells in systemic lupus erythematosus. J. Clin. Invest. 74:1948–1960.

42. Morimoto, C., Distaso, J.A., Borel, Y., Schlossman, S.F., and Reinherz, E.L.

(1982). Communicative interactions between subpopulations of human T lymphocytes required for generation of suppressor effector function in a primary antibody response. J. Immunol. 128:1645–1650.

43. Shoenfeld, Y., Rauch, J., Massicotte, H., Datta, S.K., Andre-Schwartz, J., Stollar, B.D., and Schwartz, R.S. (1983). Polyspecificity of monoclonal lupus autoantibodies produced by human-human hybridomas. N. Engl. J. Med. 308:414–420.

44. Shoenfeld, Y., Zamir, R., and Joshua, H. (1985). Human monoclonal anti-DNA antibodies react as lymphocytotoxic antibodies. Eur. J. Immunol. 15:1024–1028.

45. Andre-Schwartz, J., Datta, S.K., Shoenfeld, Y., Isenberg, D.A., Stollar, B.D., and Schwartz, R.S. (1984). Binding of cytoskeletal proteins by monoclonal anti-DNA lupus antibodies. Clin. Immunol. Immunopathol. 31:261–271.

46. Shoenfeld, Y., Vilner, Y., Coates, A.R.M., Rauch, J., Lavie, G., Shaul, D., and Pinkhas, J. (1986). Monoclonal anti-TB antibodies react with DNA and monoclonal anti-DNA autoantibodies react with Mycobacterium tuberculosis. Clin. Exp. Immunol. 66:255–261.

47. Casali, P., Burastero, S.E., Nakamura, M., Inghirami, G., and Notkins, A.L. (1987). Human lymphocytes making rheumatoid factor and antibody to ssDNA belong to Leu-1+ B-cell subset. Science 236:77–81.

48. Suzuki, N., Sakane, T., and Engleman, E.G. (1990). Anti-DNA antibody production by CD5+ and CD5– B cells of patients with systemic lupus erythematosus. J. Clin. Invest. 85:238–247.

49. Huse, W.D., Sastry, L., Iverson, S.A., Kang, A.S., Alting-Mees, M., Burton, D.R., Benkovic, S.J., and Lerner, R.A. (1989). Generation of a large combinatorial library of the immunoglobulin repertoire in phage lambda. Science 246:1275–1281.

5

Biologic Therapies for Rheumatoid Arthritis: Concepts from Considerations on Pathogenesis

Ian R. Mackay and Merrill J. Rowley
Centre for Molecular Biology and Medicine, Monash University, Clayton, Victoria, Australia

Claude C. A. Bernard
Brain-Behaviour Research Institute, LaTrobe University, Bundoora, Victoria, Australia

I. INTRODUCTION: THE CAUSE OF RHEUMATOID ARTHRITIS

Rheumatoid arthritis is an immune-mediated and antigen-driven disease of the articular tissues. Naturally, rational treatment of this disease requires insight into causation. Although the source of the antigen drive in rheumatoid arthritis is not established, the lymphocyte and cytokine interactions that dictate progression of the disease offer good prospects for intervention with biologic agents—biotherapy. As for many other autoimmune diseases, there is a high degree of "immunogenetic predeterminism," based on major histocompatibility complex (MHC; HLA) alleles; this could be seen as a constraint to modulatory treatment, yet this same genetic system offers one of the promising prospects for biotherapy. The assumption that rheumatoid arthritis is an immune-mediated articular disease is the premise for the scheme in Fig. 1, which is used in this chapter to analyze its multifactorial causation and to identify likely points of intervention with biotherapy. Also, two well-studied experimental autoimmune diseases, autoimmune encephalomyelitis (EAE) and collagen-induced arthritis (CIA), are cited to illustrate the experimental background to biotherapy with monoclonal antibodies (MAbs).

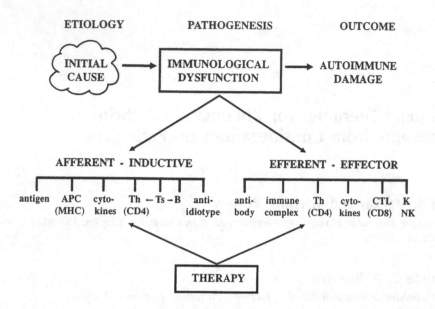

Figure 1 A perspective applicable to an immunopathologic basis for rheumatoid arthritis. The top sequence shows *etiology*, the as-yet unknown primary initiating event; *pathogenesis*, including immunoregulatory abnormalities, defective suppression, and class II MHC induction on synovial cells; and *outcome*, the expression of tissue damage and/or functional lesions. The middle sequence indicates that the ongoing immune process requires an *afferent* and *efferent* arm, each with multiple interactive components. The bottom line, therapy, can be directed at any of the components in either limb. Not shown is the vascular endothelial component, also a possible target for immunotherapy (see text). [Reproduced with permission from Springer Seminars in Immunopathology (107)].

II. THE ETIOLOGY → PATHOGENESIS → OUTCOME SEQUENCE

It is postulated that there is a sequence of etiology → pathogenesis → outcome for autoimmune disease and that there are afferent and efferent limbs of the self-perpetuating immune response (Fig. 1). However, various biologic agents, particularly cytokines, operate in both the afferent and efferent limbs of the response.

Etiology refers to the inciting agents or process, whether infectious, physical, toxic, or other, that operates on "day 1" of the disease. For rheumatoid arthritis, possible infectious agents include Epstein-Barr virus (EBV), a retrovirus, or a bacterium, as reviewed elsewhere (1). The postulated initiating infection could be transient or persistent and, if persistent, could be cytopathic per se or act by providing antigens that either provoke a damaging immune response or interfere with normal self tolerance by molecular mimicry.

Pathogenesis represents the combination of immunologic regulatory derangements that result in self-perpetuating rheumatoid synovitis. These derangements include defects in immune suppression and other immunoregulatory processes that could lead to uncontrolled responses to an intrasynovial antigen, perhaps collagen or other cartilage components, cytokine imbalance, and increased expression of MHC class II molecules on antigen-presenting cells. The result is activation of the various "downstream" effector processes (see Fig. 1), among which are cytokine molecules acting as potentiators of the immune response and as effectors of the local damage and systemic effects of rheumatoid disease.

Outcome is the final effect of the unregulated immunologic response within joints. The acute inflammatory phase is expressed initially as an exudative synovitis. This is followed by a proliferative reaction (pannus), fibrogenesis, and destruction of bone and cartilage, which proceed under the influence of cytokines, inflammatory products, and immune complexes generated during the course of the progressive phase of rheumatoid arthritis.

III. BIOLOGIC THERAPY: THE AFFERENT LIMB

A. The Antigen

Bacteria

There are experimental models that depend on the presence in joint tissues of foreign immunostimulatory antigenic particles; these include intra-articular injection of antigen into a previously sensitized animal (2) and the arthritis produced in rats by intraperitoneal injection of bacterial cell wall fragments, which after becoming localized in synovial tissues generate a continued antigenic stimulus (3). However, these models resemble more the reactive arthropathies that depend on an intrasynovial response to persisting immunogenic fragments of such microorganisms as *Yersinia*, *Chlamydia*, or *Borrelia* (4).

Virus

The Epstein-Barr virus has long been suspected as an etiologic agent, based particularly on high titers of virus-specific antibody in patients with rheumatoid arthritis (5). EBV could provide an intrasynovial rheumatogenic antigen or determine the rheumatoid process indirectly by molecular mimicry. The EB viral glycoprotein gp110 has an aminoacid sequence QKRRA which has homology with part of the hypervariable region of the DRβ molecule of HLA-DR4 (6), leading to two eventualities: either natural tolerance for the autologous HLA DR4 molecule could attenuate reactivity to the EB viral capsid antigen and so influence the course of EB virus infection, or the gp 110 could generate an autoimmune response by

T cells to HLA-Dw4 on intrasynovial B cells, so establishing a continuing autologous mixed lymphocyte reaction within joints.

As another type of mimicry involving EBV, we can cite the sequence homology and cross-reactivity between the EBV-encoded EBNA-1 and denatured collagen (7). This was claimed to be yet another route by which EBV could contribute to the pathogenesis of rheumatoid arthritis.

If an infectious background were to be established, then biotherapy could take the form of a vaccine rather than the interventions discussed in the remainder of this chapter.

Autoantigen

The alternative for the rheumatogenic antigen is that this is an autoantigen to which an immune response arises de novo or following synovial infection or trauma. The four candidate autoantigens are the Fc piece of the IgG molecule to which rheumatoid factors are directed, type II collagen, an as-yet unidentified synovial constituent, or an MHC molecule expressed on B cells or macrophages that stimulates CD4 T cells, as in the autologous mixed lymphocyte reaction in vitro. It is not within the scope of this chapter to review the evidence for the participation of these candidate autoantigens in rheumatoid arthritis, but there is an evident bias here toward a role for collagen type II, based on serologic evidence, including serum antibodies to collagen (8–13), intrasynovial sequestration of such antibodies (14–16), and the animal model of collagen-induced arthritis (CIA) (17–19). If an autoantigen can be convincingly shown to be relevant to pathogenesis, then tolerogenic procedures (see later) may be possible.

B. The Antigen Presenting Cell

MHC Class II Molecules

According to the rules, the postulated rheumatogenic antigen should be displayed to T cells within the synovium in association with major histocompatibility class II molecules on the surface of antigen presenting cells; these include macrophages, B lymphocytes and synovial lining cells. Also, this antigenic display should be augmented by increased expression in such cells of MHC molecules under the influence of lymphokines released by activated T lymphocytes.

There are sequences on the hypervariable region of the β chain of MHC class II molecules that have binding affinity for antigens, and it is suspected that disease associations with MHC class II (DR loci) are determined by this effect. In the case of rheumatoid arthritis, there is a genetic risk conferred by the susceptibility alleles HLA DR4, and the linked D locus specificities Dw4 and Dw14 (20). This risk may be attributed to molecular configurations associated with the hypervariable regions of DRβ1 in particular, allowing affinity of binding of the rheumatogenic antigen and facilitation of presentation of this antigen to "helper" CD4 T lymphocytes (21). Accordingly biotherapy, as in other autoimmune diseases associated with HLA alleles, could be directed to blockade of antigen presentation by MHC class II (Ia) molecules, by injection of anti-Ia monoclonal antibody raised to the appropriate MHC specificity. Therapy with anti-Ia rests on the premise that such antibody in a heterozygote would *selectively* suppress the response to antigens under the control of the relevant Ia molecule without causing complete immunosuppression; in particular, the blocking MAb should be specific for a single chain of the class II molecule so that, in heterozygotes, there would be two unblocked heterodimers to permit a normal response to foreign antigens.

Therapy with Monoclonal Anti-MHC Class II: Experimental Data

Studies in experimental autoimmune disease have validated immunotherapy with anti-Ia directed to blocking antigen presentation. For example, in experimental autoimmune encephalomyelitis (EAE) in the susceptible SJL mouse, the injection of a MAb to an Ia molecule before immunization with brain emulsion prevented EAE in 25 of 28 treated mice, and treatment with MAb after the appearance of lesions, or in mice with chronic relapsing EAE, reduced the frequency of relapses (7 of 18 versus 18 of 18 in controls) and the frequency of deaths (22). There are equivalent data for EAE in monkeys, although acute deaths are recorded in some monkeys given MAb (23). Various other experimentally induced autoimmune diseases have been attenuated by anti-Ia MAb, including myasthenia gravis induced by immunization with acetylcholine receptor (24). This therapy is also effective in spontaneously developing autoimmunity exemplified by thyroiditis or diabetes in the BB rat (25) or lupus in mice when MAb to the appropriate Ia molecule is used over months 4–8 of life (26). Moreover, since collagen may be an antigen relevant to rheumatoid arthritis, it is of interest that monoclonal and polyclonal antisera to Ia suppressed the occurrence of collagen-induced arthritis in mice after immunization with type II collagen (27).

Monoclonal MHC Class II: Clinical Prospects

It is worth commenting that rheumatoid arthritis in humans may be a final expression of responses provoked by different antigens or one antigen, such as collagen type II, with several pathogenic epitopes, each of which could engage one of several "rheumatogenic" sequences on DRβ chains, so accounting for the genetic diversity of the disease. Clearly, there is an element of nonspecificity in this therapy compared with other procedures, and the MAb used would need to be carefully tailored.

As yet, no clinical experience is available. As a first assessment, intrasynovial treatment of "pauciarticular" human rheumatoid arthritis with anti-MHC Class II MAb could be visualized in patients who have an HLA DR4 allele. Eventually the MAb should be directed against sequences on the DRβ chain that are shown to have binding affinity for the rheumatogenic antigen.

Competitive Mimotope

As another possibility for therapy directed at the antigen-presenting cell, we can refer to analogs of the culprit antigen, designated mimotopes. This of course depends on knowing the identity and structural sequence of the antigen, particularly the sequence that binds to the MHC class II molecule. This sequence is known as the agretope. The idea is that an analog of the agretope, the mimotope, competes with the agretope for the binding site on the MHC class II molecule and so interferes with presentation of the antigen to the T cell receptor. This approach to immunotherapy may appear conceptual rather than applicable, but we draw attention to the demonstrated competition in vivo in mice between self peptides and foreign antigens for MHC class II binding, with resulting interference in T cell activation (28). This has led to studies in experimental models to show that a mimotope can indeed block the expression of an autoimmune disease by competing with autoantigen at the level of the antigen presenting cell (29).

As an illustrative prototype, there is the successful use of a synthetic structural analog of the basic protein of myelin (BPM), the autoantigen that induces EAE in animals. This analog, copolymer 1, inhibits the development of EAE whether injected before or during the induction phase of the disease (30). Trials have been instituted with the use of copolymer 1 for multiple sclerosis, on the basis that EAE is a model for that disease, with claimed success (31). In the case of rheumatoid arthritis a mimotope strategy will not be applicable until the provoking antigen has been identified.

Cytokines: Interleukin-1

There is release of cytokines, particularly interleukin-1 (IL-1), after uptake of antigen by macrophages. Il-1 and the related cytokine tumor necrosis factor (TNF) aid the immune response by activating T cells but also cause various local and sytemic adverse effects of rheumatoid inflammation. Interference with the secretion of IL-1 by antibody blockade or by other cytokines would obviously damp the afferent limb of the autoimmune response. However, it is more convenient to consider biotherapy based on cytokines in Sec. IV.D dealing with the efferent (effector) limb.

C. The "Helper" T Lymphocyte

T Cell Activation

The helper CD4 T lymphocyte is activated by the engagement of its specific binding receptor by the display on the surface of an antigen presenting cell of a composite antigenic complex. This consists of a peptide derived from the endocytosis and intracellular degradation of an antigen that associates with an MHC class II molecule within the cell. Intracellular processing of antigen may not be mandatory, since peptide antigens in the milieu of the antigen presenting cell may associate with MHC class II molecules on the cell surface. Recognition of this complex by the receptor of the CD4 T cell activates other surface molecules and causes signals to be transduced. The effects of signal transduction include mitogenesis and production of IL-2, which acts in an autocrine manner to upregulate the expression of IL-2 receptors on the T cell surface, so amplifying the mitogenic stimulus and providing for further rounds of helper T cell proliferation.

The various surface structures on the CD4 T cell that facilitate the transduction of the signal generated by activation of the T cell receptor include the CD3 complex, the CD4 and the CD2 molecules, and the IL-2 receptor. All these molecules on CD4 T cells have been exploited in biotherapy with monoclonal antibodies in experimental and human settings. As a general consideration, therapy that potentially ablates or inactivates major subsets of the T cell population clearly should be used only for acute therapy, to avoid the complications of protracted pan immunosuppression. Preferentially, of course, biotherapy should be antigen specific, that is, directed at the T cell antigen receptor (TCR), and prototypes for this are already available.

"Pan-T Cell" Antibodies

Antibodies with pan-T cell reactivity have been used experimentally and clinically as "anti-immune" agents in various settings. Citations are listed of the experimental use of antibodies to the Thy-1 and Thy 1-2 antigens to suppress murine autoimmune disease (32), and these are of most benefit when given in the inductive stage of experimental autoimmunity. Although no analog of Thy-1 is identified in the human, the earlier heterologous antilymphocyte serum used to suppress allograft rejection could exemplify use of a pan-T cell antibody. Subsequently, targeting has become far more specific.

CD3 Molecule

The CD3 molecular complex transduces activation signals after occupancy of the T cell antigen receptor. MAbs to CD3 have long been used successfully as anti-immune agents for attenuation of acute rejection of organ allografts—kidney, liver, or heart. Antibody to CD3 is not cytotoxic and appears to act by steric blockade of the T cell receptor for antigen. MAb to CD3 has not proven successful in the therapy of chronic immune-mediated disease, and the potential of anti-CD3 for total rather than selective immunosuppression requires that short-term courses be used in acute relapses. Hence anti-CD3 would not be judged as suitable for sustained systemic treatment of rheumatoid arthritis, although intrasynovial injection could be effective.

CD4 Molecule

The CD4 molecule mediates the restricted recognition of MHC class II products on antigen presenting cells. Hence monoclonal antibodies against CD4 have been used to block antigen recognition by CD4-bearing T cells. Such antibodies have been shown to suppress various types of immune response, including responses to soluble antigens, responses causing allograft rejection, various immune-mediated diseases (cited in Refs. 32 and 33), and relapsing multiple sclerosis (34). Since this chapter is concerned with rheumatoid arthritis, the example is taken of collagen arthritis as a close experimental model. The suppression of collagen-induced arthritis in DBA/1 mice was achieved by a MAb raised to L3T4 (CD4) (35). Treatment with anti-L3T4 resulted in a >90% depletion of L3T4$^+$ T cells in lymph nodes and spleen, and administration of anti-L3T4 before immunization with type II collagen reduced the incidence of arthritis from 14 of 20 in the control group to 3 of 25 in the treated mice and delayed the onset of the disease (35). However, treatment begun after a strong anticollagen IgG humoral response was underway, but before the onset of arthritis, did not alter disease expression.

There is one promising report on the use of an anti-CD4 MAb for rheumatoid arthritis; eight patients were treated for 7 days with a daily injection of 10 mg (36). There was improvement in clinical indices lasting from 3 weeks to 5 months. There was depletion of CD4$^+$ cells from blood, but this was incomplete and transient. Of interest, the depleted subset of CD4 was CD4$^+$CDw29$^+$, the "helper-inducer" or memory subset. There was an associated and transient decrease in indices of cell-mediated immune reactivity. The authors discussed the several ways in which anti-CD4 MAb might act on the rheumatoid autoimmune process (36).

T Cell Antigen Receptor

It has been shown, for given antigens and autoantigens, that there is preferential usage of certain T cell receptor genes by immune T cells, and MAbs have been raised to particular T cell receptors by immunization of mice or rats with T cells of the appropriate clonotype. Such MAbs provide a highly specific type of T cell suppression. In EAE produced in both mice and rats, the T cell receptor V gene products involved in encephalitogenicity display a remarkable homology as well as restricted heterogeneity despite that both species recognize different epitopes on the BPM molecule. Thus, in the PL mouse strain, at least 80% of the encephalitogenic T cells directed against BPM peptide 1–9 utilize V_β 8.2, and 100% utilize the V_α 4 family (37). In B10PL mice, 79% utilized V_β 8.2, 58% V_α 2.3, and 42% V_α 4.2 (38). In the Lewis rat, 100% of the encephalitogenic T cells that recognized the MBP peptide 72–86 expressed the T cell receptor β chain homologous to the mouse V_β 8.2 and 73% had the rat homolog of V_α 2 (39). Taking advantage of the limited heterogeneity of the T cell receptors used by encephalitogenic T cell clones, it has been possible to prevent and treat EAE using antireceptor monoclonal antibodies prepared against the V_β 8 chain (37,38). An even more precise protocol is described in which Lewis rats were immunized with a synthetic peptide representing a hypervariable region of the

T cell receptor V_β 8 molecule to obtain protection against EAE by induction of V_β-specific regulatory T cells (40).

In collagen-induced arthritis, certain V_β T cell receptor gene segments are necessary for the development of the disease (19,41), and it can be expected that similar "vaccination" strategies would be effective for this experimental disease. In human rheumatoid arthritis, oligoclonal T cells with limited types of rearrangement of receptor genes have been recovered from joints (42); this allows the idea that MAbs could be raised to the appropriate T cell receptor gene products to provide a disease-specific T cell suppression, equivalent to that demonstrable in the experimental setting.

The Interleukin-2 (IL-2) Receptor

The receptor for IL-2 on T cells is upregulated by various cytokines, including IL-2 itself, as part of the inductive amplification of the immune response. This receptor was characterized initially by a MAb to an antigen known as Tac. Receptor binding studies have identified receptor molecules for IL-2: low-affinity receptor molecule (55 kD) is recognized by anti-Tac and there is a sparsely distributed high-affinity heterodimer that binds IL-2 with a 1000-fold greater avidity than the 55 kD molecule but comprises only about 3% of all IL-2R molecules (43).

Since the IL-2R is uniquely expressed during the inductive phase of the immune response, there is good logic in the use of MAb to IL-2R to eliminate the critical inductive T cell population and, in support of this, the effectiveness of various MAbs to IL-2R in abrogating delayed-type hypersensitivity, graft-versus-host (GVH) disease, and allograft rejection is well documented (32,44). The activity of MAbs to IL-2R, at least in the transplantation setting, appears to depend on actual elimination of IL-2R-positive T cells (44). We note that MAbs directed to the IL-2R suppress the development of collagen-induced arthritis (45) and passively transferred adjuvant arthritis (46), although MAb did not suppress the development of the arthritis after active immunization (46). Further citations of biotherapy directed to the IL-2R are given in Sec. IV.D, Interleukin-2.

T Cell Adhesion Molecules

The migration of leukocytes across endothelial surfaces and into inflammatory lesions, a critical function in health and disease, is effected by specific ligand-receptor interactions involving "adhesion molecules" (47–51). A long-recognized adhesion molecule is the leukocyte functional antigen 1 (LFA-1/MAC-1), the two chains of which are now called CDIIa and CD18; this is the major member of the integrin family of adhesion molecules. An important ligand for LFA-1 is the intercellular adhesion molecule 1 (ICAM-1). Other adhesion or homing molecules include MEL-14/Leu-8 and CD44 (Pgp-1 and HERMES 1). Ligands for adhesion molecules have important functions in immune responses. Thus their expression on antigen presenting cells facilitates engagement of CD4 T cells with cognate peptide antigens, and another function is to promote the binding of cells to receptors on vascular endothelium, so facilitating cellular extravasation. The ligands that are recognized by the MEL-14/Leu-8 and CD44 molecules are relevant to normal lymphocyte recirculation, whereas ICAM-1 is upregulated by inflammatory stimuli and cytokines, particularly IL-1, tumor necrosis factor (TNF), and interferon-γ, and is therefore more relevant to the "emergency exodus" of T cells into inflammatory sites (47).

The ligand-receptor interactions between cell adhesion molecules have been examined in relation to synovial inflammation (48a–50). The enhanced expression on synovial fluid T lymphocytes of the adhesion molecules LFA-1 and VLA-1 was considered to facilitate localization of T cells to the inflamed synovium (49). Moreover ICAM-1, the "partner" for LFA-1, is expressed on all major components of the synovial microenvironment in rheumatoid arthritis, particularly on synovial lining (type A) cells and on vascular endothelium, further indicating the importance of the LFA-1–ICAM-1 adhesion pathway in maintaining immuno-inflammatory activity (50). Finally, ICAM-1 mediates neutrophil transfer and influx into inflammatory sites; it has been shown that MAbs to either LFA-1 or to ICAM-1 inhibit granulocyte infiltration into an inflammatory site, at least in a model situation (51). It is therefore evident that LFA-1 or ICAM-1 could become targets for biotherapy in situations in which cellular extravasation should be inhibited, so that MAbs to these structures given by intrasynovial injection could be visualized for anti-inflammatory effects in exacerbations of rheumatoid arthritis.

Another adhesion-mediated pathway is via leukocyte functional antigen 3 (LFA-3), now called CD58, for which the ligand is the CD2 molecule (47[a]). In preliminary studies on the use of anti-CD2 in cases of chronic relapsing multiple sclerosis (34), there was a progressive decline in the count of CD2[+] cells during administration. No effect on the disease could be recorded in these short-term studies.

D. The Suppressor T Lymphocyte

Immune Suppression

The function of the suppressor subset of T cells is the down-regulation of immune responses, although there is yet to be a clear identification of the cell type(s) responsible for this effect or a clear understanding of the nature of immune suppression. As evidence for the reality of immune suppression, there is the inhibitory effect of putative suppressor T cells on the expression of various experimentally induced autoimmune diseases. For example, it has long been known from studies in EAE that when normally encephalitogenic preparations of BPM are injected with Freund's incomplete rather than complete adjuvant, the animal develops a resistant (protected) state to subsequent induction of EAE, and this resistance can be induced even during the developmental phase of EAE. Moreover, this resistance can be transferred to syngeneic animals by inoculating spleen cells, which presumably contain the suppressor population (52).

Suppressogenic Epitopes

It is proposed that multideterminant antigens contain some epitopes that are immunogenic and others that are suppressogenic (53); the latter are particularly represented on autoantigens and tumor antigens. An example of an autoantigen for which suppressogenic epitopes are postulated is the liver-specific F antigen (54). F antigen (M_r 42,000) occurs in mice in two allelic forms, F1 and F2. There is tolerance to self F, and the response to allo F is under immunogenetic control in that only mice that possess the class II MHC molecule A^k can respond to allo F. In responder-nonresponder hybrids, nonresponsiveness is dominant and due to MHC-linked suppression. The explanation offered is that T suppressor epitopes are distributed over the part of the molecule common to the two allelic forms of F and outnumber the single T helper epitope (54).

In collagen-induced arthritis, it has been shown that injection with poorly arthritogenic forms of collagen II, either before immunization or within 1–2 weeks after immunization, can prevent the induction of arthritis (55,56). Thus, although chick collagen type II is relatively ineffective at inducing collagen-induced arthritis, IV injection of chick type II collagen significantly decreased the incidence of arthritis induced by immunization with bovine type II collagen (55). Similarly, rats exposed parenterally or pergastrically to polymerized type II collagen became resistant to subsequent induction of disease (56). In a recent study, suppression of collagen-induced arthritis in DBA/1 mice was obtained by IV injection of a 26 amino acid synthetic peptide corresponding to the cyanogen bromide-derived peptide CB11 112–147 (56a); moreover, the critical determinant residues were mapped to the region CB11 137–147, an 11 amino acid stretch.

Reference was made earlier to the use of copolymer I as an analog of the neural antigen BPM to confer protection against induction of EAE; its use as a biotherapy for multiple sclerosis depends on the long-term administration to patients. It is not certain whether copolymer I acts by competing at the level of the antigen presenting cell (see earlier) or by inducing a state of immune suppression by presentation of suppressogenic epitopes. If such epitopes are recognized by suppressor T cells, this represents one mechanism for maintenance of extrathymic (peripheral) tolerance of T cells. For rheumatoid arthritis, there is still the need to identify the rheumatogenic antigen and suppressogenic epitopes to use these as a "negative" vaccine to re-establish failed tolerance. The induction of suppressor T cells through the anti-idiotype network is discussed later (Sec. III.F, Idiotypes of T Cells).

In the setting of suppression we can draw attention to suppressogenic lymphokines that can downregulate immune responses, illustrated by the blocking effect of IL-4 on release of IL-1 (Sec. IV.D, Interleukin-1 and Tumor

Necrosis Factor) and the inhibitory cytokine contra-IL-2 (Sec. IV.D, Interleukin-2).

E. The B Lymphocyte

The CD5 B Cell

There is a pronounced activation of B lymphocytes in the diseased synovium in rheumatoid arthritis, and these particular B cells bear an interesting surface marker, CD5 (Leu-1). This marker is normally present on T lymphocytes but is also associated with an early stage of B cell differentiation; CD5-positive B cells are highly represented among fetal B cells and B cells of lymphocytic leukemia (57). In rheumatoid arthritis, the proportion of CD5 B cells is increased in the blood, and these B cells are the source of rheumatoid factor (57). Moreover there is a high representation of CD5 B cells among synovial lymphocytes (58). It is suggested that the CD5 population is less susceptible to normal regulatory controls over B cell proliferation. We are unaware of any reports on the use of MAb to the CD5 antigen as a therapy for experimental or human disease.

Monoclonal Antibodies to B Cells

The course of murine lupus in BXSB mice was ameliorated by treatment with a MAb to a non-exclusive B cell molecule, Ly-5 (CD45), and the authors visualized extrapolation of their finding to the treatment of human autoimmune disease (59). In another study, MRL/1pr autoimmune mice were treated for 12 weeks with a MAb to the B220 cell marker, with an ensuing reduction in the B220$^+$ and Thy-1.2$^+$ subpopulation and, correspondingly, a decrease in levels of anti-DNA and anti-Sm and degree of lymphadenopathy (60). A pathogenic role for lymphocytes carrying B220 was suggested, but since this marker is present on naive T cells (pre-T) as well as B cells, the mode of intervention by the MAb to B220 is uncertain.

There have been no attempts in human autoimmune disease to direct biotherapy to autoreactive B cells, whether of the conventional or CD5 phenotype, even in situations in which a truly pathogenic autoantibody is demonstrable.

F. The Idiotype Network

Idiotypes of Autoantibodies

The concept of internal regulation of immune responsiveness by an idiotype network has enthusiastic adherents and has led to interesting experiments on the regulation of autoimmune responses. Anti-idiotypic antibodies have been shown to exist for idiotypes of autoantibodies in various experimental and human autoimmune diseases, for example to anti-DNA in murine and in human lupus and to anti-IgG (rheumatoid factor) (61,62). Considering rheumatoid arthritis, we note that anti-idiotypic antibodies to rheumatoid factor (RF) occur spontaneously in serum and were held to account for seronegativity in a patient with rheumatoid arthritis, and anti-idiotypic antibody (Ab_2) raised in animals against RF suppressed synthesis of RF by human B cell in vitro (63). Antiidiotypes can be raised using synthetic peptides corresponding to the variable region binding sites of RF (see Ref. 61); whether these would have any therapeutic application depends on the view taken on the pathogenicity of rheumatoid factor itself (see Ref. 64, pp. S184–185).

In a more general way, comment can be made on some remarkable successes in treating autoimmune disease with plasma exchange or high doses of intravenous polyspecific IgG. A good case has been made that benefit results from the presence in multiple-donor IgG of anti-idiotypes against pathogenic autoantibodies (62). Since IV IgG is usually given as crisis therapy there are no reports on systematic trials in rheumatoid arthritis; an assessment of effectiveness in acute exacerbations would be of interest.

Idiotypes of T Cells

Of much interest for anti-idiotype therapy are the extensive studies reported on "vaccination" with primed attenuated T cells, which presumably elicit an anti-idiotypic T cell response. The initial experiments, reported in the setting of EAE, showed that T cells cultured from rats or mice inoculated for EAE would, on transfer, induce EAE in syngenic animals, but such T cells when "attenuated" by irradiation or hydrostatic pressure induced resistance to subsequent induction of EAE (65).

Of relevance for arthritis, an equivalent protocol was developed in rats for protection against experimental adjuvant arthritis, an experimental arthritic disease induced by immunization with antigens of *Mycobacterium tuberculosis* (MT) and transferable with cultured T cells. There are critical antigens of MT that are cross-reactive with a cartilage proteoglycan (66). As for EAE, inoculation of attenuated (non-pathogenic) lines of cells reactive with a relevant epitope of MT induced protection against subsequent challenge for adjuvant arthritis (67). Various other experimental autoimmune diseases can be attenuated by a similar protocol, including collagen-induced arthritis (68).

The process of "T cell vaccination" remains to be clarified. It seems likely that the immunogen is the configuration of the T cell receptor on the cultured cell line and the responding protective T cell is anti-idiotypic to this. However, in addition to immunity to T cell receptors there may be an "antiergotypic" response to activation molecules on the surface of the immunogenic T cells (69). Of note, there are already some observations in humans of the therapeutic use of T cell vaccination (69a).

IV. BIOLOGIC THERAPY: THE EFFERENT LIMB

A. Autoantibody

The role of antibodies as effectors of rheumatoid synovial damage is unsettled since the antibodies that are demonstrable in rheumatoid arthritis to IgG Fc (rheumatoid factor) and collagen type II are not apparently pathogenic, and there is no clear relationship between levels of antibody and articular damage. However, in one study, arthritis was passively transferred to mice using the IgG fraction of serum from a patient with high levels of collagen antibodies (70).

B. Immune Complexes

In rheumatoid arthritis, there is an impressive formation of immune complexes containing rheumatoid factor (71) and collagen antibodies (14,15,72) and complement consumption in the synovial cavity. Although immune complexes to not appear to be the direct cause of articular destruction, the development of collagen-induced arthritis in animals has been shown to be complement dependent (73), with susceptibility linked to the ability to produce high levels of complement-activating IgG antibodies (74,75). Thus, it may be relevant that antibodies to collagen in rheumatoid arthritis are also predominantly of complement fixing subclasses (76,77). The main biologic therapy relevant to this effector process would be plasmaphesis.

C. The CD4 T Cell

The CD4 T cell has an important role in both the afferent and efferent limbs of immune response. On the efferent side, the CD4 T cell may have cytotoxic potential per se but more probably mediates effects, including tissue damage, through the release of inflammatory cytokines, as exemplified by the cutaneous delayed-type hypersensitivity reaction. Biologic therapy directed to the CD4 T cell could limit both afferent and efferent processes. The containment of afferent activity of CD4 T cells is referred to in Sec. III.C, T Cell Antigen Receptor. Biologic therapy relevant to cytokines is discussed in the next section.

D. Cytokines

Properties of Cytokines

The cytokines are a complex family of intercellular hormones with a primary structure of up to several hundred amino acids. The activated CD4 T lymphocyte is a major source of most lymphokines. The macrophage is the classic source of IL-1, but this lymphokine may, under the appropriate stimulus, be produced by various cells, including chondrocytes, fibroblasts, and endothelial cells. Except for IL-1, tumor necrosis factor, interferon-α (IFN-α) and IFN-γ, the cytokines do not have primary sequence homologies, and their structural dissimilarities are matched by the specificity of their ligand-receptor interactions. On the other hand, the cytokines do have interactive and overlapping functions and can cross-modulate the expression of the alternate receptors.

It is not within the scope of this chapter to survey the physiologic properties and pathologic roles of cytokines in inflammatory diseases, including rheumatoid arthritis, as these are covered in contemporary reviews (78–81). We can annotate that there are interrelated groups of cytokines, such as the following: (1) the inflammatory-catabolic cytokines, which include IL-1α and β and TNF-α and β; (2) lymphoid cell growth factors, which include IL-2, IL-4, IL-5, and IL-6; (3) myeloid growth factors, which include the colony-stimulating factors (CSFs) and IL-3; and (4) the interferons-α, β, and γ. The sharing of properties by cytokines is illustrated by potentiation of inflammatory reactions mediated by IL-1, TNF, and CSFs, catabolic degradation by IL-1 and TNF, amplification of B cell activity at the site of an inflammatory response by IL-2, IL-4, IL-5, and IL-6, and increase of expression of MHC molecules on cells by IFN-γ, TNF, IL-4, and IL-6. It is clearly evident that the action of a number of conventional and experimental therapies for rheumatoid arthritis can be explained by modulation of one or another of these various cytokine effects.

Interleukin-1 and Tumor Necrosis Factor

Interleukin-1 and tumor necrosis factor are structurally analogous cytokines with overlapping properties. IL-1 potentiates immune responses by inducing the proliferation of B and T lymphocytes. However, of importance in rheumatoid arthritis, IL-1 is responsible for various of the systemic "acute-phase" effects of inflammation (82), and in rheumatoid arthritis, raised serum concentrations of IL-1 correlate well with indices of activity (83). Moreover, of relevance to local pathology, IL-1 originates from stimulated intrasynovial monocytes-macrophages (84). Activities of IL-1 and TNF include the destruction of articular bone and cartilage (85), the inhibition of synthesis of proteoglycan in cartilage (86,87), and stimulation of secretion of collagenase and prostaglandin E_2 (PGE$_2$) from synovial lining cells (84). Synoviocytes in rheumatoid cell cultures possess IL-1 receptors that are of high affinity, and the potent bioactivities of IL-1α and β are mediated through this single class of receptors (88). Accordingly, a possibly useful biotherapy for rheumatoid arthritis would be a MAb that inhibits the activity of IL-1 or blocks the IL-1 receptor (IL-1R). Further possibilities include use of a soluble form of IL-1R (88a) or the recently characterized IL-1R antagonist (88b).

Another potential biotherapy for rheumatoid arthritis arises from the observations that although purified human monocytes can be stimulated in vitro with lipopolysaccharide to produce TNF-α, IL-1, and PGE$_2$, cotreatment of the stimulated cells with interleukin-4 blocks the release of these three cytotoxic mediators (89). These effects of IL-4 on human monocytes simulate those of

dexamethasone, indicating that IL-4 may of itself have anti-inflammatory properties. Thus IL-4 or IL-4 receptor agonists could be effective as "steroid-sparing"
agents in rheumatoid arthritis (89).

Interleukin-2

IL-2 is produced exclusively by T cells and has the important functions of promoting the growth and function of T and B cells and activating natural killer (NK)
cells and macrophages. Binding studies have shown that there are two IL-2 receptor
molecules with low and medium affinities that, as a heterodimer, form the high-
affinity receptor. The low-affinity receptor is recognized by the MAb anti-Tac;
the high-affinity receptor binds IL-2 with a 1000-fold greater avidity than the
low-affinity receptor but comprises only about 3% of all IL-2R molecules (43).
The very low expression of high-affinity IL-2R on T lymphocytes in blood and
synovial fluid could be a limiting factor for biotherapy directed to the IL-2R in
rheumatoid arthritis.

The actual role(s) of IL-2 in the pathogenesis of rheumatoid arthritis is unclear.
Thus the histologic appearance of synovial tissue in RA suggests an excess production of IL-2, yet there are low amounts demonstrable by bioassays of synovial
tissue, attributable in part to a soluble inhibitor that may be shed IL-2 receptor.
Moreover, T cells of patients with rheumatoid arthritis are deficient in their ability
to produce IL-2 (43). Nonetheless, therapy directed at IL-2 in rheumatoid arthritis is being actively explored. One avenue is the use of the hybridoma-derived
cytokine, contra-IL-2, described elsewhere in this volume as inhibitory to collagen-
induced arthritis. The other avenue is the use of Mab to the IL-2R, which was
shown experimentally to reduce the incidence of collagen-induced arthritis in mice
(46) and rats (47). In a limited study on three cases of rheumatoid arthritis, a
rat IgG_{2b} MAb to IL-2R (Campath 6) was infused IV for 10 days, and benefit
was evident in each case (90).

Interferons

The interferons are immunoregulatory cytokines that are produced by various
cells, including T lymphocytes, in response to viral, bacterial, or mitogenic stimuli.
The three major IFN species α, β, and γ are grouped by reason of sequence
homologies and some common properties. However, the activities of IFN-α and
β, and IFN-γ, differ in many respects, different receptors (types I and II) are
used, and the major cell sources differ, from myeloid cells for IFN-α to fibroblasts
for IFN-β and T cells for IFN-γ. The common properties of the IFNs include
the ability to render cells refractory to viral infection, the inhibition of cell proliferation, and modulation of various functions of the immune system. In addition, IFN-γ has the capacity for upregulation of MHC class II molecules on lymphoid and tissue cells.

A detailed study on IFN-α in rheumatoid arthritis revealed several aberrations

(91). IFN-α activity was not detected by antiviral bioassays using two indicator cell lines in any of the 23 serum samples and in only 1 of the 12 synovial fluids, yet peripheral blood leukocytes (PBL) from patients with inactive (but not active) rheumatoid arthritis had high activity of the enzyme 2',5'-oligoadenylate synthetase (OAS), which reflects an influence of IFN on cells, and PBL were hyperresponsive to inducers of IFN. Presumably, induction of 2',5'-OAS occurred by exposure locally to IFN at sites of rheumatoid inflammation, without such IFN reaching detectable levels in the circulation. The interpretation was that active rheumatoid arthritis is associated with hyperstimulation of IFN-α with an ensuing refractory state, analogous to that presumed to hold for IL-2 in systemic autoimmune diseases, with recovery (remission) followed by an overswing to a hyperinducible state. Alternatively, the occurrence of rheumatoid arthritis depends on a primary failure, for whatever reason, of lymphocytes to produce IFN and this is one factor in precipitating active phases of the disease. For either explanation, an action of disease-modifying drugs, such as gold or D-penicillamine, could be to restore, directly or indirectly, the normal regulation of IFN responses.

Given our evidence that remission is associated with evidence of increased IFN production, therapy with IFN-α could be beneficial. However, if the defects in IFN production and response described in rheumatoid arthritis occur as a natural protective reaction, therapy with IFN-α could exacerbate the disease. In any event, there are some mildly encouraging reports on the effects of IFN-α in rheumatoid arthritis (92,93). One recommendation at present is for well-monitored observations on intermittent intrasynovial therapy with IFN-α.

Interferon-γ has been examined in serum and synovial fluids with results differing according to the assay used, but in general levels in joint fluids are low and lymphocytes are less rather than more sensitive to IFN-γ (94). Hence cytokines other than IFN-γ must act in synergy to increase class II MHC expression on synovial cells (94,95). Even though IFN-γ upregulates MHC class II expression on synovial cells and would presumably facilitate presentation of the hypothetical rheumatoid autoantigen, this cytokine is being considered for therapy of rheumatoid arthritis. Initial reports that arthritis improved in patients undergoing treatment with IFN-γ have prompted several clinical trials. Although results in these trials have been variable (96–99), there appears to be a subset of patients who may respond to IFN-γ. However, until the mechanism of any immunologic effect is understood, it is appropriate to proceed with caution, as interferons can induce acute synovitis when injected intra-articularly into rats (100) and IFN-γ triggers the onset of collagen arthritis in immunized mice (101). Moreover, in rheumatoid arthritis, IFN-γ may stimulate the production of antinuclear antibodies or more severe disease (96).

The more logical approach of inhibiting the effects of IFN-γ in autoimune disease is illustrated by a study on the blockade of its effects by use of a MAb raised to IFN-γ. This induced significant remission in lupus in NZB $\times$ NZW mice (102), but such an antibody has not been used in humans. Inhibition of the effect of IFN-γ could also be achieved by blockade of the cell surface receptor for IFN-γ by MAb to the receptor, but there are no reports on this so far.

E. Cytotoxic Lymphocytes (CD8 T Cells)

If there were involvement of cytotoxic T cells in the effector phase of rheumatoid arthritis, then depletion of this subset by MAb to the CD8 molecule seems rational. However, studies on the effects of a MAb to the equivalent CD8 (Lyt-2) subset in mice, based on the capacity of MAb to Lyt-2 to influence skin graft rejection, showed that depletion of this subset did not greatly affect graft survival (103). Similar results are cited for the use of anti-CD8 MAb (OX8) in various experimental autoimmune diseases in rats, including EAE, experimental autoimmune neuritis, and collagen-induced arthritis; despite "total elimination" of circulating CD8 T cells, there was no modification of disease expression (32).

Anti-CD4 and anti-CD8 MAB's have been given together to achieve a synergistic action, and this regimen prevented EAE in rats and insulitis in prediabetic NOD mice (32). These results underscore the cooperative effects of CD4 and CD8 cells in the induction of autoimmune disease, but clinical benefit from this therapy would be outweighted by the risk of profound immunosuppression unless intrasynovial therapy were used.

V. CONCLUSIONS

We have reviewed in this chapter the general considerations applicable to the use of biologic therapy in autoimmune disease, with particular attention to rheumatoid arthritis in the human and the model, collagen-induced arthritis in animals. The approach taken was to analyze each of the components of the afferent and efferent limbs of the autoimmune response in terms of access to these with biotherapeutic agents, monoclonal antibodies, or cytokine antagonists.

We excluded any reference to technical aspects of monoclonal antibody therapy. However, there must be awareness of the self-limiting nature of therapy with intact murine MAb, in terms of "antimouse" responses to the antibody or anti-idiotypic responses to the active site of the antibody. These limitations can be overcome by the use of hybrid human-mouse MAbs or by linkage to the MAb of toxins, which can thereby be directed to sites of relevance (104). A particular limitation for rheumatoid arthritis, referred to throughout this review, is the unknown nature of the rheumatogenic antigen. We draw attention to the "conformational equivalence" hypothesis, which reviews the new knowledge on disease susceptibility sites on DR molecules; this is presented in the context of the rheumatogenic "antigen X" that currently eludes characterization (21).

On the other hand there is the advantage, as emphasized frequently in this chapter, that the rheumatologist enjoys a singular access to the major site of disease, the synovial cavity, allowing avoidance of problems associated with systemic use of biotherapies.

We should note again an optimism that therapy with mimotopes may become a reality in the 1990s. So far, the relevant experimental studies have been based on the model disease EAE (29,105,106), but the principle of peptide immunotherapy could be widely applicable for the therapy of autoimmune disease. The aim is to design synthetic peptides that compete for recognition of self antigens either at the site of attachment of antigen to the MHC molecule or at the level of recognition by the T cell receptor.

Cytokines have been the "debutantes" of the 1980s and by the 1990s will have a more clearly identified role in autoimmune inflammation than at present. The accumulating knowledge of the biochemical character, immunologic function, and pathologic effects of cytokines is not yet matched by knowledge of interventional strategies that could attenuate their unwanted effects. However, the already available description of "contracytokine" agents points to reasonable expectations for the future.

REFERENCES

1. Phillips, P.E. (1986). Infectious agents in the pathogenesis of rheumatoid arthritis. Semin. Arthritis Rheum. 16:1–10.
2. Brackertz, D., Mitchell, G.F., and Mackay, I.R. (1977). Studies on antigen-induced arthritis in mice. I Induction of arthritis in various strains of mice. Arthritis Rheum. 20:841–850.
3. Cromartie, W.J., Craddock, J.G., Schwab, J.H., Anderle, S.K., and Yang, C.H. (1977). Arthritis in rats after systemic injection of streptococcal cells or cell walls. J. Exp. Med. 146:1585–1602.
4. Arnett, F.C. (1989). The Lyme spirochaete: Another cause of Reiter's syndrome. Arthritis Rheum. 32:1182–1184.
5. Yokochi, T., Yanagawa, A., Kimura, Y., and Mizushima, Y. (1989). High titer of antibody to the Epstein-Barr virus membrane antigen in sera from patients with rheumatoid arthritis and systemic lupus erythematosus. J. Rheumatol. 16:1029–1032.
6. Roudier, J., Rhodes, G., Peterson, J., Vaughan, J.H., and Carson, D.A. (1988). The Epstein-Barr virus glycoprotein gp110, a molecular link between HLA DR4, HLA DR1 and rheumatoid arthritis. Scand. J. Immunol. 27:367–371.
7. Birkenfeld, P., Haratz, N., Klein, G., and Sulitzeanu, D. (1990). Cross-reactivity between the EBNA-1 p.107 peptide, collagen, and keratin: Implications for the pathogenesis of rheumatoid arthritis. Clin. Immunol. Immunopathol. 54:14–25.
8. Andriopoulos, N.A., Mestecky, J., Miller, E.J., and Bradley, E.L. (1976). Antibodies to native and denatured collagens in sera of patients with rheumatoid arthritis. Arthritis Rheum. 19:613–617.
9. Menzel, J., Steffen, C., Kolarz, G., Kojer, M., and Smolen, J. (1978). Demonstration of anticollagen antibodies in rheumatoid arthritis synovial fluid by ^{14}C-radioimmunoassay. Arthritis Rheum. 21:243–248.

10. Clague, R.B., Shaw, M.J., and Holt, P.J.L. (1981). Incidence and correlation be-
     tween serum IgG and IgM antibodies to native type II collagen in patients with chronic
     inflammatory arthritis. Ann. Rheum. Dis. 40:6–10.

11. Stuart, J.M., Huffstutter, E.H., Townes, A.S., and Kang, A.H. (1983). Incidence
     and specificity of antibodies to types I, II, III, IV, and V collagen in rheumatoid
     arthritis and other arthritic diseases as measured by ^{125}I-radioimmunoassay. Ar-
     thritis Rheum. 26:832–840.

12. Rowley, M., Tait, B., Mackay, I.R., Cunningham, T., and Phillips, B. (1986).
     Collagen antibodies in rheumatoid arthritis. Significance of antibodies to denatured
     collagen and their association with HLA-DR4. Arthritis Rheum. 29:174–184.

13. Rowley, M.J., Gershwin, M.E., and Mackay, I.R. (1988). Collagen antibodies
     in juvenile arthritis: Differences in levels and type-specificity. J. Rheumatol.
     15:289–293.

14. Clague, R., and Moore, L.J. (1984). IgG and IgM antibody to native type II collagen
     in rheumatoid arthritis serum and synovial fluid. Evidence for the presence of
     collagen-anticollagen immune complexes in synovial fluid. Arthritis Rheum.
     27:1370–1377.

15. Jasin, H. (1985). Autoantibody specificities of immune complexes sequestered in
     articular cartilage of patients with rheumatoid arthritis and osteoarthritis. Arthritis
     Rheum. 28:241–248.

16. Rowley, M., Williamson, D.J., and Mackay, I.R. (1988). Local synthesis of anti-
     bodies to collagen in the synovium in rheumatoid arthritis. Arthritis Rheum.
     30:1420–1425.

17. Trentham, D.E., Townes, A.S., and Kang, A.H. (1977). Autoimmunity to type
     II collagen: An experimental model of arthritis. J. Exp. Med. 146:857–868.

18. Yoo, T.J., Kim, S.-Y., Stuart, J.M., Floyd, R.A., Olson, G.A., Cremer, M.A.,
     and Kang, A.H. (1988). Induction of arthritis in monkeys by immunization with
     type II collagen. J. Exp. Med. 168:777–782.

19. Banerjee, S., Haqqi, T.M., Luthra, H.S., Stuart, J.M., and David, C.S. (1988).
     Possible role of Vβ T cell receptor genes in susceptibility to collagen induced ar-
     thritis in mice. J. Exp. Med. 167:832–839.

20. Nepom, G.T., Hansen, J.A., and Nepom, B.S. (1987). The molecular basis for
     HLA class II associations with rheumatoid arthritis. Clin. Immunol. 7:1–7.

21. Winchester, R.J., and Gregersen, P.K. (1988). The molecular basis of susceptibility
     to rheumatoid arthritis: the conformational equivalence hypothesis. Springer Semin.
     Immunopathol. 10:119–140.

22. Steinman, L., Waldor, M.K., Zamvel, S.S., Lim, M., Herzenberg, L., Herzenberg,
     L., McDevitt, H.O., Mitchell, D., and Sriram, S. (1986). Therapy of autoimmune
     disease with antibody to immune response gene products or to T-cell surface markers.
     Ann. N.Y. Acad. Sci. 475:274–283.

23. McDevitt, H.O., Perry, R., and Steinman, L.A. (1987). Monoclonal anti-Ia an-
     tibody therapy in animal models of autoimmune disease. In: Autoimmunity and
     Autoimmune Disease. Ciba Foundation Symposium 129. Evered, D. and Whelan,
     J., eds. Wiley, Chichester, pp. 184–190.

24. Waldor, M., Sriram, S., McDevitt, H.O., and Steinman, L. (1983). In vivo therapy
     with monoclonal anti I-A antibody suppresses immune responses to AchR. Proc.
     Natl. Acad. Sci. USA 80:2713–2717.

25. Biotard, C., Nickie, S., Serrurier, P., Butcher, G.W., Larkins, A.P., and McDevitt, H.O. (1985). In vivo prevention of thyroid and pancreatic autoimmunity in the BB rat by antibody to class II major histocompatibility complex gene products. Proc. Natl. Acad. Sci. USA 82:6627–6631.

26. Adelman, N., Watling, D., and McDevitt, H.O. (1983). Treatment of NZB/W F_1 disease with monoclonal anti-I-A monoclonal antibodies. J. Exp. Med. 158:1350–1355.

27. Wooley, P.M., Luthra, H.S., Lafuse, W.P., Huse, A., Stuart, J., and David, C.S. (1985). Type-II collagen-induced arthritis in mice. III. Suppression of arthritis by using monoclonal and polyclonal anti-Ia antisera. J. Immunol. 134:2361–2371.

28. Adorini, L., Muller, S., Cardinaux, F., Lehmann, P.V., Falconi, F., and Nagy, Z.A. (1988). In vivo competition between self peptides and foreign antigens in T cell activation. Nature 334:623–625.

29. Wraith, D.C., Smilek, D.E., Mitchell, D.J., Steinman, L., and McDevitt, H.O. (1989). Antigen recognition in autoimmune encephalomyelitis and the potential for peptide-mediated immunotherapy. Cell 59:247–255.

30. Teitelbaum, D., Aharoni, R., Arnon, R., and Sela, M. (1988). Specific inhibition of the T-cell response to myelin basic protein by the syntheic copolymer Cop 1. Proc. Natl. Acad. Sci. USA 85:9724–9728.

31. Bornstein, M., Miller, A, Slagle, S., et al. (1987). A pilot trial of Cop 1 in exacerbating-remitting multiple sclerosis. N. Engl. J. Med. 317:408–414.

32. Mackay, I.R., and Rowley, M.J. (1988). Premises for immune interventional therapy in rheumatoid arthritis. Postgrad. Med. J. 64:522–530.

33. Pankewycz, O., Strom, T.B., and Kelley, V.E. (1989). Therapeutic strategies using monoclonal antibodies in autoimmune disease. Curr. Opinion Immunol. 1:757–763.

34. Hafler, D.A., Ritz, J., Schlossman, S.F., and Weiner, H.L. (1988). Anti-CD4 and anti-CD2 monoclonal antibody infusions in subjects with multiple sclerosis. J. Immunol. 141:131–138.

35. Ranges, G.E., Sriram, S., and Cooper, S.M. (1985). Prevention of type II collagen-induced arthritis by in vivo treatment with anti-L3T4. J. Exp. Med. 162:1105–1110.

36. Herzog, C., Walker, C., Muller, W., Ricker, P., Reiter, C., Riethmuller, G., Wassmer, P., Stockinger, H., Madic, O., and Pichler, W.J. (1989). Anti-CD4 antibody treatment of patients with rheumatoid arthritis. 1. Effects on clinical course and circulating T cells. J. Autoimmun. 2:627–642.

37. Acha-Orbea, H., Mitchell, D.J., Timmerman, L., Wraith, D.C., Tausch, G.S., Waldor, M.K., Zamvil, S.S., McDevitt, H.O., and Steinman, L. (1988). Limited heterogeneity of T cell receptors from lymphocytes mediating autoimmune encephalomyelitis allows specific immune intervention. Cell 54:263–273.

38. Urban, J.L., Kumar, V., Kono, D.H., Gomez, C., Horvath, S.J., Clayton, J., Ando, D.G., Sercarz, E.E., and Hood, L. (1988). Restricted use of T cell receptor V genes in murine autoimmune encephalomyelitis raises possibilities for antibody therapy. Cell 54:577–592.

39. Chluba, J., Steeg, C., Becker, A., Wererle, H., and Epplen, J.T. (1989). T cell receptor chain usage in myelin basic protein-specific rat T lymphocytes. Eur. J. Immunol. 19:279–284.

40. Vandenbark, A.A., Hashim, G., and Offner, H. (1989). Immunization with a synthetic T-cell receptor V-region peptide protects against experimental autoimmune

encephalomyelitis. Nature 341:541–544.

41. Haqqi, T.M., Banerjee, S., Jones, W.L., Anderson, G., Behlke, M.A., Loh, D.Y., Luthra, H.S., and David, C.S. (1989). Identification of T-cell receptor Vβ deletion mutant mouse strain AU/ssJ (H-2^q) which is resistant to collagen-induced arthritis. Immunogenetics 29:180–185.

42. Stamenkovic, I., Stegagno, M., Wright, K.A., Krane, S.M., Amento, E.P., Colvin, R.B., Duquesnoy, R.J., and Kurnick, J.T. (1988). Clonal dominance among T-lymphocyte infiltrates in arthritis. Proc. Natl. Acad. Sci USA 85:1179–1183.

43. Emery, P., Wood, N., Gentry, K., Stockman, A., Mackay, I.R., and Bernard, O. (1988). High affinity IL-2 receptors on blood lymphocytes are decreased in active rheumatoid arthritis. Arthritis Rheum. 31:1176–1181.

44. Tanaka, K., Hancock, W.W., Osawa, H., Stunkel, K.G., Alverghini, T.V., Diamantstein, T., Tilney, N.L., and Kupiec-Weglinski, J.W. (1989). Mechanism of action of anti-IL-2R monoclonal antibodies. ART-18 prolongs cardiac allograft survival in rats by elimination of IL-2R+ mononuclear cells. J. Immunol. 143:2873–2879.

45. Banerjee, S., Wei, B.-Y., Hillman, K., Luthra, H.S., and David, C.S. (1988). Immunosuppression of collagen-induced arthritis in mice with an anti-IL-2 receptor antibody. J. Immunol. 141:1150–1154.

46. Stunkel, K.G., Theisen, P., Mouzaki, A., Diamantstein, T., and Schlumberger, H.D. (1988). Monitoring of interleukin-2 receptor (IL-2R) expression in vivo and studies on an IL-2R–directed immunosuppressive therapy of active and adoptive adjuvant-induced arthritis in rats. Immunology 64:683–689.

47. Warwyk, S.O., Novotny, J.R., Wicks, I.P., Wilkinson, D., Maher, D., Salvaris, E., Welch, K., Fecondo, J., and Boyd, A.W. (1988). The role of the LFA-1/ICAM-1 interaction in human leucocyte homing and adhesion. Immunol. Rev. 108:135–161.

47a. Makgoba M.W., Sanders, M.E. and Shaw, S.(1989). The CD2-LFA-3 and LFA-1-ICAM pathways: relevance to T cell recognition. Immunol. Today 12:417–428.

48. Patarroyo, M., and Makgota, M.W. (1989). Leucocyte adhesion to cells in immune and inflammatory responses. Lancet 2:1139–1142.

48a. Haynes, B.F., Hale, L.P., Denning, S.M., Le, P.T., and Singer, K.H. (1989). The role of adhesion molecules in cellular interactions: Implications for the pathogenesis of inflammatory synovitis. Springer Semin. Immunopathol. 11:163–185.

49. Cush, J.J., and Lipsky, P.E. (1988). Phenotypic analysis of synovial tissue and peripheral blood lymphocytes isolated from patients with rheumatoid arthritis. Arthritis Rheum. 31:1230–1238.

50. Hale, L.P., Martin, M.E., McCollum, D.E., Nunley, J.A., Springer, T.A., Singer, K.H., and Haynes, B.F. (1989). Immunohistologic analysis of the distribution of cell adhesion molecules within the inflammatory synovial microenvironment. Arthritis Rheum. 32:22–30.

51. Barton, R.W., Rothlein, R., Ksiazek, J., and Kennedy, C. (1989). The effect of anti-intercellular adhesion molecule-1 on phorbol-ester-induced rabbit lung inflammation. J. Immunol. 143:1278–1282.

52. Bernard, C.C.A. (1977). Suppressor T cells prevent experimental autoimmune encephalomyelitis in mice. Clin. Exp. Immunol. 29:100–109.

53. Sercarz, E.E., Yowell, R.L., Turkin, D., Miller, A., Araneo, B.A., and Adorini,

L. (1978). Different functional specificity repertoire for suppressor and helper T cells. Immunol. Rev. 39:108–136.

54. Oliveira, D.B.G., and Nardi, N.B. (1987). Immune suppression genes control the anti-F antigen response in F1 hybrids and recombinant inbred sets of mice. Immunogenetics 26:359–365.

55. van Vollenhoven, R.F., Nagler-Anderson, C., Soriano, A., Siskind, G.W., and Thorbecke, G.J. (1988). Tolerance induction by a poorly arthritogenic collagen II can prevent collagen-induced arthritis. Cell. Immunol. 115:146–155.

56. Thompson, H.S.G., Henderson, B., Spencer, J.M., Hobbs, S.M., Peppard, J.V., and Staines, N.A. (1988). Tolerogenic activity of polymerized type II collagen in preventing collagen-induced arthritis in rats. Clin. Exp. Immunol. 72:20–25.

56a. Myers, L.K., Stuart, J.M., Seyer, J.M., and Kang, A.H. (1989). Identification of an immunosuppressive epitope of type II collagen that confers protection against collagen-induced arthritis. J. Exp. Med. 170:1999–2010.

57. Hardy, R.R., Hayakawa, K., Shimizu, M., Yamasaki, K., and Kishimoto, T. (1987). Rheumatoid factor secretion from human Leu-1 B cells. Science 236:81–83.

58. Brennan, F., Plater-Zyberk, C., Maini, R.N., and Feldmann (1989). Coordinate expansion of "fetal type" lymphocytes (TCR$\gamma\delta$ +ve T and CD5$^+$B) in rheumatoid arthritis and primary Sjogren's syndrome. Clin. Exp. Immunol. 77:175–178.

59. Yakura, H., Ashida, T., Kawabata, I., and Katagiri, M. (1989). Alleviation of autoimmunity in BXSB mice by monoclonal alloantibody to Ly-5 (CD45). Europ. J. Immunol. 19:1505–1508.

60. Aseni, V., Kimeno, K., Kawamura, I., Sakumoto, M., and Nomoto, K. (1989). Treatment of autoimmune MLR/1pr mice with anti-B220 monoclonal antibody reduces the level of anti-DNA antibodies and lymphadenopathies. Immunology 68:204–208.

61. Mackay, I.R. (1988). The idiotype network: Implications for autoimmunity, infections, cancer, aging and vaccines. In: The Liver: Biology and Pathobiology, 2nd ed. Arias, I.M., Jakoby, W.B., Popper, H., Schachter, D., and Shafritz, D.A., eds., Raven Press, New York, pp. 1259–1268.

62. Rossi, F., Dietrich, G., and Kazatchkine, D. (1989). Anti-idiotypes against autoantibodies in normal immunoglobulins: Evidence for network regulation of human autoimmune responses. Immunol. Rev. 110:135–149.

63. Takeuchi, T., Hosono, O., Koide, J., Homma, M., and Abe, T. (1985). Suppression of rheumatoid factor synthesis by anti-idiotype antibody in rheumatoid arthritis patients with cross-reactive idiotypes. Arthritis Rheum. 28:873–881.

64. Gelfand, E.W., Ochs, H.D., and Stiehm, E.R., eds. (1989). Symposium on autoimmunity and immunointervention. Clin. Immunol. Immunopathol. 53:S1–S185.

65. Lider, O., Reshef, T., Beraud, E., Ben-Nun, A., and Cohen, I.R. (1988). Anti-idiotype network induced by T cell vaccination against experimental autoimmune encephalomyelitis. Science 239:181–183.

66. Van Eden, W., Holoshitz, J., Nevo, Z., Frenkel, A., Klajman, A., and Cohen, I.R. (1985). Arthritis induced by a T-lymphocyte clone that responds to *Mycobacterium tuberculosis* and to cartilage proteoglycans. Proc. Natl. Acad. Sci. USA 82:5117–5120.

67. Van Eden, W., Holoshitz, J., and Cohen, I. (1987). Antigenic mimicry between mycobacteria and cartilage proteoglycans: The model adjuvant arthritis. Concepts Immunopathol. 4:144–170.

68. Kakimoto, K., Katsuki, M., Hirofuji, T., Iwata, H., and Koga, T. (1988). Isolation of a T cell line capable of protecting mice against collagen-induced arthritis. J. Immunol. 140:78-83.

69. Lohse, A.W., Mor, F., Karin, N., and Cohen, I.R. (1989). Control of experimental autoimmune encephalomyelitis by T cells responding to activated T cells. Science 244:820-822.

69a. Cohen, I.R., and Weiner, H.L. (1988). Conference report. Immunol. Today 9:332-335.

70. Wooley, P.H., Luthra, H.S., Singh, S.K., Huse, A.R., Stuart, J.M., and David, C.S. (1984). Passive transfer of arthritis to mice by injection of human anti-type II collagen antibody. Mayo Clin Proc. 59:737-743.

71. Mannik, M., Nardella, F.A., and Sasso, E.H. (1988). Rheumatoid factors in immune complexes of patients with rheumatoid arthritis. Springer Semin. Immunopathol. 10:215-230.

72. Kerwar, S.S., Englert, M.E., McReynolds, R.A., Landes, M.J., Lloyd, J.M., Oronsky, A.L., and Wilson, F.J. (1983). Type II collagen-induced arthritis. Studies with purified anti-collagen immunoglobulin. Arthritis Rheum. 26:1120-1131.

73. Morgan, K., Clague, R.B., Shaw, M.J., Firth, S.A., Twose, T.M., and Holt, P.J.L. (1981). Native type II collagen induced arthritis in the rat: The effect of complement depletion by cobra venom factor. Arthritis Rheum. 24:1356-1362.

74. Watson, W.C., and Townes, A.S. (1985). Genetic susceptibility to murine collagen II autoimmune arthritis: Proposed relationship to the IgG_{2a} autoantibody response, complement C5, MHC and non-MHC loci. J. Exp. Med. 162:1878-1891.

75. Firth, S.A., Morgan, K., Evans, H.B., and Holt, P.J.L. (1984). IgG subclasses in collagen-induced arthritis in the rat. Immunol. Lett. 7:243-247.

76. Watson, W.C., Cremer, M.A., Wooley, P.H., and Townes, A.S. (1986). Assessment of the potential pathogenicity of type II collagen autoantibodies in patients with rheumatoid arthritis. Evidence of restricted IgG_3 subclass expression and activation of complement C5 to C5a. Arthritis Rheum. 29:1316-1321.

77. Collins, I., Morgan, K., Clague, R.B., Brenchley, P.E.C., and Holt, P.J.L. (1988). IgG subclass distribution of anti-native type II collagen and anti-denatured type II collagen antibodies in patients with rheumatoid arthritis. J. Rheumatol. 15:770-774.

78. Harrison, L.C., and Campbell, I.L. (1988). Cytokines: An expanding network of immuno-inflammatory hormones. Mol. Endocrinol. 2:1151-1156.

79. Balkwill, F.R., and Burke, F. (1989). The cytokine network. Immunol. Today 10:299-304.

80. Mizel, S.B. (1988). The interleukins. FASEB J. 3:2379-2388.

81. Emery, P., Williamson, D.J., and Mackay, I.R. (1987). Role of cytokines in rheumatological inflammation. Concepts Immunopathol. 4:171-199.

81a. Lipsky, P.E., Davis, L.S., Cush, J.J., and Oppenheimer-Marks, N. (1989). The role of cytokines in the pathogenesis of rheumatoid arthritis. Springer Semin. Immunopathol. 11:123-162.

82. Le, J., and Vilcek, J. (1987). Biology of disease. Tumour necrosis factor and interleukin 1: Cytokines with multiple overlapping biological activities. Lab. Invest. 56:234-248.

83. Eastgate, J.A., Symons, J.A., Wood, N.G., Grinlinton, F.M., Digiovine, F.S., and Duff, G.W. (1988). Correlation of plasma interleukin 1 levels with disease activity in rheumatoid arthritis. Lancet 2:706-709.

84. Miyasaki, N., Sato, K., Goto, M., Sasano, M., Matsuyama, M., Inoue, K., and Nishioka, K. (1988). Augmented interleukin-1 production and HLA-DR expression in the synovium of rheumatoid arthritis patients. Possible involvement in joint destruction. Arthritis Rheum. 31:480–486.

85. Shinmei, M., Masuda, K., Kikuchi, T., and Shimomura, Y. (1989). Interleukin 1, tumor necrosis factor, and interleukin 6 as mediators of cartilage destruction. Semin. Arthritis Rheum. 18(Suppl.):27–32.

86. Ikebe, T., Hirata, M., and Koga, T. (1988). Effects of human recombinant tumor necrosis factor α and interleukin 1 on the synthesis of glycosaminoglycan and DNA in cultured rat costal chondrocytes. J. Immunol. 140:827–831.

87. Yaron, I., Meyer, F.A., Dayer, J.M., Bleiberg, I., and Yaron, M. (1989). Some recombinant human cytokines stimulate glycosaminoglycan synthesis in human synovial fibroblast cultures and inhibit it in human articular cartilage cultures. Arthritis Rheum. 32:173–180.

88. Chin, J., Rupp, E., Cameron, P.M., MacNaul, K.L., Lotke, P.A., Tocci, M.J., and Schmidt, J.A. (1988). Identification of a high affinity receptor for interleukin 1α and interleukin 1β on cultured human rheumatoid synovial cells. J. Clin. Invest. 82:420–426.

88a. Fanslow W.C., Sims J.E., Sassenfled H., Morrissey, P.J., Gillis, S., Dower, S.K., and Widmer, M.B. (1990). Regulation of alloreactivity by a soluble form of the interleukin-1 receptor. Science 243:739–742.

88b. Carter, D.B., Deibel M.R. Jr., Dunn C.J., et al. (1990). Purification, cloning, expression, and biological characterization of an interleukin-1 receptor antagonist protein. Nature 344:633–638.

89. Hart, P.H., Vitti, G.F., Burgess, D.R., Whitty, G.A., Piccoli, D.S., and Hamilton, J.A. (1989). Potential antiinflammatory effects of interleukin 4: Suppression of human monocyte tumor necrosis factor α, interleukin 1, and prostaglandin E_2. Proc. Natl. Acad. Sci. USA 86:3803–3807.

90. Kyle V., Coughlan, R.J., Tighe, H., Waldmann, H., and Hazleman, B.L. (1989). Beneficial effect of monoclonal antibody to interleukin receptor on activated T cells in rheumatoid arthritis. Ann. Rheum. Dis. 48:428–429.

91. Hertzog, P.J., Emery, P., Cheetham, B.F., Mackay, I.R., and Linnane, A.W. (1988). Interferons in rheumatoid arthritis: Alterations in production and response related to disease activity. Clin. Immunol. Immunopathol. 48:192–201.

92. Peddinani, M.V., Savery, F., and Hang, L.M. (1979). Human leukocyte interferon in the treatment of rheumatoid arthritis. Clin. Ther. 9:39–43.

93. Kajander, A., von Essen, R., Isomaki, H., and Cantell, K. (1979). Interferon treatment of rheumatoid arthritis. Lancet 1:984–985.

94. Bergroth, V., Zvaifler, N.J., and Firestein, G. (1989). Cytokines in chronic inflammatory arthritis III. Rheumatoid arthritis monocytes are not unusually sensitive to γ-interferon, but have defective γ-interferon mediated HLA-DQ and HLA-DR induction. Arthritis Rheum. 32:1074–1079.

95. Hessian, P.A., Highton, J., and Palmer, D.G. (1989). Quantification of macrophage cell surface molecules in rheumatoid arthritis. Clin. Exp. Immunol. 77:47–51.

96. Lemmel, E.M., Franke, M., Gaus, W., Hartl, P.W., Hofschneider, P.H., Miehlke, K., Machalke, K., and Obert, H.J. (1987). Results of a phase II clinical trial on treatment of rheumatoid arthritis with recombinant interferon-gamma. Rheumatol. Int. 7:127–132.

97. Cannon, G.W., Pincus, S.H., Emkey, R.D., Denes, A., Cohen, S.A., Wolfe, F.,
     Saway, P.A., Jaffer, A.M., Weaver, A.L., Cogen, L., and Schindler, J.D. (1989).
     Double-blind trial of recombinant γ-interferon versus placebo in the treatment of
     rheumatoid arthritis. Arthritis Rheum. 32:964–973.
98. Veys, E.M., Mielants, H., Verbruggen, G., Girosclaude, J.-P., Meyer, W.,
     Galazka, A., and Schindler, J. (1988). Interferon gamma in rheumatoid arthritis—a
     double blind study comparing human recombinant interferon gamma with placebo.
     J. Rheumatol. 15:570–574.
99. Lemmel, E.M., Brackertz, D., Franke, M., Gaus, W., Hartl, P.W., Machalke,
     K., Mielke, H., Obert, H.J., Peter, H.H., Sieper, J., Sprekeler, R., and Stierle,
     H. (1988). Results of a multicenter placebo-controlled double-blind randomized phase
     II clinical study of treatment of rheumatoid arthritis with recombinant interferon-
     gamma. Rheumatol. Int. 8:87–93.
100. Rosenbach, T.O., Zor, U., Baratz, M., and Yaron, M. (1987). Induction of acute
     synovitis in the rat by human interferon. Clin. Exp. Rheumatol. 5:35–40.
101. Mauritz, N.J., Holmdahl, R., Jonsson, R., Van der Meide, P.H., Scheynius, A.,
     and Klareskog, L. (1988). Treatment with gamma-interferon triggers the onset of
     collagen arthritis in mice. Arthritis Rheum. 31:1297–1304.
102. Jacob, C.O., Van der Meide, P.H., and McDevitt, H.O. (1987). In vivo treatment
     of (NZBxNZW)F$_1$ lupus-like nephritis with monoclonal antibody to γ interferon.
     J. Exp. Med. 165:798–803.
103. Waldmann, H., Cobbold, S., Qin, S., Benjamin, R., Nash, T., Welsh, J., and
     Tarnesby, G. (1987). Monoclonal antibodies for the depletion of specific popula-
     tions of lymphocytes. In: Autoimmunity and Autoimmune Disease. Ciba Founda-
     tion Symposium 129, Evered, D. and Whelan, J. eds. Wiley, Chichester, pp.
     194–206.
104. Byers, V.S., and Baldwin, R.W. (1988). Therapeutic strategies with monoclonal
     antibodies and immunoconjugates. Immunology 65:329–335.
105. Sakai, K., Zamvil, S.S., Mitchell, D.J., Hodgkinson, S., Rothbard, J.B. and Stein-
     man, L. (1989). Prevention of experimental encephalomyelitis with peptides that
     block interaction of T cells with major histocompatibility complex proteins. Proc.
     Natl. Acad. Sci. USA 86:9470–9474.
106. Janeway, C.A. (1989). Immunotherapy by peptides? Nature 341:482–483.
107. Mackay I.R. and Gershwin, M.E. (1990). Primary biliary cirrhosis: considerations
     on pathogenesis based on identification of the M2 autoantigens. Springer Semin.
     Immunopathol. 12:101–119.

6

Cellular and Molecular Interactions in the Induction of Inflammation in Rheumatic Diseases

Sharon M. Wahl

National Institute of Dental Research, National Institutes of Health, Bethesda, Maryland

I. INTRODUCTION

Rheumatoid arthritis is a chronic inflammatory disease that progresses to destruction of bone and cartilage in the peripheral joints (1). The pathologic changes in the tissues include, but are not limited to, increased production of synovial fluid, extensive infiltration of inflammatory cells, proliferation of cells in the synovial membrane, tissue destruction, tissue repair, and fibrosis (2). Although the etiology and pathogenic mechanisms are incompletely understood, similarities exist between the immunologic processes represented in rheumatoid synovial tissue and those characteristic of delayed hypersensitivity reactions (1). Notably, the tissues are infiltrated by significant numbers of activated T lymphocytes expressing interleukin-2 receptors (IL-2R) and class II MHC antigens (3,4) and by phenotypically activated constituents of the mononuclear phagocyte lineage (5). Numerous B lymphocytes and plasma cells are found in the synovium of arthritis patients (6), but it is the T cells that appear to orchestrate the evolution of the active lesions.

The most compelling evidence for the contribution of T lymphocytes and their products in the pathogenesis of arthritis is the ability of T cell-specific immunosuppressive therapy to ameliorate the disease process (1,7,8). Accumulating evidence also favors a pivotal role for cells of the mononuclear phagocyte lineage in the complex cellular network in these tissues. A plethora of interacting T lymphocyte-

Table 1 Cytokines Identified in Rheumatoid Synovial Fluid and Tissues

	mRNA Levels	Protein levels
T lymphocytes		
IFN-γ	+ +	±
IL-2	+ +	±
TNF-β (LT)	+ +	±
IL-6	?	+ + +
IL-3	−	−
GM-CSF	+ +	+ +
TGF-β	+ +	+ +
Monocyte-macrophages		
IL-1α	+ +	+
IL-1β	+ +	+
TNF-α (cachectin)	+	+ + +
IL-6	?	+ + +
PDGF	?	+ +
TGF-β	+ +	+ + +
GM-CSF	+ +	+ +
M-CSF	+ +	+ +

and monocyte-derived peptide mediators (cytokines) have been identified in the synovium that contribute to the cascade of events leading to destruction of the joint (Table 1) (9,10). Recent studies have focused on the multifunctional roles of these cytokines, which are synthesized by, and act upon, the various cell types involved in inflammatory and immune processes. Although the advent of recombinant cytokines has facilitated the definition of the unique biologic activities of individual mediators, the complex interactions among these inflammatory products continue to be unraveled. Several of the cytokines that have been identified in inflamed synovium and their potential roles in rheumatoid arthritis are reviewed in this chapter.

II. ROLE OF T LYMPHOCYTES

Although the inciting antigen(s) has not yet been identified in rheumatoid arthritis, the infiltrating T lymphocytes, in association with antigen-presenting accessory cells, are presumably triggered to proliferate and to synthesize and secrete cytokines that contribute to the recruitment, activation, proliferation, and functional response of additional inflammatory cells. Although the synovial T cells appear activated by morphologic and immunocytochemical parameters (1-4), a paradox exists in that many of the soluble mediators normally produced by activated T cells are often found to be deficient in the synovial milieu. Interleukin-2 (IL-2), tumor necrosis factor β (TNF-β), and interferon γ (IFN-γ) levels are unexpectedly low in these tissues despite the demonstration of elevated gene expression for some of these cytokines, as discussed later. Whether this deficit of anticipated mediators is the consequence of absence or decreased production, increased utilization, the presence of binding proteins or soluble shed receptors, the existence of membrane-bound forms of the cytokines, or the presence of antagonists remains to be defined.

A. Interleukin-2

Upon activation, T lymphocytes normally produce interleukin-2, a 133 amino acid glycoprotein with a molecular weight of 15 kD (11). Required for the transition of activated T cells from the G_1 to the S phase of the cell cycle (11), IL-2 is thought to play a crucial role in the generation and maintenance of immune cells and their products necessary for an immune response. Thus, the low or nondetectable levels of IL-2 in the inflamed synovial tissues of rheumatoid arthritis patients appear inconsistent with an active immune response (12–17). However, recent studies examined freshly isolated and cultured synovial lymphocytes for IL-2-specific mRNA and identified high levels of IL-2 mRNA expression (18,19). Although it is unknown whether the cells actually secrete IL-2, these studies favor the concept that persistent T cell activation and cytokine generation contribute to the disease process. In a related hypothesis, it has been suggested that the initial T cell activation in the synovium results in a transient exhaustion of IL-2 secretion (20) and that, in fact, a hyperactive IL-2–IL-2R system is involved in autoimmune tissue injury (21). Thus, the decreased levels of detectable IL-2 may be due to an inhibitor of IL-2 (22) or to the increased polyamines in arthritis patients that inhibit T cell function (23). Moreover, transforming growth factor β, a potent T cell inhibitor (24–26) that has been identified in rheumatoid synovium, may contribute to the modulation of T cell function in these tissues, as described in a later section.

Once generated, the action of IL-2 on its target cells is dependent upon its binding to a specific, high-affinity membrane receptor (IL-2R) (27) composed of the IL-2R β chain (p55, Tac antigen) and the α chain (p75) (28,29). Not present on resting T cells, the IL-2R is rapidly expressed on antigen-activated T cells (30). Following the binding of IL-2 to the IL-2R on the cell surface, the IL-2–IL-2R complex is internalized and cellular proliferation commences. Synovial T lymphocytes have been demonstrated to express both IL-2R mRNA and IL-2R protein (16,17,19).

In addition to the T lymphocytes, stimulated monocytes also express IL-2R (31–33), and IL-2R-positive monocytes have been identified in synovial fluids of arthritis patients (34). IL-2R expression on monocytes provides another level of

T cell regulation of monocyte effector function and cytokine secretion (33). Furthermore, elevated binding and internalization of IL-2 by the IL-2R-positive macrophages may contribute to the decreased levels of IL-2 detectable in synovial preparations. Shed, soluble IL-2R detected in rheumatoid arthritis patients (35) may also contribute to IL-2 depletion.

B. Tumor Necrosis Factor β

Activated T lymphocytes are also a source of tumor necrosis factor β (lymphotoxin), a glycoprotein that exhibits structural and functional similarities to the macrophage product, TNF-α (cachectin) (36). The genes for TNF-β and TNF-α are closely linked to the major histocompatibility complex on chromosome 6, and the proteins encoded by these genes share approximately 30% homology at the amino acid level (37–40). Moreover, TNF-α and β appear to bind to a common cell surface receptor (40). However, in the inflamed synovium of rheumatoid arthritis patients TNF-β protein is absent, even though TNF-β mRNA levels are reportedly high in synovial cell cultures (18). Presumably, the TNF activity that has been demonstrated in synovitis is derived from activated macrophages (41, Table 1).

C. Interferon-γ

Interferon-γ Levels in Arthritis

Interferon-γ is another cytokine commonly associated with activated T cell populations that provides important effector cell regulatory activity (42). However, within the inflamed synovium and in synovial cell cultures, IFN-γ levels are minimal (15,43–45). Interestingly, IFN-γ gene expression is apparent in synovial preparations, again suggesting a defect in posttranscriptional mechanisms (18,45). Since IL-2 has been shown to regulate IFN-γ production (46), the paucity of IL-2 may in turn impede the production of IFN-γ.

In inflammation, IFN-γ is thought to have a wide range of effects on both the evolution and resolution of the host response. The effects of IFN-γ on macrophages are extensive, and macrophages exposed to IFN-γ display numerous enhanced functions, including increased phagocytosis, respiratory burst, and antimicrobial and antitumor activity (42). Moreover, in response to IFN-γ these cells demonstrate increase surface expression of class II HLA antigens and IL-2R and an enhanced ability to secrete a number of mediators, including IL-1, TNF-α, granulocyte-macrophage colony stimulating factor (GM-CSF), proteases, and arachidonic acid metabolites. However, in the absence of significant levels of IFN-γ in the inflamed synovium, activation of the mononuclear phagocyte population must occur by other mechanisms and this cytokine appears not to play a major role in the pathogenesis of rheumatoid arthritis.

Interferon-γ Therapy

In light of the paucity of IFN-γ in rheumatoid synovial lesions and based on its potent antiproliferative and immunomodulatory effects, recent studies have addressed the potential clinical application of IFN-γ in arthritis. In an experimental animal model with clinical, radiologic, and histologic features that resemble those of human rheumatoid arthritis, IFN-γ was found to ameliorate the disease process (47). In this model, the systemic administration of cell wall fragments from group A streptococci (SCW) induces a biphasic pattern of polyarthritis (48). The SCW are deposited and persist in the phagocytic cells of the synovium, inducing joint pathology that begins as an acute, leukocyte-mediated inflammatory response. As the acute response subsides, a chronic T cell-dependent response occurs in which synovial lining cell hyperplasia, mononuclear cell infiltration, and eventual erosive destruction of the bone and cartilage are apparent.

Administration of recombinant IFN-γ in this model reduced not only the acute inflammatory response but had an even greater suppressive effect on the chronic mononuclear cell-mediated destructive phase of the disease (47). Histopathologic evaluation of the joints demonstrated that IFN-γ-treated animals had significantly fewer inflammatory cells and less synovial hyperplasia and erosions than the control arthritic animals. IFN-γ was shown to selectively suppress mononuclear cell prostaglandin synthesis, but not cytokine production, to inhibit monocyte chemotaxis and to inhibit synovial fibroblast proliferation (47). These data indicate that the pathophysiology of antigen-induced erosive polyarthritis is subject to regulatory control at several levels by IFN-γ and that these mechanisms of suppression may be relevant in the treatment of rheumatoid arthritis.

In this regard, recently conducted trials of recombinant human IFN-γ in the treatment of rheumatoid arthritis have revealed improvement in disease activity as assessed by multiple measures (49–54). In the two trials that were placebo controlled, one demonstrated significant IFN-γ-mediated improvement (50); the other showed improvement that did not reach significance (49). Administration of IFN-γ was associated with minimal adverse drug reactions. Taken together, these initial clinical trials suggest that IFN-γ may offer a new approach to management of the pathophysiology of rheumatoid arthritis.

D. Colony Stimulating Factors

Similar to IL-2, TNF-β, and IFN-γ, inflammatory joint fluids are deficient in the T cell-derived colony stimulating factor known as IL-3 or multi-CSF. However, in contrast to IL-3, the synovial preparations are a rich source of certain other colony stimulating factors (55). Four distinct human CSFs have been characterized, including granulocyte-CSF (G-CSF), macrophage CSF (M-CSF or CSF-1), granulocyte-macrophage CSF, and IL-3 (56,57). Whereas IL-3 is primarily a T cell product, GM-CSF is produced not only by T cells but also by macrophages and fibroblasts (58,59). G-CSF is produced by monocytes and fibroblasts, and similarly, monocytes, fibroblasts, and endothelial cells all synthesize M-CSF (60).

Although IL-3 may be an important immunoregulatory cytokine (56), its role in synovitis is questionable, since neither the protein nor the mRNA for IL-3 was found in rheumatoid synovial tissues (17). The activities of IL-3, including promotion of early steps in T cell maturation, differentiation of bone marrow progenitors into various hematopoietic cells, and activation of monocyte genes coding for such monokines as IL-1 and TNF-α (61–63) may be replaced by other CSFs in the synovium. Both GM-CSF and CSF-1 are present in inflamed synovium (17,55). Although the specific role of these factors in the arthritic process is unclear, it must extend beyond the promotion of hematopoietic colony formation since these cytokines exhibit a spectrum of other immunomodulatory activities on mature cells (64,65). GM-CSF, a 22 kD glycoprotein, shares with IL-3 the ability to stimulate myeloid and erythroid progenitor cells (56,57). Additionally, GM-CSF augments monocyte effector functions, including phagocytosis, interleukin-1 and superoxide anion production, class II MHC expression, and cytotoxicity (62,64,66). In fact, recent studies indicate that GM-CSF, rather then IFN-γ, may be the primary cytokine in rheumatoid synovium responsible for monocyte activation and for induction of class II MHC antigen on these cells and on macrophagelike synovial lining cells and tissue macrophages (67). All these biologic activities are initiated by the binding of GM-CSF to specific and saturable high-affinity (10^{-9}–10^{-10} M) cell surface receptors (100–500 receptors per cell) (68,69).

E. Interleukin-6

In contrast to certain other T cell products, IL-6 levels are very high in synovial fluid and cells (50–22,000 U/ml) (70–74). Other cells in addition to T lymphocytes produce IL-6, including both synovial cells and infiltrating cells of monocyte lineage. The overproduction of IL-6 in the synovium likely contributes to the localized characteristic immunopathology, including plasma cell accumulation, autoantibody production, and T cell activation, and may also influence certain systemic symptoms due to elevated serum levels (74).

Originally characterized as a T cell product that regulated B lineage cell differentiation into antibody producing cells (75), this 184 amino acid 26 kD phosphoglycoprotein has subsequently been shown to provide a wide variety of biologic signals to various tissues and cells that express IL-6 receptors (100–1000 per cell) (76). The IL-6R, a member of the immunoglobulin superfamily, appears to consist of two polypeptide chains: a ligand-binding and a signal-transducing chain (77). The IL-6R is expressed on resting T cells, and IL-6 can in turn induce IL-2R expression and IL-2 production to mediate T cell activation (78).

After molecular cloning, the proteins, interferon-β2 (IFN-β_2), B cell differentiation factor (BCDF/BSF2), and IL-6 were found to be identical (75). Although the initially reported antiviral activity was not confirmed (79), this protein plays an important role in various aspects of the immune response, including T cell activation, induction of acute-phase protein synthesis by hepatocytes and fever (80). In addition, IL-6 increases the expression of class I HLA antigens on fibroblasts (81,82) and IL-6 production by fibroblasts is induced by IL-1, TNF-α, and TNF-β (72,83), suggesting an autocrine control loop in fibroblast activity.

F. Transforming Growth Factor β

Activated T cells of both CD4 and CD8 subsets express mRNA for TGF-β and secrete TGF-β, and these cells also possess receptors for TGF-β (24), implicating another autocrine and/or paracrine regulatory loop (84,85). Discovered by its ability to stimulate the anchorage-independent growth in soft agar of cells that are otherwise anchorage dependent (review, Ref. 86), TGF-β consists of two disulfide-linked identical chains each containing 112 amino acids (87). TGF-β is secreted in an inactive precursor form that requires activation before exerting its biologic effects (88). Considering the ubiquity of TGF-β and of cells possessing TGF-βR (86), activation of the latent TGF-β must represent an important regulatory step in TGF-β action.

Recently identified in synovial fluids of arthritis patients (89,90), TGF-β may be an important early trigger in synovial inflammation. This cytokine is an extremely potent chemoattractant for monocytes, with optimal concentrations in the femtomolar range (91). Because the cells responsible for synovial inflammation must be recruited to the synovium from the circulation and/or surrounding areas, TGF-β-directed cellular migration and accumulation is likely an essential first step in the pathogenic process. Furthermore, the ability of TGF-β to inhibit lymphocyte proliferative responses may contribute in both an autocrine and paracrine fashion to the apparent paradox of the activated T cell population in the synovium, which is in many ways suppressed (see earlier). The multifunctional capabilities of this cytokine (86), which is produced by nearly all cells, suggest its central role in arthritis and other inflammatory lesions. In fact, direct administration of TGF-β to the joint space induces synovitis in experimental animals, as described in a later section.

G. Inhibition of T Cells Inhibits Arthritis

The role of T cells in arthritis is clear, even though certain anticipated cytokines are absent within the synovium of patients. Although most forms of immunosuppressive therapy that benefit arthritis inhibit several aspects of immune function (1), specific inhibition of T cell function, in particular inhibition of lymphokine synthesis, ameliorates the disease process. In this regard, cyclosporin A (CsA), which acts specifically during T lymphocyte activation to inhibit the transcription of a limited set of early activation genes, including IL-2, IL-3, IFN-γ, TNF, and c-*myc* (92,93), effectively modulates the pathogenic events in certain subsets of rheumatoid arthritis patients (7). CsA binds to and inhibits cyclophilin, a peptidyl-prolyl isomerase responsbile for catalyzing the refolding of proteins and peptides into their native conformations during T cell activation (94,95). Comparison of high-dose (10 mg/kg) and low-dose (1 mg/kg) oral regimens in a prospective 6 month randomized, double-blind trial revealed that CsA significantly reduced disease activity by several parameters and improved function in a dose-related manner. Although drug-related toxicities occurred, these toxicities were often reversible with a reduction in the dose (7). These studies confirm the pivotal role of lymphocytes in the pathogenic process and point to additional related avenues of selective therapy.

III. MONOCYTE-MACROPHAGES IN SYNOVIAL INFLAMMATION

A. Recruitment and Activation

Adherence and Migration

Monocytes are recruited into the synovial tissue, where they become activated, differentiate into macrophages, and participate in the synovial inflammatory response. This emigration of monocytes from the blood to the tissues and their subsequent activities there may be a primary event in rheumatoid arthritis. Triggered by adherence and chemotactic signals, monocytes adhere to and cross the endothelial cell barrier, moving toward the site of inflammation. Monocytes express a family of cell adhesion molecules, including Mac-1 (CR3) and p150,95, which not only mediate adhesion to endothelial cells (96) but also promote their movement through inflamed tissues (97). Upregulation of p150,95 and to a lesser extent CR3 on synovial macrophages has been reported in hyperplastic rheumatoid synovial membranes, and the pattern of cellular expression of these adhesion proteins was consistent with trafficking of the cells from the synovial vessels through the synovial membrane and finally to the joint surface (98).

During this process of adhesion and migration, peripheral blood monocytes acquire the capacity to generate type IV collagenase, which binds to and degrades type IV collagen, the major structural component of vessel basement membranes (99). Collagenase release enables disruption of the basement membrane to facilitate monocyte entry into the inflamed tissues. Movement into the tissues occurs in response to chemoattractants, including complement fragments, cytokines, and other mediators (100). Detected levels of the cytokine TGF-β in synovial fluid and tissues are sufficient for promoting monocyte chemotaxis (89,90). During the chronic phases of synovial inflammation, multiple mechanisms probably account for the sustained accumulation of mononuclear phagocytes, including an increase in proliferative capacity and mobilization of locally derived cells, as well as increased recruitment from the circulation.

Monocyte Activation

Maturation of the newly recruited monocytes evoked by any of a number of inflammatory stimuli is apparent by morphologic, functional, and biochemical criteria (1,5). Localized within the synovial tissue, the monocytes become macrophages and exhibit enhanced phagocytic and lysosomal activity, phenotypic markers characteristic of the activated state, release of reactive oxygen intermediates (ROI) and arachidonic acid products, and generation of cytokines important in the maintenance and amplification of the host response (101). Within the tissues, the cells of the mononuclear phagocyte lineage represent a heterogeneous population of cells in various stages of activation intermixed with newly recruited, less mature monocytes.

Enhanced monocyte phagocytosis occurs via complement and Fc receptors (FcγR), which are increased during maturation induced by such inflammatory stimuli as IFN-γ (102). However, the reported absence of IFN-γ in the rheumatoid synovium suggested other mechanisms of augmented FcγR expression and phagocytosis. In this regard, another cytokine, TGF-β, has recently been shown to selectively augment the expression of FcγRIII, an important receptor for immunophagocytosis (103). During FcγR-mediated phagocytosis, monocytes as well as neutrophils experience an oxidative burst that causes the release of reactive oxygen species (102,104). The initial product of the respiratory burst, superoxide anion (O_2^-), is formed at the membrane of monocytes by NADPH oxidase and is converted by superoxide dismutase (SOD) to H_2O_2. This H_2O_2 subsequently forms toxic hypohalous acids with potent oxidizing potential. These products can be extremely toxic to adjacent cells and tissues if released to the external milieu (105).

Inhibition of ROI Inhibits Arthritis

The potential role of these leukocyte-derived ROI, which are an early, and potentially continuous, product of monocyte activation in destructive joint lesions, was recently evaluated in an experimental arthritis model. As described earlier, injection of group A SCW fragments induces acute and chronic erosive polyarthritis in inbred susceptible Lewis rats. To determine whether ROI contribute to the development of joint pathology in this model, superoxide dismutase was injected into one of the hind joints on day 0 or day 10 following SCW administration (106). The contralateral joint received saline only, and the articular indices were monitored for 4–6 weeks. A single injection of SOD given immediately following the SCW was found to dramatically suppress not only acute synovitis but also the chronic destructive phase of the disease. Furthermore, intraarticular administration of SOD to animals already arthritic (day 10) suppressed the subsequent mononuclear cell-mediated pathology (106). These studies suggest that the toxic oxygen species of the respiratory burst are central to the evolution of joint pathology and that inhibition of their production modulates the course of the disease. Further studies on the mechanisms of action of these antioxidants may enable selective suppression of acute and chronic phases of inflammation.

Chronic Activation

Continued activation of the mononuclear cell infiltrate, apparently due to persistence of the inflammatory stimulus, causes the chronic secretion of monocyte-derived neutral proteases, hydrolases, complement components, coagulation factors, and polypeptide hormones that interact with various target tissues and cells in an endocrine, paracrine and/or autocrine fashion (107). The accumulation of these molecules due to persistent secretion contributes to the detrimental aspects of the inflammatory response. In light of the paucity of certain T cell products in the rheumatoid joint, many of these soluble inflammatory mediators responsible for joint pathology must be products of activated macrophages within the synovium (Table 1).

B. Transforming Growth Factor β

Production and Autoregulation

In addition to T cells, monocytes also generate the polypeptide hormone TGF-β. However, monocytes constitutively express TGF-β mRNA, and, when activated, synthesize and secrete this cytokine (108). TGF-β may be an important autoregulator of monocyte function in that it appears to upregulate its own gene expression and induces monocytes to produce other growth factors (85,109). TGF-β at picomolar concentrations induces monocyte gene expression for TNF-α, IL-1, basic fibroblast growth factor (bFGF), and c-sis (PDGF) (85,91,109), each of which participates in a wide variety of inflammatory processes.

Although many cells in the inflamed synovium and surrounding connective tissue may generate TGF-β (107), synovial mononuclear cells appear to be an important source of this inflammatory mediator (90). Adherent macrophages isolated from synovial fluid of rheumatoid arthritis patients not only constitutively express mRNA for TGF-β, but they also secrete and activate latent TGF-β (90) similar to macrophages activated in vitro (110). The levels of TGF-β constitutively secreted by synovial macrophages are higher than have been described for stimulated peripheral blood monocytes in vitro and are sufficient to mediate numerous cellular functions in this lesion.

In addition to promoting many aspects of the immune response, TGF-β has also been shown to be one of the most potent immunosuppressive agents yet described. TGF-β inhibits lymphocyte proliferation in vivo and in vitro (24–26) and can deactivate macrophage ROI metabolism (111). The events within the synovium are consistent with many of the in vitro activities attributed to TGF-β, in that synovially derived TGF-β inhibits IL-1-dependent lymphocyte proliferation while enhancing the production of IL-1 (90).

Induction of Synovitis

Although the identification of TGF-β in arthritic synovial effusions provided circumstantial evidence for its role in arthritis, recent studies directly evaluated the effect of this peptide in synovial inflammation (112). Injection of TGF-β directly into the synovial space of naive animals induced clinically apparent synovitis. Within hours after the initial injection, macrophages were the dominant infiltrating cell, with fewer lymphocytes. This extensive monocytic cell recruitment into the synovium after intra-articular injection of TGF-β is consistent with the chemotactic activity of this peptide demonstrated in vitro (91). Furthermore, TGF-β is chemotactic for fibroblasts (113), which also increase in number soon after TGF-β administration (112).

The increased cellularity of the synovial lining layer was also the consequence of local fibroblast proliferation. Since fibroblast and endothelial cell proliferation are reportedly inhibited by TGF-β in vitro (86), additional signals induced in situ by TGF-β most probably contribute to the development of TGF-β-induced synovial pathology. In this regard, gene expression for the growth-promoting cytokine IL-1, as well as TGF-β itself, was elevated in the synovial tissue after TGF-β administration (112).

Discontinuance of the TGF-β resulted in reversal of the joint inflammation and fibroplasia. Repeated cycles of TGF-β administration reinitiated the inflammatory response. No evidence of pannus invasion or destruction of cartilage and bone characteristic of arthritis was apparent. However, the transient nature of the TGF-β stimulus (three injections) did not rule out the possibility that the continued presence of TGF-β and/or other cytokines, as occurs in chronic lesions, may promote pannus formation and tissue erosion.

C. Interleukin-1

As already described, TGF-β can induce monocyte IL-1 gene expression and synthesis both in vitro and in the synovium. IL-1 is an important regulatory cytokine with many proinflammatory functions (114) and is considered a key player in the evolution of destructive joint lesions. Well known for its interaction with lymphocytes of the helper-inducer (CD4) phenotype through a high-affinity receptor (115,116), IL-1 stimulates these T cells to release IL-2 and to express increased IL-2R (117). These IL-2R-positive cells then become responsive to the IL-2 signal, undergoing clonal expansion critical for an immune response. Although two distinct IL-1 genes encode two proteins (IL-1α and IL-1β) with similar size and biologic activity (118,119), both IL-1α and IL-1β bind to the

T cells or other target cells through the same 80–85 kD glycoprotein receptor sites (120).

IL-1 has probably been studied more than any other cytokine for its role in arthritis. Produced by synovial cells (121) as well as inflammatory cells, IL-1 is found in the synovial fluid of arthritis patients (122–125). TNF-α has been shown to induce IL-1 synthesis in the synovium (18), and IL-1 itself induces both IL-1α and β protein secretion by synovial fibroblasts (126). IL-1 protein levels in synovial cell cultures are high (18), but activity levels in biologic assays frequently are not. The low levels of IL-1 bioactivity are thought to be due to the presence of IL-1-specific inhibitors (127), one of which has been recently identified as TGF-β (90).

In addition to its important role in immunoregulation, IL-1 is instrumental in modulating many of the connective tissue changes characteristic of arthritis. Importantly, IL-1 has been associated with both disease induction and progression in arthritis models (128,129). Intra-articular injection of nanogram quantities of recombinant IL-1α or IL-1β into naive rat joints initiated an acute transient arthritis, but similar to TGF-β-induced synovitis, there was no evolution into erosive disease (130). On the other hand, IL-1 injection directly into already inflamed joints (130) or administered subcutaneously in arthritic animals (129) promoted a more rapid and severe response, with pannus formation and some marginal erosion of cartilage and subchondral bone. Similarly, in rabbits IL-1 caused only a transient loss of proteoglycan from the articular cartilage (131). Given the multifunctional aspects of the biologic activity of IL-1, other mediators and cell types may also be necessary to elicit chronic arthritogenic effects.

D. Tumor Necrosis Factor β

Another monocyte-derived cytokine that plays an important role in mediating the host response to injury is tumor necrosis factor α (cachectin), a 157 amino acid nonglycosylated 17 kD molecule (132). TNF-α has been identified in synovial fluids (133), and its production in rheumatoid synovial cell cultures reportedly ranges from 82 to 2000 pg/ml (18). Although the cellular source of the TNF in the inflamed synovium is unknown, in situ hybridization studies implicate the synovial macrophage population (18).

Initially shown to promote cytotoxicity and cachexia, numerous other biologic activities have been demonstrated for TNF-α, including many that overlap with IL-1 even though these two cytokines have minimal sequence homology and distinct receptor systems (120). TNF-α can induce IL-1 production, and IL-1 can induce the release of TNF-α from mononuclear cells (114,134), setting in motion a cycle of cytokine induction and regulation. TNF-α promotes the early stages of an inflammatory response through its ability to increase endothelial cell production of arachidonic acid metabolites, platelet activating factor, and IL-1

(135,136). Furthermore, TNF-α augments leukocyte adhesion, procoagulant activity, and release of plasminogen activator inhibitor (137,138). In further contributing to the cytokine network, TNF-α augments GM-CSF transcription and translation in endothelial cells and fibroblasts (139,140) to promote the local proliferation and differentiation of granulocytes and macrophages.

E. Platelet-Derived Growth Factor

Synovial fluids from arthritis patients contain high levels of platelet-derived growth factor (PDGF) (141), and the local release of this peptide may be crucial in regulating the migration and proliferation of synovial cells. PDGF is a potent mitogen, chemoattractant, and stimulator of protein synthesis, particularly for mesenchymal cell populations (review, Ref. 142). Once thought to be a potent chemoattractant for both neutrophils and monocytes (143–145), recent evidence indicates that purified or recombinant PDGF does not have leukocyte chemotactic activity (146). Thus the primary target of PDGF appears to be mesenchymal cells, somewhat at variance with many of the other cytokine growth factors, which interact with various cell types in a cascadelike fashion.

Released during platelet adherence and/or aggregation (142), PDGF is also synthesized and secreted by monocytes following activation (147,148). Tissue macrophages as well as monocytes undergoing maturation in culture spontaneously release low levels of PDGF (147,149). Continued activation of monocytes could provide a persistent source of PDGF in a chronic inflammatory site. In addition to platelets and monocytes, PDGF is produced by vascular endothelial cells (150,151) and smooth muscle cells (152).

A dimeric glycoprotein, PDGF consists most often of an A chain (14 kD) and a B chain (17 kD) linked by two disulfide bonds (153–155). However, biologically active AA and BB dimers are also synthesized by certain cell types. It is the B chain, coded for by the c-*sis* proto-oncogene, which is expressed by activated monocytes and tissue macrophages (147–149), suggesting that activation of this particular proto-oncogene contributes to diseases characterized by mesenchymal cell proliferation. The biologic action of PDGF is initiated by binding to a high-affinity cell surface receptor (PDGF-R), which is a tyrosine-specific protein kinase (156–158). The PDGF-R is itself a dimer composed of α and/or β subunits (159), providing selectivity of binding of the A and B chains of the PDGF protein. Expression of PDGF-R is clearly upregulated in rheumatoid synovium (160).

F. Fibroblast Growth Factor

Additional potent mitogens for fibroblasts and endothelial cells are the fibroblast growth factors (FGF), which stimulate both angiogenesis and granulation tissue formation in vivo (161,162). An acid and a basic FGF have been characterized that are similar in size (140 and 146 amino acid residues) and share >50%

sequence homology, heparin affinity, and biologic activity (163,164). An important source of this activity in inflammatory sites is the macrophage population (165). Following activation, monocytes express the gene for FGF and synthesize biologically active FGF (108,165). Interestingly, posttranslationally processed aFGF and bFGF exhibit similarities in sequence homology to IL-1α and IL-1β (164), suggesting that FGF and IL-1 are members of a family of homologous growth factors.

G. Interleukin-6

In the ongoing cytokine cascade, TNF, IL-1, and PDGF can promote the synthesis of yet another monocyte-derived cytokine, interleukin-6 (81,166,167). IL-6 is produced much more rapidly by monocytes than T cells in culture, suggesting that T cell- and monocyte-derived IL-6 may have distinct roles in different phases of the immune response (168). As shown for certain other monocyte products, IL-6 shares a significant homology with monocyte-derived G-CSF (75), and the genes for these two cytokines may be evolutionarily derived from a common ancestral gene. Based on its ability to regulate immune responses, hematopoiesis, and acute-phase reactions as described earlier, this multifunctional cytokine identified in high levels in inflamed synovium may be pivotal in synovial immunopathogenesis. Attempts to antagonize IL-6 activity will facilitate the unraveling of its contribution to synovial pathology.

IV. SYNOVIAL HYPERPLASIA AND CONNECTIVE TISSUE DEGRADATION

A. Synovial Fibroblast Recruitment and Proliferation

The infiltration of lymphocytes and monocyte-macrophages into the synovium and their release of inflammatory mediators, including the cytokines described in this chapter, are associated with the recruitment and proliferation of synovial fibroblastlike cells and synovial tissue neovascularization (1,2,10,169). These observations suggest that immune cell-synovial cell interactions are involved in the formation and function of the pannus, which is composed of proliferating fibroblasts, numerous small blood vessels, collagen, and inflammatory cells. This hyperplasia of synovial lining cells and fibroblastlike cells is an early and characteristic feature of the synovitis associated with rheumatoid arthritis. The pathologic fibroplasia in arthritis, as well as normal tissue repair, is intimately linked to processes that recruit mesenchymal cells and stimulate them to proliferate at local sites (10,169–171). The inflammatory cell-derived products mediate this cellular accumulation, leading to the excessive levels of collagenase and prostaglandins, which in turn are responsible for connective tissue destruction. Erosion of bone, cartilage, and soft connective tissue occurs primarily in areas adjacent to the pannus.

Although synovial lining cells possess the innate ability to migrate and to proliferate, they are normally quiescent unless exposed to mediators that trigger these processes through specific cell surface receptors (review, Ref. 172). Among these mediators are the products of lymphocytes and monocytes-macrophages, some of which are recruitment signals and others, or the same ones, that induce proliferative responses (Table 2). Although the proliferative response is influenced by many factors, the polypeptide growth factors are the most critical. Interestingly, epidermal growth factor, insulinlike growth factor, and substance P, which stimulate fibroblasts from other tissue sites, do not stimulate the proliferation of synovial fibroblasts in culture (173). Consequently, the macrophage-derived growth factors IL-1α and β, TNF-β, PDGF, and FGF may be among the most important fibroproliferative mediators in synovial lesions (173–176).

In this regard, synovial fibroblasts express high-affinity receptors for IL-1α and IL-1β (177) and fibroblasts proliferate following exposure to IL-1 (178). However, IL-1 is not directly mitogenic for fibroblasts, but rather, IL-1 induces fibroblasts to produce PDGF, which then, in an autocrine manner, triggers a proliferative response (179). In these studies, growth of fibroblasts occurred after a lag phase required for PDGF synthesis, release, and action. In confirmation of this regulatory loop, treatment with a PDGF-specific neutralizing antibody completely inhibited fibroblast proliferation following exposure to IL-1. In a potentially similar fashion, TGF-β induces fibroblast c-*sis* mRNA expression followed by a corresponding increase in PDGF B chain release, which promotes the mitogenic response (180). Thus, a commonality of pathways is emerging in which certain cytokines modulate mesenchymal cell growth via the induction of oncogenes, such as PDGF. Whether IL-1, TNF-α, and TGF-β act as progression factors after PDGF confers competence is not known.

Modulation of receptor expression may also favor susceptibility to certain growth factors. Expression of growth factor receptors has been shown to be increased on connective tissue cells in inflamed synovium, and in particular, elevated expression of PDGF-R on fibroblasts in pannus tissue adjacent to resorbing bone and cartilage has been demonstrated (160).

Most cytokines have additional effects on mesenchymal cells, including differentiation, motility, and protein and matrix synthesis (Table 2). The role of the expanded fibroblast population in rheumatoid disease is likely extensive since these cells contribute to cytokine release, bone and cartilage resorption, and fibrosis (169). The inducible expression of class II MHC antigens on fibroblasts (181) also plays an important role in the regulation and exacerbation of the ongoing immune response. Moreover, fibroblasts release GM-CSF, IL-6, arachidonic acid metabolities, and collagenase in response to IL-1 and TNF-α, contributing further to the molecular signaling network. These factors may act synergistically and/or may regulate the functions of each other. For example, stimulation of proliferation by TNF and IL-1, but not PDGF or FGF, is associated with increased

Table 2 Inflammatory Cell Mediators That May Modulate Synovial Cell Function

Chemotactic factors	Mitogenic factors
TGF-β	IL-1β
PDGF	IL-1α
LDCF-F	TNF-α
C5	TNF-β
Fibronectin	bFGF
LTB$_4$	PDGF
	IL-6
	TGF-β
Protease-inducing factors	Matrix-inducing factors
IL-1α	IL-1α
IL-1β	IL-1β
TNF-α	TNF-α
PDGF	TGF-β

PGE$_2$ synthesis, which serves as a negative feedback mechanism and may enable some control of the proliferative response (173).

B. Connective Tissue Degradation

Synovial fibroblasts stimulated to proliferate by T cell and monocyte products also exhibit heightened enzymatic activity in response to these and other biologic mediators (Table 2). A correlation exists between the degree of hyperplasia and the severity of cartilage erosion (182). The augmented release of proteolygic enzymes and mediators has a significant role in degradation of the connective tissue matrix. Among these products are PGE$_2$, elastase, proteoglycanase, collagenase, and plasminogen activator, which have been identified in inflammatory synovial cells and fluids (183–185). The tissue destructive component of an inflammatory process may be mediated, in part, by the ability of IL-1 to stimulate other cells, such as chondrocytes, synovial cells, and fibroblasts, to secrete prostaglandins and collagenase (186–188).

Enzymes, such as collagenase, a product of both macrophages and mesenchymal cells, are released and break down matrix components into peptide fragments (review, Ref. 189). Collagenase, the only enzyme that can cleave helical collagen, is a major secretory product of synovial fibroblasts stimulated with PDGF, IL-1, and TNF (190–192). The abundance of macrophages at the inflammatory site implicates these cells in the secretion of this rate-limiting collagenolytic enzyme. The ability of macrophages to synthesize and secrete collagenase is dependent upon activation of PGE$_2$ synthesis and elevation of the intracellular levels of cyclic adenosine monophosphate (cAMP) (189). This enzyme seems to be responsible in a major way for the extensive joint destruction seen in rheumatoid arthritis. Stimulation of fibroblasts by IL-1 causes increased mRNA for pro-collagenase (193), which is regulated by the protein product of the proto-oncogene c-*jun* (194). Associated with and preceding collagenase production, stimulated synovial fibroblasts release serum amyloid A and β_2-microglobulinlike proteins, which appear to regulate collagenase production (195). The mechanism of control is unclear, but these proteins may function as autocrine regulators or as paracrine products of activated macrophages (196) to amplify other signals. Stromelysin, coordinately released with procollagenase after stimulation by IL-1, is responsible for activating the collagenolytic enzyme (197,198). Tissue inhibitor of metalloproteinases (TIMP) has been identified in human cartilage (199) and may play a major role in modulating the activity of collagenase and other metalloproteinases (200). IL-1 coordinately enhances both collagenase and TIMP production by fibroblasts (201). The cytokine induction of collagenase disproportionately to TIMP could conceivably alter the rate of collagen turnover. At least in osteoarthritis, TIMP has been shown to not be elevated whereas proteinase levels were elevated. This imbalance in enzymes and inhibitors, with the proteinases escaping control by the inhibitor, favors excessive matrix degradation (199). Conversely, TGF-β stimulates the production of proteinase inhibitors, including plasminogen activator inhibitor and TIMP (202,203), while inhibiting the metalloproteinases stromelysin and collagenase (203–205). Thus, control of enzymes and/or their inhibitors is likely pivotal to the net degradative processes in arthritic lesions.

Accompanying chronic inflammatory synovitis are other changes in mesenchymal tissues. Although this is speculative, IL-1 is thought to be a key mediator of cartilage matrix degradation in arthritis (131,206), again through its ability to stimulate the production of the metalloproteinases (207). In addition to the loss of cartilagenous connective tissue, inflammatory cells also influence the resorption of subchondral bone. In this regard, monocytes and fibroblasts, through the elaboration of prostaglandins, mediate the release of an osteoclast-activating factor (208), subsequently identified as interleukin 1β (209), that can also promote the destruction of bone constituents. Osteoclasts are multinucleated cells that become engaged in the synthesis and apical secretion of lysosomal enzymes in an acidified compartment (review, Ref. 210). Within the acidified environment of the bone-resorbing lacuna formed by the osteoclast, the mineral phase dissolves and the organic matrix is exposed to the action of the secreted enzymes. Exposure of osteoclasts to an acid microenvironment initiates a series of rapid intracellular events involving ion transport, morphologic changes, and enzyme synthesis (211). This is an incompletely understood multistep process that may be controlled at several levels by peptide mediators. In this regard, IL-1 and TNF cause osteoclastic bone resorption and inhibit bone collagen synthesis (212–214). The mechanism of this cytokine-induced bone resorption involves induction of osteoblast production of another factor that stimulates osteoclastic activity (215,216). In addition, both TNF and IL-1 stimulate the release of collagenase and PGE_2, important mediators of tissue destruction (190,191). As is becoming more evident, the mononuclear cells appear to mediate joint destruction through an interconnecting network of cytokines and other secreted products.

V. CONCLUSIONS

The evolving significance of peptide mediators or cytokines in the pathogenesis of rheumatoid arthritis suggests that the source of these peptides, the peptides themselves, and also their target cells may provide potential sites for interrupting the network of cellular and molecular interactions that otherwise culminates in synovial destruction. This cellular communication by peptide signals encompasses a complex set of events involving receptor-ligand interactions, intracellular signal transduction, gene expression, and protein synthesis and secretion. This dynamic sequence of events must occur in a coordinated pattern before the effects of the cytokines are exerted on any given biologic target. The normally controlled synthesis, secretion, and action of the cytokines likely becomes dysregulated in such chronic diseases as arthritis. Continued efforts to decipher these dysregulated events will provide the basis for determining the actions of antirheumatic drugs and for developing appropriate new drugs. In addition to the long-standing therapeutic modalities, including nonsteroidal anti-inflammatory drugs, corticosteroids, slow-acting drugs, and immunosuppressants, a variety of novel synthetic compounds as well as a variety of immunomodulatory agents produced by recombinant technology are being evaluated in the treatment of this disease. Modulation of the pathogenic cellular and molecular pathways, some of which are described in this review, offers new insights into potential avenues of interventional treatment of chronic inflammatory disorders.

REFERENCES

1. Decker, J.L., Malone, D.G., Haraoui, B., Wahl, S.M., Schrieber, L., Klippel, J.H., Steinberg, A.D., and Wilder, R.L. (1984). Rheumatoid arthritis: Evolving concepts of pathogenesis and treatment. Ann. Intern. Med. 101:810.
2. Zvaifler, N.J. (1984). Immunopathology and inflammatory diseases. Rheumatoid arthritis as an example. Adv. Inflamm. Res. 7:1.
3. Klareskog, L., Forsum, U., Malmnas Tjernlund, U., Kabelitz, D., and Wigren, A. (1981). Appearance of anti-HLA-DR-reactive cells in normal and rheumatoid synovial tissue. Scand. J. Immunol. 14:183.
4. Burmester, G.R., John, B., Gramatzi, M., Zacher, J., and Kalden, J.R. (1984). Activated T cells in vivo and in vitro: Divergence in expression of Tac and antigens in the non-blastoid small T cells of inflammation and T cells activated in vitro. J. Immunol. 133:1230.

5. Firestein, G., and Zvaifler, N. (1987). Peripheral blood and synovial fluid monocyte activation in inflammatory arthritis. I. A cytofluorographic study of monocyte differentiation antigens and class II antigens and their regulation by gamma interferon. Arthritis Rheum. 30:857.
6. Petersen, J. (1988). B lymphocyte function in patients with rheumatoid arthritis: Impact of regulatory T lymphocytes and macrophages—modulation by antirheumatic drugs. Danish Med. Bull. 35:140.
7. Yocum, D.E., Klippel, J.H., Wilder, R.L., Gerber, N.L., Austin, H.A., Wahl, S.M., Lesko, L., Minor, J.R., Preuss, H.G., Yarboro, C., Berkebile, C., and Dougherty, S. (1988). Cyclosporin A in severe, treatment-refractory rheumatoid arthritis. A randomized study. Ann. Intern. Med. 109:863.
8. Wahl, S.M., Katona, I.M., Wahl, L.M., Allen, J.B., Decker, J.L., Scher, I., and Wilder, R.L. (1983). Leukaperesis in rheumatoid arthritis. Association of clinical improvement with reversal of anergy. Arthritis Rheum. 26:1076.
9. Dayer, J.M., and Demczuk, S. (1984). Cytokines and other mediators in rheumatoid arthritis. Springer Semin. Immunopathol. 7:387.
10. Wahl, S.M. (1988). Inflammatory cell regulation of connective tissue metabolism. Rheumatology 10:404.
11. Smith, K.A. (1980). T-cell growth factor. Immunol. Rev. 51:337.
12. Lemm, G., and Warnatz, H. (1986). Evidence for enhanced interleukin 2 (IL-2) secretion and IL-2 receptor presentation by synovial fluid lymphocytes in rheumatoid arthritis. Clin. Exp. Immunol. 64:71.
13. Nouri, A.M.E., Panayi, G.S., and Goodman, S.M. (1984). Cytokines and the chronic inflammation of rheumatic disease. II. The presence of interleukin 2 in synovial fluids. Clin. Exp. Immunol. 58:402.
14. Wilkins, J.A., Warrington, R.J., Sigurdson, S.I., and Rutherford, J. (1983). The demonstration of an interluein 2-like activity in the synovial fluids of rheumatoid arthritis. J. Rheumatol. 10:109.
15. Husby, G., and Williams, R.C., Jr. (1985). Immunohistochemical studies of interleukin-2 and γ-interferon in rheumatoid arthritis. Arthritis Rheum. 28:174.
16. Egeland, T., and Lund, H. (1987). Immunoregulatory lymphokines in rheumatoid joints. I. Search for interleukin 2 in synovial fluid. Scand. J. Immunol. 25:101.
17. Firestein, G.S., Xu, X., Townsend, K., Broide, D., Alvaro-Gracia, J., Glasebrook, A., and Zvaifler, N.J. (1988). Cytokines in chronic inflammatory arthritis. I. Failure to detect T cell lymphokines (interleukin 2 and interleukin 3) and presence of macrophage colony-stimulating factor (CSF-1) and a novel mast cell growth factor in rheumatoid synovitis. J. Exp. Med. 168:1573.
18. Brennan, F.M., Chantry, D., Jackson, A.M., Maini, R.N., and Feldman, M. (1989). Cytokine production in culture by cells isolated from the synovial membrane. J. Autoimmun. 2:177.
19. Buchan, G., Barrett, K., Fujita, T., Taniguchi, T., Maini, R.N., and Feldman, M. (1988). Detection of activation T-cell products in the rheumatoid joint using cDNA probes to interleukin-2 (IL-2), IL-2 receptor and IFN-γ. Clin. Exp. Immunol. 71:295.
20. Huang, YiP., Perrin, L.H., Miescher, P.A., et al. (1988). Correlation of T and B cell activities in vitro and serum IL-2 levels in systemic lupus erythematosus. J. Immunol. 141:827.

20. Huang, YiP., Perrin, L.H., Miescher, P.A., et al. (1988). Correlation of T and B cell activities in vitro and serum IL-2 levels in systemic lupus erythematosus. J. Immunol. 141:827.

21. Kroemer, G., and Wick, G. (1989). The role of interleukin 2 in autoimmunity. Immunol. Today 10:246.

22. Miossec, P., Kashiwado, T., and Ziff, M. (1987). Inhibitor of IL-2 in rheumatoid synovial fluid. Arthritis Rheum. 30:121.

23. Flescher, E., Bowlin, T.L., Ballester, A., Houk, R., and Talal, N. (1989). Increased polyamines may downregulate interleukin 2 production in rheumatoid arthritis. J. Clin. Invest. 83:1356.

24. Kehrl, J.H., Wakefield, L.M., Roberts, A.B., Jakolew, S., Alvarez-Mon, M., Derynck, R., Sporn, M.B., and Fauci, A.S. (1986). Production of transforming growth factor-beta by human T lymphocytes and its potential role in the regulation of T cell growth. J. Exp. Med. 163:1037.

25. Wahl, S.M., Hunt, D.A., Wong, H.L., Dougherty, S., McCartney-Francis, N., Wahl, L.M., Ellingsworth, L., Schmidt, J.A., Hall, G., Roberts, A.B., and Sporn, M.B. (1988). Transforming growth factor-β is a potent imunosuppressive agent that inhibits IL-1-dependent lymphocyte proliferation. J. Immunol. 140:3026.

26. Wahl, S.M., Hunt, D.A., Bansal, G., McCartney-Francis, N., Ellingsworth, L., and Allen, J.B. (1988). Bacterial cell wall-induced immunosuppression: role of transforming growth factor beta. J. Exp. Med. 168:1403.

27. Robb, R.J., Munck, A., and Smith, K.A. (1981). T-cell growth factor receptors: Quantification, specificity, and biological relevance. J. Exp. Med. 154:1455.

28. Sharon, M., Siegel, J.P., Tosato, G., Yodoi, J., Gerrard, T.L., and Leonard, W.J. (1988). The human interleukin 2 receptor β chain (p70). Direct identification, partial purification and patterns of expression on peripheral blood mononuclear cells. J. Exp. Med. 167:1265.

29. Smith, K.A. (1988). Interleukin-2: Inception, impact, and implications. Science 240:1169.

30. Depper, J.M., Leonard, W.J., Drogula, C., Krönke, M., Waldmann, T.A., and Greene, W.C. (1985). Interleukin 2 (IL-2) augments transcription of the IL-2 receptor gene. Proc. Natl. Acad. Sci. USA 82:4230.

31. Herrmann, F., Cannistra, S.A., Levine, H., and Griffin, J.D. (1985). Expression of interleukin 2 receptors and binding of interleukin 2 by gamma interferon-induced human leukemic and normal monocytic cells. J. Exp. Med. 162:1111.

32. Holter, W., Goldman, C.I., Casabo, L., Nelson, D.L., Greene, W.C., and Waldmann, T.A. (1987). Expression of functional IL-2 receptors by lipopolysaccharide and interferon-gamma stimulated human monocytes. J. Immunol. 138:2917.

33. Wahl, S.M., McCartney-Francis, N., Hunt, D.A., Smith, P.D., Wahl, L.M., and Katona, I.M. (1987). Monocyte interleukin 2 receptor gene expression and interleukin 2 augmentation of microbicidal activity. J. Immunol. 139:1342.

34. Wahl, S.M., Allen, J.B., and Katona, I.M. (1990). Expression of IL-2 receptors on synovial monocytes. (Submitted)

35. Wood, N.C., Symons, J.A., and Duff, G.W. (1988). Serum interleukin-2-receptor in rheumatoid arthritis: A prognostic indicator of disease activity? J. Autoimmun. 1:353–361.

36. Pennica, D., Nedwin, G.E., Hayflick, J.S., Seeburg, P.H., Derynck, R., Palladino, M.A., Kohr, W.J., Aggarwal, B.B., and Goeddel, D.V. (1984). Human tumor necrosis factor: Precursor structure, expression, and homology to lymphotoxin. Nature 312:724.

37. Gray, P.W., Aggarwal, B.B., Benton, C.V., Bringman, T.S., Henzel, W.J., Jarrett, J.A., Leung, D.W., Moffat, B., Ng, P., Svendersky, L.P., Palladino, M.A., and Nedwin, G.E. (1984). Cloning and expression of cDNA for human lymphotoxin, a lymphokine with tumour necrosis activity. Nature 312:721.

38. Aggarwal, B.B., Henzel, W.J., Moffat, B., Kohr, W.J., and Harkins, R.N. (1985). Primary structure of human lymphotoxin derived from 1788 lymphoblastoid cell line. J. Biol. Chem. 260:2334.

39. Spies, T., Morton, C.C., Nedospasov, S.A., Fiers, W., Pious, D., and Strominger, J.L. (1986). Genes for the tumor necrosis factors alpha and beta are linked to the human major histocompatibility complex. Proc. Natl. Acad. Sci. USA 83:8699.

40. Nedwin, G.E., Naylor, S.L., Sakaguchi, A.Y., Smith, D., Jarrett-Nedwin, J., Pennica, D., Goeddel, D.V., and Gray, P.W. (1985). Human lymphotoxin and tumor necrosis factor genes: Structure, homology and chromosomal localization. J. Cell Biochem. 29(3):171.

41. Old, L.J. (1985). Tumor necrosis factor (TNF). Science 230:630.

42. Nathan, C., and Yoshida, R. (1988). Cytokines: Interferon-γ. In: Inflammation: Basic Principles and Clinical Correlates. Gallin, J.I., Goldstein, I.M., and Snyderman, R., Raven Press, New York, p. 229.

43. Cesario, T.C., Andrews, B.S., Martin, D.A., Jason, M., Treadwell, T., Friou, G., and Tilles, J.G. (1983). Interferon in synovial fluid and serum of patients with rheumatic disease. J. Rheumatol. 10:647.

44. Degre, M., Mellbye, O.J., and Clarke-Jenssen, O. (1983). Immune interferon in serum and synovial fluid in rheumatoid arthritis and related disorders. Ann. Rheum. Dis. 42:672.

45. Firestein, G.S., and Zvaifler, N.J. (1987). Peripheral blood and synovial fluid monocyte activation in inflammatory arthritis. II. Low levels of synovial fluid and synovial tissue interferon suggest that gamma-interferon is not the primary macrophage activating factor. Arthritis Rheum. 30:857.

46. Torres, B.A., Farrar, W.L., and Johnson, H.M. (1982). Interleukin 2 regulates immune interferon (IFNγ) production by normal and suppressor cell cultures. J. Immunol. 128:2217.

47. Allen, J.B., Bansal, G., Hand, A., Feldman, G.M., Wahl, L., and Wahl, S. (1990). Interferons suppress bacterial cell wall-induced polyarthritis. Cytokines. In Press.

48. Wilder, R.L., Allen, J.B., Wahl, L.M., Calandra, G.B., and Wahl, S.M. (1983). The pathogenesis of group A streptococcal cell wall induced polyarthritis in the rat: Comparative studies in arthritis resistant and susceptible inbred rat strains. Arthritis Rheum. 26:1442.

49. Cannon, G.W., Pincus, S.H., Emkey, R.D., Denes, A., Cohen, S.A., Wolfe, F., Saway, P.A., Jaffer, A.M., Weaver, A.L., Cogen, L., and Schindler, J.D. (1989). Double-blind trial of recombinant γ-interferon versus placebo in the treatment of rheumatoid arthritis. Arthritis Rheum. 32:8.

50. Lemmel, E.M., Brackertz, D., Franke, M., Gaus, W., Hartl, P.W., Machalke, K., Meikle, H., Obert, H.J., Peter, H.H., Sieper, J., Sprekeler, R., and Stierle, H. (1988). Results of a multicenter placebo-controlled double-bind randomized phase III clinical study of treatment of rheumatoid arthritis with recombinant interferon-gamma. Rheumatol. Int. 8:87.

51. Veys, E.M., Mielants, H., Verbruggen, G., Grosclaude, J.P., Merner, M., Galazka, A., and Schindler, J. (1988). Interferon gamma in rheumatoid arthritis: a double bind study comparing human recombinant interferon gamma with placebo. J. Rheumatol. 15:570.

52. Wolfe, F., Cathey, M.A., Hawley, D.J., Balser, J.P., and Schindler, J.D. (1986). Clinical trial with R-IFN-g in rheumatoid arthritis. In: Biologically Based Immunomodulators in the Therapy of Rheumatic Diseases. Pincus, S.H., Pisetsky, D.S., and Rossenwasser, L.J., eds. Elsevier, New York.

53. Seitz, M., Manz, G., and Franke, M. (1986). Use of recombinant human gamma interferon in patients with rheumatoid arthritis. J. Rheumatol. 45:93.

54. Obert, H.J., and Hofschneider, P.H. (1985). Interferon in chronic polyarthritis: Positive effect in clinical evaluation. Dtsch. Med. Wochenschr. 110:1766.

55. Xu, W.D., Firestein, G.S., Taetle, T., Kaushanksy, K., and Zvaifler, N.J. (1989). Cytokines in chronic inflammatory arthritis. II. Granulocyte-macrophage colony-stimulating factor in rheumatoid synovial effusions. J. Clin. Invest. 83:876.

56. Metcalf, D. (1985). The granulocyte-macrophage colony-stimulating factors. Science 229:16.

57. Clark, S.C., and Kamen, R. (1987). The human hematopoietic colony-stimulating factors. Science 236:1229.

58. Piacibello, W., Lu, L., Wachter, M., Rubin, B., and Broxmeyer, H.E. (1985). Release of granulocyte-macrophage colony-stimulating factors from major histocompatibility complex class II antigen-positive monocytes is enhanced by human gamma interferon. Blood 66:1343.

59. Zucali, J.R., Dinarello, C.A., Oblon, D.J., Gross, M.A., Anderson, L., and Weiner, R.S. (1986). Interleukin 1 stimulates fibroblasts to produce granulocyte-macrophage colony-stimulating activity and prostaglandin E_2. J. Clin. Invest. 77:1857.

60. Rambaldi, A., Young, D.C., and Griffin, J.D. (1987). Expression of M-CSF (CSF-1) gene by human monocytes. Blood 69:1409.

61. Ihle, J.N., Rebal, L., Keller, J., Lee, J.C., and Happel, A.J. (1982). Interleukin 3: Possible roles in the regulation of lymphocyte differentiation and growth. Immunol. Rev. 63:5.

62. Wong, H., Hunt, D.A., Dougherty, S., and Wahl, S.M. (1990). CSF modulate monocyte phenotype and function. Submitted.

63. Sieff, C.A. (1987). Hematopoietic growth factors. J. Clin. Invest. 79:1549.

64. Smith, P.D., Lamerson, C., and Wahl, S.M. (1989). Granulocyte-macrophage colony-stimulating factor augmentation of leukocyte effector function. J. Cell Biochem. 105:137.

65. Smith, P.D., and Wahl, S.M. (1989). Cytokines. In: Natural Immunity. Nelson, D., ed. Academic Press, New York, p. 241.

66. Morrissey, P.J., Bressler, L., Park, L.S., Alpert, A., and Gillis, S. (1987). Granulocyte-macrophage colony-stimulating factor augments the primary antibody

response by enhancing the function of antigen-presenting cells. J. Immunol. 139:
1113.

67. Alvaro-Garcia, J.M., Zvaifler, N.J., and Firestein, G.S. (1989). Cytokines in chronic
inflammatory arthritis. IV. Granulocyte/macrophage colony-stimulating factor-
mediated induction of class II MHC antigen on human monocytes: A possible role
in rheumatoid arthritis. J. Exp. Med. 170:865.

68. Walker, F., and Burgess, A.W. (1985). Specific binding of radioiodinated granulocyte-
macrophage colony-stimulating factor to hemopoietic cells. EMBO J. 4:933.

69. Park, L.S., Friend, D., Gillis, S., and Urdal, D.L. (1986). Characterization of the
cell surface receptor for a multi-lineage colony-stimulating factor (CSF-2 alpha).
J. Biol. Chem. 26:205.

70. Miyasaka, N., Sato, K., Hashimoto, J., Kohsaka, H., Yamamoto, K., Goto, M.,
Inoue, K., Matsuda, T., Hirano, T., Kishimoto, T., and Nishioka, K. (1989).
Constitutive production of interleukin 6/B cell stimulatory factor-2 from inflammatory
synovium. Clin. Immunol. Immunopathol. 52:238.

71. Hirano, T., Matsuda, T., Turner, M., Miyasaka, N., Buchan, G., Tang, B., Sato,
K., Shimizu, M., Maini, R., Feldman, M., and Kishimoto, T. (1988). Excessive
production of interleukin 6/B cell stimulatory factor-2 in rheumatoid arthritis. Eur.
J. Immunol. 18:1797.

72. Guerne, P.-A., Zuraw, B.L., Vaughan, J.H., Carson, D.A., and Lotz, M. (1989).
Synovium as a source of interleukin 6 in vitro. Contribution to local and systemic
manifestations of arthritis. J. Clin. Invest. 83:585.

73. Waage, A., Kaufmann, C., Espevik, T., and Husby, G. (1989). Interleukin-6 in
synovial fluid from patients with arthritis. Clin. Immunol. Immunopathol. 50:394.

74. Houssiau, F.A., DeVogelaer, J.P., van Damme, J., Nagant de Deuxchaisnes, C.,
and van Snick, J. (1988). Interleukin 6 in synovial fluid and serum of patients with
rheumatoid arthritis and other inflammatory arthritides. Arthritis Rheum. 31:784.

75. Hirano, T., Yasukawa, K., Harada, H., Taga, T., Watanabe, Y., Matsuda, T.,
Kashiwamura, S., Nakajima, K., Koyama, K., Iwamatus, A., Tsunasawa, S.,
Sakiyama, F., Matsui, H., Takahara, Y., Taniguchi, T., and Kishimoto, T. (1986).
Complementary DNA for a novel human interleukin (BSF-2) that induces B
lymphocytes to produce immunoglobulin. Nature 324:73.

76. Kishimoto, T. (1989). The biology of interleukin-6. Blood 74:1.

77. Yamasaki, K., Taga, T., Hirata, Y., Ywata, H., Kawanishi, Y., Seed, B., Taniguchi,
T., Hirano, T., and Kishimoto, T. (1988). Cloning and expression of the human
interleukin-6 (BSF-2/IFNβ) receptor. Science 241:825.

78. Taga, T., Kawanishi, K., Hardy, R.R., Hirano, T., and Kishimoto, T. (1987).
Receptors for B cell stimulatory factor 2 (BSF-2): Quantitation, specificity, distribution
and regulation of the expression. J. Exp. Med. 166:967.

79. Hirano, T., Matsuda, T., Hosoi, K., Okano, A., Matsui, H., and Kishimoto, T.
(1988). Absence of antiviral activity in recombinant B cell stimulatory factor 2
(BSF-2). Immunol. Lett. 17:41.

80. Helle, M., Brakenhoff, J.P.J., DeGroot, E.R., and Aarden, L.A. (1988). Interleukin
6 is involved in interleukin 1-induced activities. Eur. J. Immunol. 18:957.

81. May, L.T., Ghrayeb, J., Santhanam, U., Tatter, S.B., Sthoeger, Z., Helfgott, D.C.,
Chiorazzi, N., Grieninger, G., and Sehgal, P.B. (1988). Synthesis and secretion

of multiple forms of "β_2-interferon/B-cell differentiation factor BSF-2/hepatocyte stimulating factor" by human fibroblasts and monocytes. J. Biol. Chem. 263:7760.

82. May, L.T., Helfgott, D.C., and Seghal, P.B. (1986). Anti-β-interferon antibodies inhibit the increased expression of HLA-B7 mRNA in tumor necrosis factor-treated human fibroblasts: Structural studies of the $\beta2$ interferon involved. Proc. Natl. Acad. Sci. USA 83:8957.

83. Zilberstein, A., Ruggieri, R., Korn, J.H., and Revel, M. (1986). Structure and expression of cDNA and genes for human interferon-beta-2, a distinct species inducible by growth-stimulating cytokines. EMBO J. 5:2529.

84. Wahl, S.M., McCartney-Francis, N., and Mergenhagen, S.E. (1989). Inflammatory and immunomodulatory role of transforming growth factor beta. Immunol. Today 10:258.

85. Wahl, S.M., Wong, H., and McCartney-Francis, N. (1988). Role of growth factors in inflammation and repair. J. Cell Biochem. 12:8.

86. Roberts, A.B., and Sporn, M.B. (1990). The transforming growth factors beta. In: Handbook of Experimental Pharmacology: Peptide Growth Factors and Their Receptors. Sporn, M.B., and Roberts, A.B., eds. Springer-Verlag, Berlin, p. 425.

87. Derynck, R., Jarrett, J.A., Chen, E.Y., Eaton, D.H., Bell, J.R., Assoian, R.K., Roberts, A.B., Sporn, M.B., and Goeddel, D.V. (1985). Human transforming growth factor-beta cDNA sequence and expression in tumor cell lines. Nature 316:701.

88. Wakefield, L.M., Smith, D.M., Masui, T., Harris, C.C., and Sporn, M.B. (1987). Distribution and modulation of the cellular receptor for transforming growth factor-beta. J. Cell. Biol. 105:965.

89. Fava, R., Olsen, N., Keski-Oja, J., Moses, H., and Pincus, T. (1989). Active and latent forms of transforming growth factor β activity in synovial effusions. J. Exp. Med. 169:291.

90. Wahl, S.M., Allen, J.B., Wong, H., and Ellingsworth, L. (1990). Antagonistic and agonistic effects of transforming growth factor β and IL-1 in rheumatoid synovium. J. Immunol. 145: In press..

91. Wahl, S.M., Hunt, D., Wakefield, L., McCartney-Francis, N., Wahl, L.M., Roberts, A., and Sporn, M.B. (1987). Transforming growth factor beta (TGF-β) induces monocyte chemotaxis and growth factor production. Proc. Natl. Acad. Sci. USA 84:5788.

92. Elliot, J.F., Lin, Y., Mizel, S.B., Bleackley, R.C., Harnish, D.G., and Paetku, V. (1984). Induction of interleukin 2 messenger RNA inhibited by cyclosporin A. Science 226:1439.

93. Kronke, M., Leonard, W.J., Depper, J.M., Arya, S.K., Wong-Staal, F., Gallo, R.C., Waldmann, T.A., and Greene, W.C. (1984). Cyclosporin A inhibits T-cell growth factor gene expression at the level of mRNA transcription. Proc. Natl. Acad. Sci. USA 81:5214.

94. Takahashi, N., Hayano, T., and Suzuki, M. (1989). Peptidyl-prolyl *cis-trans* isomerase is the cyclosporin A-binding protein cyclophilin. Nature 337:473.

95. Fischer, G., Wittman-Liebold, B., Lang, K., Keifhaber, T., and Schmid, F.X. (1989). Cyclophilin and peptidyl-prolyl *cis-trans* isomerase are probably identical proteins. Nature 337:476.

96. Te Velde, A.A., Keizer, G.D., and Figdor, C.G. (1987). Differential function of LFA-1 family molecules (CD11 and CD18) in adhesion of human monocytes to melanoma and endothelial cells. Immunology 61:261.

97. Springer, T.A., Dustin, M.L., Kishimoto, T.K., and Marlin, S.D. (1987). The lymphocyte function-associated LFA-1, CD2, and LFA-3 molecules: Cell adhesion receptors of the immune system. Annu. Rev. Immunol. 5:223.

98. Allen, C.A., Highton, J., and Palmer, D.G. (1989). Increased expression of p150,95 and CR3 leukocyte adhesion molecules by mononuclear phagocytes in rheumatoid synovial membranes. Comparison with osteoarthritic and normal synovial membranes. Arthritis Rheum. 32:947.

99. Garbisa, S., Ballin, M, Daga-Gordini, D., Fastelli, G., Naturalc, M., Negro, A., Semenzato, G., and Liotta, L.A. (1986). Transient expression of type IV collagenolytic metalloproteinase by human mononuclear phagocytes. J. Biol. Chem. 261:2369.

100. Snyderman, R., and Uhing, R.J. (1988). Phagocytic cells: Stimulus-response coupling mechanisms. In: Inflammation: Basic Principles and Clinical Correlates. Gallin, J.I., Goldstein, I.M., and Snyderman, R., eds. Raven Press, New York, p. 343.

101. Nathan, C.F. (1987). Secretory products of macrophages. J. Clin. Invest. 79: 319.

102. Unkeless, J.C., and Wright, S.D. (1988). Phagocytic cells: Fcγ and complement receptors. In: Inflammation: Basic Principles and Clinical Correlates. Gallin, J.I., Goldstein, I.M., and Snyderman, R., eds. Raven Press, New York, p. 343.

103. Welch, G., and Wahl, S.M. (1990). Modulation of monocyte Fc receptors by transforming growth factor beta. Ann. N.Y. Acad. Sci. 593:374.

104. Henson, P.M., and Johnston, R.B., Jr. (1987). Tissue injury in inflammation. Oxidants, proteinases, and cationic proteins. J. Clin. Invest. 79:669–674.

105. Halliwell, B. (1987). Oxidants and human disease: Some new concepts. FASEB J. 1:358–364.

106. Skaleric, U., Allen, J.B., Mergenhagen, S.E., and Wahl, S.M. (1990). Inhibitors of reactive oxygen intermediates inhibit erosive polyarthritis. (submitted).

107. Centrella, M., McCarthey, T.L., and Canalis, E. (1988). Skeletal tissue and transforming growth factor β. FASEB J. 2:3066.

108. Assoian, R.K., Fleurdelys, B.E., Stevenson, H.C., Miller, P.J., Madtes, D.K., Raines, E.W., Ross, R., and Sporn, M.B. (1987). Expression and secretion of type β transforming growth factor by activated human macrophages. Proc. Natl. Acad. Sci. USA 84:6020.

109. McCartney-Francis, N., Mizel, D., Wong, H., Wahl, L.M., and Wahl, S.M., (1990). TGF-β regulates production of growth factors and TGF-β by human peripheral blood monocytes. Growth Factors. In press.

110. Twardzik, D.R., Mikovits, J., Ranchalis, J., Purchio, T., Ellingsworth, L., and Ruscetti, F.W. (1990). γ-Interferon-induced activation of latent transforming growth factor-β by human monocytes. Ann. N.Y. Acad. Sci. 593:276.

111. Tsunawaki, S., Sporn, M.B., Ding, A., and Nathan, C. (1988). Deactivation of macrophages by transforming growth factor-β. Nature 334:260.

112. Allen, J.B., Manthey, C.L., Hand, A.R., Ohura, K., Ellingsworth, L., and Wahl, S.M. (1990). Rapid onset synovial inflammation and hyperplasia induced by TGF-β. J. Exp. Med. 171:231.

113. Postlethwaite, A.E., Keski-Oja, J., Moses, H.L., and Kang, A.H. (1987). Stimulation of the chemotactic migration of human fibroblasts by transforming growth factor β. J. Exp. Med. 165:251.

114. Dinarello, C.A. (1986). Il-1: Amino acid sequences, multiple biological activities and comparison with tumor necrosis factor (cachectin). Year Immunol. 2:68.

115. Dower, S.K., and Urdal, D.L. (1987). The interleukin-1 receptor. Immunol. Today 8:46.

116. Irlé, C., Piquet, P.F., and Vassalli, P. (1978). In vitro maturation of immature thymocytes into immunocompetent T cells in the absence of direct thymic influence. J. Exp. Med. 148:32.

117. Gillis, S., and Mizel, S.B. (1981). T-cell lymphoma model for the analysis of interleukin 1-mediated T cell activation. Proc. Natl. Acad. Sci. USA. 78:1133.

118. Gubler, U., Chua, A.O., Stern, A.S., Hellman, C.P., Vitek, M.P., DeChiara, T.M., Benjamin, W.R., Collier, K.J., Dukovich, M., Familletti, P.C., Fiedler-Nagy, C., Jenson, J. Kaffka, K., Kilian, P.L., Stremlo, S., Wittreich, B.H., Wohle, D., Mizel, S.B., and Lomedico, P.T. (1986). Recombinant human interleukin 1 alpha: Purification and biological characterization. J. Immunol. 136:2492.

119. March, C.J., Mosley, B., Larsen, A., Cerretti, D.P., Braedt, G., Price, V., Gillis, S., Henney, C.S., Kronheim, S.R., Grabstein, K., Conlon, P.J., Hopp, T.P., and Cosman, D. (1985). Cloning, sequence and expression of two distinct human interleukin-1 complementary DNAs. Nature 315:641.

120. Gubler, U., Farrar, J.J., Mizel, S.B., and Lomedico, P.T. (1986). Interleukin-1-alpha and interleukin-1-beta bind to the same receptor on T-cells. J. Immunol. 136:4509.

121. Goto, M., Sasano, M., Yamanaka, H., Miyasaka, N., Kamatani, N., Inoie, K., Nishioka, K., and Miyamoto, T. (1987). Spontaneous production of an IL-1-like factor by cloned rheumatoid synovial cells in long-term culture. J. Clin. Invest. 80:786.

122. Fontana, A., Hengartner, H., Weber, E., Fehr, K., Grob, P.J., and Cohen, G. (1982). IL-1 activity in the synovial fluid of patients with rheumatoid arthritis. Rheumatol. Int. 2:49.

123. Nouri, A.M.E., Panayi, G.S., and Goodman, S.M. (1984). Cytokines and the chronic inflammation of rheumatic disease. I. The presence of interleukin 1 in synovial fluids. Clin. Exp. Immunol. 58:402.

124. Wood, D.D., Ihrie, E.J., Dinarello, C.A., and Cohen, P.L. (1983). Isolation of an IL-1-like factor from human joint effusions. Arthritis Rheum. 26:975.

125. Hopkins, S.J., Humphreys, M., and Jayson, M.I.V. (1988). Cytokines in synovial fluid. I. The presence of biologically active and immunoreactive IL-1. Clin. Exp. Immunol. 72:422.

126. Dalton, B.J., Connor, J.R., and Johnson, W.J. (1989). IL-1 induces IL-1α and β gene expression in synovial fibroblasts and peripheral blood monocytes. Arthritis Rheum. 32:279.

127. Lotz, M., Tsoukas, C.D., Robinson, C.A., Dinarello, C.A., Carson, D.A., and Vaughan, J.H. (1986). Basis for defective responses of rheumatoid arthritis synovial fluid lymphocytes to anti-CD3 (T3) antibodies. J. Clin. Invest. 78:713.

128. Johnson, W.J., Muirhead, K.A., Meunier, P.C., Votta, B.J., Schmitt, T.C., DiMartino, M.J., and Hanna, N. (1986). Macrophage activation in rat models of inflammation and arthritis. Systemic activation precedes arthritis induction and progression. Arthritis Rheum. 29:1122.

129. Horn, J.T., Bendele, A.M., and Carlson, D.G. (1988). In vivo administration with IL-1 accelerates the development of collagen-induced arthritis in mice. J. Immunol. 141:834.

130. Stimpson, S.A., Dalldorf, F.G., Otterness, I.G., and Schwab, J.H. (1988). Exacerbation of arthritis by IL-1 in rat joints previously injured by peptidoglycan-polysaccharide. J. Immunol. 140:2964–2969.

131. Pettipher, E.R., Higgs, G.A., and Henderson, B. (1986). IL-1 induces leukocyte infiltration and cartilage proteoglycan degradation in the synovial joint. Proc. Natl. Acad. Sci. USA 83:8749–8753.

132. Kunkel, S.L., Remick, D.G., Strieter, R.M., and Larrick, J.W. (1989). Mechanisms that regulate the production and effects of tumor necrosis factor-α. Crit. Rev. Immunol. 9:93–117.

133. Di Giovine, F.S., Nuki, G., and Duff, G.W. (1988). Tumour necrosis factor in synovial exudates. Ann. Rheum. Dis. 47:768.

134. Philip, R, and Epstein, L.B. (1986). Tumor necrosis factor as immunomodulator and mediator of monocyte cytotoxicity induced by itself, γ-interferon and interleukin-1. Nature 323:86.

135. Nawroth, P.P., Bark, I., Handley, D., Cassimeris, J., Chess, L., and Stern, D. (1986). Tumor necrosis factor/cachectin interacts with endothelial cell receptors to induce release of interleukin 1. J. Exp. Med. 163:1363.

136. Beutler, B.A., and Cerami, A. (1986). Cachectin and tumor necrosis factor as two sides of the same biological coin. Nature 320:584.

137. Bevilacqua, M.P., Pober, J.S., Majeau, G.R., Fiers, W., Cotran, R.S., and Gimbrone, M.A., Jr. (1986). Recombinant tumor necrosis factor induces procoagulant activity in cultured human vascular endothelium: Characterization and comparison with the actions of interleukin 1. Proc. Natl. Acad. Sci. USA 83:4533.

138. Gamble, J.R., Harlan, J.M., Klebanoff, S.J., and Vadas, M.A. (1985). Stimulation of the adherence of neutrophils to umbilical vein endothelium by human recombinant tumor necrosis factor. Proc. Natl. Acad. Sci. USA 82:8667.

139. Munker, R., Gasson, J., Ogawa, M., and Koeffler, H.P. (1986). Recombinant human necrosis factor induces production of granulocyte-macrophage colony stimulating factor mRNA and protein from lung fibroblasts and vascular endothelial cells in vitro. Nature 323:79.

140. Broudy, V.C., Kaushansky, K., Segal, G.M., Harlan, J.M., and Adamson, J.W. (1987). Tumor necrosis factor stimulates human endothelial cells to produce granulocyte/macrophage colony-stimulating factor. Proc. Natl. Acad. Sci. USA 83:7467.

141. Ross, R. (1988). Personal communication.

142. Ross, R., Raines, E.W., and Bowen-Pope, D.F. (1986). The biology of platelet-derived growth factor. Cell 46:155.

143. Deuel, T.F., Senior, R.M., Huang, J.S., and Griffin, G.L. (1982). Chemotaxis of monocytes and neutrophils to platelet-derived growth factor. J. Clin. Invest. 69:1046.

144. Williams, L.T., Antoniades, H.N., and Goetzl, E.J. (1983). Platelet-derived growth factor stimulates mouse 3T3 cell mitogenesis and leukocyte chemotaxis through different structural determinants. J. Clin. Invest. 72:1759.

145. Senior, R.M., Huang, J.S., Griffin, G.L., and Deuel, T.F. (1985). Dissociation of the chemotactic and mitogenic activities of platelet-derived growth factor by human neutrophil elastase. J. Cell. Biol. 100:351.

146. Graves, D.T., Grotendorst, G.R, Antoniades, H.N., Schwartz, C.J., and Valente, H.A. (1989). Platelet-derived growth factor is not chemotactic for human peripheral blood monocytes. Exp. Cell Res. 180:497.

147. Shimokado, K., Raines, E.W, Madtes, D.K., Barrett, T.B., Benditt, E.P., and Ross, R. (1985). A significant part of macrophage-derived growth factor consists of at least two forms of PDGF. Cell 43:277.

148. Martinet, Y., Bitterman, P.B., Mornex, J., Grotendorst, G.R., Martin, G.R., and Crystal, R.G. (1986). Activated human monocytes express the c-sis proto-oncogene and release a mediator showing PDGF-like activity. Nature 319:158.

149. Mornex, J.-F., Martinet, Y., Yanauchi, K., Bitterman, P.B., Grotendorst, G.R., Chytil-Weir, A., Martin, G.R., and Crystal, R.G. (1986). Spontaneous expression of the c-sis gene and release of a platelet-derived growth factor-like molecule by human alveolar macrophages. J. Clin. Invest. 78:61.

150. DiCorleto, P.E., and Bowen-Pope, D.F. (1983). Cultured endothelial cells produce a platelet-derived growth factor-like protein. Proc. Natl. Acad. Sci. USA 80:1919.

151. Barret, T.B., Gajdusek, C.M., Schwartz, S.M., McDougall, J.K., and Benditt, E.P. (1984). Expression of the sis gene by endothelial cells in culture and in vivo. Proc. Natl. Acad. Sci. USA 81:6772.

152. Walker, L.N., Bowen-Pope, D.F. Ross, R., and Reidy, M.A. (1986). Production of platelet-derived growth factor-like molecules by cultured arterial smooth muscle cells accompanies proliferation after arterial injury. Proc. Natl. Acad. Sci. USA 83:7311.

153. Deuel, T.F., and Huang, J.S. (1984). Platelet-derived growth factor: Structure, function and roles in normal and transformed cells. J. Clin. Invest. 74:669.

154. Raines, E.W., and Ross, R. (1985). Purification of human platelet-derived growth factor. Methods Enzymol. 109:749.

155. Westermark, B., Heldin, C.-H., Ek, B., et al. (1983). Biochemistry and biology of platelet-derived growth factor. Growth Maturation Factors. 1:73.

156. Bowen-Pope, D.F., and Ross, R. (1982). Platelet-derived growth factor. II. Specific binding to cultured cells. J. Biol. Chem. 257:5161.

157. Ek, B., Westermark, B., Wasteson, A., and Heldin, C.-H. (1982). Stimulation of tyrosine-specific phosphorylation by platelet-derived growth factor. Nature 295:419.

158. Huang, J.S., Huang, S.S., Kennedy, B., and Deuel, T.F. (1982). Platelet-derived growth factor. Specific binding to target cells. J. Biol. Chem. 257:8130.

159. Heldin, C.H., Ernlund, A., Rorsman, C., and Rönnstrand, L. (1989). Dimerization of B-type platelet-derived growth factor receptors occurs after ligand binding and is closely associated with receptor kinase activation. J. Biol. Chem. 264:8905.

160. Rubin, K., Terracio, L., Ronnstrand, L., Heldin, C.-H., and Klareskog, L. (1988). Expression of platelet-derived growth factor receptors is induced on connective tissue cells during chronic synovial inflammation. Scand. J. Immunol. 27:285.

161. Gospodarowicz, D., Ferrara, N., Schweigerer, L., and Neufeld, G. (1987). Structural characterization and biological functions of fibroblast growth factor. Endocrinol. Rev. 8:95.

162. Folkman, J., and Klagsbrun, M. (1987). Angiogenic factors. Science 235:442.

163. Esch, F., Baird, A., Ling, N., Ueno, N., Hill, D., Denoroy, L., Klepper, R., Gospodarowicz, D., Böhlen, P., and Guillemin, R. (1985). Primary structure of bovine pituitary basic fibroblast growth factor and comparison with the amino-terminal sequence of bovine brain acidic FGF. Proc. Natl. Acad. Sci. USA 82:6507.

164. Gimenez-Gallego, G.L., Rodkey, J., Bennett, C., Rios-Caldelore, M., DiSalvo, J., and Thomas, K. (1985). Brain-derived acidic fibroblast growth factor: complete amino acid sequence and homologies. Science 230:1385.

165. Baird, A., Mormede, P., and Bohlen, P. (1985). Immunoreactive fibroblast growth factor in cells of peritoneal exudate suggests its identity with macrophage-derived growth factor. Biochem. Biophys. Res. Commun. 126:358.

166. Van Damme, J., Opdenakker, G., Shimpson, R.J., Rubira, M.R., Cyphas, S., Vink, A, Billiau, A., and Snick, J.V. (1987). Identification of the human 26-KD protein, interferon β2 (IFNβ 2), as a B cell hybridoma/plasmacytoma growth factor induced by interleukin 1 and tumor necrosis factor. J. Exp. Med. 615:914.

167. Tosato, G., Seamon, K.B., Goldman, N.D., Sehgal, P.B., May, L.T., Washington, G.C., Jones, K.D., and Pike, S.E. (1988). Monocyte-derived human B-cell growth factor identified as interferon-β_2 (BSF-2, IL-6). Science 239:5021.

168. Horii, Y., Muraguchi, A., Suematsu, S., Matsuda, T., Yoshizaki, K., Hirano, T., and Kishimoto, T. (1988). Regulation of BSF-2/IL-6 production by human mononuclear cells: Macrophage-dependent synthesis of BSF-2/IL-6 by T cells. J. Immunol. 141:1529.

169. Harris, E.D., Jr. (1986). Pathogenesis of rheumatoid arthritis. In: Textbook of Rheumatology. Kelley, W.N., Harris, E.D., Ruddy, S., and Sledge, C.B., eds. W.B. Saunders, Philadelphia, p. 886.

170. Wahl, S.M., Malone, D.G., and Wilder, R.L. (1985). Spontaneous production of fibroblast activating factor(s) by synovial inflammatory cells. A potential mechanism for enhanced tissue destruction. J. Exp. Med. 161:210.

171. Postlethwaite, A.E., and Kang, A.H. (1988). Fibroblasts. In: Inflammation: Basic Principles and Clinical Correlates. Gallin, J.I., Goldstein, I.M., and Snyderman, R. Raven Press, New York, p. 577.

172. Henderson, B., and Pettipher, E.R. (1985). The synovial lining cell: Biology and pathobiology. Semin. Arthritis Rheum. 15:1.

173. Butler, D.M., Leizer, T., Hamilton, J.A. (1989). Stimulation of human synovial fibroblast DNA synthesis by platelet-derived growth factor and fibroblast growth factor: Differences to the activation by IL-1. J. Immunol. 142:3098–3103.

174. Butler, D.M., Piccoli, D.S., Hart, P.H., and Hamilton, J.A. (1988). Stimulation of human synovial fibroblast DNA synthesis by recombinant cytokines. J. Rheumatol. 15:1463.

175. Sugarman, B.J., Aggarwal, B.B., Hass, P.E., Figari, I.S., Palladino, M.A., Jr., Shepard, H.M. (1985). Recombinant human tumor necrosis factor-α: Effects on proliferation of normal and transformed cells in vitro. Science 230:943.

176. Vilcek, J., Palombella, V.J., Henriksen-DeStefano, D., Swenson, C., Feinman, R., Hirai, M., and Tsujimoto, M. (1986). Fibroblast growth-enhancing activity of tumor necrosis factor and its relationship to other polypeptide growth factors. J. Exp. Med. 163:632.

177. Chin, J., Rupp, E., Cameron, P.M., MacNaul, K.L., Lotke, P.A., Tocci, M.J., Schmidt, J.A., and Bayne, E.K. (1988). Identification of a high-affinity receptor for interleukin 1α and interleukin 1β on cultured human rheumatoid synovial cells. J. Clin. Invest. 82:420.

178. Schmidt, J.A., Mizel, S.B., Cohen, D., and Green, I. (1982). Interleukin 1, a potential regulator of fibroblast proliferation. J. Immunol. 128:2177.

179. Raines, E.W., Dower, S.K., and Ross, R. (1989). IL-1 mitogenic activity for fibroblasts and smooth muscle cells is due to PDGF-AA. Science 243:393.

180. Leof, E.B., Proper, J.A., Goustin, A.S., Shipley, G.D., DiCorleto, P.E., and Moses, H.L. (1986). Induction of c-sis mRNA and activity similar to platelet-derived growth factor by transforming growth factor β: A proposed model for indirect mitogenesis involving autocrine activity. Proc. Natl. Acad. Sci. USA 83:2453–2457.

181. Burmester, G.R., Jahn, B., Rohwer, P., Zacher, J., Winchester, R.J., and Kalden, J.R. (1987). Differential expression of Ia antigens by rheumatoid synovial lining cells. J. Clin. Invest. 80:595.

182. Muirden, K.D. (1982). Lysosomal enzymes in synovial membrane in rheumatoid arthritis. Relationship to joint damage. Ann. Rheum. Dis. 31:265.

183. Robinson, D.R., Tashjian, A.H., Jr., and Levine, L. (1975). Prostaglandin-stimulated bone resorption by rheumatoid synovia. A possible mechanism for bone destruction in rheumatoid arthritis. J. Clin. Invest. 56:1181.

184. Breedveld, F.C., Lafeber, G.J.M., Seigert, C.E.H., Vlemming, L.-J., and Cats, A. (1987). Elastase and collagenase activities in synovial fluid of patients with arthritis. J. Rheumatol. 14:1008.

185. Mochan, E., Uhl, J., and Newton, R. (1986). Evidence that interleukin-1 induction of synovial cell plasminogen activator is mediated via prostaglandin E_2 and cyclic AMP. Arthritis Rheum. 29:1078.

186. Mizel, S.B., Dayer, J.M., Krane, S.M., and Mergenhagen, S.E. (1981). Stimulation of rheumatoid synovial cell collagenase and prostaglandin by partially purified lymphocyte-activating factor (interleukin-1). Proc. Natl. Acad. Sci. USA 78:2474.

187. McGuire, M.K., Meats, J.E., Ebsworth, N.M., Gowen, M., Murphy, G., Reynolds, J.J., and Russell, R.G. (1982). Interactions in connective tissue involving monocyte/macrophages and control of production of proteinases and proteinase inhibitors. Agents Actions (Suppl.) 11:131.

188. Postlethwaite, A.E., Lachman, L.B., Mainardi, C.L., and Kang, A.H. (1983). Stimulation of fibroblast collagenase production by human interleukin-1. J. Exp. Med. 157:801.

189. Wahl, L.M., and Mergenhagen, S.E. (1989). Regulation of monocyte-macrophage collagenase. J. Oral Pathol. 17:452.

190. Dayer, J.M., de Rochemonteix, B., Burrus, B., Demczuk, S., and Dinarello, C.A. (1986). Human recombinant interleukin 1 stimulates collagenase and prostaglandin E_2 production by human synovial cells. J. Clin. Invest. 77:654.

191. Dayer, J.M., Beutler, B., and Cerami, A. (1985). Cachectin/tumor necrosis factor stimulates collagenase and prostaglandin E_2 production by human synovial cells and dermal fibroblasts. J. Exp. Med. 162:2163.

192. Bauer, E.A., Cooper, T.W., Huang, J.S., Altman, J., and Deuel, T.F. (1985). Stimulation of in vitro human skin collagenase expression by platelet-derived growth factor. Proc. Natl. Acad. Sci. USA 82:4132.

193. Brinckerhoff, C.E. (1987). Regulation of collagenase gene expression in synovial cells. J. Rheumatol. 14:61.

194. Conca, W., Kaplan, P.B., and Krane, S.M. (1989). Increases in levels of procollagenase messenger RNA in cultured fibroblasts induced by human recombinant interleukin 1β or serum follow c-*jun* expression and are dependent on new protein synthesis. J. Clin. Invest. 83:1753.

195. Brinckerhoff, C.E., Mitchell, T.I., Karmilowicz, M.J., Kluve-Beckerman, B., and Benson, M.D. (1989). Autocrine induction of collagenase by serum amyloid A-like and B_2-microglobulin-like proteins. Science 243:655.

196. Ramadori, G., Sipe, J.D., and Colten, H.R. (1985). Expression and regulation of the murine serum a myloid A(SAA) gene in extrahepatic sites. J. Immunol. 135:3645.

197. Fini, E.M., Karmilowiez, M.J., Ruby, P.L., Beeman, A.M., Borges, K.A., and Brinckerhoff, C.E. (1987). Cloning of a complementary DNA for rabbit proactivator. A metalloproteinase that activates synovial cell collagenase, shares homology with stromelysin and transin and is coordinately regulated with collagenase. Arthritis Rheum. 30:1254.

198. Murphy, G., Cockett, M.I., Stephens, P.E., Smith, B.J., and Docherty, A.J.P. (1987). Stromelysin is an activator of procollagenase. A study with natural and recombinant enzymes. Biochem. J. 248:265.

199. Dean, D.D., Martel-Pelletier, J., Pelletier, J.-P., Howell, D.S., and Woessner, J.F., Jr. (1989). Evidence for metalloproteinase and metalloproteinase inhibitor imbalance in human osteoarthritic cartilage. J. Clin. Invest. 84:678.

200. Welgus, H.G., and Stricklin, G.P. (1983). Human skin fibroblast collagenase inhibitor: Comparative studies in human connective tissues, serum, and amniotic fluid. J. Biol. Chem. 258:12259.

201. Murphy, G., Reynolds, J.J., and Werb, Z. (1983). Biosynthesis of tissue inhibitor of metalloproteinases by human fibroblasts in culture: Stimulation by 12-O-tetra-decanoylphorbol 13-aetate and interleukin-1 in parallel with collagenase. J. Biol. Chem. 260:3079.

202. Laiho, M., Saksela, O., and Keski-Oja, J. (1987). Transforming growth factor-β induction of type 1 plasminogen activator inhibitor. J. Cell. Biol. 262:17467.

203. Edwards, D.R., Murphy, G., Reynolds, J.J., Whitham, S.E., Docherty, A.J.P., Angel, P., and Heath, J.K. (1987). Transforming growth factor beta modulates the expression of collagenase and metalloproteinase inhibitor. EMBO J. 6:1899.

204. Matrisian, L.M., Leroy, P., Ruhlmann, C., Gesnel-M.-C., and Breathnach, R. (1986). Isolation of the oncogene and epidermal growth factor-induced transin gene: Complex control in rat fibroblasts. Mol. Cell. Biol. 6:1679.

205. Chandrasekhar, S., and Harvey, A.K. (1988). Transforming growth factor-beta is a potent inhibitor of IL-1 induced protease activity and cartilage proteoglycan degradation. Biochem. Biophys. Res. Commun. 157:1352.

206. Saklatvala, J., Pilsworth, L.M., Sarsfield, S.J., Gavrilovic, J., and Heath, J.K. (1984). Pig catabolin is a form of interleukin 1. Cartilage and bone resorb, fibroblasts make prostaglandin and collagenase, and thymocyte proliferation is augmented in response to one protein. Biochem. J. 224:461.

207. Bunning, R.A., Richardson, H.J., Crawford, A., Skjodt, H., Hughes, D., Evans, D.B., Gowen, M., Dobson, P.R., Brown, B.L., and Russell, R.G. (1986). The effect of interleukin-1 on connective tissue metabolism and its relevance to arthritis. Agents Actions (Suppl.) 18:131.

208. Horton, J.E., Oppenheim, J.J., Mergenhagen, S.E., and Raisz, L.G. (1974). Macrophage-lymphocyte synergy in the production of osteoclast activating factor. J. Immunol. 113:1278.

209. Dewhirst, F.E., Stashenko, P.P., Mole, J.E., and Tsurumachi, T. (1985). Purification and partial sequence of human osteoclast-activating factor: Identity with interleukin 1β. J. Immunol. 135:2562.

210. Baron, R. (1989). Molecular mechanisms of bone resorption by the osteoclast. Anat. Rec. 224:317–324.

211. Teti, A., Blair, H.C., Schlesinger, P., Grano, M., Zambonin-Zallone, A., Kahn, A.J., Teitelbaum, S.L., and Hruska, K.A. (1989). Extracellular protons acidify osteoclasts, reduce cytosolic calcium, and promote expression of cell-matrix attachment structures. J. Clin. Invest. 84:773.

212. Bertolini, D.R., Nedwin, G.E., Bringman, T.S., Smith, D.D., and Mundy, G.R. (1986). Stimulation of bone resorption and inhibition of bone formation in vitro by human tumor necrosis factors. Nature 319:516.

213. Gowen, M., Wood, D.D., Ihrie, E.J., McGuire, M., and Russell, R.G.G. (1983). Stimulation by human interleukin 1 of cartilage breakdown and production of collagenase and proteoglycanase by human chondrocytes but not by human osteoblasts in vitro. Nature 306:378.

214. Heath, J.K., Saklatvala, J., Meikle, M.C., Atkinson, S.J., and Reynolds, J.J. (1985). Pig interleukin 1 (catabolin) is a potent stimulator of bone resorption in vitro. Calif. Tissue Int. 37:95.

215. Thomson, B.M., Saklatvola, J., and Chambers, T.J. (1986). Osteoblasts mediate interleukin 1 responsiveness of bone resorption by rat osteoclasts. J. Exp. Med. 164:104.

216. Thomson, B.M., Mundy, G.R. and Chambers, T.J. (1987). Tumor necrosis factors α and β induce osteoblastic cells to stimulate osteoclastic bone resorption. J. Immunol. 138:775.

7

Interleukin-1 Inhibitors and Their Significance in Rheumatoid Arthritis

Gloria C. Higgins
University of Tennessee, Memphis, Tennessee

Arnold E. Postlethwaite
University of Tennessee and Veterans' Administration Medical Center, Memphis, Tennessee

I. INTRODUCTION

Interleukin-1 (IL-1), an immunoregulatory cytokine present in rheumatoid synovium and synovial fluids (1,2), is likely to play an important role in the immunopathogenesis of rheumatoid arthritis. This product of activated synovial mononuclear cells (2,3) participates in the process of inflammation and repair through a variety of mechanisms. For example, IL-1 participates in the breakdown of cartilage (4,5) by stimulating the production of collagenase and other neutral proteinases by synovial cells (6,7), fibroblasts (8), and chondrocytes (5). The osteoclast-activating property of IL-1 promotes bone resorption (9). The effects of IL-1 on endothelial cells include 1) increased superoxide anion release (10) and synthesis of procoagulants (11), which may contribute to microvascular injury; 2) increased adhesiveness for neutrophils (12), monocytes (13), and lymphocytes (14); and 3) release of other mediators and induction of other surface changes leading to increased permeability and transendothelial passage of leukocytes (15,16). These vascular effects contribute to the accumulation of inflammatory cells within synovium and in synovial effusions. Activation of T and B lymphocytes by IL-1 itself and in conjunction with other lymphokines results in lymphocyte proliferation, immunoglobulin synthesis, and release of additional soluble mediators of inflammation (reviewed in Ref. 17). IL-1 is likely to participate in pannus formation and in cartilage repair by stimulating fibroblast proliferation (8,18,19) and synthesis of hyaluronic acid and glycosaminoglycans (20,21). Its ability to alter the synthesis of various types of collagen by chondrocytes (22) and to decrease the production of sulfated glycosaminoglycans in cartilage (21) may lead to defective cartilage repair. In addition to its local effects, the systemic effects of IL-1 associated with rheumatoid arthritis include fever, induction of acute-phase reactants, and suppression of erythropoiesis (17,23,24). IL-1 induces the release of multiple inflammatory mediators, including other cytokines and prostaglandins, which may either augment or antagonize various actions of IL-1. Thus, IL-1 seems to participate in nearly every aspect of the elaborate regulatory network of cells, receptors, and soluble factors that modulate inflammation. A more complete description of the cytokine network and its participants is found in other chapters of this volume.

Over the past decade, there have been numerous reports of factors that inhibit the action of IL-1. When the source of these inhibitors can be identified, many are (like IL-1 itself) produced by cells of the monocyte-macrophage lineage. Other cells that produce IL-1, including lymphocytes and endothelial cells, are additional potential sources of IL-1 inhibitors. Thus, the production of inhibitors may be one process in the immunoregulatory network whereby cells that secrete IL-1 also modulate the effects of this cytokine. In this chapter we critically survey the current literature on IL-1 inhibitors and attempt to place them in the context of the known effects and postulated mechanisms of action of IL-1. We discuss inhibitors with special relevance to rheumatoid arthritis and speculate on how they may contribute to future therapeutic modalities.

II. IL-1: PROPERTIES AND MECHANISMS OF ACTION

To provide a conceptual framework for discussing IL-1 inhibitors, it is necessary to summarize the physical properties of this cytokine and its cellular receptor. More thorough reviews of these topics have recently been published (17,25).

A. Production

Interleukin-1 is a family of polypeptide cytokines consisting, in humans, of an acid molecule (IL-1α, pI 5.0) and a neutral molecule (IL-1β, pI 7.0). Other, less well characterized forms of IL-1 also exist (26,27). The cDNAs for human IL-1α and β (28) and for the murine equivalents (29,30) have been cloned. Human recombinant IL-1α and β have less than 30% amino acid identity but probably have similar tertiary structures (17). In many in vitro systems they are functionally identical. However, recent reports have shown that different forms of IL-1α and β are not equivalent in their ability to elicit certain biologic responses (31) or to bind IL-1 receptors (27,32,33). Furthermore, the preferentially secreted form of IL-1 may be either α or β depending on cell type (34,35). These studies suggest a dissociation in the biologic functions of the different forms of IL-1.

IL-1α and β are both translated as precursors of approximately 31 kD, which lack the usual signal cleavage sequence for secreted proteins (27,36,37). The mechanism for processing and export of IL-1 has not been completely worked out. It appears that an intermediate 23 kD peptide, the C-terminal 17.5 kD secreted peptide, and smaller fragments are generated by serine proteases (17,36,37). Although cells of the monocyte-macrophage lineage probably account for most of the circulating IL-1, many other kinds of cells, including synovial mononuclear cells (2,3), B lymphocytes (35), T lymphocytes (34, and vascular endothelial cells (38), produce IL-1. IL-1β is the major extracellular form released by macrophages (17) and B lymphocytes (35). A biologically active membrane-associated IL-1, predominantly the α form, has been described by numerous investigators (39–44), but the validity of some of these findings has been questioned (45). It is likely that IL-1 produced in tissues and released into the local microenvironment or presented on cell surfaces is of primary importance in regulating cell-cell interactions in immunologic and inflammatory processes.

B. The IL-1 Receptor(s)

The in vitro binding of [^{125}I]IL-1 has been demonstrated for many types of cells, including rheumatoid synovial cells (46), fibroblasts (47), lymphocytes (33,48–50), and neutrophils (51). Although early evidence suggested that IL-1α and β bound the same receptor with similar affinity (46,49,52), recent reports have shown differences in affinity and apparent number of binding sites for IL-1α and β (32,33). An IL-1 receptor of 80 kD was demonstrated on cells of the EL4-6.1 mouse thymoma line by cross-linking radiolabeled IL-1β to cell surface molecules (53). The receptor has been purified (54), and the cDNA for the protein portion has been cloned, sequenced, and expressed (55). The three-dimensional conformation of the cloned 64.5 kD protein places it in the immunoglobulin supergene family and predicts extracellular, transmembrane, and cytoplasmic domains. Glycosylation accounts for the increase in molecular weight to 80 kD. The cloned IL-1 receptor expressed in COS cells (55) and natural IL-1 receptors on many kinds of cells have relatively low affinity for IL-1 (apparent $K_d > 5 \times 10^{-10}$ M). Other binding studies have suggested that presence of a second higher affinity receptor (apparent K_d 10^{-11}–10^{-12} M) (46,50,56). In some cross-linking experiments, proteins of various sizes in addition to the 80 kD receptors have been specifically bound to IL-1β (25,32,57). These could represent other IL-1 receptors, additional subunits of a multichain receptor, and/or proteins that are associated with the receptor and involved in signal transduction. Some investigators have proposed a two-chain model of the IL-1 receptor, similar to the two components of the IL-2 receptor, which would account for both low- and high-affinity binding (25,32,57). In some cells, IL-1 produces a biologic effect but receptor binding cannot be demonstrated (58), suggesting that the number of IL-1 receptors is extremely low or that IL-1 may act through non-receptor-mediated events (a controversial hypothesis).

C. Postreceptor Signal Transduction

The signal transduction events by which IL-1 exerts its effects are poorly understood. In analogy to known mechanisms of hormone action, it is reasonable to postulate that a "second messenger" system is involved. The adenylate cyclase-cyclic AMP system has been implicated in some studies of IL-1 mediated activation. In one study, IL-1 rapidly increased cAMP levels in human fibroblasts (59,60). A concomitant increase in the ability of cell extracts to phosphorylate histone HII-B suggested activation of cAMP-dependent protein kinase. In addition, synthesis messenger RNA for IL-6 was increased by either IL-1 or a cAMP-inducing agent. Others have shown that fibroblasts exposed to IL-1 increase their expression of IL-1 receptor by a mechanism involving prostaglandin synthesis and increased cAMP (61). In another report, treatment of mouse thymocytes with IL-1α also resulted in a rise in cAMP (62). Analogs of cAMP, or cAMP-inducing agents, could replace IL-1 in the mouse thymocyte costimulation assay and in induction of IL-2 receptors on a human natural killer cell line. It was later shown that the IL-1α-induced synthesis of immunoglobulin light chain in a pre-B cell line, IL-2 receptor expression in a natural killer cell line, and PGE$_2$ production by rheumatoid synovial cells were all accompanied by increased levels of cAMP (63). Pertussis toxin markedly inhibited all three actions of IL-1, as well as an IL-1-induced GTPase activity, suggesting that the IL-1 receptor and adenylate cyclase may be linked by a GTP binding protein (G protein). In opposition to these findings, treatment of human T cells with prostaglandins or with other agents that increased intracellular cAMP resulted in a decrease in phytohemagglutin (PHA)-induced IL-2 receptor synthesis (64). This apparent contradiction calls attention to the complex relationships among IL-1, cAMP, and prostaglandins.

Prostaglandins are believed to be feedback inhibitors of IL-1 production. The synthesis of prostaglandins in response to IL-1 has been studied mainly in synovial cells and fibroblasts (6,7,65,66). IL-1 amplifies receptor-mediated activation of phospholipase A$_2$, resulting in increased release of arachidonic acid, and induces the synthesis of cyclo-oxygenase (65,67), the first enzyme in the pathway from arachidonate to prostaglandins. Because of the requirement for new protein synthesis, the increase in prostaglandins is a late event after IL-1 treatment. PGE$_2$ was shown to suppress the production of IL-1 by macrophages (68). The proposed mechanism of this suppression was through activation of adenylate cyclase and formation of cAMP (26). In another study, however, no effect of PGE$_2$ on macrophage IL-1 production was demonstrated (69). In some cases prostaglandins antagonize the actions, as well as the synthesis, of IL-1. Physiologic concentrations of PGE_2 inhibited mouse thymocyte PHA/IL-1 comitogenesis (69) and IL-1 induced IL-2 synthesis by a mouse thymoma cell line (70).

The interactions of cAMP and prostaglandins in producing or modulating the biologic effects of IL-1 are poorly understood. It is likely that various kinds of IL-1 responsive cells differ in their biologic response to the same second messenger, cAMP. Alternatively, the timing of the increase in intracellular cAMP or the presence of signals generated by other mediators may be important in determining the ultimate cellular response.

Another "second messenger" system that may be involved in IL-1 signal transduction is the phosphatidylinositol-protein kinase C pathway. T lymphocytes require a T cell receptor-mediated stimulus, such as presentation of antigen by accessory cells, binding of anti-T cell receptor antibody, or binding of lectins, for activation or proliferation to occur (71,72). T cell receptor binding results in a cascade of signal transduction events: activation of phospholipase C, stimulation of phospholipid turnover, liberation of diacylglycerol, which binds and activates protein kinase C, release of inositol triphosphate, and increased intracellular calcium levels (73–75). These events may result in little or no cellular response unless a second signal, such as IL-1, is also present (72), but the reason for this requirement is unknown. Abraham and coworkers showed that activation of a mouse T cell line by the lectin phytohemagglutinin and IL-1 could be mimicked by the combination of a calcium ionophore and a phorbol ester (75). The calcium ionophore reproduced all three events associated with PHA binding: increased turnover of phospholipids, including phosphatidylinositol bisphosphate hydrolysis, calcium mobilization, and protein kinase C activation. The phorbal ester, an analog of diacylglycerol, seemed to stabilize cell membrane-associated protein kinase C. In contrast, IL-1 did not alter the subcellular distribution of protein kinase C or increase phosphoinositide breakdown. These investigators suggested that the mechanism of action of IL-1 is either independent of protein kinase C or distal to its activation. Others have also failed to detect the activation of protein kinase C by IL-1 (60,76). Nevertheless, membrane phospholipase Cs have been implicated in IL-1 signal transduction by reports of IL-1 induced increases in diacylglycerol production from phosphatidylcholine in human T cell line (58) and phosphatidylethanolamine in glomerular mesangial cells (76). Whether the diacylglycerol generated from these substrates participates in protein kinase C activation or in other, yet unknown, effector pathways has not been determined. Involvement of a serine-threonine protein kinase in signal transduction is supported by the detection of phosphorylation of cytosolic (77,78) and membrane (79) proteins at these amino acids, after IL-1 treatment of peripheral blood mononuclear cells (PBMC), fibroblasts, and glomerular mesangial cells, respectively.

An alternative mechanism by which IL-1 may produce biologic effects is ligand-receptor complex internalization and activation of a tyrosine kinase activity, analogous to the mechanism of action of several other polypeptide growth factors (80). Internalization of surface-bound ^{125}I-labeled IL-1 has been demonstrated in fibroblasts and lymphocytes from several sources (56,81–83). Appearance of labeled IL-1 in lysosomal fractions (81,82) and re-expression of receptor in the absence of de novo protein synthesis, suggesting reutilization of receptors (82), were also demonstrated. A role for IL-1 receptor internalization in cell activation is supported by observations of membrane protein tyrosine phosphorylation after IL-1 binding (79,84). The demonstration of nuclear localization of internalized [^{125}I]IL-1 (83) raises the possibility of direct regulation of transcription by the receptor or IL-1-receptor complex (17).

It is conceivable that a number of these proposed mechanisms of IL-1 action are correct. IL-1 receptors may be linked to different effector systems in different cells or to more than one effector system in the same cell, depending upon stage of development or the influence of other cytokines or mediators.

III. POSSIBLE MECHANISMS OF IL-1 INHIBITOR ACTION

Given the complexity of signal transduction in IL-1-mediated responses, it is clear that a plethora of possibilities exists for inhibition of these responses. As shown in Fig. 1, an inhibitor could bind IL-1 or bind the IL-1 receptor, thereby preventing the formation of the IL-1-receptor complex, or suppress the ability of the IL-1-receptor complex to transmit its signal. This may involve rendering the complex unable to activate a G protein, phosphorylate membrane proteins, translocate to the nucleus, and so on. Inhibitors could interfere with the same signal transduction events by binding to components of the pathway distal to the IL-1 receptor. In cells that require an activation signal in addition to IL-1, an inhibitor could interfere with generation of the second signal; for example, it could inhibit the protein kinase C pathway at one of many steps. Alternatively, an IL-1 inhibitor could act indirectly to counteract signals generated by IL-1, perhaps by downregulating the expression of IL-1 receptors or augmenting prostaglandin synthesis. Such events could be mediated by the binding of the inhibitor to its own receptor on the cell surface. Most previously described putative IL-1 inhibitors have not been studied in sufficient detail to elucidate their mechanism of action.

IV. ASSAYS FOR IL-1 INHIBITORS

The assay most commonly used to detect IL-1 inhibitors has been the thymocyte costimulation or comitogenesis assay (85,86). The basis for this assay is the ability of IL-1α or β to enhance the in vitro proliferation of mouse thymocytes stimulated with a suboptimal dose of plant lectin. Proliferation is measured by incorporation of tritiated thymidine into DNA. The lectins concanavalin A (ConA) and

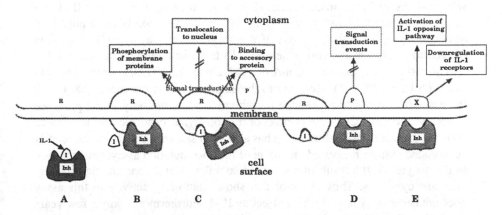

Figure 1 Possible mechanisms of IL-1 inhibition. The cell surface receptor (R) for IL-1 is depicted as a transmembrane protein. Inhibition of formation of the IL-1–receptor complex is accomplished by binding of inhibitor (Inh) to IL-1 (I) or to the IL-1 receptor as shown in A and B. (C) The inhibitor does not prevent IL-1 binding but interacts with the receptor to block a signal transduction event (for example, protein kinase activation or transloca-tion of the complex to the nucleus) or to prevent binding of the receptor to an accessory protein (P) required for signal transduction. (D) The inhibitor binds such an accessory protein and blocks either its interaction with the IL-1–receptor complex or its ability to transduce the signal generated by IL-1 receptor binding. (E) The inhibitor binds its own cell surface receptor (X) and induces a state of decreased IL-1 responsiveness, for example by downregulating IL-1 receptor expression or by activating intracellular pathways that oppose those activated by IL-1.

phytohemagglutinin are usually employed. These mitogens, which have binding specificity for oligosaccharides, are presumed to bind glycosylated moieties on the cell surface and signal activation and proliferation (87). The specific binding sites and signal transduction mechanisms are not well understood, but cross-linking of T cell receptors is probably involved (72,75,88). With large (mitogenic) doses, binding of lectin is sufficient to cause activation, proliferation, and concomitant production of and/or responsiveness to lymphokines (89). With small (sub-mitogenic) doses of lectin, exogenous IL-1 must be supplied to give comparable proliferation.

The enhancement of T cell proliferation by IL-1 is believed to be the result of both increased IL-2 production and IL-2 receptor expression (72,86,90,91). However, IL-2 is not the only cytokine likely to be involved in thymocyte pro-liferation. Activation of a subset of T lymphocytes through antigen receptors leads to the synthesis of IL-4 (92–94). This cytokine in turn augments T cell prolifera-tion in response to a variety of stimuli (95,96). Culture of mouse thymocytes with IL-1 results in the production of IL-6 (97), which synergizes with IL-1 and IL-2 to promote proliferation (97,98). A further complication is the requirement of accessory cells for the response of thymocytes in this assay (99). Depletion of accessory (IA$^+$, nylon wool adherent) cells from the mouse thymocyte population abolishes the response to ConA or PHA alone (85,100,101) or in combination with IL-1 (100,101). Relevant to this phenomenon is the report that ConA increases IL-1 receptor expression on human T cells, but only in the presence of accessory cells (102). A direct effect of IL-1 on thymic dendritic cells to enhance their in vitro accessory cell function has also been shown (101). It can be readily appreciated that the measured end point of the costimulation assay, proliferation of thymocytes, is the result of a series of complex interactions among different cells and cytokines. Thus, a factor that shows inhibitory activity in this assay does not necessarily have a direct effect on IL-1. Furthermore, only a few years ago before the widespread availability of highly purified or recombinant IL-1, crude or partially purified IL-1 from culture supernatants of various kinds of cells was used in the thymocyte costimulation assay. These preparations contained variable amounts of other cytokines that could be the actual target of "IL-1" inhibitors in earlier studies.

To substantiate the claims of inhibitor specificity for IL-1, more stringent assays are necessary. A simpler assay system, which contains a single type of cell, is proliferation of the murine helper T cell line D10.G4.1 in response to IL-1 plus specific anti-T cell receptor monoclonal antibody or lectins (103). Costimulation results in both the production of IL-4 and induction of responsiveness to this autocrine growth factor (104). However, this assay, like the thymocyte assay, suffers from the requirement for a costimulus.

To exclude binding and inactivation of ConA or PHA as the mechanism for inhibition of proliferation, inhibitors should be tested in mitogen-independent assays of IL-1. (The absence of inhibition of mitogenesis in the presence of large doses of lectin alone does not completely rule out such an interaction, since the concentration of lectin may be sufficient to saturate both inhibitor and cellular binding sites.) Some investigators have described inhibition of thymocyte proliferation in response to large doses of IL-1 without mitogen (105,106), but this assay is not very sensitive as a result of the weakness of the response to IL-1 alone. At least one IL-1 inhibitor (107) has shown activity in the assay developed by Falk et al. (108), in which proliferation of thymocytes in response to IL-1 is measured in the presence of saturating amounts of IL-2. In this assay, proliferation is postulated to be mainly the result of increased IL-2 receptor expression. A human astrocytoma cell line that proliferates in response to IL-1 alone (109) has been used to test another IL-1 inhibitor (110). Sublines of D10.G4.1 that respond to IL-1 in the absence of lectin have been reported (111,112) but have not been used for assays of IL-1 inhibitors. Some inhibitors have been shown to inhibit mitogen-independent events, such as IL-1 induced fibroblast proliferation (113), collagenase production (114,115), and prostaglandin synthesis (115,116). Other inhibitors of T cell proliferation have paradoxically stimulated fibroblasts (117,118).

The ability of IL-1 to stimulate the production of other cytokines forms the basis for additional assays of IL-1 and its inhibitors. In this method, culture supernatants from cells that produce other cytokines in response to IL-1 are assayed for cytokine content by their ability to induce proliferation of an IL-1-unresponsive indicator cell line. Indicator cell lines generally employed include the T cell lines CTLL-2 and HT-2, which respond to both IL-2 and IL-4, and CT6, which is IL-2 specific (119). For the purpose of demonstrating inhibition of cytokine production, the most useful IL-1 responder cell is the mouse thymoma cell line EL4 or the subline EL4-6.1. In the presence of IL-1 and the calcium ionophore A23187, these cells produce increased cytokine activity, initially attributed to IL-2 (120), but now known to include IL-4 (121). A subclone of EL4 that requires no costimulus has recently been described (122) but has not been used for inhibitor assays. Some inhibitors of IL-1 have been shown to suppress lymphokine production by a T cell line or by thymocytes (106,123,124). As for all proliferation assays, care must be taken to ensure that decreased proliferation of indicator cells is not artifactual. In one instance, excess thymidine released by inhibitor-treated thymocytes accounted for much of the observed suppression of indicator cell proliferation (124).

To prove specificity for IL-1, it is obviously necessary to investigate the effects of inhibitors on other cytokines. Proliferation assays using purified or recombinant IL-2 and mouse thymocytes, IL-2-responsive mouse T cell lines, such as those already discussed, or IL-2-dependent human T cell lines (CTL) have been used to rule out the effects of IL-1 inhibitors on IL-2. Not surprisingly, some factors that are suppressive in the mouse thymocyte costimulation assay for IL-1 also suppress IL-2-induced proliferation (125,126) and thereby cannot be considered specific for IL-1. Most inhibitors have not been tested for their effects on IL-4 or IL-6, since knowledge of these cytokines is relatively recent.

Finally, one must exclude the effects of nonspecific factors that may be responsible for inhibition of proliferation assays. For example, contamination of a cell line with mycoplasma was said to be the source of IL-1 inhibition in one previously published study (26,127). Nonspecific cytotoxic substances, prostaglandins, or excess free nucleotides are other possibilities that should be excluded.

Binding studies offer a direct method of assessing specificity for those IL-1 inhibitors that interfere with this initial phase of IL-1 action. Inhibitor binding to IL-1 using solid-phase radioimmunoassays has been demonstrated (128), but this method has been criticized by others (129). Binding of a serum factor to IL-1 has been revealed by a shift in mobility of [^{125}I]IL-1 on gel filtration (130). Another class of inhibitors has been shown to interfere with the binding of radiolabeled IL-1 to cells (114,123) and thus may have specificity for the IL-1 receptor.

V. REVIEW OF IL-1 INHIBITORS

The literature on IL-1 inhibitors is rather confusing. Most inhibitors have only been partially purified, and the effects described may be due to more than one active moiety. In addition, the limitations of commonly used assay systems, as described earlier, and the use of crude or partially purified cytokines in earlier studies further cloud the issue of specificity. The apparent large number of different inhibitors, based on approximate molecular weight by gel filtration or isoelectric point, may be due to artifacts produced by protein aggregation, differences in glycosylation, and other factors that can influence these measurements. Although cell-specific or tissue-specific inhibitors are likely to exist, many of the proposed IL-1 inhibitors may turn out to be the same. Summaries of inhibitors that are probably specific for IL-1 and those that appear to inhibit other cytokines in addition to IL-1 are shown in Tables 1 and 2, respectively.

In the discussion to follow, we have attempted to organize the literature on IL-1 inhibitors by dividing them into categories. The three different IL-1 inhibitors that have been best characterized are discussed first. The next section includes inhibitors that may be specific for IL-1 but have not been studied in detail. A discussion of inhibitors that are probably not specific for IL-1 but appear relevant to biologic effects of IL-1 follows. The final section describes lymphokine inhibitors found in synovial tissues and fluid of patients with rheumatoid arthritis, which may have special significance in the pathogenesis of this disorder.

A. Uromodulin

Uromodulin, an 85 kD glycoprotein, was purified from the urine of pregnant women by Muchmore and Decker (131). Purified uromodulin was initially shown to inhibit assays of three populations of lymphocytes in human peripheral blood mononuclear cells, namely, T cell proliferation in response to tetanus toxoid, B cell reverse hemolytic plaque formation in response to pokeweed mitogen, and monocyte spontaneous cytotoxic response against ^{51}Cr-labeled chicken erythrocytes. Subsequently it was shown that uromodulin decreased the proliferation of mouse thymocytes in response to PHA and mouse or human recombinant IL-1 but enhanced the response to human recombinant IL-2 (132).

The proposed mechanism of action of uromodulin was binding of IL-1. Using an indirect radiolabeled antibody technique, uromodulin was shown to bind enzyme-linked immunosorbent assay (ELISA) plates coated with mouse IL-1α but not to uncoated plates or plates coated with a variety of other proteins.

Table 1 Inhibitors That Appear Specific for IL-1[a]

Name of inhibitor	Source	Molecular weight (kD)	Assay	Mechanism/comments	References
Uromodulin	Urine, pregnant women	85	Thymocyte comitogenesis	May bind IL-1	128, 131–136
Febrile Inhibitor	Urine, febrile patients	38	Thymocyte comitogenesis	Has DNAse activity	105, 118, 132, 140–142
—	Urine, monocyte leukemia	25	Thymocyte comitogenesis; fibroblast PGE_2 and collagenase synthesis	Blocks receptor binding ↑ Probably identical →	115, 123, 143
—	Human PBMC culture supernatants	25	Thymocyte comitogenesis; fibroblast collagenase synthesis; cytokine production by EL4-6.1	Blocks receptor binding	114, 144
—	LPS-stimulated human PBMC culture supernatants	5–9	Thymocyte comitogenesis		106, 117, 145
Contra-IL-1	HIV-infected human macrophages	9	Thymocyte comitogenesis	Does not inhibit IL-1 binding	148
—	Virus-infected human macrophages	99	Thymocyte comitogenesis		149
—	Stimulated human alveolar macrophages	40–50	Thymocyte comitogenesis	Not a prostaglandin	150
—	LPS-stimulated mouse P388D1 cells	160	Thymocyte comitogenesis	Not a protease	107

(continued)

Table 1 *Continued*

Name of inhibitor	Source	Molecular weight (kD)	Assay	Mechanism/comments	References
—	LPS-stimulated rat Kupffer's cells	27	Thymocyte comitogenesis		151
Contra-IL-1	EBV-transformed human lymphoblast line ROHA-9	95	Thymocyte comitogenesis	May bind receptor	152
—	Human myelomonocyte line M20	51–53	Thymocyte comitogenesis; fibroblast proliferation		153
—	Human polymorphonuclear leukocytes	> 160 and 45–70	Thymocyte comitogenesis	Not a protease	154
EC–contra–IL-1	UV-irradiated mouse epidermal cells; mouse keratinocyte line Pam 212	40	Thymocyte comitogenesis; fibroblast proliferation		113, 155
SMG-ISF	Rat submandibular glands	59–96	Thymocyte comitogenesis	May decrease IL-2 production	156, 157
—	Serum, JRA patients		Fibroblast PGE_2 production		116
—	Normal human urine		Thymocyte comitogenesis		
Natural antibody	Normal human serum	100–200	Thymocyte comitogenesis	Inhibits IL-1α binding to EL4 cells, binds IL-1α	130
IL-1α inhibitor	Rheumatoid synovial fluid	100	T cell proliferation; cytokine production by EL4-6.1	Not a protease, DNAse, or prostaglandin inducer	186–188

aPGE$_2$, prostaglandin E$_2$; PBMC, peripheral blood mononuclear cell; LPS, lipopolysaccharide; HIV, human immunodeficiency virus; EBV, Epstein-Barr virus; JRA, juvenile rheumatoid arthritis.

Table 2 Some Inhibitors That Do Not Appear to Be Specific for IL-1

Name of inhibitor	Source	Molecular weight (kD)	Assay	Mechanism/comments	References
IDS	U937 cells	45–75	Proliferation of PBMC, T and B cell lines	Inhibits spontaneous proliferation	158
—	U937 cells	67–130	T-cell proliferation, IL-2 production	Inhibits response to IL-2 and mitogens	125, 159
TGF-β	U937 cells; synovial fluid	12.5			177, 178, 180
ILS	Gingival organ culture	97	Thymocyte comitogenesis, CD-1 antigen expression	Inhibits IL-1 and IL-2	126, 161
p15E and related peptides	Retroviral envelope	15	T-cell proliferation; tumor cell lysis; astrocytoma proliferation	Inhibits IL-1 and IL-2	110, 162–165
α-MSH	Synthetic pituitary hormone	1.3	Thymocyte comitogenesis; fibroblast prostaglandin synthesis; acute-phase reaction	Inhibits IL-1 and TNF-α	168, 169
Endopeptidase 24.11	Kidney and other nonlymphoid cells	95	Thymocyte comitogenesis	Metalloproteinase, cleaves numerous neuropeptides	170
—	Rheumatoid synovial fluid	150–180	T-cell proliferation	Inhibits IL-2	171–173
Soluble IL-2 receptor	Rheumatoid synovial fluid and sera	40	IL-2-dependent cell proliferation	Binds IL-2	174
	Synovial fluid	65–70	IL-2-dependent cell proliferation		175

Conversely, IL-1α was shown to bind to uromodulin-coated ELISA plates (128). In a direct assay, ^{125}I-labeled uromodulin bound to IL-1-coated plates and was displaced by cold uromodulin but not by a variety of other proteins. In addition, [^{125}I]uromodulin coprecipitated with IL-1 using an antibody specific for IL-1. Extension of these studies revealed binding of uromodulin to human recombinant IL-1α and β and to human recombinant tumor necrosis factor (TNF) (133,134). The active site for both IL-1 binding and immunosuppression appeared to reside in the carbohydrate portion of uromodulin, since both functions were decreased by digestion or biochemical modification of carbohydrate. In addition, oligosaccharides derived from uromodulin were immunosuppressive in vitro and blocked the binding of the intact molecule to IL-1 (135,136).

The protein portion of uromodulin has been shown, by comparison of actual and derived amino acid sequences, to be identical to the previously described Tamm-Horsfall urinary glycoprotein (133,137). However, several batches of Tamm-Horsfall protein, isolated by the technique of salt precipitation, consistently gave significantly less immunosuppression than uromodulin isolated by lectin adherence. It was proposed that this discrepancy was due to differences in the carbohydrate portions of these glycoproteins, which in turn could have resulted from differences in the isolation method (133). If this proposal is true, it may partially explain the conflicting findings of Moonen et al. (129). These investigators isolated both Tamm-Horsfall protein from urine of males and uromodulin from urine of pregnant females by the technique of salt precipitation. The binding of their preparations to immobilized human recombinant TNF depended upon both the type of microtiter plates used and the pH at which the plates were coated and was not blocked by TNF in the liquid phase. They observed binding of uromodulin to human recombinant IL-1α-coated plates with an affinity of less than one-tenth that reported by Muchmore and Decker, no binding of IL-1α to uromodulin-coated plates, and no binding of ^{125}I]IL-1α to uromodulin in liquid phase as assayed by migration on gel filtration. They contended that 1) uromodulin does not specifically bind IL-1 or TNF; 2) uromodulin supplied by Muchmore behaved similarly to their preparation; and 3) the binding observed by Muchmore and coworkers was the result of protein denaturation. They also questioned whether the in vivo function of uromodulin is the inhibition of IL-1 and suggested that its effect in the thymocyte costimulation assay is the result of its ability to bind PHA (138).

The uromodulin controversy remains undecided. However, the recent observation by Brody and Durum (139) that IL-1α precursor is bound to macrophage cell membranes by a lectinlike interaction and can be solubilized by mannose further suggests that carbohydrate interactions between IL-1 and other molecules may be biologically significant.

B. The Urine-Derived (DNAse-like) IL-1 Inhibitor

Liao and coworkers identified a substance from the urine of febrile patients that inhibited the proliferation of mouse thymocytes in response to IL-1 and PHA (105,140) or to IL-1 alone (105). Initial purification steps included precipitation with 40–60% saturated ammonium sulfate and elution from DE-52 with 100–250 mM NaCl. The inhibitor migrated on gel filtration with an apparent molecular weight of 25–45 kD and was heterogenous in its affinity for ConA-Sepharose. The portion that bound to the lectin and could be eluted by α-methyl-D-glucose was further studied. The febrile inhibitor had no effect on proliferation of thymocytes in response to ConA (141) or human recombinant IL-2 (105) and was antigenetically distinct from uromodulin (132). These investigators presented evidence that their inhibitor was affecting a late stage of activation, rather than IL-1 binding. The febrile inhibitor was still active when thymocytes were incubated with IL-1 for 24 h, washed, and then exposed to either PHA alone or PHA plus inhibitor (141). Paradoxically, this inhibitor preparation augmented fibroblast PGE_2 synthesis in response to IL-1 (118). However, increased prostaglandin synthesis did not appear to account for its inhibition of thymocyte comitogenesis, since addition of indomethacin to thymocyte cultures did not alter the activity of inhibitor in this assay (141). Subsequently, the febrile inhibitor was purified to homogeneity, and partial amino acid sequence was performed on this 38 kD protein (142). Of the first 70 amino acids, 46 were sequenced and found to have 78% identity with bovine DNAse I. The purified inhibitor was also shown to degrade ^{14}C-labeled DNA with a potency equal to that of bovine DNAse I. The cellular events in response to this DNAse-like molecule have not been determined. Bovine DNAse does not affect in vitro proliferation of T cells in response to IL-1 (Higgins and Postlethwaite, unpublished observation). If the effect of the DNAse-like inhibitor is simply that of increasing the pool of free nucleotides, thereby decreasing the uptake of radiolabeled thymidine in the proliferation assay, then it is not apparent how one may account for its specificity for the IL-1-induced proliferation or stimulation of PGE_2 synthesis described in earlier studies.

C. The 25 kD Monocyte-Derived IL-1 Inhibitor

An IL-1 inhibitor was identified in the urine of patients with monocytic leukemia by Balavoine and coworkers (143), which appeared to be distinct from uromodulin and the febrile urine inhibitor. This inhibitor was partially purified by 40–80% ammonium sulfate precipitation, ion-exchange chromatography, hydroxyapatite chromatography, and gel filtration. It had an apparent molecular weight of 18–25 kD and, in contrast to uromodulin and febrile inhibitor, did not bind ConA-Sepharose. This preparation equally inhibited the proliferation of mouse thymocytes in response to PHA plus human recombinant IL-1α or β. Unlike uromodulin or the urine-derived (DNAse-like) inhibitor, it suppressed collagenase and PGE_2 production by human fibroblasts and synovial cells, as well as fibroblast proliferation, in response to IL-1α and β (115). The inhibitor was specific for IL-1 in that it did not interfere with TNF-α stimulation of fibroblast proliferation or PGE_2 production. It was subsequently shown that this inhibitor blocked the binding of IL-1 to its receptor (123). The specific binding of [^{125}I]IL-1 to the mouse thymoma cell line EL4-6.1 was inhibited in a dose-dependent manner by the partially purified inhibitor. When cells were preincubated with inhibitor and washed, binding of [^{125}I]IL-1 was virtually abolished at 4 °C and substantially reduced at 37 °C, suggesting that the inhibitor may bind the IL-1 receptor. This effect was not due to contaminating IL-1 in the preparation, since no IL-1 was detected by Western blot analysis. Furthermore, the inhibitor also decreased the production of "IL-2" (IL-4) by EL4-6.1 cells in response to IL-1 and a calcium ionophore.

An inhibitor with virtually identical characteristics was produced in vitro by Arend and coworkers (144). These investigators found that supernatants from human peripheral blood monocytes, cultured on immune complex-coated plates, produced a factor that inhibited the mouse thymocyte IL-1β comitogenesis assay and collagenase production in response to IL-1β by fibroblasts and chondrocytes. It had no effect on IL-2-induced proliferation of CTLL and HT-2 cells and a small effect on IL-2-induced proliferation of thymocytes (114). The inhibitor blocked the binding of [^{125}I]IL-1α and β to EL4-6.1 cells in a competitive manner but was negative for IL-1 by Western blot analysis. It was shown to be different from TGF-β because of the failure of TGF-β to inhibit fibroblast PGE_2 synthesis or T cell binding of IL-1. Furthermore, anti-TGFβ did not reduce the biologic effects of this factor. Based on similarities in molecular weight and apparent mechanism of action, this inhibitor and that of Dayer and coworkers are probably closely related or identical. (See Addendum, p. 159.)

D. IL-1 Inhibitor Candidates

The inhibitors described in this section have only been partially purified and characterized. Based on data presented to date, they appear to specifically antagonize IL-1-induced responses. However, further investigation is required to elucidate their true relationship to IL-1.

Inhibitors from Macrophages or Macrophagelike Cells

A low-molecular-weight inhibitor of IL-1 activity produced by human peripheral blood mononuclear cells stimulated with bacterial cell wall lipopolysaccharide (LPS) was described by Berman and coworkers (106). This product of the adherent population of PBMC had an apparent molecular weight of 5–9 kD by gel filtration and a pI of 4.5–5.6 by chromatofocusing. It inhibited mouse thymocyte proliferation in response to partially purified human IL-1 alone and comitogenesis with PHA plus IL-1. It had no effect on PBMC proliferation in response to PHA, ConA, or pokeweed mitogen or on CTLL-2 proliferation in response to IL-2. The inhibitor decreased the production of IL-2 by thymocytes, but not to the same degree that it inhibited proliferation. Since the addition of recombinant IL-2 to thymocyte cultures did not overcome the inhibition of proliferation, the mechanism of action did not appear to be inhibition of IL-2 synthesis. Indomethacin suppressed the ability of PBMC to produce inhibitor; however, it did not appear to be a prostaglandin since no PGE was detected in inhibitor fractions by radioimmunoassay. In subsequent reports, PBMC from scleroderma patients made 3-fold more inhibitor (117), and PBM from patients infected with human immunodeficiency virus 1 (HIV-1) made 20-fold more inhibitor (145) than those from normal controls. In contrast to its effect on T cell proliferation, the partially purified factor, alone or with IL-1, stimulated fetal dermal fibroblast proliferation (117). Factors of similar molecular weight and isolectric point that stimulate fibroblast proliferation have been described by other investigators (146,147). Whether both the thymocyte inhibitory and the fibroblast stimulatory activities reside in a single molecule has not been determined.

Contra-IL-1, described by Locksley et al., is an approximately 9 kD factor produced by human monocyte-derived macrophages infected in vitro with HIV (148). This low-molecular-weight material was partially purified by gel filtration and found to be protease and acid sensitive. Contra-IL-1 inhibited mouse thymocyte comitogenesis in response to PHA and recombinant human IL-1β. It also reduced the proliferative response of normal human peripheral blood mononuclear cells to ConA and to tetanus toxoid. Addition of IL-1β could partially overcome this effect. No decrease in proliferation of CTLL cells in response to purified human IL-2 or HT-2 cells in response to crude mouse IL-2 was observed. Contra-IL-1 did not inhibit the binding of [^{125}I]IL-1β to a mouse fibroblast cell line, so it probably acts at a site distal to IL-1 receptor binding. Cultured spleen macrophages from HIV-infected patients also produced contra-IL-1 activity, indicating that this factor was not an artifact of in vitro infection. The relationship of contra-IL1 to the low-molecular-weight inhibitor of Berman and coworkers has not been investigated. Such IL-1 inhibitors may play an important role in the profound immunosuppression seen in HIV-infected patients. They may be viral products, like p15E (see Sec. V.E.), or cellular products induced by viral infection.

In the report of Roberts et al., macrophages derived from human PBMC and infected in vitro with influenza or respiratory syncytial virus (RSV) produced IL-1 and two inhibitory factors (149). The high-molecular-weight factor, approximately 99 kD by gel filtration, inhibited mouse thymocyte costimulation with PHA and purified IL-1 but not proliferation of the HT-2 cell line in response to IL-2. The low-molecular-weight factor, 3–5 kD on gel filtration, had inhibitory activity in the thymocyte assay but was not further investigated.

Gosset et al. have described an inhibitor of IL-1 released from alveolar macrophages of asthmatic and control patients after stimulation with IgE or antigen in vitro (150). This factor suppressed thymocyte comitogenesis in response to purified IL-1 and PHA but was unable to suppress the proliferation of the mouse cytotoxic T cell line CTLL in response to IL-2. The molecular weight of this inhibitor by gel filtration was 40–50 kD. The inhibitor was insensitive to treatment with heat, trypsin, or neuraminidase. Activity was not reduced by the addition of protease inhibitors, suggesting that the mechanism of action was not enzymatic degradation of IL-1. Induction of the inhibitor was not reduced by pretreatment of alveolar macrophages with indomethacin, suggesting that it was not a prostaglandin.

An inhibitor of IL-1 was demonstrated in culture supernatants of LPS-stimulated P388D$_1$ cells, a mouse macrophage line, by Nishihara and coworkers (107). The inhibitor could be separated from IL-1 activity by gel filtration and appeared in fractions corresponding to approximately 160 kD. This partially purified inhibitor suppressed the costimulation of mouse thymocytes by ConA and crude mouse IL-1 or human recombinant IL-1α and β. Greater inhibition was seen with IL-1β than with α. In contrast, the response to ConA alone was augmented by inhibitor fractions. To further show that the inhibitor was not interacting with ConA in the thymocyte assay, costimulation was carried out with crude IL-1 and saturating amounts of crude IL-2. The inhibitor still suppressed the IL-1-augmented proliferation. Absence of IL-2 inhibition was demonstrated using the IL-2-sensitive CTLL-2 cell line. The inhibitor was not inactivated by soybean trypsin inhibitor or aprotinin and thus probably was not an IL-1 protease.

Shirahama and collaborators have demonstrated the presence of two immunosuppressive factors produced by rat Kupffer's cells stimulated with LPS (151). After ammonium sulfate precipitation and gel filtration of culture supernatants, inhibitory fractions of approximately 27 and 6 kD were separated from IL-1. Both fractions inhibited the comitogenesis assay of mouse thymocytes with PHA and partially purified human IL-1. Suppression by the 27 kD fraction could be partially overcome by excess IL-1. The 6 kD inhibitor also suppressed thymocyte proliferation in response to IL-2, but the 27 kD inhibitor did not. The low-molecular-weight inhibitor appears to be different from that of Berman et al., and from the 9 kD macrophage-derived contra-IL-1, in its lack of specificity for IL-1. This apparent difference could be due to the use of two different responding cells in the IL-2 assays: thymocytes in this study, CTLL-2 in the others. The 27 kD inhibitor shares a common size and cell lineage of origin with that found in urine from monocytic leukemia patients (143) and in monocyte culture supernatants (144).

Inhibitors from Other Leukocytes or Cell Lines

Scala and coworkers have described an inhibitor produced by the EBV-transformed human lymphoblastoid cell line ROHA-9 (152). This "contra-IL-1" was separated from IL-1 by gel filtration, and migrated at an approximate molecular weight of 95 kD. It was able to suppress costimulation of mouse thymocytes with ConA and partially purified human IL-1. It also inhibited the proliferative response of human PBMC to suboptimal, but not optimal, doses of ConA, to streptolysin O, and to allogeneic monocytes in a one-way mixed lymphocyte reaction. The factor had no effect on proliferation in response to IL-2 by mouse thymocytes or the IL-2-dependent cell line CT6. Contra-IL-1 was absorbed by thymocytes but not by CT6 cells. Furthermore, thymocytes that were treated with this inhibitor and thoroughly washed were then suppressed in their ability to respond to IL-1 in the costimulation assay. These results suggest that this inhibition may bind to the IL-1 receptor or to some other surface molecule involved in IL-1-induced T cell activation. Subsequent purification steps revealed that the inhibitor eluted from anion exchange with the major protein peak and migrated as a single species with pI 4.75 on isoelectric focusing.

An IL-1 inhibitor produced by the human myelomonocytic cell line M20 has been described by Barak et al. (153). The response of mouse thymocytes to PHA and several preparations of crude IL-1 was suppressed by this inhibitor, which was partially purified by anion-exchange chromatography and gel filtration. This 51–53 kD factor also inhibited the proliferation of human fibroblasts in response to crude IL-1 and of human PBMC depleted of adherent cells in response to PHA and PPD. It had no effect on the proliferation of the IL-2-dependent cell lines CTL-1 and CTL-2 in response to crude IL-2.

Tiku and coworkers (154) have reported a factor from lysates and culture supernatants of human polymorphonuclear leukocytes (PMN) that suppresses the response of mouse thymocytes to partially purified human IL-1 and PHA. Inhibition could be partially overcome by increasing amounts of IL-1. Synthesis of this inhibitor was increased by zymosan stimulation of PMN and occurred in the absence of serum. Addition to protease inhibitors to PMN lysate did not alter its ability to inhibit IL-1. When ConA was used in place of PHA in the co-mitogenesis assay, the PMN inhibitor was active in the presence or absence of IL-1. When thymocytes were maximally stimulated by higher concentrations of ConA, however, the inhibitor was inactive. No inhibition of IL-2-induced proliferation of the CTLL-2 cell line was observed. When zymosan-stimulated PMN lysates or supernatants were fractionated on gel filtration, the IL-1 inhibitor appeared in two peaks: one greater than 160 kD, possibly representing aggregates, and one at about 70 kD (supernatant) or 45–70 kD (lysate). This inhibitor has not been further characterized.

Tissue-Derived Inhibitors

Schwarz et al. have described EC–contra-IL-1, and inhibitory factor in culture supernatants from mouse epidermal cells or the keratinocyte cell line Pam 212 after ultraviolet (UV) irradiation (113). Crude supernatants containing both IL-1 and inhibitor activity were separated by HPLC gel filtration. The partially purified EC–contra-IL-1, approximately 40 kD, inhibited costimulation of mouse thymocytes with ConA and purified mouse IL-1 but not mitogenesis by ConA alone. It also inhibited the IL-1-induced proliferation of mouse dermal fibroblasts. EC–contra-IL-1 failed to suppress the proliferation of CTLL cells in response to purified mouse IL-2, the IL-3-dependent cell line 32 DCL in response to crude IL-3, or the spontaneous proliferation of four other cell lines, suggesting that it was specific for IL-1. On further purification, EC–contra-IL-1 eluted at a pH of 8.8 on chromatofocusing and was resolved into three separate peaks of activity by reversed-phase high performance liquid chromatography (HPLC). In a subsequent report, serum from UV-irradiated mice contained an inhibitor with properties identical to those of EC–contra-IL-1 (155). Further purification and characterization of this inhibitor have not been reported.

Kemp and coworkers partially purified an immunosuppressive factor from rat submandibular glands (SMG-ISF) by gel filtration and chromatofocusing (156,157). This 50–96 kD factor blocked the proliferation of mouse lymphoid cells in response to ConA, PHA, and LPS. It also inhibited the proliferation and cell-mediated cytotoxicity induced in mixed lymphocyte culture. These effects could be reversed by the addition of IL-2 (156). SMG-ISF also inhibited costimulation of mouse thymocytes with ConA and recombinant human IL-1α or β or purified mouse IL-1. This effect was partly overcome by addition of excess IL-1. On the other hand, the proliferation of CTLL-2 cells in response to crude rate IL-2 was not affected (157). These studies suggest that SMG-ISF in some way decreases IL-2 production in response to various stimuli, possibly by inhibition of IL-1 action.

Other Inhibitors

Prieur and colleagues found that serum and urine from several children with systemic juvenile rheumatoid arthritis contained a substance that suppressed PGE$_2$ production by cultured synovial fibroblasts in response to human recombinant IL-1β (116). This activity tended to occur during episodes of fever. Further purification or characterization of this inhibitor has not been reported.

Svenson and Bendtzen have reported that urine from healthy human volunteers inhibited mouse thymocyte proliferation and IL-2 synthesis in response to PHA and purified human IL-1 (124). The same urine failed to suppress IL-1-induced cytokine synthesis by the EL4 cell line. The reason for this discrepancy was partly due to excess thymidine released by urine-treated thymocytes. However, when assays were conduced to remove the effect of free thymidine, the difference between thymocytes and EL4 in susceptibility to inhibition remained. Further studies on this activity, to elucidate its relationship to uromodulin or the DNAse-like urine inhibitor, have not been reported.

Svenson et al. recently reported that normal human serum reduced the binding of ^{125}I-labeled human recombinant IL-1α to EL4 cells (130). The factor in serum that inhibited binding had an apparent molecular weight of 100–200 kD by gel filtration. When [^{125}I]IL-1α was preincubated with human serum and subjected to gel filtration, radiolabel appeared in two peaks, one in the retained volume and one in the void volume, indicating binding of [^{125}I]IL-1α to a high-molecular-weight ligand. This binding could be displaced by excess unlabeled IL-1α, but not IL-1β. Furthermore, a significant portion of [^{125}I]IL-1α in serum-containing media could be precipitated by antihuman IgG or bound to Protein A-Sepharose, suggesting that it was complexed to immunoglobulin. These investigators proposed the presence of naturally occurring antibodies against IL-1α in human serum.

E. Inhibitors Lacking IL-1 Specificity

The factors discussed in this section antagonize the effects of IL-1 but also antagonize other cytokines or hormones. They may participate in modulating in vivo processes that involve IL-1.

Several immunosuppressive activities have been demonstrated in culture supernatants of U937 cells, a human macrophagelike line. Wilkins and coworkers described IDS (inhibitor of DNA synthesis), a product of ConA- or PHA-stimulated U937 cells (158). This inhibitor suppressed both the spontaneous and the induced proliferation of human PBMC and several T and B lymphoid cell lines. On gel filtration, the activity migrated in the 45–75 kD range. In a later report, Fujiwara and Ellner described an immunosuppressive factor constitutively produced by U937 cells (125). This factor inhibited the proliferation of mouse thymocytes in response to PHA, crude human IL-1 both alone and with PHA, and crude human IL-2 with PHA. Inhibition was not overcome by increasing the concentration of IL-1 or PHA. The U937 supernatants also suppressed proliferation, IL-2 production, and IL-2 receptor expression by human blood T lymphocytes in response to PHA or tuberculin purified protein derivative (PPD). PHA-stimulated IL-2 production by the human leukemic cell line Jurkat was also inhibited (159). These inhibitory activities resided in the 67–130 kD protein peak on gel filtration. Since both the constitutively produced and the mitogen-induced inhibitors were inactivated at pH 2 and were of higher molecular weight, they did not appear to be related to transforming growth factor β (TGF-β), which is another product of U937 cells (see Sec. V.F, Transforming Growth Factor β). Subsequently, it has been shown that TGF-β, unlike the constitutively produced U937 factor, does not alter T cell IL-2 production or IL-2 receptor expression

(160). These partially characterized U937 inhibitors appear to affect mulitple cytokine-induced T cell responses, rather than IL-1 specifically.

Walsh and coworkers have described a substance termed ILS from human gingival organ cultures (126,161). When gingival tissue was cultured in serum-free media for 6 h, they detected only two proteins in the supernatants by sodium dodecyl sulfate-polyacrylamide gel electrophoresis (SDS-PAGE). These were separated by ion-exchange chromatography and gel filtration. The 70 kD molecule had IL-1-like activity. The 97.4 kD molecule, ILS, inhibited the proliferation of mouse thymocytes in response to crude mouse IL-1 and PHA and also in response to crude mouse IL-2. Inhibition in each case could be reduced by addition of excess cytokine. ILS treatment also reduced both basal and IL-1-induced expression of CD-1 antigen by gingival Langerhans' cells. Thus, ILS does not appear to be specific for IL-1. Its mechanism of action is unknown.

A retroviral transmembrane envelope protein, p15E, inhibits a variety of immune functions of lymphocytes, monocytes, and macrophages. A portion of this protein is conserved among murine and feline retroviruses, and homologous regions have been found in envelope proteins of human T cell leukemia virus types I (HTLV-I) and II (110,162). Studies of the effects of p15E on immune function have been hindered by its low solubility. The major hydrophilic region of p15E, prepared using recombinant DNA techniques, was shown by Schmidt et al. to inhibit the anti-CD3-driven proliferation of human T cells and the proliferation of CTLL-2 in response to IL-2 (163). The synthetic peptide CKS-17, corresponding to the first 17 amino acids of the highly conserved region of p15E, was synthesized and coupled to bovine serum albumin (BSA) by Cianciolo and coworkers (162). This peptide-carrier conjugate significantly suppressed the proliferation of the mouse cytotoxic T cell line CTLL-2 in response to recombinant IL-2. It also inhibited the proliferation of mouse splenocytes and of human PBMC in two-way mixed lymphocyte reactions. In other studies, the CKS-17–BSA conjugate suppressed polyclonal activation of feline B cells (164) and the lysis of tumor cells by activated human monocytes (110). In the tumor lysis assay, CKS-17–BSA exhibited its effect in the killing phase, not during the activation phase, and appeared to inhibit the action rather than the synthesis of IL-1. Furthermore, the proliferation of mouse thymocytes and of the astrocytoma line U373 in response to IL-1 alone, and the proliferation of the mouse helper T cell line D10.G4.1 in response to IL-1 plus ConA, were all significantly depressed (110). No inhibitory activity of CKS-17–BSA against the cytotoxic activity of TNF-α was found. Thus, this retroviral peptide, when coupled to a protein carrier, appears to inhibit the effects of IL-1 and IL-2 and perhaps other cytokines but exhibits some specificity since TNF-α activity was not affected. Recently it was shown that CKS-17–BSA did not bind IL-1 itself or affect IL-1 receptor number, affinity, or internalization in EL4-6.1 cells (165). It did decrease IL-2 production by a mechanism that appeared to involve the inhibition of protein kinase C activity.

An inhibitor of leukocyte chemotaxis antigenically related to p15E is produced by human endothelial cells stimulated with IL-1 (166). In addition, mitogen-transformed human lymphocytes express a protein that reacts with antibody to p15E (167). These studies suggest that the existence of a class of naturally occurring cytokine inhibitors related to retroviral membrane proteins, perhaps encoded by endogenous retroviral sequences in the human genome.

α-Melanocyte-stimulating hormone (α-MSH) is one of several neuropeptides with imunomodulatory as well as endocrine activity. Cannon et al. showed that synthetic α-MSH (13 amino acids) inhibited the ability of human recombinant IL-1β to augment the proliferation of PHA-stimulated mouse thymocytes and prostaglandin synthesis by a human fibroblast cell line (168). IL-2-induced proliferation of CTLL cells was not affected. Nle^4,D-$phe^7\alpha$-MSH, an analog that is more potent than α-MSH in assays of melanotropic activity, failed to inhibit IL-1. This result suggested that the inhibition of IL-1 action on thymocytes and fibroblasts did not occur through the classic α-MSH receptor. On the other hand, Robertson and coworkers demonstrated that in vivo injection of either α-MSH or Nle^4,D-$phe^7\alpha$-MSH antagonized the ability of simultaneously administered recombinant IL-1β or TNF-α to induce fever, acute-phase reactants, and neutrophilia in mice (169). Thus, the mechanisms of α-MSH interaction with cytokines or their target cells have not yet been elucidated.

Cleavage of IL-1 by membrane-bound enzymes could represent a mechanism by which IL-1 effects are regulated. Endopeptidase 24.11 (enkephalinase) is a 95 kD membrane-bound metalloproteinase found in a wide variety of cell types, including neutrophils and reticular cells of lymphoid organs (170), but not in lymphocytes. This enzyme cleaves numerous neuropeptides and hormones in vitro. Recently Pierart and coworkers (170) have shown that pretreatment with endopeptidase 24.11 reduced the activity of crude or purified human IL-1β in the mouse thymocyte comitogenesis assay. Phosphoramidon, a specific endopeptidase 24.11 inhibitor, prevented the inactivation of IL-1. No effect on recombinant or crude IL-2, as measured by CTLL-2 proliferation, was found. Thus, one possible class of soluble IL-1 inhibitors may be proteases, such as endopeptidase 24.11, shed or secreted from cells.

F. Synovial Fluid-Derived Inhibitors

Most of the previously discussed IL-1 inhibitors could conceivably be involved in modulating inflammation in arthritic joints. Since monocytes, macrophages, and neutrophils are abundant in inflamed synovial tissues and fluids, inhibitors from these cellular sources may be particularly relevant. However, direct demonstration of inhibitory factors in synovial fluid may be most significant to rheumatoid arthritis, since this fluid should reflect what is being produced in synovial tissue.

IL-2 Inhibitors from Synovial Fluid

An inhibitor of IL-2 in rheumatoid synovial fluid has been described (171) and partially purified (172) by Miossec and Kashiwado and coworkers. The 150–180 kD gel filtration fraction from rheumatoid, but not traumatic, synovial fluids inhibited PHA–IL-1 comitogenesis of mouse thymocytes but failed to inhibit IL-1-stimulated fibroblast proliferation. This preparation also decreased the proliferation of the HT-2 cell line in response to recombinant IL-2. Inhibition was not due to a nonspecific cytopathic effect. Removal of IgG from the inhibitor preparation by immunoaffinity chromatography did not alter its activity. This preparation also decreased the production of IL-2 by PHA-activated human PBMC. Thus, the synovial fluid IL-2 inhibitor appeared to decrease both the production of and the response to IL-2. Antibody against macrophage-derived suppressor factor (MDSF), an IL-2 inhibitor with similar properties produced by the THP-1 cell line, neutralized the activity of the synovial fluid IL-2 inhibitor (172). In a later report, normal human macrophages and endothelial cells stimulated with LPS in vitro produced a 150–180 kD IL-2 inhibitor that was also neutralized by anti-MDSF (173). Therefore, all three inhibitors appear to be identical or closely related.

Symons and coworkers have detected significantly higher levels of soluble IL-2 receptor (sIL-2R) in synovial fluids and sera from rheumatoid arthritis patients than in control sera (174). Receptor was detected by an ELISA using monoclonal antibodies to the α chain of the IL-2 receptor. The level of sIL-2R correlated with the level of IL-1β, measured by radioimmunoassay (RIA), in synovial fluids. Levels also correlated with the ability of synovial fluids to inhibit the IL-2-induced proliferation of CTLL-2 cells. The proposed mechanism of this inhibition was competition by sIL-2. Synovial fluid mononuclear cells spontaneously released high levels of sIL-2R into serum-free culture fluids. On gel filtration, the sIL-2R produced in vitro migrated at approximately 40 kD, which corresponds to the molecular weight of the released α chain. However, both sIL-2R and functional IL-2 inhibitor from synovial fluid comigrated at approximately 100 kD. The hypothesis that sIL-2R was forming aggregates or binding to another protein in synovial fluid was tested by incubating synovial fluid mononuclear cell (SFMC) culture supernatant and synovial fluid together before gel filtration. There was a decrease in the amount of sIL-2R migrating at 40 kD, which could be accounted for by an increase in sIL-2R migrating in the 50–200 kD range. These results suggest that soluble IL-2 receptor in synovial fluid may bind IL-2 and modulate its activity in vivo.

Another IL-2 inhibitory activity was identified in synovial fluids by Emery and coworkers (175). These investigators observed inhibition of proliferation of

CTLL-2 cells in response to IL-2 by synovial fluids from patients with seropositive rheumatoid arthritis and with other arthritides (osteoarthritis, seronegative RA, psoriatic arthritis, and traumatic arthritis). The activity was lower in the fluids from seropositive RA patients than in fluids from the second group. In individual RA patients, active disease seemed to be associated with lower IL-2 inhibitory activity. The inhibitor was found in the fractions of approximately 65–70 kD on gel filtration, with no inhibitory activity in higher molecular weight fractions that would correspond to the IL-2 inhibitor of Miossec et al. The relationship of both these IL-2 inhibitors to the soluble IL-2 receptors demonstrated by Symons et al. is unclear.

Transforming Growth Factor β

In an early report, Zembala and Lemmel (176) described inhibition of PHA mitogenesis of normal human PBMCs by synovial fluids from rheumatoid arthritis patients and by SFMC supernatants. This activity has an apparent molecular weight of 50–100 kD by ultrafiltration. The suppression of mitogenesis by exogenous inhibitor depended on the presence of adherent cells in the normal PBMC population. Later, Lotz and coworkers (177) described decreased proliferative responses of rheumatoid SFMC compared to autologous PBMC, which in turn showed lower responses than PBMC from normal controls. They identified an activity in culture supernatants of rheumatoid SFMC and PBMC that decreased the response of mouse thymocytes to purified human IL-1 and PHA and of normal PBMC to anti-CD3 antibody and IL-1. Inhibition could be overcome by excess IL-1. No effect was seen on the proliferation of thymocytes in response to PHA alone or on the proliferation of the CTLL-2 cell line in response to human recombinant IL-2. Production of this inhibitory activity depended upon the presence of adherent cells in the rheumatoid mononuclear cell cultures. In a second report (178) these investigators found that supernatants from adherent rheumatoid PBMC inhibited the synthesis of IL-2 and interferon-γ by normal PBMC in response to in vitro Epstein-Barr virus infection.

Since the IL-1 inhibitory activity from rheumatoid synovial cell cultures appeared to be produced by adherent cells, these workers then turned to U937 cells as a source of IL-1 inhibitor. They confirmed an earlier observation that supernatants from U937 cells contained a factor that inhibited the IL-1 comitogenesis assay of mouse thymocytes. This inhibitory activity had been previously separated from IL-1 by gel filtration by Amento and coworkers (179) and had an apparent molecular weight of greater than 23 kD. Using anion- and cation-exchange chromatography, Lotz and Carson (180) partially purified an inhibitory factor from U937 culture supernatants that was neutralized by antibodies against TGF-β (molecular weight 12.5 kD). They also demonstrated the production of biosynthetically labeled TGF-β by U937 cells. The relationship of TGF-β to the apparently higher molecular weight U937-derived inhibitors of Amento et al. and of Fujiwara and Ellner (see Sec. V.E) has not been clarified.

Lotz and Carton have suggested that the IL-1 inhibitor in rheumatoid synovial fluids and culture supernatants is TGF-β. In support of this proposal, they note that the IL-1 inhibitory activity of synovial fluids is partially neutralized by anti-TGFβ (180). Indeed, TGF-β is produced by synovial fibroblasts from rheumatoid arthritis patients (181) and has been found in both latent and active forms in inflammatory synovial fluids by other investigators (182). Both TGF-β_1 and β_2 are potent suppressors of IL-1-induced T cell proliferation, as measured in mouse thymocyte (183) and human tonsillar T lymphocyte assays (184). The effect of TGF-β on IL-1 mediated events is not straightforward, however, since it is also a potent stimulator of IL-1 production by monocytes and possesses many other proinflammatory properties (185). TGF-β is likely to play an important role in the cytokine network modulating inflammatory responses in the rheumatoid joint, inducing inhibition of some IL-1-induced responses. It is clear, however, that TGF-β is not the only IL-1 inhibitor in rheumatoid tissues.

The Synovial Fluid IL-1α Inhibitor

An inhibitor of IL-1 from synovial fluids of rheumatoid arthritis patients has been partially purified in the authors' laboratory by differential ammonium sulfate precipitation, gel filtration, and anion-exchange chromatography (186–188). This trypsin-sensitive, acid-labile factor has an approximate molecular weight of 100 kD. It inhibits the proliferation of mouse thymocytes and of the D10.G4.1 cell line in response to PHA plus human recombinant IL-1α but has minimal effects on IL-1β. It also suppresses the less vigorous proliferative response to IL-1α alone but has no effect on proliferation in response to PHA alone. In a two-stage assay, there is little suppression of proliferation if cells are incubated with inhibitor and PHA for the first 24 h, washed, and then exposed to IL-1α. On the other hand, significant inhibition occurs if cells are incubated with PHA alone for the first 24 h, washed, and then treated with IL-1α plus inhibitor. These results, as well as its minimal effect on IL-1β, indicate that the inhibitor is not interacting with the costimulus PHA. Furthermore, the synovial fluid inhibitor suppresses the synthesis of IL-4 by EL4-6.1 cells in response to the calcium ionophore A23187 plus IL-1α, but not IL-1β. The inhibitor preparation does not degrade [^{125}I]IL-1α or β, and its activity in the D10.G4.1 costimulation assay is not reduced by phosphoramidon, suggesting that it is not a protease. It also has no DNAse activity when assayed for its ability to nick supercoiled plasmid DNA.

Specificity for IL-1 has been shown by the absence of inhibition of proliferation of mouse thymocytes, D10.G4.1, and CTLL-2 cells in response to human recombinant IL-2. The inhibitor also fails to suppress the response of human peripheral blood mononuclear PHA-induced blasts to human recombinant IL-4. It is unlikely to be working through IL-6, since contrary to the report of Mizutani et al. (189), we are unable to demonstrate any effect of human recombinant IL-6, alone or in combination with PHA and/or IL-1α or β, on the proliferation of D10.G4.1 cells. Its major mechanism of action does not appear to be through stimulation of prostaglandin synthesis, since addition of indomethacin has no effect on its ability to inhibit D10.G4.1 proliferation and little effect on its ability to inhibit thymocyte proliferation. This inhibitor is not TGF-β, since neither human recombinant TGF-β_1 nor β_2 had any effect on D10.G4.1 proliferation but both suppressed thymocyte proliferation in response to IL-1α and β equally.

Further purification and characterization of the synovial fluid IL-1 inhibitor, including binding studies, are in progress. Its selectivity for IL-1α suggests that it may be specifically binding IL-1α or the IL-1α–receptor complex. On the other hand, this inhibitor may counteract a postreceptor signal transduction event unique to IL-1α in the responding cells studied.

VI. IMPLICATIONS FOR FUTURE THERAPEUTIC STRATEGIES

Theoretically, IL-1 is a very attractive target for pharmacologic intervention, since this cytokine produces so many proinflammatory responses directly and indirectly through its induction of other mediators. Nonsteroidal anti-inflammatory drugs and glucocorticoids are examples of currently used therapies for rheumatoid arthritis that derive at least part of their efficacy from their ability to antagonize the effects of IL-1. The nonsteroidals are cyclo-oxygenase antagonists that inhibit prostaglandin synthesis induced by IL-1 and other cytokines. Glucocorticoids inhibit the synthesis of both IL-1 (190) and IL-2 (70,191). Thus, there is good precedent for the therapeutic approach of developing IL-1 inhibitors for the treatment of inflammation. The therapeutic use of an endogenous protein inhibitor of IL-1 would require that it be purified and cDNA clones be isolated and that sufficient quantities of protein be produced by recombinant techniques. It is clear from the previous discussion of IL-1 inhibitors that in some cases the requirement for large amounts of pure material has been, or is close to being, fulfilled. Since there appear to be at least several different natural inhibitors of IL-1, some may exist that are, by virtue of their mechanism of action, relatively selective for certain target cells or tissues. Therefore, it is important to proceed with characterization and purification of different IL-1 inhibitors. The administration of such substances or synthetic analogs, by either a parenteral or an intra-articular route, may become a useful adjunct to treatment of rheumatoid arthritis and other inflammatory arthritides.

Addendum: Complementary DNAs for the 25 kD monocyte-derived IL-1 inhibitor have been cloned and expressed in two separate laboratories (Hannum, C.H. et al., 1990, Nature 343:336; Eisenberg, S.P.. et al., 1990, Nature 343:341; Carter, D.B. et al., 1990, Nature 344:633). This inhibitor is an IL-1 receptor antagonist which competes with IL-1 for receptor binding and does not induce postreceptor signal events.

REFERENCES

1. Hopkins, S.J., Humphreys, M., and Jayson, M.I. (1988). Cytokines in synovial fluid. I. The presence of biologically active and immunoreactive IL-1. Clin. Exp. Immunol. 72:422.

2. Ruschen, S., Lemm, G., and Warnatz, H. (1989). Spontaneous and LPS-stimulated production of intracellular IL-1 beta by synovial macrophages in rheumatoid arthritis is inhibited by IFN-gamma. Clin. Exp. Immunol. 76:246.

3. Bhardwaj, N., Lau, L.L., Rivelis, M., and Steinman, R.M. (1988). Interleukin-1 production by mononuclear cells from rheumatoid synovial effusions. Cell. Immunol. 114:405.

4. Saklatvala, J. (1987). Interleukin 1: Purification and biochemical aspects of its action on cartilage. J. Rheumatol. 14 (Spec. No.):52.

5. Campbell, I.K., Piccoli, D.S., Butler, D.M., Singleton, D.K., and Hamilton, J.A. (1988). Recombinant human interleukin-1 stimulates human articular cartilage to undergo resorption and human chondrocytes to produce both tissue- and urokinase-type plasminogen activator. Biochim. Biophys. Acta 967:183.

6. Dayer, J.M., de Rochemonteix, B., Burrus, B., Demczuk, S., and Dinarello, C.A. (1986). Human recombinant interleukin 1 stimulates collagenase and prostaglandin E2 production by human synovial cells. J. Clin. Invest. 77:645.

7. Leizer T., Clarris, B.J., Ash, P.E., van Damme, J., Saklatvala, J., and Hamilton, J.A. (1987). Interleukin-1 beta and interleukin-1 alpha stimulate the plasminogen activator activity and prostaglandin E_2 levels of human synovial cells. Arthritis Rheum. 30:562.

8. Postlethwaite, A.E., Raghow, R., Stricklin, G.P., Poppleton, H., Seyer, J.M., and Kang, A.H. (1988). Modulation of fibroblast functions by interleukin 1: Increased steady-state accumulation of type I procollagen messenger RNAs and stimulation of other functions but not chemotaxis by human recombinant interleukin 1 alpha and beta. J. Cell Biol. 106:311.

9. Thomson, B.M., Saklatvala, J., and Chambers, T.J. (1986). Osteoblasts mediate interleukin 1 stimulation of bone resorption by rat osteoclasts. J. Exp. Med. 164:104.

10. Matsubara, T., and Ziff, M. (1986). Increased superoxide anion release from human endothelial cells in response to cytokines. J. Immunol. 137:3295.

11. Nawroth, P.P., Handley, D.A., Esmon, C.T., and Stern, D.M. (1986). Interleukin 1 induces endothelial cell procoagulant while suppressing cell-surface anticoagulant activity. Proc. Natl. Acad. Sci. USA 83:3460.

12. Schleimer, R.P., and Rutledge, B.K. (1986). Cultured human vascular endothelial cells acquire adhesiveness for neutrophils after stimulation with interleukin 1, endotoxin, and tumor-promoting phorbol diesters. J. Immunol. 136:649.

13. Wheeler, M.E., Luscinskas, F.W., Bevilacqua, M.P., and Gimbrone, M.J. (1988). Cultured human endothelial cells stimulated with cytokines or endotoxin produce an inhibitor of leukocyte adhesion. J. Clin. Invest. 82:1211.

14. Cavender, D.E., Haskard, D.O., Joseph, B., and Ziff, M. (1986). Interleukin 1 increases the binding of human B and T lymphocytes to endothelial cell monolayers. J. Immunol. 136:203.

15. Goldblum, S.E., Yoneda, K., Cohen, D.A., and McClain, C.J. (1988). Provocation of pulmonary vascular endothelial injury in rabbits by human recombinant interleukin-1 beta. Infect. Immun. 56:2255.

16. Moser, R., Schleiffenbaum, B., Groscurth, P., and Fehr, J. (1989). Interleukin 1 and tumor necrosis factor stimulate human vascular endothelial cells to promote transendothelial neutrophil passage. J. Clin. Invest. 83:444.

17. Dinarello, C., and Savage, N. (1989). Interleukin-1 and its receptor. In: Critical Reviews in Immunology. Atassi, M.Z., ed. CRC Press, Boca Ration, FL, p. 1.

18. Postlethwaite, A.E., Lachman, L.B., and Kang, A.H. (1984). Induction of fibroblast proliferation by interleukin-1 derived from human monocytic leukemia cells. Arthritis Rheum. 27:995.

19. Butler, D.M., Piccoli, D.S., Hart, P.H., and Hamilton, J.A. (1988). Stimulation of human synovial fibroblast DNA synthesis by recombinant human cytokines. J. Rheumatol. 15:1463.

20. Butler, D.M., Vitti, G.F., Leizer, T., and Hamilton, J.A. (1988). Stimulation of the hyaluronic acid levels of human synovial fibroblasts by recombinant human tumor necrosis factor alpha, tumor necrosis factor beta (lymphotoxin), interleukin-1 alpha, and interleukin-1 beta. Arthritis Rheum. 31:1281.

21. Yaron, I., Meyer, F.A., Dayer, J.M., Bleiberg, I., and Yaron M. (1989). Some recombinant human cytokines stimulate glycosaminoglycan synthesis in human synovial fibroblast cultures and inhibit it in human articular cartilage cultures. Arthritis Rheum. 32:173.

22. Goldring, M.B., Birkhead, J., Sandell, L.J., Kimura, T., and Krane, S.M. (1988). Interleukin 1 suppresses expression of cartilage-specific types II and IX collagens and increases types I and III collagens in human chondrocytes. J. Clin. Invest. 82:2026.

23. Ramadori, G. Sipe, J.D., Dinarello, C.A., Mizel, S.B., and Colten, H.R. (1985). Pretranslational modulation of acute phase hepatic protein synthesis by murine recombinant interleukin 1 (IL-1) and purified human IL-1 J Exp. Med. 162:930.

24. Maury, C.P., Andersson, L.C., Teppo, A.M., Partanen, S., and Juvonen, E. (1988). Mechanism of anaemia in rheumatoid arthritis: Demonstration of raised interleukin 1 beta concentrations in anaemic patients and of interleukin 1 mediated suppression of normal erythropoiesis and proliferation of human erythroleukaemia (HEL) cells in vitro. Ann. Rheum. Dis. 47:972.

25. Dinarello, C.A., Clark, B.D., Puren, A.J., Savage, N., and Rosoff, P.M. (1989). The interleukin 1 receptor. Immunol. Today 10:49.

26. Larrick, J. (1989). Native interleukin 1 inhibitors. Immunol. Today 10:61.

27. Mosley, B., Urdal, D.L., Prickett, K.S., Larsen, A., Cosman, D., Conlon, P.J., Gillis, S., and Dower, S.K. (1987). The interleukin-1 receptor binds the human interleukin-1 alpha precursor but not the interleukin-1 beta precursor. J. Biol. Chem. 262:2941.

28. March, C.J., Mosley, B., Larsen, A., Cerretti, D.P., Braedt, G., Price, V., Gillis, S., Henney, C.S., Kronheim, S.R., Grabstein, K., et al. (1985). Cloning, sequence and expression of two distinct human interleukin-1 complementary DNAs. Nature 315:641.

29. Lomedico, P.T., Gubler, U., Hellman, C.P., Dukovich, M., Giri, J.G., Pan, Y.C., Collier, K., Semionow, R., Chua, A.O., and Mizel, S.B. (1984). Cloning and expression of murine interleukin-1 cDNA in Escherichia coli. Nature 312:458.

30. Gray, P.W., Glaister, D., Chen, E., Goeddel, D.V., and Pennica, D. (1986). Two interleukin 1 genes in the mouse: Cloning and expression of the cDNA for murine interleukin 1 beta. J. Immunol. 137:3644.

31. Dejana, E., Breviario, F., Erroi, A., Bussolino, F., Mussoni, L., Gramse, M., Pintucci, G., Casali, B., Dinarello, C.A., Van Damme, J., and Mantovani, A. (1987).

Modulation of endothelial cell functions by different molecular species of interleukin 1. Blood 69:695.

32. Bird, T.A., Gearing, A.J., and Saklatvala, J. (1987). Murine interleukin-1 receptor: Differences in binding properties between fibroblastic and thymoma cells and evidence for a two-chain receptor model. FEBS Lett. 225:21.

33. Scapigliati, G., Ghiara, P., Bartalini, M., Tagliabue, A., and Boraschi, D. (1989). Differential binding of IL-1 alpha and IL-1 beta to receptors on B and T cells. FEBS Lett. 243:394.

34. Acres, R.B., Larsen, A., and Conlon, P.J. (1987). Il 1 expression in a clone of human T cells. J. Immunol. 138:2132.

35. Bonnefoy, J.-Y., Denoroy, M.-C., Guillot, O., Martens, C.L., and Banchereau, J. (1989). Activation of normal human B cells through their antigen receptor induces membrane expression of IL-1 alpha and secretion of IL-1 beta. J. Immunol. 143: 864.

36. Matsushima, K., Taguchi, M., Kovacs, E.J., Young, H.A., and Oppenheim, J.J. (1986). Intracellular localization of human monocyte associated interleukin 1 (IL 1) activity and release of biologically active IL 1 from monocytes by trypsin and plasmin. J. Immunol. 136:2883.

37. Hazuda, D., Webb, R.L., Simon, P., and Young, P. (1988). Purification and characterization of human recombinant precursor interleukin 1 beta. J. Biol. Chem. 264:1689.

38. Miossec, P., Cavender, D., and Ziff, M. (1986). Production of interleukin 1 by human endothelial cells. J. Immunol. 136:2486.

39. Zlotnik, A., Daine, B., and Smith, C.A. (1985). Activation of an interleukin-1-responsive T-cell lymphoma by fixed P388D1 macrophages and an antibody against the Ag:MHC T-cell receptor. Cell. Immunol. 94:447.

40. Kurt-Jones, E.A., Beller, D.I., Mizel, S.B., and Unanue, E.R. (1985). Identification of a membrane-associated interleukin 1 in macrophages, Proc. Natl. Acad. Sci. USA 82:1204.

41. Kurt-Jones, E.A., Fiers, W., and Pober, J.S. (1987). Membrane interleukin 1 induction on human endothelial cells and dermal fibroblasts. J. Immunol. 139: 2317.

42. Bakouche, O., Brown, D.C., and Lachman, L.B. (1987). Subcellular localization of human monocyte interleukin 1: Evidence for an inactive precursor molecule and a possible mechanism for IL-1 release. J. Immunol. 138:4249.

43. Beuscher, H.U., Fallon, R.J., and Colten, H.R. (1987). Macrophage membrane interleukin 1 regulates the expression of acute phase proteins in human hepatoma Hep 3B cells. J. Immunol. 139:1896.

44. Conlon, P.J., Grabstein, K.H., Alpert, A., Prickett, K.S., Hopp, T.P., and Gillis, S. (1987). Localization of human mononuclear cell interleukin 1. J. Immunol. 139:98.

45. Minnich, C.L., Suttles, J., and Mizel, S.B. (1989). Evidence against the existence of a membrane form of murine IL-1 alpha. J. Immunol. 142:526.

46. Chin, J., Rupp, E., Cameron, P.M., MacNaul, K.L., Lotke, P.A., Tocci, M.J., Schmidt, J.A., and Bayne, E.K. (1988). Identification of a high-affinity receptor for interleukin 1 alpha and interleukin 1 beta on cultured human rheumatoid synovial cells. J. Clin. Invest. 82:420.

47. Bird, T.A., and Saklatvala, J. (1986). Identification of a common class of high affinity receptors for both types of porcine interleukin-1 on connective tissue cells. Nature 324:263.

48. Dower, S.K., Kronheim, S.R., March, C.J., Conlon, P.J., Hopp, T.P., Gillis, S., and Urdal, D.L. (1985). Detection and characterization of high affinity plasma membrane receptors for human interleukin 1. J. Exp. Med. 162:501.

49. Kilian, P.L., Kaffka, K.L., Stern, A.S., Woehle, D., Benjamin, W.R., Dechiara, T.M., Gubler, U., Farrar, J.J., Mizel, S.B., and Lomedico, P.T. (1986). Interleukin 1 alpha and interleukin 1 beta bind to the same receptor on T cells. J. Immunol. 136:4509.

50. Bensimon, C., Wakasugi, N., Tagaya, Y., Takakura, K., Yodoi, J., Tursz, T., and Wakasugi, H. (1989). Two distinct affinity binding series for IL-1 on human cell lines. J. Immunol. 143:1168.

51. Parker, K.P., Benjamin, W.R., Kaffka, K.L., and Kilian, P.L. (1989). Presence of IL-1 receptors on human and murine neutrophils. Relevance to IL-1-mediated effects in inflammation. J. Immunol. 142:537.

52. Matsushima, K., Akahoshi, T., Yamada, M., Furutani, Y., and Oppenheim, J.J. (1986). Properties of a specific interleukin 1 (IL 1) receptor on human Epstein-Barr virus-transformed B lymphocytes: Identity of the receptor for IL 1 alpha and IL 1-beta. J. Immunol. 136:4496.

53. Bron, C., and MacDonald, H.R. (1987). Identification of the plasma membrane receptor for interleukin-1 on mouse thymoma cells. FEBS Lett. 219:365.

54. Bird, T.A., Gearing, A.J., and Saklatvala, J. (1988). Murine interleukin 1 receptor. Direct identification by ligand blotting and purification to homogeneity of an interleukin 1-binding glycoprotein. J. Biol. Chem. 263:12063.

55. Sims, J.E., March, C.J., Cosman, D., Widmer, M.B., MacDonald, H.R., McMahan, C.J., Grubin, C.E., Wignall, J.M., Jackson, J.L., Call, S.M., Friend, D., Alpert, A.R., Gillis, S., Urdal, D.L., and Dower, S.K. (1988). cDNA expression cloning of the IL-1 receptor, a member of the immunoglobulin superfamily. Science 241:585.

56. Lowenthal, J.W., and MacDonald, H.R. (1986). Binding and internalization of interleukin 1 by T cells. Direct evidence for high- and low-affinity classes of interleukin 1 receptor. J. Exp. Med. 164:1060.

57. Kroggel, R., Martin, M., Pingoud, V., Dayer, J.M., and Resch, K. (1988). Two-chain structure of the interleukin 1 receptor. FEBS Lett. 229:59.

58. Rosoff, P.M., Savage, N., and Dinarello, C.A. (1988). Interleukin-1 stimulates diacylglycerol production in T lymphocytes by a novel mechanism. Cell 54:73.

59. Zhang, Y., Lin, J.X., and Vilcek, J. (1988). Synthesis of interleukin 6 (interferon-beta 2/B cell stimulatory factor 2) in human fibroblasts is triggered by an increase in intracellular cyclic AMP. J. Biol. Chem. 263:6177.

60. Zhang, Y.H., Lin, J.X., Yip, Y.K., and Vilcek, J. (1988). Enhancement of cAMP levels and of protein kinase activity by tumor necrosis factor and interleukin 1 in human fibroblasts: Role in the induction of interleukin 6. Proc. Natl. Acad. Sci. USA 85:6802.

61. Akahoshi, T., Oppenheim, J.J., and Matsushima, K. (1988). Interleukin 1 stimulates its own receptor expression on human fibroblasts through the endogenous production of prostaglandin(s). J. Clin. Invest. 82:1219.

62. Shirakawa, F., Yamashita, U., Chedid, M., and Mizel, S.B. (1988). Cyclic AMP—an intracellular second messenger for interleukin 1. Proc. Natl. Acad. Sci. USA 85: 8201.

63. Chedid, M., Shirakawa, F., Naylor, P., and Mizel, S.B. (1989). Signal transduction pathway for IL-1. Involvement of a pertussis toxin-sensitive GTP-binding protein in the activation of adenylate cyclase. J. Immunol. 142:4301.

64. Rincon, M., Tugores, A., Lopez-Rivas, A., Silva, A., Alonson, M., De Landazuri, M.O., and Lopez-Botet, M. (1988). Prostaglandin E_2 and the increase of intracellular cAMP inhibit the expression of interleukin 2 receptors in human T cells. Eur. J. Immunol. 18:1791.

65. Burch, R.M., Connor, J.R., and Axelrod, J. (1988). Interleukin 1 amplifies receptor-mediated activation of phospholipase A_2 in 3T3 fibroblasts. Proc. Natl. Acad. Sci. USA 85:6306.

66. Zucali, J.R., Dinarello, C.A., Oblon, D.J., Gross, M.A., Anderson, L., and Weiner, R.S. (1986). Interleukin 1 stimulates fibroblasts to produce granulocyte-macrophage colony-stimulating activity and prostaglandin E_2. J. Clin. Invest. 77:1857.

67. Raz, A., Wyche, A., Siegel, N., and Needleman, P. (1988). Regulation of fibroblast cyclooxygenase synthesis by interleukin-1. J. Biol. Chem. 263:3022.

68. Kunkel, S.L., Chensue, S.W., and Phan, S.H. (1986). Prostaglandins as endogenous mediators of interleukin 1 production. J. Immunol. 136:186.

69. Otterness, I.G., Bliven, M.L., Eskra, J.D., Reinke, M., and Hanson, D.C. (1988). The pharmacologic regulation of interleukin-1 production: The role of prostaglandins. Cell. Immunol. 114:385.

70. Tracey, D.E., Hardee, M.M., Richard, K.A., and Paslay, J.W. (1988). Pharmacological inhibition of interleukin-1 activity on T cells by hydrocortisone, cyclosporine, prostaglandins, and cyclic nucleotides. Immunopharmacology 15: 47.

71. Kaye, J., Porcelli, S., Tite, J., Jones, B., and Janeway, C.A., Jr. (1983). Both a monoclonal antibody and antisera specific for determinants unique to individual cloned helper T cell lines can substitute for antigen and antigen-presenting cells in the activation of T cells. J. Exp. Med. 158:836.

72. Meuer, S.C., and Meyer zum Buschenfelde, K.H. (1986). T cell receptor triggering induces responsiveness to interleukin 1 and interleukin 2 but does not lead to T cell proliferation. J. Immunol. 136:4106.

73. Berridge, M.J. (1984). Inositol trisphosphate and diacylglycerol as second messengers. Biochem. J. 220:345.

74. Farrar, W.L., and Ruscetti, F.W. (1986). Association of protein kinase C activation with IL 2 receptor expression. J. Immunol. 136:1266.

75. Abraham, R.T., Ho, S.N., Barna, T.J., and McKean, D.J. (1987). Transmembrane signaling during interleukin 1-dependent T cell activation. Interactions of signal 1- and 2-type mediators with the phosphoinositide-dependent signal transduction mechanism. J. Biol. Chem. 262:2719.

76. Kester, M., Simonson, M.S., Mene, P., and Sedor, J.R. (1989). Interleukin-1 generates transmembrane signals from phospholipids through novel pathways in cultured rat mesangial cells. J. Clin. Invest. 83:718.

77. Matsushima, K., Kobayashi, Y., Copeland, T.D., Akahoshi, T., and Oppenheim, J.J. (1987). Phosphorylation of a cytosolic 65-kDa protein induced by interleukin 1 in glucocorticoid pretreated normal human peripheral blood mononuclear leukocytes. J. Immunol. 139:3367.

78. Kaur, P., and Saklatvala, J. (1988). Interleukin 1 and tumor necrosis factor increase phosphorylation of fibroblast proteins. FEBS Lett. 241:6.

79. Lovett, D.H., Martin, M., Bursten, S., Szamel, M., Gemsa, D., and Resch, K. (1988). Interleukin 1 and the glomerular mesangium. III. Il-1-dependent stimulation of mesangial cell protein kinase activity. Kidney Int. 34:26.

80. James R., and Bradshaw, R.A. (1984). Polypeptide growth factors. Annu. Rev. Biochem. 53:259.

81. Matsushima, K., Yodoi, J., Tagaya, Y., and Oppenheim, J.J. (1986). Downregulation of interleukin 1 (IL 1) receptor expression by IL 1 and fate of internalized ^{125}I-labeled IL 1 beta in a human large granular lymphocyte cell line. J. Immunol. 137:3183.

82. Bird, T.A., and Saklatvala, J. (1987). Studies on the fate of receptor-bound ^{125}I-interleukin 1 beta in porcine synovial fibroblasts. J. Immunol. 139:92.

83. Mizel, S.B., Kilian, P.L., Lewis, J.C., Paganelli, K.A., and Chizzonite, R.A. (1987). The interleukin 1 receptor. Dynamics of interleukin 1 binding and internalization in T cells and fibroblasts. J. Immunol. 138:2906.

84. Martin, M., Lovett, D.H., Szamel, M., and Resch, K. (1989). Characterization of the interleukin-1-induced tyrosine phosphorylation of a 41-kDa plasma membrane protein of the human tumor cell line K 562. Eur. J. Biochem. 180:343.

85. Gery, I., and Waksman, B.H. (1972). Potentiation of the T-lymphocyte response to mitogens. II. The cellular source of potentiating mediator(s). J. Exp. Med. 136:143.

86. Smith, K.A., Lachman, L.B., Oppenheim, J.J., and Favata, M.F. (1980). The functional relationship of the interleukins. J. Exp. Med. 151:1551.

87. Serke, S., Serke, M., and Brudler, O. (1987). Lymphocyte activation by phytohaemagglutinin and pokeweed mitogen. Identification of proliferating cells by monoclonal antibodies. J. Immunol. Methods 99:167.

88. Williams, J.M., Deloria, D., Hansen, J.A., Dinarello, C.A., Loertscher, R., Shapiro, H.M., and Strom, T.B. (1985). The events of primary T cell activation can be staged by use of Sepharose-bound anti-T3 (64.1) monoclonal antibody and purified interleukin 1. J. Immunol. 135:2249.

89. Paetkau, V., Mills, G., Gerhart, S., and Monticone, V. (1976). Proliferation of murine thymic lymphocytes in vitro is mediated by the concanavalin A-induced release of a lymphokine (costimulator). J. Immunol. 117:1320.

90. Conlon, P.J., Henney, C.S., and Gillis, S. (1982). Cytokine-dependent thymocyte responses: Characterization of IL-1 and IL-2 target subpopulations and mechanism of action. J. Immunol. 128:797.

91. Lowenthal, J.W., Cerottini, J.C., and MacDonald, H.R. (1986). Interleukin 1-dependent induction of both interleukin 2 secretion and interleukin 2 receptor expression by thymoma cells. J. Immunol. 137:1226.

92. Kurt-Jones, E.A., Hamberg, S. Ohara, J., Paul, W.E., and Abbas, A.K. (1987). Heterogeneity of helper/inducer T lymphocytes. I. Lymphokine production and lymphokine responsiveness. J. Exp. Med. 166:1774.

93. Lichtman, A.H., Chin, J., Schmidt, J.A., and Abbas, A.K. (1988). Role of interleukin 1 in the activation of T lymphocytes. Proc. Natl. Acad. Sci. USA 85:9699.
94. Lewis, D.B., Prickett, K.S., Larsen, A., Grabstein, K., Weaver, M., and Wilson, C.B. (1988). Restricted production of interleukin 4 by activated human T cells. Proc. Natl. Acad. Sci. USA 85:9743.
95. Spits, H., Yssel, H., Takebe, Y., Arai, N., Yokota, T., Lee, F., Arai, K., Banchereau, J., and de Vries, J.E. (1987). Recombinant interleukin 4 promotes the growth of human T cells. J. Immunol. 139:1142.
96. Mitchell, L.C., Davis, L.S., and Lipsky, P.E. (1989). Promotion of human T lymphocyte proliferation by IL-4. J. Immunol. 142:1548.
97. Helle, M., Boeije, L., and Aarden, L.A. (1989). IL-6 is an intermediate in IL-1-induced thymocyte proliferation. J. Immunol. 142:4335.
98. Le, J.M., Fredrickson, G., Reis, L.F., Diamantstein, T., Hirano, T., Kishimoto, T., and Vilcek, J. (1988). Interleukin 2-dependent and interleukin 2-independent pathways of regulation of thymocyte function by interleukin 6. Proc. Natl. Acad. Sci. USA 85:8643.
99. Rock, K.L., and Benacerraf, B. (1984). The role of Ia molecules in the activation of T lymphocytes. IV. The basis of the thymocyte IL 1 response and its possible role in the generation of the T cell repertoire. J. Immunol. 132:1654.
100. Hurme, M. (1988). Both interleukin 1 and tumor necrosis factor enhance thymocyte proliferation. Eur. J. Immunol. 18:1303.
101. Inaba, K., Witmer, P.M., Inaba, M., Muramatsu, S., and Steinman, R.M. (1988). The function of Ia$^+$ dendritic cells and Ia- dendritic cell precursors in thymocyte mitogenesis to lectin and lectin plus interleukin 1. J. Exp. Med. 167:149.
102. Shirakawa, F., Tanaka, Y., Ota, T., Suzuki, H., Eto, S., and Yamashita, U. (1987). Expression of interleukin 1 receptors on human peripheral T cells. J. Immunol. 138:4243.
103. Kaye, J., Gillis, S., Mizel, S.B., Shevach, E.M., Malek, T.R., Dinarello, C.A., Lachman, L.B., and Janeway, C.J. (1984). Growth of a cloned helper T cell line induced by a monoclonal antibody specific for the antigen receptor: Interleukin 1 is required for the expression of receptors for interleukin 2. J. Immunol. 133:1339.
104. Kupper, T., Horowitz, M., Lee, F., Robb, R., and Flood, P.M. (1987). Autocrine growth of T cells independent of interleukin 2: Identification of interleukin 4 (IL 4, BSF-1) as an autocrine growth factor for a cloned antigen-specific helper T cell. J. Immunol. 138:4280.
105. Liao, Z., Grimshaw, R.S., and Rosenstreich, D.L. (1984). Identification of a specific interleukin 1 inhibitor in the urine of febrile patients. J. Exp. Med. 159:126.
106. Berman, M.A., Sandborg, C.I., Calabia, B.S., Andrews, B.S., and Friou, G.J. (1986). Studies of an interleukin 1 inhibitor: Characterization and clinical significance. Clin. Exp. Immunol. 64:136.
107. Nishihara, T., Koga, T., and Hamada, S. (1988). Production of an interleukin-1 inhibitor by cell line P388D1 murine macrophages stimulated with *Haemophilus actinomycetemcomitans* lipopolysaccharide. Infect. Immuno. 56:2801.
108. Falk, W., Krammer, P.H., and Mannel, D.N. (1987). A new assay for interleukin-1 in the presence of interleukin-2. J. Immunol. Methods 99:47.

109. Lachman, L.B., Brown, D.C., and Dinarello, C.A. (1987). Growth-promoting effect of recombinant interleukin 1 and tumor necrosis factor for a human astrocytoma cell line. J. Immunol. 138:2913.

110. Kleinerman, E.S., Lachman, L.B., Knowles, R.D., Snyderman, R., and Cianciolo, G.J. (1987). A synthetic peptide homologous to the envelope proteins of retroviruses inhibits monocyte-mediated killing by inactivating interleukin 1. J. Immunol. 139:2329.

111. Lacey, D.L., Chappel, J.C., and Teitelbaum, S.L. (1987). Interleukin 1 stimulates proliferation of a nontransformed T lymphocyte line in the absence of a co-mitogen. J. Immunol. 139:2649.

112. Helle, M., Boeije, L., and Aarden, L.A. (1988). Functional discrimination between interleukin 6 and interleukin 1. Eur. J. Immunol. 18:1535.

113. Schwarz, T., Urbanska, A., Gschnait, F., and Luger, T.A. (1987). UV-irradiated epidermal cells produce a specific inhibitor of interleukin 1 activity. J. Immunol. 138:1457.

114. Arend, W.P., Joslin, F.G., Thompson, R.C., and Hannum, C.H. (1989). An IL-1 inhibitor from human monocytes. Production and characterization of biologic properties. J. Immunol. 143:1851.

115. Seckinger, P., Williamson, K., Balavoine, J.F., Mach, B., Mazzei, G., Shaw, A., and Dayer, J.M. (1987). A urine inhibitor of interleukin 1 activity affects both interleukin 1 alpha and 1 beta but not tumor necrosis factor alpha. J. Immunol. 139:1541.

116. Prieur, A.M., Kaufmann, M.T., Griscelli, C., and Dayer, J.M. (1987). Specific interleukin-1 inhibitor in serum and urine of children with systemic juvenile chronic arthritis. Lancet 2:1240.

117. Sandborg, C.I., Berman, M.A., Andrews, B.S., Mirick, G.R., and Friou, G.J. (1986). Increased production of an interleukin 1 (IL-1) inhibitor with fibroblast stimulating activity by mononuclear cells from patients with scleroderma. Clin. Exp. Immunol. 66:312.

118. Korn, J.H., Brown, K.M., Downie, E., Liao, Z.H., and Rosenstreich, D.L. (1987). Augmentation of IL 1-induced fibroblast PGE_2 production by a urine-derived IL 1 inhibitor. J. Immunol. 138:3290.

119. Ho, S.N., Abraham, R.T., Gillis, S., and McKean, D.J. (1987). Differential bioassay of interleukin 2 and interleukin 4. J. Immunol. Methods 98:99.

120. Simon, P.L., Laydon, J.T., and Lee, J.C. (1985). A modified assay for interleukin-1 (IL-1). J. Immunol. Methods 84:85.

121. Ohara, J., Coligan, J.E., Zoon, K., Maloy, W.L., and Paul, W.E. (1987). High-efficiency purification and chemical characterization of B cell stimulatory factor-1/interleukin 4. J. Immunol. 139:1127.

122. Gearing, A.J., Bird, C.R., Bristow, A., Poole, S., and Thorpe, R. (1987). A simple sensitive bioassay for interleukin-1 which is unresponsive to 10^3 U/ml of interleukin-2. J. Immunol. Methods 99:7.

123. Seckinger, P., Lowenthal, J.W., Williamson, K., Dayer, J.M., and MacDonald, H.R. (1987). A urine inhibitor of interleukin 1 activity that blocks ligand binding. J. Immunol. 139:1546.

124. Svenson, M., and Bendtzen, K. (1988). Inhibitor of interleukin 1 in normal human urine. Different effects on mouse thymocytes and on a murine T-cell line. Scand. J. Immunol. 27:593.

125. Fujiwara, H., and Ellner, J.J. (1986). Spontaneous production of a suppressor factor by the human macrophage-like cell line U937. I. Suppression of interleukin 1, interleukin 2, and mitogen-induced blastogenesis in mouse thymocytes. J. Immunol. 136:181.

126. Walsh, L.J., Lander, P.E., Seymour, G.J., and Powell, R.N. (1987). Isolation and purification of ILS, an interleukin 1 inhibitor produced by human gingival epithelial cells. Clin. Exp. Immunol. 68:366.

127. Rodgers, B.C., Scott, D.M., Mundin, J., and Sissons, J.G. (1985). Monocyte-derived inhibitors of interleukin 1 induced by human cytomegalovirus. J. Virol. 55:527.

128. Muchmore, A.V., and Decker, J.M. (1986). Uromodulin. An immunosuppressive 85-kilodalton glycoprotein isolated from human pregnancy urine is a high affinity ligand for recombinant interleukin 1 alpha. J. Biol. Chem. 261:13404.

129. Moonen, P., Gaffner, R., and Wingfield, P. (1988). Native cytokines do not bind to uromodulin (Tamm-Horsfall glycoprotein). FEBS Lett. 226:314.

130. Svenson, M., Poulsen, L.K., Fomsgaard, A., and Bendtzen, K. (1989). IgG autoantibodies against interleukin 1 alpha in sera of normal individuals. Scand. J. Immunol. 29:489.

131. Muchmore, A.V., and Decker, J.M. (1985). Uromodulin: A unique 85-kilodalton immunosuppressive glycoprotein isolated from urine of pregnant women. Science 229:479.

132. Brown, K.M., Muchmore, A.V., and Rosenstreich, D.L. (1986). Uromodulin, an immunosuppressive protein derived from pregnancy urine, is an inhibitor of interleukin 1. Proc. Natl. Acad. Sci. USA 83:9119.

133. Hession, C., Decker, J.M., Sherblom, A.P., Kumar, S., Yue, C.C., Mattaliano, R.J, Tizard, R., Kawashima, E., Schmeissner, U., Heletsky, S., Chow, E.P., Burne, C.A., Shaw, A., and Muchmore, A.V. (1987). Uromodulin (Tamm-Horsfall glycoprotein): A renal ligand for lymphokines. Science 237:1479.

134. Sherblom, A.P., Decker, J.M., and Muchmore, A.V. (1988). The lectinlike interaction between recombinant tumor necrosis factor and uromodulin. J. Biol. Chem. 263:5418.

135. Muchmore, A.V., and Decker, J.M. (1987). Evidence that recombinant IL 1 alpha exhibits lectin-like specificity and binds to homogeneous uromodulin via N-linked oligosaccharides. J. Immunol. 138:2541.

136. Muchmore, A.V., Shifrin, S., and Decker, J.M. (1987). In vitro evidence that carbohydrate moieties derived from uromodulin, an 85,000 dalton immunosuppressive glycoprotein isolated from human pregnancy urine, are immunosuppressive in the absence of intact protein. J. Immunol. 138:2547.

137. Pennica, D., Kohr, W.J., Kuang, W.J., Glaister, D., Aggarwal, B.B., Chen, E.Y., and Goeddel, D.V. (1987). Identification of human uromodulin as the Tamm-Horsfall urinary glycoprotein. Science 236:83.

138. Serafini-Cessi, F., Franceschi, C., and Sperti, S. (1979). Specific interaction of

human Tamm-Horsfall glycoprotein with leucoaggluninin, a lectin from *Phaseolus vulgaris* (red kidney bean). Biochem. J. 183:381.

139. Brody, D.T., and Durum, S.K. (1989). Membrane IL-1: IL-1 alpha precursor binds to the plasma membrane via a lectin-like interaction. J. Immunol. 143:1183.

140. Liao, Z., Haimovitz, A., Chen, Y., Chan, J., and Rosenstreich, D.L. (1985). Characterization of a human interleukin 1 inhibitor. J. Immunol. 134:3882.

141. Brown, K.M., and Rosenstreich, D.L. (1987). Mechanism of action of a human interleukin 1 inhibitor. Cell. Immunol. 105:45.

142. Rosenstreich, D.L., Tu, J.H., Kinkade, P.R., Mauerer, F.I., Kahn, J., Barton, R.W., and Farina, P.R. (1988). A human urine-derived interleukin 1 inhibitor. Homology with deoxyribonuclease I. J. Exp. Med. 168:1767.

143. Balavoine, J.F., de Rochemonteix, B., Williamson, K., Seckinger, P., Cruchaud, A., and Dayer, J.M. (1986). Prostaglandin E$_2$ and collagenase production by fibroblasts and synovial cells is regulated by urine-derived human interleukin 1 and inhibitor(s). J. Clin. Invest. 78:1120.

144. Arend, W.P., Joslin, F.G., and Massoni, R.J. (1985). Effects of immune complexes on production by human monocytes of interleukin 1 or an interleukin 1 inhibitor. J. Immunol. 134:3868.

145. Berman, M.A., Sandborg, C.I., Calabia, B.S., Andrews, B.S., and Friou, G.J. (1987). Interleukin 1 inhibitor masks high interleukin 1 production in acquired immunodeficiency syndrome (AIDS). Clin. Immunol. Immunopathol. 42:133.

146. Dohlman, J.G., Payan, D.G., and Goetzl, E.J. (1984). Generation of a unique fibroblast-activating factor by human monocytes. Immunology 52:577.

147. Dohlman, J.G., Cooke, M.P., Payan, D.G., and Goetzl, E.J. (1985). Structural diversity of the fibroblast-activating factors generated by human blood monocytes and U937 cells. J. Immunol. 134:3185.

148. Locksley, R.M., Crowe, S., Sadick, M.D., Heinzel, F.P., Gardner, K.J., McGrath, M.S., and Mills, J. (1988). Release of interleukin 1 inhibitory activity (contra-IL-1) by human monocyte-derived macrophages infected with human immunodeficiency virus in vitro and in vivo. J. Clin. Invest. 82:2097.

149. Roberts, N.J., Prill, A.H., and Mann, T.N. (1986). Interleukin 1 and interleukin 1 inhibitor production by human macrophages exposed to influenza virus or respiratory syncytial virus. Respiratory syncytial virus is a potent inducer of inhibitor activity. J. Exp. Med. 163:511.

150. Gosset, P., Lassalle, P., Tonnel, A.B., Dessaint, J.P., Wallaert, B., Prin, L., Pestel, J., and Capron, A. (1988). Production of an interleukin-1 inhibitory factor by human alveolar macrophages from normals and allergic asthmatic patients. Am. Rev. Respir. Dis. 138:40.

151. Shirahama, M, Ishibashi, H., Tsuchiya, Y., Kurokawa, S., Hayashida, K., Okumura, Y., and Niho, Y. (1988). Kupffer cells may autoregulate interleukin 1 production by producing interleukin 1 inhibitor and prostaglandin E$_2$. Scand. J. Immunol. 28:719.

152. Scala, G., Kuang, Y.D., Hall, R.E., Muchmore, A.V., and Oppenheim, J.J. (1984). Accessory cell function of human B cells. I. Production of both interleukin 1-like activity and an interleukin 1 inhibitory factor by an EBV-transformed human B cell line. J. Exp. Med. 159:1637.

153. Barak, V., Treves, A.J., Yanai, P., Halperin, M., Wasserman, D., Biran, S., and Braun, S. (1986). Interleukin 1 inhibitory activity secreted by a human myelomonocytic cell line (M20). Eur. J. Immunol. 16:1449.
154. Tiku, K., Tiku, M.L., Liu, S., and Skosey, J.L. (1986). Normal human neutrophils are a source of a specific interleukin 1 inhibitor. J. Immunol. 136:3686.
155. Schwarz, T., Urbanski, A., Kirnbauer, R., Kock, A., Gschnait, F., and Luger, T.A. (1988). Detection of a specific inhibitor of interleukin 1 in sera of UVB-treated mice. J. Invest. Dermatol. 91:536.
156. Kemp, A., Mellow, L., and Sabbadini, E. (1985). Suppression and enhancement of in vitro lymphocyte reactivity by factors in rat submandibular gland extracts. Immunology 56:261.
157. Kemp, A., Mellow, L., and Sabbadini, E. (1986). Inhibition of interleukin 1 activity by a factor in submandibular glands of rats. J. Immunol. 137:2245.
158. Wilkins, J.A., Sigurdson, S.L., Rutherford, W.J., Jordan, Y., and Warrington, R.J. (1983). The production of immunoregulatory factors by a human macrophage-like cell line. I. Characterization of an inhibitor of lymphocyte DNA synthesis. Cell. Immunol. 75:328.
159. Fujiwara, H., Toossi, Z., Ohnishi, K., Edmonds, K., and Ellner, J.J. (1987). Spontaneous production of a suppressor factor by a human macrophage-like cell line U937. II. Suppression of antigen- and mitogen-induced blastogenesis, IL 2 production and IL2 receptor expression in T lymphocytes. J. Immunol. 138:197.
160. Wahl, S.M., Hunt, D.A., Wong, H.L., Dougherty, S., McCartney-Frances, N., Wahl, L.M., Ellingsworth, L., Schmidt, J.A., Hall, G., Roberts, A.B., and Sporn, M.B. (1988). Transforming growth factor-beta is a potent immunosuppressive agent that inhibits IL-1-dependent lymphocyte proliferation. J. Immunol. 140:3026.
161. Walsh, L.J., Seymour, G.J., and Powell, R.N. (1986). Modulation of gingival Langerhans cell T6 antigen expression in vitro by interleukin 1 and an interleukin 1 inhibitor. Clin. Exp. Immunol. 64:334.
162. Cianciolo, G.J., Copeland, T.D., Oroszlan, S., and Snyderman, R. (1985). Inhibition of lymphocyte proliferation by a synthetic peptide homologous to retroviral envelope proteins. Science 230:453.
163. Schmidt, D.M., Sidhu, N.K., Cianciolo, G.J., and Snyderman, R. (1987). Recombinant hydrophilic region of murine retroviral protein p15E inhibits stimulated T-lymphocyte proliferation. Proc. Natl. Acad. Sci. USA 84:7290.
164. Mitani, M., Cianciolo, G.J., Snyderman, R., Yasuda, M., Good, R.A., and Day, N.K. (1987). Suppressive effect on polyclonal B-cell activation of a synthetic peptide homologous to a transmembrane component of oncogenic retroviruses. Proc. Natl. Acad. Sci. USA 84:237.
165. Gottlieb, R.A., Lennarz, W.J., Knowles, R.D., Cianciolo, G.J., Dinarello, C.A., Lachman, L.B., and Kleinerman, E.S. (1989). Synthetic peptide corresponding to a conserved domain of the retroviral protein p15E blocks IL-1-mediated signal transduction. J. Immunol. 142:4321.
166. Wang, J.M., Chen, Z.G., Cianciolo, G.J., Snyderman, R., Breviario, F., Dejana, E., and Mantovani, A. (1989). Production of a retroviral P15E-related chemotaxis inhibitor by IL-1-treated endothelial cells. A possible negative feedback in the regulation of the vascular response to monokines. J. Immunol. 142:2012.

167. Cianciolo, G.J., Phipps, D., and Snyderman, R. (1984). Human malignant and mitogen-transformed cells contain retroviral P15E-relted antigen. J. Exp. Med. 159:964.

168. Cannon, J.G., Tatro, J.B., Reichlin, S., and Dinarello, C.A. (1987). Alpha melanocyte stimulating hormone inibits immunostimulatory and inflammatory actions of interleukin 1. J. Immunol. 137:2232.

169. Robertson, B., Dostal, K., and Daynes, R.A. (1988). Neuropeptide regulation of inflammatory and immunologic response. The capacity of alpha-melanocyte-stimulating hormone to inhibit tumor necrosis factor and IL-1-inducible biologic responses. J. Immunol. 140:4300.

170. Pierart, M.E., Najdovski, T., Appelboom, T.E., and Deschodt, L.M. (1988). Effect of human endopeptidase 24.11 ("enkephalinase") on IL-1-induced thymocyte proliferation activity. J. Immunol. 140:3808.

171. Miossec, P., Kashiwado, T., and Zif, M. (1987). Inhibitor of interleukin-2 in rheumatoid synovial fluid. Arthritis Rheum. 30:121.

172. Kashiwado, T., Miossec, P., Oppenheimer, M.N., and Ziff, M. (1987). Inhibitor of interleukin-2 synthesis and response in rheumatoid synovial fluid. Arthritis Rheum. 30:1339.

173. Kashiwado, T., Oppenheimer-Marks, N., and Ziff, M. (1988). T cell inhibitor secretd by macrophages and endothelial cells. Arthritis Rheum. 31:s60.

174. Symons, J.A., Wood, N.C., Di Giovine, F.S., and Duff, G.W. (1988). Soluble IL-2 receptor in rheumatoid arthritis. Correlation with disease activity, IL-1 and IL-2 inhibition. J. Immunol. 141:2612.

175. Emery, P., Gentry, K.C., Kelso, A., and Mackay, I.R. (1988). Interleukin 2 inhibitor in synovial fluid. Clin. Exp. Immunol. 72:60.

176. Zembala, M., and Lemmel, E.-M. (1980). Inhibitory factor(s) of lymphoproliferation produced by synovial fluid mononuclear cells from rheumatoid arthritis patients: The role of monocytes in suppression. J. Immunol. 125:1087.

177. Lotz, M., Tsoukas, C.D., Robinson, C.A., Dinarello, C.A., Carson, D.A., and Vaughan, J.H. (1986). Basis for defective responses of rheumatoid arthritis synovial fluid lymphocytes to anti-CD3 (T3) antibodies. J. Clin. Invest. 78:713.

178. Lotz, M., Tsoukas, C.D., Fong, S., Dinarello, C.A., Carson, D.A., and Vaughan, J.H. (1986). Release of lymphokines after infection with Epstein-Barr virus in vitro. II. A. monocyte-dependent inhibitor of interleukin 1 downregulates the production of interleukin 2 and interferon-gamma in rheumatoid arthritis. J. Immunol. 136:3643.

179. Amento, E.P., Kurnick, J.T., and Krane, S.M. (1982). Interleukin-1 production by a monocyte cell line is induced by a T lymphocyte product. Immunobiology 163:276.

180. Lotz, M., and Carson, D.A. (1989). Transforming growth factor beta (TGFbeta) and cellular immune responses in synovial fluids. Arthritis Rheum. 32:s42.

181. Lafyatis, R., Thompson, N.L., Remmers, E.F., Flanders, K.C., Roche, N.S., Kim, S.-J., Case, J.P., Sporn, M.B., Roberts, A.B., and Wilder, R.L. (1989). Transforming growth factor-beta production by synovial tissues from rheumatoid patients and streptococcal cell wall arthritic rats. Studies on secretion by synovial fibroblast-like cells and immunohistologic localization. J. Immunol. 143:1142.

182. Fava, R., Olsen, N., Keski, O.J., Moses, H., and Pincus, T. (1989). Active and latent forms of transforming growth factor beta activity in synovial effusions. J. Exp. Med. 169:291.

183. Ellingsworth, L.R., Nakayama, D., Segarini, P., Dasch, J., Carrillo, P., and Waegell, W. (1988). Transforming growth factor-betas are equipotent growth inhibitors of interleukin-1-induced thymocyte proliferation. Cell. Immunol. 114:41.

184. Kehrl, J.H., Wakefield, L.M., Roberts, A.B., Jakowlew, S., Alvarez, M.M., Derynck, R., Sporn, M.B., and Fauci, A.S. (1986). Production of transforming growth factor beta by human T lymphocytes and its potential role in the regulation of T cell growth. J. Exp. Med. 163:1037.

185. Wahl, S.M., McCartney-Francis, N., and Mergenhagen, S.E. (1989). Inflammatory and immunomodulatory roles of TGF-beta. Immunol. Today 10:258.

186. Aelion, J.A., Endres, R.O., and Postlethwaite, A.E. (1985). Characterization of an interleukin-1 inhibitor derived from human synovial fluid. Arthritis Rheum. 28:s79.

187. Higgins, G.C., and Postlethwaite, A.E. (1989). Partial purification of an inhibitor of interleukin-1 from synovial fluid of patients with rheumatoid arthritis. Arthritis Rheum. 32:s57.

188. Higgins, G.C., Aelion, J.A., Endres, R.O., and Postlethwaite, A.E. (1990). Manuscript in preparation.,

189. Mizutani, H., May, L.T., Pravinkumar, B.S., and Kupper, T.S. (1989). Synergistic interactions of IL-1 and IL-6 in T cell activation. Mitogen but not antigen receptor-induced proliferation of a cloned T helper cell line is enhanced by exogenous IL-6. J. Immunol. 143:896.

190. Lew, W., Oppenheim, J.J., and Matsushima, K. (1988). Analysis of the suppression of IL-1 alpha and IL-1 beta production in human peripheral blood mononuclear adherent cells by a glucocorticoid hormone. J. Immunol. 140:1895.

191. Culpepper, J., and Lee, F. (1987). Glucocorticoid regulation of lymphokine production by murine T lymphocytes. In: Lymphokines. Webb, D.R, and Goeddel, D., eds. Academic Press, New York, p. 275.

8

Interleukins and Metalloproteinases in Arthritis

Gene DiPasquale
CIBA-GEIGY, Summit, New Jersey

I. INTRODUCTION

Rheumatoid arthritis and osteoarthritis are diseases of unknown etiology that are clinically characterized by pain, stiffness, limitation of motion, and deformity of articulating joints (1-3). Etiopathologic evaluations of arthritis have implicated multiple processes regulating cartilage degradation, including genetic predisposition, aging, and immunologic, endocrine, biochemical, and biomechanical mechanisms (3,4).

One of the main biochemical changes occurring in cartilage appears to be related to structural alterations of proteoglycans and collagen and the total content of these macromolecules in cartilage. The structural integrity of these macromolecules is necessary to maintain the unique biomechanical characteristics of diarthrodial joints.

The rheumatoid joint is usually associated with a marked synovitis and growth of a pannus (synovial membrane) over the articular cartilage (1,5). The cartilage degradation in rheumatoid arthritis appears to take place both at the synoviocartilage junction and on the free surface of cartilage (6,7).

Early alterations in osteoarthritic cartilage include a reduction of proteoglycans, increased water content, hypercellularity (chondrocyte cloning), and an increased synthesis of matrix (reparative response) (8-10). As the disease progresses, cartilage ulcers, fibrillations, fissuring, osteophyte formation, and subchondral bone sclerosis are observed. The degradation of osteoarthritic cartilage is initially focal but may in advanced stages involve diffuse areas of the cartilage surface.

Chondrocytes, synoviocytes (fibroblasts and dendritic cells), and inflammatory cells (macrophages, neutrophils, and lymphocytes) have been reported to release cartilage matrix-degrading proteinases (11–17). In addition, cartilage matrix-degrading proteinases, which are significantly elevated in rheumatoid and osteoarthritic cartilage, appear to correlate with the severity of the arthritis (18–21).

It has been reported that synovial fluid obtained from joints with arthritis contain cartilage debris (22,23). These degradation products (chemical inflammogens) have been reported to induce synovitis and pain when injected intraarticularly in experimental animals (24–27). These products may contribute to the chronicity of the inflammation and the severity of the cartilage degradation by recruiting additional cells into the synovial fluid that are also capable of releasing proteinases and inflammatory mediators. In addition, cartilage matrix-degrading metalloproteinase inhibitors (e.g., EDTA and EGTA) appear to inhibit the severity of experimentally induced arthritis in rabbits and dogs (28,29). These and other observations, which are listed in Table 1, suggest a "matrix-degrading enzyme" mechanism in the developing arthritis. Neutral metalloproteinases and other degradative proteinases appear to play a central role in the cartilage destruction and inflammation associated with arthritis (1,29–31]. However, basal production and secretions of neutral proteinases by chondrocytes is important in the physiologic turnover of cartilage matrix. Possibly, chondrocytes are "turned on" by at present unknown etiologic factor(s) that increase the synthesis, release, and activation of degradative proteinases.

II. INTERLEUKIN AND TUMOR NECROSIS FACTOR

During the past several years an increasing number of investigators and research organizations have identified (purified and synthesized by genetic technology) biologically active proteins that are released from activated monocyte-macrophages and lymphocytes. These multifunctional cytokines, commonly referred to as monokines or lymphokines, have been associated with biologic activities ranging from disease modifying (e.g., antiarthritic) to mediators of pathophysiologic states (e.g., arthritis) (32–39). Table 2 lists the various research organization(s) and the specific cytokines and cell-stimulating proteins that have been targeted for development. The potential of these proteins (or their inhibitors) as disease modifiers, diagnostic agents, or research tools is emphasized by the increasing number of publications during recent years. At the recent national meeting of the American College of Rheumatology approximately 55 abstracts were presented.

Table 1 Evidence Suggesting a Central Role for Neutral Metalloproteinases in the Development of Osteoarthritis and Rheumatoid Arthritis

1. Neutral metalloproteinases extracted from animal and human articular cartilage can degrade cartilage matrix.
2. Neutral metalloproteinases have been isolated from animal and human cartilage, animal and human chondrocyte culture, and animal and human synovial cells.
3. Mediators from monocytes (IL-1) induce chondrocyte and synovial cells to snythesize collagen- and proteoglycan-degrading enzymes.
4. Elevations in proteoglycan- and collagen-degrading proteinases have been reported in rheumatoid arthritic and osteoarthritic cartilage.
5. Neutral metalloproteoglycan- and collagen-degrading enzyme(s) activity correlates with the pathologic evaluation of arthritic cartilage.
6. Potent endogenous inhibitors of neutral metalloproteinases have been demonstrated in intact cartilage and synovial fluid.
7. Epitopes of proteoglycan have been found in synovial fluid obtained from patients with arthritis.
8. Proteoglycans from arthritic cartilage are smaller and more easily extractable than those from normal cartilage.
9. Interleukin-1 has been identified in synovial fluid obtained from patients with arthritis.
10. Animal or human articular cartilage cultured in the presence of IL-1 or TNF release proteoglycan fragments into the culture medium.
11. Proteoglycan fragments and cartilage particles may provoke much of the pathophysiology occurring in arthritic joints (identified in synovial fluid of arthritic patients).
12. Proteoglycanases have been immunolocalized in cartilage obtained from collagen-induced arthritis rat.
13. EDTA and EGTA improved a surgically induced osteoarthritis in animals.
14. IL-1 induced a dose-dependent increase in inflammatory leukocytes and cartilage degradations when injected intra-articularly in mice and rabbits.
15. Di- and tripeptides with thiol, carboxylic, and hydroxamic acid functions inhibit chondrocyte-derived proteoglycan- and collagen-degrading enzymes and stimulate cartilage autolysis.

Several of these cell-stimulating proteins have been reported to stimulate chondrocytes and synoviocytes to release cartilage matrix-degrading metalloenzymes and induce cartilage and bone resorption and fibroblast proliferation (40–44]. Interleukin-1 (IL-1) and several other cytokines have been identified in synovial fluid obtained from arthritic patients (45–48). Plasma levels of IL-1β in rheumatoid arthritic patients correlated positively with the Ritchie joint index, pain score, and erythrocyte sedimentation rate (49). Endogenous inhibitors of IL-1 have also

Table 2 Research Organizations Active in Cytokine Research[a]

Organization(s)	Product(s)
Amgen, Johnson & Johnson	IL-2
Biogen, Schering-Plough	Interferon (Introma), interferon-γ, IL-2, IFN, IL-4
Biogen, BASF	IL-2, TNF
Biogen, Glaxo	Uromodulin, bioleukin, GM-CSF, IL-I, IL-4, IL-5, IL-6, IL-1 inhibitors
Cetus, Biotherapeutics	IL-2
Chemex, Yale	Topical drugs controlling IL-1, IL-2, growth factors
Chugai	IL-6 receptor
Cistrom, DuPont	IL-1
Genentech	Uromodulin, IL-1 inhibitors-antagonists, angiogenesis factor, epidermal growth factor, nerve growth factor, insulin growth factor
Imclone	Natural inhibitors of IL-1
Immunex, Kodak, Syntex, Roche, Hoechst	Synthetic inhibitors of IL-1, IL-α and β, IL-2, IL-3, IL-4, IL-7, IL-1β receptor GM-CSF
Immunotherapeutics	IL-2
Janssen	T cell growth factor, IL-2, interferon-α and β, hibridoma growth factor
Knoll	TNF, IL-1
Nippon Shinyakii	Synthetic RNA with promotes production of interferon, TNF, IL-1, IL-2
Roche	IL-I agonists-antagonists, IL-2 receptor, teceleukin (IL-2), IL-2 agonists-antagonists, RO-31-3948 (IL-1 inhibitor)
Sanofi	SR-41319 (IL-1 function inhibitor)
Shawa Denko	Protein A absorption gel (removes IL-2 inhibitors from blood)
SmithKline	IL-I antagonists
Toso	IL-6
Xenova	IL-1 inhibitors-antagonists

[a]IL, interleukin; GM-CSF, granulocyte-macrophage colony stimulating factor; TNF, tumor necrosis factor; IFN, interferon.

been detected in urine, serum, and cell culture supernatants and appear to function as physiologic modulators of IL-1 (50–52).

Synergy and more profound biologic activities are observed with combination treatments (IL-1 and IL-6; acute-phase proteins; IL-1 and tumor necrosis factor, TNF; thymocyte proliferation) (32,53–57). In addition, several monokines induce similar biologic activities and/or induce the release of other monokines. One of the more interesting monokines associated with many of the characteristics of arthritis and inflammation is IL-1. The cloning of IL-1 genes and the purification of IL-1 reveal that there are two major classes of IL-1 protein, designated IL-1α and IL-1β. The cloning and expression of the cDNA for human IL-1α and IL-1β also reveals that these proteins are synthesized as a precursor molecule and that the mature forms of the protein are located in the carboxyl terminus of the precursor (32,58,59).

Studies have also shown that a relatively large portion of the mature IL-1 protein is required for activity and that a small region of either IL-1α or IL-1β alone is not able to bind to the IL-1 receptor (59).

Despite major differences in amino acid sequences both classes appear to have similar biologic activities. (60,61). The diverse biologic actions (immunologic and nonimmunologic) that have been attributed to IL-1, as previously mentioned, appear to be associated with many physiologic and immunologic responses to inflammation, infection, and trauma (13,21,25,32,37,40,61). It appears that IL-1 and other monokines are associated with initiation or exacerbation of chronic inflammatory diseases, such as arthritis. Table 3 describes the multiple biologic activities of IL-1 associated with chronic inflammation, tissue damage, and arthritis, whereas Table 4 lists other important biologic activities that may represent potential safety considerations (62). However, IL-6, which regulates the expression of all the endogenous antiproteinases and clotting factors, may be considered an anti-inflammatory agent (56).

Tumor necrosis factor (TNF-α and TNF-β) also acts as a mediator of many pathophysiologic states, including inflammation and arthritis. IL-1 and TNF (α and β) do not share any apparent structural homology or recognize the same cellular receptors; however, they do share many biologic activities (54,63,64). TNF is the second macrophage-derived monokine whose production during arthritic or inflammatory processes could contribute to tissue destruction and chronicity (12). TNF, like IL-1, increases caseinate activity (proteoglycanase and stromolysin) in articular chondrocytes and induces resorption of human articular cartilage. These appear to be important events leading to tissue destruction and arthritis. In addition, TNF induces neutrophil superoxide production. However, unlike IL-1, TNF is not required for lymphocyte function.

Many of these studies suggest that TNF-α, along with TNF-β, IL-1, and other polypeptide mediators, forms part of a network of coordinating cellular signals that control many inflammatory and immunologic events.

Table 3 Biologic Activities of Cytokines (IL-1) Associated with Arthritis and Inflammation

1. Stimulates secretion of collagenase, proteoglycanase, plasminogen activator, and PGE$_2$ from cultured chondrocytes and synovial cells
2. Increased proteoglycan release from cartilage explants (cartilage degradation)
3. Induces bone resorption (osteoclast activating factor)
4. High levels of IL-1 are found in synovial fluids obtained from patients with arthritis
5. IL-1 enhances lymphokine production and induction of lymphocyte growth factors (e.g., IL-2, IL-3, IL-4, IL-6, and interferon-α)
6. Intra-articular injections of IL-1 in rabbits or mice induce synovitis, leukocytosis, and cartilage degradation
7. Induces synovial neovascularizations (angiogenesis)
8. Induces proliferation of synovial fibroblasts
9. Chemoattractant for neutrophils, monocytes, and lymphocytes
10. Increases the adhesion of leukocytes to vascular endothelium
11. Increases acute-phase proteins (IL-6 necessary to obtain a full acute-phase protein response)
12. Pyrogenicity
13. Induces histamine release and granule release from basophils, eosinophils and neutrophils
14. Enhances thymocyte proliferation in response to lectins
15. Stimulates B lymphocytes and synthesis of immunoglobulins, including rheumatoid factor
16. Synovial tissue, synovial cells, dendritic cells, and peripheral blood mononuclear cell from rheumatoid arthritic patients display an increased production of IL-1
17. Induces IFN-β_2 and GM-CSF production
18. Stimulates CRF and ACTH release
19. Increase plasma corticosteroid level

III. EFFECT OF IL-1 ON CHONDROCYTES AND CARTILAGE

Experimentally, four important events appear to be central to the pathogenesis of arthritis: (1) the stimulated release and activation of catabolic metalloproteinase (proteoglycan- and collagen-degrading proteinases); (2) cartilage degradation or autolysis; (3) synovitis and inflammation induced by cartilage degradation product; (4) release of cell stimulating factors that modulate immunologic and inflammatory events and perpetuate the catabolic processes.

A. Effect of IL-1 on Chondrocytes

The source of IL-1 is no longer restricted to mononuclear phagocytes but can be expressed by an increasing number of cell types, now approximately 15 (see

Table 4 Additional Biologic Activities Attributed to IL-1

1. Muscle proteolysis (induces protein catabolism in muscles)
2. Induces slow-wave sleep
3. Induces neutrophilia
4. Decreases hepatic albumin synthesis
5. Induces diuresis and natriuresis
6. Protects animals against lethal radiation, oxygen toxicity, and bacterial sepsis
7. Inhibits lipoprotein lipase
8. Induces toxicity in β cells of the islets of Langerhans
9. Modulates Leydig's cell steroidogenesis (inhibited stimulated testosterone formation)
10. Stimulates hepatic synthesis of fibrinogen
11. Stimulates pituitary cells to secrete ACTH, LH, GH, and TSH
12. Protects mice against cyclophosphamide-induced granulocytopenia
13. Induces anorexia

Table 5). Likewise, the target for these monokines is no longer solely restricted to lymphocytes but also includes modifying the function of several nonimmunologic cells, including chondrocytes, fibroblasts, synoviocytes, and osteoclasts (65,66).

Mediators from monocytes induce chondrocytes to synthesis and release latent collagen- and proteoglycan-degrading proteinases (11,45). This monokine(s), which also augment the production of collagenase by cultured human synovial

Table 5 IL-1-Producing Cells

Lymphocytes
Macrophages
PMN leukocytes
Epidermal cells
Chondrocytes
Osteoclasts
Synovial dendritic cells
Fibroblasts
Keratinocytes
Glomerular mesangial cells
Langerhans' cells
Corneal epithelial cells
Astrocytes
Endothelial cells
Vascular smooth muscle cells

membrane cells (15), has similar physical properties to IL-1 and porcine synovial tissue-derived catabolin (67,68). Chondrocyte and synoviocyte proteinase production was ablated in the presence of protein synthesis inhibitors, such as cycloheximide or puromycin (40). Table 6 lists various agents that induce cellular release of IL-1.

Unstimulated rabbit articular chondrocytes in culture also produce latent matrix-degrading metalloproteinases, but detection requires the concentration of the culture medium (12).

Murine purified human IL-1 and human IL-1 stimulate normal rabbit and human chondrocytes to release latent collagen- and proteoglycan-degrading enzymes (16). The latent enzymes require aminophenylmercuric acetate (APMA) activation. Table 7 lists other effects of IL-1 on articular chondrocytes, such as increasing proteoglycan and collagen synthesis and increasing phospholiphase A activity (69).

IL-1 stimulated chondrocytes derived from bovine, rat, rabbit, and human normal and osteoarthritic cartilage release matrix-degrading metalloproteinases (16). However, chondrocytes from the various species did not appear to be equally sensitive to human IL-1. Rat and bovine chondrocytes appear to release minimal amounts of collagenase (see Table 8), whereas chondrocytes derived from swarm rat chondrosarcoma did not respond to IL-1 stimulation (70).

Human chondrocytes derived from normal-appearing or osteoarthritic cartilage release matrix-degrading metalloproteinase when stimulated with IL-1.

Table 6 Factors That Induce Cellular Release of IL-1

Collagen types II and III
Proteoglycan subunits
Cartilage and bone breakdown particles (fragments)
Microcrystals (e.g., urate)
Hyaluronic acid
Lymphokines
Tumor necrosis factor
Immune complexes (aggregated IgG)
Microorganisms (microbial products)
Lipopolysaccharide
Muramyl dipeptide
Zymosan
Bleomycin
Retinoic acid
UV irradiation (epidermal cells)
Bile salts
Neurotensin stimulates the effects of muramyl dipeptide or zymosan

Table 7 Effect of IL-1 on Articular Chondrocytes and Cartilage in Culture

Increased collagenase, proteoglycanase, and plasminogen activator activity
Decreased proteoglycan and collagen synthesis
Increased proteoglycan release from cartilage explants
Increased PGE_2 concentrations
Increased phospholipase A_2 activity
Cytostatic effect on chondrocytes

Osteoarthritic cartilage-derived chondrocytes appear to be more sensitive to IL-1 stimulation and release more proteoglycan- and collagen-degrading enzymes than normal human or rabbit articular chondrocytes (71). In addition, unlike normal rabbit, bovine, dog, rat, or human articular cartilage chondrocytes, human osteoarthritic (OA) cartilage chondrocytes produced measurable metalloproteinases without IL-1 stimulation. These results suggest that chondrocytes obtained from osteoarthritic cartilage have been "primed" to release increased quantities of matrix-degrading metalloproteinases. This suggestion appears to agree with that of Pelletier et al. (72,73), who reported increased proteoglycanase and collagenase activity in cartilage obtained from arthritic dogs (crusciate ligament ligation). The metalloproteinases obtained from various species and OA cartilage-derived chondrocytes were inhibited by EDTA, phenanthroline, and α_2-macroglobulin but not by PMSF, pepstatin, TLCK, or α_1-antitrypsin (see Table 9) (16,71).

An understanding of the factors that stimulate or control the synthesis and activation of catabolic enzymes is important in understanding the pathogenesis of arthritis and other inflammatory processes.

In other studies, Pasternak et al. (74) also demonstrated that human IL-1 and supernatants from P388 D murine macrophage cell line induce metalloproteinase release from chondrocytes in a concentrationlike manner. (See Table 10.) The latent proteoglycan- and collagen-degrading metalloproteinases had molecular weights of 44,000–56,000 and 34,000–44,000, whereas the activated proteinases had molecular weights of 30,000–40,000 and 22,000–36,000, respectively. Heparin-Sepharose affinity chromatography yielded two latent proteoglycan-degrading proteinase peaks, which coeluted with proteinases that degraded fibronectin, laminin, gelatin, and azocoll but not type I collagen.

The third collagenase peak also degraded proteoglycan, gelatin, fibronectin, laminin, and azocoll. More extensive purifications are required to determine whether several enzymes have coeluted in these protease peaks. All three peaks exhibited the same inhibitor profiles, suggesting that they were metalloproteinases, not serine, thiol, or carboxyproteinases.

Recently, Frisch and Ruley (75) reported the molecular cloning of cDNA

Table 8 Release of Proteoglycan- and Collagen-Degrading Enzymes From IL-1-Stimulated Chondrocytes Obtained from Several Species[a]

Chondrocyte source	Proteoglycan degradation (mg chondroitin sulfate released per h)[b]		Collagen degradation (mg collagen degraded per h)[c]	
	(−) IL-1	(+) IL-1[d]	(−) IL-2	(+) IL-1
Rabbit articular cartilage	1.8 ± 09[e] (20)[f]	420 ± 51 (20)	2.8 ± 1.0 (20)	41 ± 4.7 (14)
Bovine articular cartilage	23 ± 14 (5)	42 ± 24 (5)	1.4 ± 0.6 (4)	2.3 ± 0.6 (4)
Rat articular cartilage	<1 (1)	91 (1)	3.6 (1)	9.7 (1)
Rat chondrosarcoma	5.2 ± 3 (4)	<1 (4)	1.0 ± 09 (4)	2.3 ± 0.9 (4)
Human normal articular cartilage	<1 (2)	84 ± 3.5 (2)	1.7 ± 0.1 (2)	43.5 ± 10 (2)
Human osteoarthritis articular cartilage	24 ± 5 (2)	224 ± 12 (4)	5.8 ± 0.1 (2)	19 ± 1.5 (4)

[a]All samples were APMA activated before evaluation.
[b]Proteoglycanase assay: 1 unit of activity releases 1 mg chondroitin sulfite per h per ml at 37 °C.
[c]Collagenase assay: 1 unit of activity degrades 1 mg of collagen per h per ml at 35 °C.
[d]At 30–50 units/ml.
[e]Mean ± standard error of the mean.
[f]Number of evaluations.

encoding rabbit stromelysin, a phorbol ester-induced, secreted metalloproteinase capable of degrading cartilage matrix.

B. Effect of IL-1 on Cartilage Autolysis

The loss of cartilage extracellular matrix occurs spontaneously in vitro and can be stimulated by retinoids (76–78), lipopolysaccharide (79), IL-1 (44), TNF (64), catabolin (80), and cocultures with synovial tissue (81–83). Cocultivation of synovium or synovium-conditioned medium with articular or nasal cartilage resulted in an increased release of GAG from the explants when compared to spontaneous cartilage autolysis.

Dingle et al. (67) and Saklatvola and Dingle (84) identified the active factor in porcine synovial culture medium and named the factor catabolin. They proposed that catabolin-induced cartilage autolysis was mediated by proteinases released by chondrocytes. Neutral metalloproteinases that degrade proteoglycans and collagen have been identified in normal human and arthritic cartilage (71) and rabbit cartilage explant cultures (21).

Table 9 Inhibitor Profile of Collagen- and Proteoglycan-Degrading Proteases from IL-1-Stimulated and Nonstimulated Osteoarthritic Human and Rabbit Primary Articular Chondrocyte Cultures[a]

	% Inhibition of enzyme activity					
	Collagen degradation			Proteoglycan degradation		
Inhibitor and	Rabbit	Human		Rabbit	Human	
concentration[b]	(+) IL-1	(−) IL-1	(+) IL-1	(+) IL-1	(−) IL-1	(+) IL-1
EDTA						
(10 mM)	97	100	98	99	90	99
PMSF						
(1 mM)	0	0	0	0	0	0
Phenanthroline						
(5 mM)	92	100	91	100	99	99
Papstatin						
(0.05 mM)	0	0	0	0	0	0
TLCK						
(0.1 mM)	8	0	0	0	0	5
α_2-Macro-						
globulin						
(100 mg)	78	100	74	94	96	62
α_1-Antitrypsin						
(100 mg)	5	0	0	0	0	2

[a]Rabbit articular chondrocytes without IL-1 stimulation do not release measurable quantities of collagen- and proteoglycan-degrading enzymes in the medium (concentration necessary).
[b]EDTA, ethylenediamine tetraacetate; PMSF, phenylmethylsulfonyl fluoride; TLCK, N-α-p-tosyl-α-lysine chloromethyl ketone.

Dingle et al. (67) reported that a monocyte factor that enhanced the breakdown of articular cartilage explants had a molecular weight comparable to that of IL-1. More recently, purified human IL-1 (and recombinant human IL-1) has been shown to significantly enhanced GAG release from articular and bovine nasal cartilage explants (70,83).

Stimulation of cartilage resorption of embryonic chick limb cartilage by vitamin A was described by Dingle et al. (76). DiPasquale et al. (78) also reported that phenanthroline and cycloheximide but not pepstatin significantly inhibited retinoic acid-induced cartilage autolysis (See Table 11). The conclusions were that the autolytic stimulation was probably mediated by a neutral metalloproteinase. Chondrocyte viability and protein synthesis were required for the autolysis to occur.

Interestingly, retinoic acid has been reported to induce the cellular release of IL-1 and phenanthroline and cycloheximide also inhibit the IL-1-induced cartilage

Table 10 Human IL-1 Enhances Chondrocyte Protease Production[a]

Additions to rabbit articular chondrocyte culture	APMA activation (0.34 mM)	Units of enzyme activity ± SEM	
		Collagenase	Proteoglycanase
None	0	2.5 ± 1.8	1.2 ± 1.2
None	0	2.6 ± 0.8	2.9 ± 1.3
Human IL-1, units/ml[b]			
100	+	40 ± 1.1	727 ± 15.3
50	+	23 ± 0.6	743 ± 27.1
25	+	20 ± 0.7	731 ± 10.9
12	+	16 ± 1.0	230 ± 7.7
0	+	1 ± 0.3	8.8 ± 1.7

[a]The addition of 1 mM phenanthroline significantly inhibits the collagenase and proteoglycanase activity.
[b]Genzyme Corporation (Boston, MA).

autolysis (66). In addition, retinyl acetate has recently been reported to induce arthritis in C3H-A^{vy} mice (85).

IV. EFFECT OF PROTEOGLYCAN- AND COLLAGEN-DEGRADING NEUTRAL METALLOPROTEINASE INHIBITORS

Recently, several potent synthetic inhibitors were described for the APMA-activated form of proteoglycan- and collagen-degrading metalloproteinases obtained from IL-1-stimulated chondrocytes (16).

The design of the inhibitors was based on the premise that proteoglycanase and collagenase interactions with their substrates were similar to those of the zinc-dependent endoproteinase, thermolysin. Also considered were the analyses of the cleavage products of several small peptide substrates and the inhibitor profiles of thermolysin and proteoglycanase (86).

These synthetic peptides contained thiol, carboxyalkyl, or hydroxamic acid functional groups. Other di- and tripeptides with thiol, carboxylic, or hydroxamic acid function groups have also been shown to be reversible inhibitors of other metalloproteinases; the functional group is thought to chelate the metal at the active site of the enzyme (87–89).

The thiol, carboxyalkyl, and hydroxamic peptides were evaluated using a ^{14}C-labeled rat type I collagen (44), proteoglycan-polyacrylamide bead (42), monkey β-MSH (high-performance liquid chromatography, HPLC, was used to evaluate degradation products) (86), and radiolabeled rat proteoglycan core protein degradation assays (90). The latter two assays demonstrate the "proteinase" activity

Table 11 Effect of Phenanthroline and Cyclohexamide on the Spontaneous and Retinoic Acid-Induced Proteoglycan Release from Rabbit Articular Cartilage Explants at pH 7

Inhibitor concentration (M)	Spontaneous release[a] (% Inhibition),[b] 8 days	Retinoic acid (10^{-5} M), induced release[a] (% Inhibition)[b]	
		2 Days	8 Days
Phenanthroline			
10^{-4}	38[c]	55[c]	58[c]
10^{-5}	25[c]	25[c]	29[c]
10^{-6}	0	15	0
Cyclohexamide			
10^{-4}	53[c]	84[c]	73[c]
10^{-5}	58[c]	81[c]	73[c]

[a]Proteoglycan release.
[b]Percentage change from control.
[c]Significantly different from respective controls ($P < 0.05$). Pepstatin at concentrations ranging from (10^{-6}–10^{-4} M) had no effect on spontaneous or retionic acid-stimulated autolysis.

of proteoglycanase. Interestingly, the thiol and hydroxamic peptides inhibited both collagenase and proteoglycanase whereas the carboxyalkyl peptide inhibited solely proteoglycanase. The hydroxamic acid peptides were the most potent (IC_{50} = 10_m M). The relative potencies of the peptide inhibitors were equivalent in both the proteoglycan-polyacrylamide bead and the radiolabeled rat proteoglycan core protein degradation assays (16). (See Table 12.) As previously indicated, chondrocytes release latent enzymes that require APMA activation for at least 4 h. Reversal to latency occurs after short exposures. Exhaustive dialysis to remove the APMA was routinely done before the addition of inhibitors. Initial studies showed that the thiols were inactive when APMA was not removed.

Caputo et al. (91) also demonstrated that compound I [(R,S)-N-[2-[2-(hydroxyamino)-2-oxoethyl]-1-oxoheptyl]-L-leucyl-L-phenylalaninamide] and compound II [R,S)-N-[2-[2-(hydroxyamino)-2-oxoethyl]-1-oxoheptyl]-L-leucyl-L-alaninamide], hydroxamate inhibitors of proteoglycanase and collagenase, also inhibited the proteoglycan release from rabbit articular cartilage treated with human IL-1 or retinoic acid. IL-1 and retinoic acid (at test doses) were not cytotoxic and did not inhibit the stimulated proteoglycan synthesis.

Similarly, Mort et al. (92) reported that compound III [(R,S)-N-[2-[2-(hydroxyamino)-2-oxoethyl]-4-methyl-1-oxopentyl]-L-leucyl-L-phenyl-alaninamide], the most potent inhibitor reported by DiPasquale et al. (16), also inhibited recombinant human IL-1β-induced glycosaminoglycan-containing material release from adult human cartilage without affecting chondrocyte

Table 12 Inhibition of IL-1-Stimulated Chondrocyte-Derived Proteoglycan and Collagen Degradating Enzymes with Thiol, Carboxylic and Hydroxamic Peptides

Thiols[c]

		Proteoglycan degradation (proteoglycan/polyacrylamide bead), IC$_{50}$ (M)[a]	Collagen degradation (radiolabeled collagen), IC$_{50}$ (M)	Monkey β-MSH degradation	Proteoglycan degradation (rat-radiolabeled core protein), IC$_{50}$ (M)
Phe		$\sim 5 \times 10^{-6}$	$\sim 5 \times 10^{-6}$	+[b]	4×10^{-6}
Trp		$\sim 1 \times 10^{-6}$	1.6×10^{-6}	+	2×10^{-6}

Carboxyalkyls[d]

R$_1$	R$_1'$	R$_2'$	–X				
(R-S)Leu	Leu	Leu	Leu-COOH	5.3×10^{-6}	Inactive at 1×10^{-4}	+	4×10^{-6}
(R)Leu	Leu	Leu	Phe-NH$_2$	5.2×10^{-6}	1×10^{-4}	+	5×10^{-6}
(R)Leu	Leu	Phe	NH$_2$	1.9×10^{-6}	1×10^{-4}	+	ND

Hydroxamic acids[e]

R_1'	R_2'	R_3'		
N-Pentyl	Leu	Phe	1×10^{-7}	4.1×10^{-8}
Isobutyl	Leu	Ala	4.2×10^{-8}	6×10^{-8}
N-Pentyl	Val	Ala	3.4×10^{-8}	4.4×10^{-8}
			4.8×10^{-6}	+
			4.1×10^{-7}	+
			4.5×10^{-7}	ND

[a] Estimated concentration of inhibitor that results in 50% inhibition of enzyme (linear regression analysis). It should be noted that for some test agents, the data were out of range to derive the IC_{50} estimate.
[b] Inhibition of β-MSH degradation (HPLC Evaluation).
[c] Chemist: Dr. A. Shaw.
[d] Chemist: Dr. R. Roberts.
[e] Chemist: Dr. D. Wolanin.

metabolism or enzyme secretion. In addition, compound III also inhibited collagen degradation in situ as demonstrated by immunohistochemical procedures. These investigators concluded that activated metalloproteinases are operative in situ and that proteinase inhibitors may be useful therapeutic agents.

Cartilage removed from rabbit knees within 1 week following partial lateral meniscectomy had visible ulcers in the femora and tibiae. Cartilage from the weight-bearing areas incorporated significantly greater amounts of [^{3}H]thymidine and [^{35}S]sulfate than cartilage from nonoperated animal knees (93). These anabolic events have previously been reported to occur during the early stages of the arthritic process (9). In addition, the increased release of proteoglycanase from operated knee cartilage (in vitro and autolysis) was reduced to the nonsurgical knee cartilage by the hydroxamate inhibitor. These results suggest that proteoglycan- and collagen-degrading metalloproteinase inhibitors may directly and/or indirectly modulate the anabolic and catabolic processes occurring during the developing arthritis.

V. AGENTS THAT INHIBIT THE BIOLOGIC ACTIVITIES OF IL-1

We previously described several natural inhibitors of IL-1 (e.g., uromodulin). These agents, which have been cloned, may represent a new class of disease-modifying antiarthritic agents (see Table 2). Glucocorticoids have also been reported to inhibit IL-1 production; however, IL-1 also induces glucocorticoid biosynthesis through the stimulation of CRF and adrenocorticotropic hormone (ACTH).

Ferreira et al. reported that part of the IL-1β molecule, a Lys-Pro-Thr tripeptide, had hyperanalgesic activity, and modification of its structure to Lys-D-Pro-Thr produced a tripeptide that inhibited the bilateral hyperanalgesia effects of IL-1β. The tripeptide was not active in animal models of centrally mediated analgesia and had no effect on the synthesis or release of prostaglandins or IL-1β-induced pyrexia. The tripeptide and its congeners represent a new class of analgesic drugs that do not cause gastric lesions, which usually limits the usefulness of nonsteroidal anti-inflammatory agents. Corticosteroids effectively reduce IL-1 production by macrophages and inhibit IL-1-mediated release of proteinases by synovial cells and chondrocytes (45). Skotnicki et al. (94) reported that several 4-aminoquinolines (structurally related to chloroquine), including chloroquine and hydroxychloroquine, inhibited neutral proteinase released by IL-1-treated rabbit chondrocytes (49,90). Similar activities were observed with (((4-chlorophenyl)thio)methylene)bisphosphonic acid. Kadin et al. (95) recently reported that 3-acyl-2-oxoindole-1-carboxamides, which include a clinical candidate (CP-66,248), inhibited cyclo-oxygenase, 5-lipoxygenase, and IL-1 biosynthesis. Cyclo-oxygenase inhibitors suppress neither IL-1 production nor IL-1-induced thymocyte proliferation; however, they do inhibit IL-1-mediated responses that rely on prostaglandin synthesis, such as pyrexia.

Romazarit, a proposed DMARD, chemically related to clozic, is at present undergoing clinical evaluation. This agent inhibited a rat paw pain edema, acute-phase reactants, bone changes, and biochemical parameters in animals with experimentally induced arthritic disease (96). Romazarit also inhibited collagenase and prostaglandin E_2 (PGE_2) in talus bones obtained from collagen II-induced arthritis in rats.

Segal et al. (97) reported that methotrexate inhibits IL-1 activity without affecting IL-1 production or secretion. These activities may represent the mechanism by which methotrexate exerts its beneficial clinical effects in rheumatoid arthritis. Methotrexate caused a significant decrease in the erythrocyte sedimentations rate and the acute-phase protein levels.

Methotrexate antagonized the IL-1 induction of IL-2 secretion and the induction of IL-4 receptors on D10 cells. However, methotrexate did not show any effect on IL-1 production by murine splenic macrophages, and no information was reported on IL-1-induced proteinase release from chondrocytes, fibroblasts, or synovial cells.

VI. EFFECT OF SEVERAL AGENTS REPORTED TO BE EFFECTIVE CLINICALLY AND/OR IN EXPERIMENTAL ANIMAL MODELS OF ARTHRITIS

Several antiarthritic agents that stimulate cartilage synthesis and repair have been evaluated clinically and in experimental animal models. These agents include extracts of cartilage (Rumalon) and the synthetic heparinoids glycosaminoglycan polysulfate (Arteparon), pentosan sulfate, glucosamine sulfate, and tribenoside (98–101). EDTA and EGTA, chelating agents, inhibited cartilage degradation and the severity of an induced arthritis in animals (28). Although no common structural relationship exist between these agents they all appear to inhibit degradative proteinases.

Tissue inhibitor of metalloproteinase (TIMP), which plays a major role controlling extracellular proteoglycanase and collagenase activity, has been expressed by fibroblast tumor cells using recombinant techniques (102). TIMP may be useful in the control of arthritis and other diseases in which metalloproteinases are increased. Similarly, IL-6, the major regulator of all acute-phase proteins, induces α_2-macroglobulin, α_1-proteinase inhibitor, α_1-antichymotrypsin, and cysteine proteinase inhibitor (56). Pelletier et al. (5) have also suggested that the activity of glucocorticoids in experimentally induced arthritis in animals may be related to increased levels of α_2-macroglobulins. Other agents that may prove to be useful in arthritis include agents that stimulate chondrocytes to synthesize matrix macromolecules (e.g., fibroblast growth factor) and factors that may inhibit pannus growth and development (e.g., antiangiogenesis factors).

Several nonsteroidal anti-inflammatory agents (NSAIFA) used clinically (e.g., salicylates and indomethacin) have also been reported to suppress glycosaminoglycan synthesis in articular cartilage (62,103,104). The inhibitory effect was greater in osteoarthritic cartilage than in normal cartilage. Although NSAIFA do not appear to inhibit the degradative mechanisms, they may affect the anabolic processes operative during the arthritic process. However, NSAID do suppress synovitis, inflammation, and pain induced by cartilage degradative products and released inflammatory mediators (25–27).

VII. CHEMOTHERAPEUTIC APPROACHES TO THE TREATMENT OF ARTHRITIS

Conceptionally, the inhibition of cartilage degradation (tissue loss) and the reduction of cartilage fragments and/or matrix macromolecules in synovial fluid may reduce or inhibit synovitis, inflammation, pain, autoimmune complexes, release of inflammatory mediators (e.g., prostaglandins), and cellular stimulants (e.g., cytokines). A proposed scheme of the role of cartilage matrix-degrading enzymes in arthritis is described in Fig. 1. It appears that a degrading cartilage and the released products may be central to a developing arthritis. A network of interactions between cells, cellular factors, and matrix components appear to be involved in the destructive process that occurs in arthritis.

Inhibiting cellular stimulants like IL-1 or TNF or inhibiting their functions may also prove to be interesting approaches to control the progression of arthritis. These monokines induce many of the classic signs of inflammation and also stimulates catabolic processes in bone and cartilage, and this has focused attention on approaches to down-regulate IL-1 production or inhibit its activity (37). These agents may tilt cellular events toward catabolic mechanisms and maintain or accelerate the arthritic process. The control of these factors may indirectly decrease the release of degradative proteinases and inhibit the sequelae of events just described. Several of these monokines appear to have overlapping functions and many types of cells release similar factors, suggesting that the inhibition of cartilage matrix-degrading metalloproteinases may represent a more direct approach (see Table 13). However, a better understanding of the mechanism by which IL-1 (or TNF) stimulates the production of such proteinases may also provide a novel therapeutic approach to chronic inflammatory joint disease. Increasing or stimulating the anabolic processes would increase matrix synthesis and achieve a biochemical state in which anabolism exceeds catabolism and cartilage loss is reduced.

In the early stages of osteoarthritis, cartilage is usually hypermetabolic and further stimulation may not be required. However, the need to control the

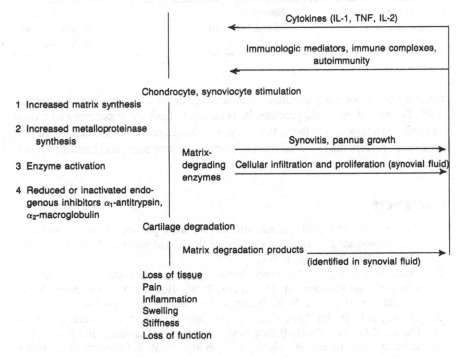

Figure 1 A proposed schema of the role of cartilage matrix-degrading enzymes in arthritis.

degradative mechanisms may still be required. Stimulation of cartilage matrix synthesis may be more useful during the later stages of a developed arthritis. Fibroblast growth factor (FGF) promotes cartilage repair in vivo. Cuevas et al. (105) administered FGF intra-articularly via an alzet osmotic pump and was able to promote the healing of intrachondral lesions.

In general it appears that the control of the catabolic mechanism or cartilage matrix degradation may be an appropriate approach to the discovery of novel therapeutic agents that may control arthritis. These agents, it is hoped, would inhibit the "spreading" cartilage degradation evident in moderate to severe

Table 13 Proteinases Associated with Cartilage Degradation

Synovial tissue (pannus)	Synovial fluid, cells (PMNs, macrophages)	Cartilage (chondrocytes)
Collagenase Neutral and acid proteinases	Elastase Neutral and acid proteinases	Collagenase Neutral and acid proteinases

arthritis and reduce the accumulation of cartilage degradation products in synovial fluid. The ideal drug would promote the synthesis of matrix components and reduce catabolic processes. Further, the drug would decrease inflammation of the synovium, restore the synovial fluid to normal, relieve pain, and inhibit progression of the arthritis.

REFERENCES

1. Zvaifler, N.J. (1984). Rheumatoid arthritis: A clinical perspective. In: Epidemiology of the Rheumatic Diseases. Reva Lawrence, R.C., and Shulman, L.E., eds. Gower Medical, New York, pp. 107–119.
2. Moskowitz, R.W. (1984). Osteoarthritis—symptoms and signs. In: Osteoarthritis Diagnosis and Management. Moskowitz, R.W., Howell, D.S., Goldberg, V.M., and Mankin, H.J., eds. W.B. Saunders, Philadelphia, pp. 149–154.
3. Howell, D.S. (1986). Etiopathogenesis of osteoarthritis. Am. J. Med. 80:24–28.
4. Harris, E.D., Jr. (1981). Pathogenesis of rheumatoid arthritis. In: Textbook of Rheumatology. Kelley, W., Harris, E.D., et al., eds. W.B. Saunders, Philadelphia, pp. 889.
5. Pelletier, J.P., and Martel-Pelletier, J. (198). Effect of steroids on neutral metalloproteinase activity in human osteoarthritic and rheumatoid arthritic cartilage. Adv. Inflamm. Res. 12:76–86.
6. Allard, S.A., Muirden, K.D., Complejohn, K.L., and Maine, R.N. (1987). Chondrocyte-derived cells and matrix at the rheumatoid cartilage-pannus junction identified with monoclonal antibodies. Rheumatol. Int. 7:153–159.
7. Kimura, H., Tateeshi, H., and Ziff, M. (1977). Surface ultrastructure of rheumatoid articular cartilage. Arthritis Rheum. 20:1085–1098.
8. Mankin, H.J., and Lippiello, L. (1970). Biochemical and metabolic abnormalities in articular human hips. J. Bone Joint Surg. 52A:424–434.
9. Mankin, N.J., Johnson, M.E., and Lippiello, L. (1981). Biochemical and metabolic abnormalities in articular cartilage osteoarthritic human hips. J. Bone Joint Surg. 63A:131–139.
10. Malemud, C.J., Goldberg, V.M., and Moskowitz, R.W. (1986). Pathological, biochemical and experimental therapeutic studies in meniscectomy models of osteoarthritis in the rabbit—its relationship to human joint pathology. Br. J. Clin. Pract. 43:21–31.

11. Deshmukh-Phadke, K., Lawrence, M., and Nander, S. (1978). Synthesis of collagenase and neutral proteases by articular chondrocytes; stimulation by a macrophage-derived factor. Biochem. Biophys. Res. Commun. 85:490–496.

12. Malemud, C.J., Weitzman, G.A., Norby, P., Sapolsky, A.I., and Howell, D.S. (1979). Metal dependent neutral proteoglycanase activity from monolayer cultured lapine articular chondrocytes. J. Lab. Clin. Med. 93:1018–1030.

13. Pujol, J.P., and Loyau, G. (1987). Interleukin-1 and osteoarthritis. Life Sci. 41:1187–1198.

14. Sandy, J.D., Sriramata, A., Brown, H.L.G., and Lowther, D.A. (1981). Evidence of polymorphonuclear leukocytes derived proteinases in arthritic cartilage. Biochem. J. 193:193–202.

15. Dayer, J.M., de Rochemonteix, B., Burrus, B., Demcjuk, S., Dinarello, C.A. (1986). Human recombinant interleukin-1 stimulates collagenase and prostaglandin E_2 production by human synovial cells. J. Clin. Invest. 77:645–648.

16. DiPasquale, G., Caccese, R., Pasternak, R., Conaty, J., Hubbs, S., and Perry, K. (1988). Proteoglycan- and collagen-degrading enzymes from human interleukin-1 stimulated chondrocytes from several species: Proteoglycanase and collagenase inhibitors as potentially new disease-modifying antiarthritic agents. Proc. Soc. Exp. Biol. Med. 183:262–267.

17. Martel-Pelletier, J., Cloutier, J.M., and Pelletier, J.P. (1986). Neutral proteases in human osteoarthritis synnovium. Arthritis Rheum. 29:1112–1121.

18. Sapolsky, A.I., Matsuta, K., Woessner, J.F., Jr., and Howell, D.S. (1979). Metal-dependent neutral proteoglycanase from normal and ulcerated human articular cartilage. Orthop. Trans. 2:119.

19. Martel-Pelletier, J., Pelletier, J.P., Cloutier, J.M., Howell, D.S., Ghandur-Mnaymneh, L., and Woessner, J.F., Jr. (1984). Neutral proteases capable of proteoglycan digesting activity in osteoarthritic and normal human articular cartilage. Arthritis Rheum. 27:305–312.

20. Martel-Pelletier, J., Clouter, J.M., Howell, D.S., and Pelletier, J.P. (1985). Human rheumatoid arthritic cartilage and its neutral proteocylycan-degrading proteases: The effect of antirheumatic drugs. Arthritis Rheum. 28:405–412.

21. Shinmei, M., Kikuchi, T., Masuda, K., and Shimonura, Y. (1988). Effect of interleukin-1 and anti-inflammatory drugs on the degradation of human articular cartilage. Drugs 35:33–41.

22. Tew, W.P., and Hockett, S.P. (1981). Identification of cartilage wear fragments in synovial fluid from equine joints. Arthritis Rheum. 24:1419–1424.

23. Witter, J.P., Roughley, P.J., Caterson, B., Poole, A.R. (1984). The isolation and characterization of proteoglycan fragments derived from articular cartilage in human arthritic synovial fluid. Orthop. Res. Soc. 9:313.

24. Chrisman, O.D., Fessel, J.M., and Southwick, W.O. (1965). Experimental production of synovitis and marginal articular exostoses in the knee joints of dogs. Yale J. Biol. Med. 37:409–412.

25. Glant, T., and Ol'ah, I. (1980). Experimental arthritis produced by proteoglycan antigens in rabbits. Scand. J. Rheumatol 9:271–279.

26. Evans, C.H., Mazzocchi, R.A., Nelson, D.D., and Rubash, H.E. (1984). Induced

experimental arthritis by intraarticular injection of allogeneic cartilage particles into rabbit knee. Arthritis Rheum. 24:200–207.

27. Bonaface, R.J., Cain, P.R., and Evans, C.H. (1988). Articular responses to purified cartilage proteoglycans. Arthritis Rheum. 31:258–266.

28. Ehrlich, M.G., Stefanich, R., Armstrong, A., and Mankin, H.J. (1983). The role of metal chelators in the management of arthritis. 29th Ann. Orth. Res. Soc. p. 78.

29. Ehrlich, M.G., Houle, P.A., Vigliani, G., and Mankin, H.J. (1978). Correlation between articular cartilage collagenase activity and osteoarthritis. Arthritis Rheum. 21:761–766.

30. Saxne, T., Heinegard, D., and Wollheim, F.A. (1978). Cartilage proteoglycans in synovial fluid and serum in patients with inflammatory joint disease: Relation to systemic treatment. Arthritis Rheum. 30:972–979.

31. DiPasquale, G. (1988). An anti-osteoarthritic drug development program. An overview. Adv. Inflamm. Res. 12:55–65.

32. Miossec, P. (1987). The role of interleukin-1 in the pathogenesis of rheumatoid arthritis. Clin. Exp. Rheumatol. 5:305–308.

33. Dinarello, C.A. (1988). Interleukin-1 Dig. Dis. Sci. 33:525–535.

34. Dinarello, C.A., Cannon, J.G., and Wolff, S.M. (1988). New concepts on the pathogenesis of fever. Rev. Infect. Dis. 10:168–189.

35. Boumpas, D.T., and Tsokos, G.C. (1985). Pathophysiologic aspects of lymphokines. Clin. Immunol. Rev. 4(2):201–240.

36. Dinarello, C.A. (1986). Biology of interleukin-1. Fed. Proc. 108–115.

37. Miller, L.C., and Dinarello, C.A. (1987). Biologic activities of interleukin-1 relevant to rheumatic diseases. Pathol. Immunopathol. Res. 6:22–36.

38. Dingle, J.T., Page Thomas, D.P., and Hazleman, B. (1987). The role of cytokines in arthritic diseases: In vitro and in vivo measurements of cartilage degradation. Int. J. Tissue React. IX(4):349–354.

39. Dinarello, C.A., Cannon, J.G., Mier, J.W., Bernheim, H.A., Lopreste, G., Lynn, D.L., Love, R.N., Webb, A.C., Auron, P.E., Reuben, R.C., Rich, A., Wolff, S.M., and Putney, S.D. (1986). Multiple biological activities of human recombinant interleukin-1. J. Clin. Invest. 77:1734–1739.

40. Hubbard, J.R., Steinberg, J.J., Bednar, M.S., and Sledge, C.B. (1988). Effect of purified human interleukin-1 on cartilage degradation. J. Orthop. Res. 6:180–187.

41. Dayer, J.M., Beutler, B., and Cerami, A. (1985). Cachectin/tumor necrosis factor stimulates collagenase and prostaglandin E_2 production by human synovial cells and dermal fibroblasts. J. Exp. Med. 162:2163–2168.

42. DiPasquale, G., Caccese, R., Pasternak, R., Perry, K., Conaty, J., and Hubbs, S. Partial characterization of collagen and proteoglycan-degrading enzymes from rabbit and human osteoarthritic chondrocytes stimulated with human IL-1. Adv. Inflamm. Res. 11:243–249.

43. Gowen, M., Wood, D., Ihrie, E.J., Meats, J.E., and Russell, R.G.G. (1984). Stimulation by human interleukin-1 of cartilage breakdown and production of collagenase and proteoglycanase by human chondrocytes but not by human osteoblasts in vitro. Biochim. Biophys. Acta 797:186–193.

44. Pasternak, R.D., Hubbs, S.J., Caccese, R.G., Marks, Rebecca L., Conaty, J.M.,

and DiPasquale, G. (1987). Interleukin-1 induces chondrocyte protease production: The development of collagenase inhibitors. Agents Actions 21:328–330.

45. Phadke, K. (1988). Role of interleukin-1 and some growth factors in the progression of arthritis. J. Sci. Ind. Res. 47:188–200.

46. Bunning, R.A.D., Richardson, H.J., Crawford, A., Skjodt, H., Hughes, D., Evans, D.B., Gowen, M., Dobson, P.R.M., Brown, B.L., and Russell, R.G.G. (1986). The effect of interleukin-1 on connective tissue metabolism and its relevance to arthritis. Agents Actions 18:131–152.

47. Bendtzen, K., Peterson, J., Halkjaer-Kristensen, J., and Ingemann-Hansen, T. (1985). Interleukin-1-like activity in synovial fluids of patients with rheumatoid arthritis and traumatic synovitis. Rheumatol. Int. 5:79–82.

48. Wood, D.D., Ihrie, E.J., Dinarello, C.A., and Cohen, R.L. (1983). Isolation of an interleukin-1-like factor from human joint effusion. Arthritis Rheum. 26: 975–983.

49. Eastgate, J.A., Wood, N.C., DiGiovine, F.S., Symons, J.A., Grinlinton, F.M., Duff, G.W. (1988). Correlations of plasma interleukin-1 levels with disease activity in rheumatoid arthritis. Lancet 2:706–709.

50. Rosenstreich, D.L., Yost, S.L., Tu, J.M., and Brown, K.M. (1987). Interleukins and interleukin inhibitors: A review. J. Biol. Med. 5:10–18.

51. Prieur, A.M., Criscelli, C., Kaufmann, M.-T., and Dayer, J.-M. (1987). Specific interleukin-1 inhibitor in serum and urine of children with systemic juvenile chronic arthritis. Lancet. 2:1240–1242.

52. Svenson, M., and Bendtzen, K. (1988). Inhibitor of interleukin-1 in normal human urine. Scand. J. Immunol. 27:593–599.

53. Ruggiero, V., and Boglioni, C. (1987). Synergistic anti-proliferative activity of interleukin-1 and tumor necrosis factor. J. Immunol. 138:661–663.

54. Mackiewicz, A., Ganapathi, M.K., Schultz, D., Samols, D., Reese, J., and Kushner, I. (1988). Relation of rabbit acute phase protein biosynthesis by monokines. Biochem. J. 253:851–857.

55. Helle, M., Brakenhoff, J.P.T., DeGroat, E.R., Aarden, L.A. (1988). Interleukin-6 is involved in interleukin-1-induced activities. Eur. J. Immunol. 18:957–959.

56. Gauldie, J. (1989). Interleukin-6 in the inflammatory response. In: Therapeutic Control of Inflammatory Control of Inflammation. In Press.

57. Dinarello, C.A. (1987). The biology of interleukin-1 and comparison to tumor necrosis factor. Immunol. Let. 16:227–233.

58. Lomedico, P.T., Hellman, G.U., Dukovich, C.P.M., Giri, J.G., Pan, Y.E., Collier, K., Semionow, R., Chua, A.O., and Mizel, S.B. (1985). Cloning and expression of murine interleukin-1 in Escherichia coli. Nature 312:458–462.

59. Gage, L.P., Benjamin, W.R., Chizzonite, R.A., DeLorenzo, W., Gubler, U., McIntyre, K.W., Stern, A.S., Unowsky, J., Lomedico, P.T., and Kilian, P.L. (1989). Interleukin-1 and the interleukin-1 receptor: Strategies for drug discovery. In: Therapeutic Control of Inflammatory Disease. In Press.

60. Wilder, R.L., Lafyates, R.T., Case, J.P., Yocum, D.E., Kumkumian, G.K., and Remmers, E.F. (1989). Cytokines in rheumatoid arthritis and streptococcal cell wall arthritis in the rat. In: Therapeutic Control of Inflammatory Disease. In Press.

61. Gray, P.W., Glaister, D., Chen, E., Goeddel, D.V., and Pennica, D. (1986). Two interleukin-1 genes in the mouse: Cloning and expression of cDNA for murine interleukin-1 beta. J. Immunol. 137:3644–3648.

62. Nojima, T., Towle, C.A., and Mankin, H.J. (1986). Secretion of higher levels of active proteoglycanases from human osteoarthritic chondrocytes. Arthritis Rheum. 29:292–295.

63. Le, J., and Vilcek, J. (1987). Tumor necrosis factor and interleukin-1: Cytokines with multiple overlapping biological activities. Lab. Invest. 56:234–245.

64. Saklatvala, J. (1986). Tumor necrosis factor α stimulates resorption and inhibits synthesis of proteoglycan in cartilage. Nature 322:547–549.

65. Maury, C.P.J. (1986). Interleukin-1 and the pathogenesis of inflammatory diseases. Acta Med. Scand. 220:291–294.

66. Emery, P., Williamson, D., James, M., Ian, R. (1987). Role of cytokines in rheumatological inflammatory. Concepts Immunopathol. 4:171–199.

67. Dingle, J.T., Page, Thomas, D.P., King, B., and Bard, D.R. (1987). In vivo studies of articular tissue damage mediated by catabolin/interleukin-1. Ann. Rheum. Dis. 46:527–533.

68. Saklatvala, J., Pilsworth, L.M., Sarsfield, S.J., Gavrilovic, J., and Heath, J.K. (1984). Pig catabolin is a form of interleukin-1. Biochem. J. 224:461–466.

69. Chang, J., Gilman, S.C., and Lewis, A.J. (1986). Interleukin-1 activates phospholipase A_2 in rabbit chondrocytes: A possible signal for IL-1 action. Am. Assoc. Immunol. 136:1283–1287.

70. DiPasquale, G., Caccese, R., Pasternak, R., Caputo, C.B., Conaty, J., and Hubbs, S. (1987). Lack of response of rat chondrosarcoma chondrocytes to IL-1 to produce proteoglycan- and collagen-degrading enzymes. Res. Commun. Chem. Pathol. Pharmacol 52:333.

71. DiPasquale, G., Caccese, R., Pasternak, R., Caputo, C.B., Conaty, J., and Hubbs, S. (1987). Partial characterization of collagen- and proteoglycan-degrading enzymes from rabbit and human osteoarthritic chondrocytes stimulated with human IL-1. (1986). Adv. Inflamm. Res. II:243–249.

72. Pelletier, J.-P., Martel-Pelletier, J., Howell, D.S., Ghandur-Mnoymneh, L., Enis, J., and Woesner, J.F., Jr. (1983). Collagenolytic activity and collagen matrix breakdown of the articular cartilage in the Pond-Nuki model of osteoarthritis. Arthritis Rheum. 26:866–874.

73. Pelletier, J.-P., and Martel-Pelletier, J. (1985). Neutral proteoglycan-degrading protease activity in the early cartilage lesions of experimental osteoarthritis. Trans. Orthop. Res. Soc. 10:128.

74. Pasternak, R., Hubbs, S.J., Caccese, R.G., Marks, R.L., Conaty, J.M., and DiPasquale, G. (1986). Interleukin-1 stimulates the secretion of proteoglycan and collagen degrading proteases by rabbit articular chondrocytes. Clin. Immunol. Immunopathol. 41:351–367.

75. Frisch, S.M., and Ruley, H.E. (1987). Transcription from the stromelysin promoter is induced by interleukin-1 and repressed by dexamethasone. J. Biol. Chem. 262:16300–16304.

76. Dingle, J.T., Lucy, J.A., and Fell, H.B. (1961). Studies on the mode of action of excess vitamin A. 1. Effect of excess of vitamin A on the metabolism and composition of embryonic chick-limb cartilage grown in organ cultures. Biochem. J. 79:497.

77. Lucy, J.A., Dingle, J.T., and Fell, H.B. (1961). Studies on the mode of action of excess vitamin A. 2. A possible role of intracellular proteases in the degradation of cartilage matrix. Biochem. J. 79:500.

78. DiPasquale, G., Perry, K.W., Dea, D, and Caccese R. (1985). Comparison of spontaneous and retinoic acid stimulated rabbit articular cartilage degradation in vitro. Int. J. Tissue React. VII:397-404.

79. Morales, T.I., and Kuettner, K.E. (1982). The properties of the neutral proteinase released by primary chondrocyte cultures and its action of proteoglycon aggregate. Biochim. Biophys. Acta 705:92-101.

80. Dingle, J.T. (1981). Catabolin—a cartilage catabolic factor from synovium. Clin. Orthop. 156:219.

81. Fell, H.B., and Jubb, R.W. (1977). The effect of synovial tissue on breakdown of articular cartilage in organ culture. Arthritis Rheum. 20:1359-1371.

82. Perry, K.W., Dea, D.M., Pasternak, R.D., and DiPasquale, G. (1983). Comparison of methods for stimulating of cartilage autolysis (abstract). Pharmacology 25(3).

83. Steinberg, J.I., Hubbard, J.R., and Sledge, C.B. (1986). In vitro models of cartilage degradation and repair. Adv. Inflamm. Res. 11:215-241.

84. Saklatvala, J., and Dingle, J.T. (1980). Identification of catabolin: A protein which induces degradation of cartilage in organ culture. Biochem. Biophys. Res. Commun. 96:1225-1231.

85. Boden, S.D., Labropoulos, P.A., Ragsdale, B.D., Gullino, P.M., and Gerber, L.H. (1989). Retinyl acetate-induced arthritis in C3H-A^{VY} mice. Arthritis Rheum. 32:625-633.

86. Shaw, A., Roberts, R.A., and Wolanin, D.J. (1988). Small substrates and inhibitors of the metalloproteoglycanase of rabbit articular chondrocytes. Adv. Inflamm. Res. 12:66-76.

87. Nishino, N., and Powers, J.C. (1979). Design of potent reversible inhibitors for thermolysin. Peptide containing zinc coordinating ligands and their use in affinity chromatography. Biochemistry 18:4340-4347.

88. Petrillo, E.W., Jr., and Ondetti, M.A. (1982). Angiotension-converting enzyme inhibitors: Medicinal chemistry and biological actions. Med. Res. Rev. 2:1-41.

89. Patchett, A.A., and Cordes, E.H. (1985). The design and properties of N-carboxyalkyldipeptide inhibitors of angiotensin-converting enzyme. Adv. Enzymol. 57:1-84.

90. Caputo, C.B., Wolanin, D.J., Roberts, R.A., Sygowski, L.A., Patton, S.P., Caccese, R.G., Shaw, A., DiPasquale, G. (1987). Proteoglycan degradation by a chondrocyte metalloprotease: Effect of synthetic protease inhibitors. Biochem. Pharmacol. 36:995-1002.

91. Caputo, C.B., Sygowski, L.A., Wolanin, D.J., Patton, S.P., Caccese, R.G., Shaw, A., Roberts, R.A., DiPasquale, G. (1987). Effect of synthetic metalloprotease inhibitors on cartilage autolysis in vitro. J. Pharmacol. Exp. Ther. 240:460-465.

92. Mort, J.S., Dodge, G.R., Roughley, J., Finch, S.J., DiPasquale, G., and Poole, A.R. (1989). Inhibition of proteoglycan and collagen degradation in interleukin-1 stimulated human articular cartilage by a metalloproteinase inhibitor. Abstract. *35th Annual Meeting, Orthop. Res. Soc.*

93. Caputo, C.B., Sygowski, L.A., Patton, S.P., Wolanin, D.J., Shaw, A., Roberts, R.A., and DiPasquale, G. (1988). Protease inhibitors decrease rabbit cartilage degradations after meniscectomy. J. Orthop. Res. 6:103–108.

94. Skotnicki, J.S., Stembaugh, B.A., Fitzgerald, J.J., Jr., Musser, J.H., Caccese, R.G., Chang, J., and Gilman, S.C. (1987). Synthesis and biological evaluation of functional inhibitors of interleukin-1. Abstract. *Fourth Intern. Conf. Inflam. Res. Assoc.*

95. Kadin, S.B., Carty, T.J., Moore, P.F., Otterness, I., Showell, J., and Weissman, A. (1989). 3-Acyl-2-oxoindole-1-carboxamides. A new class of anti-inflammatory agents inhibiting arachidonic acid metabolism and IL-1 biosynthesis. Abstract. *197th National ACS Meeting.* MEDI 67.

96. Machin, P., Barber, W.E., Bloxham, T.P., Bradshaw, P., Cashin, C.H., Dodge, P.D., Lewis, E.J., Osbond, J.M., Self, C.R., Smithen, C.E., Tong, D.T., and Westmagott, D. (1989). Ro 31-3948, A novel DMARD which acts as a functional inhibitor of IL-1. Abstract. *197th National ACS Meeting.* MEDI 66.

97. Segal, R., and Mozes, Ed., Michael, Y, and Tartakovsky, B. (1989). The effects of methotrexate on the production and activity of interleukin-1. Arthritis Rheum. 32:370–377.

98. Telhag, H. (1973). Effect of tranexamic acid on the synthesis of chondroitin sulfate and the content of hexosamine in the same fraction in normal and degenerated joint cartilage in the rabbit. Acta Orthop. Scand. 44:249–255.

99. Columbo, C., Butler, M, Hickman, L., Selwyn, M., Chart, J., and Steinetz, B. (1983). A new model of osteoarthritis in rabbits. II. Evaluation of anti-osteoarthritic effects of selected antirheumatic drugs administerd systematically. Arthritis Rheum. 26:1132–1139.

100. Howell, D.S., Manicort, D.H., Muniz, O.E., Tornero, C., and Carreno, M.R. (1984). Action of arteparon, a neutral protease inhibitor on erosions in a rabbit model of osteoarthritis. Arthritis Rheum. 24:41.

101. Altman, R.D., Dean, D.D., Muniz, O.E., Howell, D.S. (1989). Prophylactic treatment of canine osteoarthritis with glycosaminoglycan polysulfuric acid ester. Arthritis Rheum. 32:759–766.

102. Dockerty, A.J.P., Lyons, A., Smith, B.J., Wright, E.M., Stephens, P.E., and Harris, T.J.R. (1985). Sequence of human tissue inhibitor of metalloproteinases and its identity to erythroid-potentiating activity. Nature 318:66–69.

103. Palmoski, M.J., and Brandt, K.D. (1983). Relationship between matrix proteoglycan content and the effects of salicylate and indomethacin an articular cartilage. Arthritis Rheum. 26:528–531.

104. Slowman-Kovacs, S.D., Albrecht, M.E., and Brandt, K.D. (1989). Effects of salicytes on chondrocytes from osteoarthritic and contralateral knees of dogs with unilateral anterior cruciate ligament transection. Arthritis Rheum. 32:486–489.

105. Cuevas, P., Burgos, J., and Baird, A. (1988). Basic fibroblast growth factor (FGF) promotes cartilage repair in vivo. Biochem. Biophys. Res. Commun. 156:611–618.

9

T Cell Cytokines as Immunomodulators of Arthritis Disease Pathology

Thomas F. Kresina and Donna J. Spannaus-Martin

Miriam Hospital and Brown University International Health Institute, Providence, Rhode Island

I. INTRODUCTION

Chronic arthritis, an inflammation of the joints, consists of an inflammatory cell infiltration with pannus formation, culminating in cartilage and bone destruction and ultimate loss of joint function. This condition is a common and challenging medical problem. Numerous studies have suggested that the pathogenesis of arthritis is, at least in part, immunologically mediated. Noting this observation, numerous immunotherapeutic modalities haved utilized nonspecific suppressive agents, such as steroid injection and administration of nonsteroidal anti-inflammatory drugs, to reduce the pain, erythema, and edema associated with arthritis. A significant side effect of these treatments is the general compromise of the immune system. Therefore, new immunotherapeutic treatments need to be developed. The present chapter summarizes investigations of a potential specific biologic suppressive mechanism for arthritis, collagen-specific T suppressor cells, and the biologic molecules these T cells elaborate. Summarized are the initial studies from this laboratory that showed mice chronically suppressed for collagen-induced arthritis contained specific T suppressor cell populations in their lymphoid tissues. This population of suppressor cells mediates the suppression of experimentally induced arthritis. Recent studies utilized these lymphoid tissues and the technique of somatic cell hybridization with murine thymoma BW5147 and generated T cell hybridomas from the mice suppressed for collagen-induced arthritis. The T cell hybridomas were characterized with regard to cell surface phenotype and antigen specificity and tested for functional capacity to suppress the erythema and edema associated with arthritis. The data generated from these studies support the notion of an immunoregulatory circuit comprising collagen-specific T suppressor cells in the suppression of collagen-induced arthritis. The mechanism of action of the suppressor cell circuit was investigated with regard to (1) characterization of the anti-inflammatory secreted mediators of the T cell hybridomas, which represent individual members of both the afferent and efferent cell suppressor circuit, and (2) the identification of secreted mediators of these T cells that would be candidates for participants of the joint remodeling noted in this form of immunotherapy of experimental arthritis. These data represent novel information regarding two important areas detailing the use of biologic reagents for immunotherapy: (1) regulation of inflammation by mediators of T cells and (2) reconstruction of joints exhibiting arthritis pathology utilizing mediators of T cell hybridomas.

II. THE ANIMAL MODEL OF POLYARTHRITIS: COLLAGEN-INDUCED ARTHRITIS

For these studies, collagen-induced arthritis (CIA), an animal model of arthritis that exhibits many features of the human disease (1,2), was utilized. CIA provides an experimental model useful for the study of the mechanism(s) responsible for the development as well as any immunotherapy of the observed erosive inflammatory arthritis. With regard to the development of CIA, a large body of data indicates that the erosive inflammatory arthritis generated in rodents is mediated by autoimmunity to type II collagen (reviewed in Refs. 3–5). This polyarthritis can be induced in specific strains of rats (6) and mice (7) by immunization with a well-defined macromolecule of the extracellular cartilage matrix, type II collagen. This animal model of arthritis produces a chronic proliferative synovitis that secondarily destroys articular cartilage and bone (6,8). Histopathologic study (9) of joints at the onset of disease reveals a marked cellular infiltration of the synovium by neutrophils and monocytes. In addition, fibrous material is noted in the joint space around the surface of the articular cartilage.

Peritendinitis and periostitis are also noted (9). In chronic arthritis, analysis of serial sections of involved joints reveals proliferation of synoviocytes and fibroblasts resulting in synovial hypertrophy and fibrosis. Replacement of cartilage and subchondral bone is observed starting at the margin. Also observed at this disease stage is the fibrous tissue replacement of synovium and cartilage to the extent of forming adhesions between the joints (8).

Analysis of the immune response to collagen in animals with CIA shows the development of both cellular and humoral immune responses to type II collagen

(10,11). In addition, CIA can be adoptively transferred to naive rats by sensitized spleen cells (12) and passively transferred by immunoglobulin G specific for type II collagen (13). These observations are consistent with the contention that CIA results from immunologic hypersensitivity to type II collagen.

Additional studies have indicated that there is a role for T helper cell lymphocytes in the induction and pathogenesis of arthritis. In both CIA (14,15) and human rheumatoid arthritis (16–18), T lymphocytes have been shown to be increased in arthritic joint synovium and proximal to antigen-presenting Ia-bearing cells. Also, numerous laboratories have generated type II collagen-specific T helper cells of the cell surface phenotype Ly-1$^+$ L3T4$^+$ (19–22). These cell lines have been shown to functionally induce an antigen-specific delayed-type hypersensitivity response (22) and to be arthritogenic (20). In addition, an arthritogenic type II collagen-induced lymphokine has been characterized in the rat model of CIA (23). Taken together, these studies indicate that arthritis can be induced by type II collagen-reactive T helper cells.

With the observation of an immunologic basis in the pathogenesis of CIA, numerous studies detailing the suppression of CIA have utilized immunomodulating agents. Immune responses to collagen, as well as arthritic responses in rats with CIA, were shown to be modulated by administration of free collagen or anti-collagen antiserum (24). In addition, administration of collagen-coupled spleen cells (25), native type II collagen (26), or specific constituent CNBr peptides (27) before immunization with type II collagen resulted in the antigen-specific suppression of CIA. Rats administered collagen-coupled erythrocytes have been utilized as splenic cell donors in studies showing the adoptive transfer of antigen-specific suppression of CIA (28). These studies, as well as recent investigations that show the suppression of CIA by treatment with anti-L3T4 monoclonal antibody (29), intragastric administration of type II collagen (30–32), or the abrogation of suppression of CIA by cyclophosphamide treatment (33) infer a role for T cells in the suppression of CIA.

III. SUPPRESSOR T CELLS IN CIA

Recent studies from this laboratory (34) extending the latter observations and detailing a potential immunotherapeutic agent for arthritis showed that in the animals suppressed for CIA, antigen-specific T suppressor cells were present in lymphoid tissues. These T suppressor cells were noted to depress in vitro cell-mediated immune responses to type II collagen and serum anti-type II collagen antibody levels. In addition, these T cells also inhibited the generation of erythema and edema of inflammatory synovitis associated with CIA (34,35).

Noting this latter observation, somatic cell hybridization of selected T lymphocyte populations with T cell tumor lines was the method selected to establish permanent tissue culture hybridoma cell lines. These cell lines would reflect the in vivo characteristics of lymphoid cells, that is, antigen-specific suppression of CIA. Such cell lines would provide large amounts of specific subpopulations of lymphoid cells, enabling the elucidation of possible immunosuppressive mechanism(s) in arthritis. These studies could be accomplished if the T cell hybrids generated displayed the immunologic characteristics of the in vivo T lymphocytes, such as antigen reactivity, surface phenotype, and functional capacity. Studies (36) have shown that these immunologic characteristics of lymphoid cells are conserved by somatic cell fusion in T cell lymphoma cell lines with similar differentiation stages. Therefore, the AKR-derived T cell lymphoma BW5147 represents a fusion partner that can be utilized to derive murine T cell hybrids displaying different T cell functions (36). Although BW5147 cells have been noted to display nonspecific suppressor activity and produce lymphokines on stimulation (37), these properties do not affect the immunoregulation of CIA, as noted in the present studies. In addition, numerous laboratories (36–40) have used the BW5147 for the study of hapten-specific suppressor cells and lymphokines in a comparable fashion, noting a lack of immunoregulatory effects by the parental line, BW5147.

Suppressor T cells are an essential component of a homeostatic mechanism that controls the course and size of the immune response. The observation of immunologic tolerance or T cell unresponsiveness induced by the intravenous injection of high doses of soluble antigen has been hypothesized to be due to regulation of the immune response by T suppressor cells (41,42). In this regard, antigen-specific T suppressor cells have been determined to function in complex immunoregulatory circuits or suppressor T cell pathways (41,43,44). In the numerous T suppressor cell systems studied to date (reviewed in Refs. 43 and 44), common shared features are expressed. They include the utilization of multiple distinct T cell subsets; the ability of suppressor T cells to bind free antigen; soluble suppressor factors exhibiting biologic activity; a distinctive mechanism of antigen presentation to suppressor T cells; and antigen-dependent nonspecific final suppressor mechanism. With regard to the cells that comprise T suppressor cell circuits, afferent inducer T suppressor cells of phenotype Ly-1^+2^- Qa-1^+ are the earliest acting suppressor T cells and may induce another T cell subset of phenotype Ly-1^+2^+ Qa-1^+. These latter cells differentiate or activate effector Ly-1^-2^+ cells, which operate late in the course of the immune response (45–47).

Suppressor T cells secrete antigen-specific suppressor factors (43,48,49) that mediate the suppressive effects of these cells. Each suppressor T cell subpopulation produces its own suppressive factor. Inducer-suppressor T cells elaborate an inducer-suppressor factor, effector-suppressor T cells produce molecules that mediate effector cell function. These factors provide the induction, activation, and/or effector signals required for communication among the suppressor T cell populations. In addition, soluble factors permit interaction distally from the effector T cell and thereby obviate the necessity for cell-to-cell interaction for functional suppression.

Recently, numerous studies have been reported that detail the generation of T cell hybridomas that secrete immunoregulatory suppressor factors (50–55). The suppressor factors derived from these cloned cell lines have been shown to modulate antibody responses to the relevant antigens. However, studies to date have not shown an immunomodulation of antigenic responses relevant to disease states.

Cytokines with immunoregulating activity have been observed from both clonal and polyclonal populations of cells. Although antigen-specific cytokines have been noted to suppress antibody synthesis (50–59), other nonspecific suppressor factors downregulate inflammation through the inhibition of production of interleukin-2 (IL-2) (45,60,61), and still others such as lymphocyte-derived chemotactic factor (62), fibroblast inhibitory factor (63), and fibroblast activating factor (64), modulate connective tissue cell (fibroblast) function. Still other cytokines, such as collagen production factor (65–67), interferon-γ (68), and transforming growth factor β (69–73), modulate the synthesis of collagen in connective tissue cells. Therefore, it is possible that cytokines derived from specific T cell subpopulations could regulate inflammation and direct the reconstruction of connective tissue.

Initial studies designed to elucidate a role for T suppressor cells in the regulation of CIA utilized adoptive transfer experiments to detail the lymphoid cellular populations functional in the suppression of CIA by high-dose antigen tolerance (34). In these studies, animals inoculated with collagen were utilized as splenic or thymic cell donors and recipient mice were immunized with type II collagen to induce arthritis. As shown in Fig. 1, the results of these studies revealed that mice administered type II collagen to induce a state of antigen-induced tolerance possessed T cell lymphocytes that could adoptively transfer the state of suppression. In addition, these initial studies also revealed that animals chronically suppressed for collagen-induced arthritis also exhibited effector T suppressor cells reactive to antigenic epitopes of the type II collagen molecule. These data therefore indicated that mice chronically suppressed for CIA would be a rich source for T suppressor cells that may function in the immunoregulation of CIA. In this regard, the lymphoid cells of these animals and the technique of somatic cell hybridization were utilized to select T lymphocyte hybridoma cell lines. These cloned cell lines would, it was hoped, reflect the in vivo characteristics of T lymphocytes with regard to biologic function. As previously noted (74–77), numerous T cell hybridomas were generated that were initially screened for biologic function through the expression of cell surface glycoproteins associated with genetically determined function. In the murine system, cell surface markers have been designated Ly-1, Ly-2, L3T4, and Thy-1, based on cellular lineage and associated function. As shown in Table 1, T cell hybridomas were generated for the following associated function: afferent T suppressor cell Ly-1$^+$2$^-$L3T4$^-$ (CD4$^+$CD11$^-$) and effector T suppressor cell (Ly-1$^-$2$^+$L3T4$^-$(CD8$^+$). The

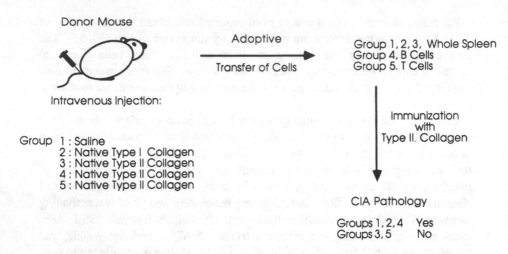

Figure 1 Adoptive transfer of CIA suppression in the mouse.

hybridomas T101N and T102V, respectively, were of these T cell lineages and also expressed the Thy-1 alloantigen (CD3$^+$). Two noteworthy hybridomas were also utilized as control cell lines for in vivo function. BW5147 is the AKR-derived parental fusion partner, and T104B1 is a T cell without high-density expression of Ly-1$^-$2$^-$L3T4$^-$ glycoproteins.

IV. T CELL HYBRIDOMAS FUNCTION IN THE IN VIVO SUPPRESSION OF THE ERYTHEMA AND EDEMA ASSOCIATED WITH CIA

Studies performed to analyze the in vivo function of hybridomas were of two types: (1) preliminary studies that examined the ability of cells to suppress the induction of athritis (i.e., cells administered before the induction of arthritis by

Table 1 Parental and Representative Generated Hybridoma Cell Lines

Cell line	Cell phenotype[a]	Associated Function
BW1547	Ly-1$^-$2$^-$L3T4$^-$Thy-1$^+$	Parental cell fusion partner
T101N	Ly-1$^+$2$^-$L3T4$^-$Thy-1$^+$	Afferent T suppressor cell
T102V	Ly-1$^-$2$^+$Thy-1$^+$	Effector T suppressor cell
T104B1	Ly-1$^-$2$^-$L3T4$^-$Thy-1$^+$	Hybridoma control cell line

[a]Cell surface phenotype determined by a direct binding radioimmunoassay (82,92).

immunization with collagen), and (2) subsequent studies that examined the ability of cells to downregulate ongoing collagen-induced arthritis (i.e., cells inoculated after the onset of collagen arthritis).

Studies examining the arthritis-suppressive ability of T cell hybridomas expressing defined cell surface glycoproteins, which recognize interstitial collagen molecules, are summarized in Table 2. The in vivo function of cell lines T101N and T102V are compared and noted to suppress the induction of CIA when administered before inoculation with native type II collagen. In arthritis control groups, parental BW5147 cell lines were administered before collagen immunization. In the BW5147-administered group, a high incidence of arthritis was noted based on gross pathology scores. Mice administered T101N cells (Lyt-1$^+$; afferent suppressor cell phenotype) or T102V cells (Ly-2$^+$ suppressor effector cell phenotype) portrayed reduced pathology scores and a lower incidence of arthritis. Concomitant with these observations was a reduction in serum anti-type II collagen antibody concentration. These mice, suppressed for CIA, were also observed to have a higher percentage of anti-type II collagen antibodies of the noncomplement-fixing IgG1 isotype. These data are consistent with the previously reported observation of reduced and restricted IgG subclass expression in mice suppressed for CIA (34,35).

T cell hybridomas of known cell surface phenotype and cellular reactivity to collagen were shown to modulate the induction of CIA in DBA/1J mice. Further studies were performed to determine if these cells could downregulate CIA (affect or regulate ongoing arthritis). To perform these experiments, breeding colonies generating F$_1$ hybrid mice (AKR × DBA and DBA × AKR) were established.

Table 2 Biologic Properties of Parental and Generated Hybridoma Cell Lines

Cell line	Function in CIA[a]	Collagen recognition[b]	Anticollagen antibody regulation[c]
BW5147	Nonsuppressive	No	No
T101N	Suppresses CIA induction and down-regulation	Yes; types I, II, III	Yes; types I, II
T102	Suppresses CIA induction	Nd[d]	Yes; type II
T104B1	Nonsuppressive	Yes; types I, II, III	No

[a]Function determined by in vivo injection of cells before (for induction studies) and after (for downregulation studies) the onset of CIA (74–76).
[b]Ability of cells to adhere to the genetically distinct collagen in a mage plate assay (76).
[c]Anticollagen antibodies measured in the serum of mice by a solid-phase radioimmunoassay (76).
[d]Not determined.

The colonies were generated because numerous previous studies had detailed a genetic linkage to CIA, and also the T cell hybridomas are F_1 cells, derived from a AKR thymoma line fused with DBA/1J lymphoid cells. In these studies, the thymoma line was generated from the AKR (H-2^k) mouse strain, which is not susceptible with regard to the generation of arthritis (78). The murine CIA model is generated in DBA/1J (H-2^q) mice, which are the donor strain for lymphoid cells in cell fusion experiments. Therefore, for histocompatibility purposes, F_1 mice were used to perform these studies.

The sex of the parental mice had an effect on the incidence of arthritis portrayed in the F_1 mice. Female mice derived from the AKR × DBA mating showed no susceptibility to CIA: male mice from the DBA × AKR mating showed a high susceptibility for CIA in both severity and incidence (77). Therefore, male F_1 mice from the latter mating were used to discern the ability of T cell hybridoma cells to downregulate CIA. F_1 mice were immunized with type II collagen to induce arthritis and, after the onset of hind paw erythema and edema, were sorted into three groups of mice. These groups were statistically indistinguishable from each other on the the the basis of incidence of arthritis, gross pathology score, and amount of foot pad swelling [measured as a change in foot width; (normal - arthritis) mice]. At this time point, 1×10^5 hybridoma cells were administered. For mice given T101N cells (Ly-1$^+$–Thy-1$^+$ fusion product of BW5147), there were a reduced incidence of arthritis, statistically significant reduced pathology scores, and reduced paw size (75). A reduction in paw size could be noted as early as 8 days after cell administration but was most notable after 18 days. A lack of suppression of CIA, as well as the flaring nature of CIA, was evident in the arthritis and arthritis + T104B1 (Ly-1$^-$–Thy-1$^+$ fusion product of BW5147) cell groups (75).

Evaluation of the joints of the arthritis, arthritis plus T104B1 cells, and arthritis plus T101N cell groups used image analysis to determine the surface area of articular cartilage in the mouse foot (75). These studies showed that the joints of animals given T101N cells had a surface area of the tibia-tarsus and intertarsal regions comparable to those of normal mice. The three arthritis groups—arthritis (day 43), arthritis (day 75), and arthritis given T104B1 cells—had elevated levels of staining within the tissue. This observation was also noted in the histologic sections of the joints. These tissue sections displayed the arthritic lesions of the joints as evidenced by joint disorganization, pannus formation, and loss of aligned articular surfaces. However, the joint structure of arthritic mice administered T101N cells were strikingly "normal" in appearance with regard to these features. These data indicate that administration of T101N cells to mice with arthritis results not only in a reduction of inflammation, but also a reorganization or remodeling of the joint to a more functional appearance.

V. SOLUBLE MEDIATORS OF IN VIVO SUPPRESSION OF CIA

Recent studies have investigated the mechanism of suppression of CIA by T cell hybridomas (75,79). In this regard, the initial studies investigated whether lethally irradiated T cell hybridomas could suppress CIA (75). Table 3 shows the summarized data indicating that lethally irradiated T101N hybridoma cells administered before the induction of arthritis were effective in reducing the erythema and edema associated with CIA. In these studies, both BW5147 and T104B1 cell lines were used as controls since these experiments did not require cell growth in the recipient mice. As shown in Table 4, in vitro cytotoxicity studies used as substrates thymocytes from normal or arthritic mice, as well as the BW5147 thymoma line. These studies showed no elevation above background levels of cytotoxicity by serum samples derived from the group of mice suppressed for CIA by administration of lethally irradiated hybridoma cells. These data indicated that generation of a cytotoxic anti-T cell immune response was not the mechanism of suppression.

It is also noteworthy that in these studies, T101N hybridoma cells administered to F_1 mice were found to migrate predominantly to the peripheral lymph nodes, in particular the popliteal lymph nodes (76). There was no observable migration to the peripheral joints, which suggests that cytokine(s) are one possible mechanism of action for the T101N hybridoma cells. Therefore, further studies utilized hybridoma ascites fluid derived from F_1 mice administered T101N cells of BW5147 cells to investigate the presence of soluble mediator(s) of suppression of CIA. A statistically significant reduction in inflammation was noted in the group of mice administered T101N ascites. These data indicate that mice can be "vaccinated" with an acellular fluid and that soluble mediator(s) can be used to induce protection from CIA.

Table 3 Suppression of CIA by T Cell Hybridoma Mediators

Cell line	Suppression of CIA by lethally irradiated cells[a]	Suppression of CIA by ascites fluid[b]	Suppression of CIA by cell culture supernatant[b]
BW5147	−	−	−
T101N	+	+	+
T104B1	−	−	−

[a]Lethally irradiated cells administered before the induction of CIA as described previously (79).
[b]Ascites fluid and cell culture supernatant as described previously (80).

Table 4 In Vitro Cytotoxicity Studies Using Sera from Mice with Arthritis or Suppressed for Arthritis

Cell line[a]	Mouse sera (cell line given IV)	Arthritis noted in serum donors	Dilution	% Cytotoxicity above complement control
Nonimmune	None	+	1:5	0
F$_1$ thymocytes	None	+	1:1000	0
	BW5147	+	1:5	1
	BW5147	+	1:100	0
	T101N	−	1:5	0
	T101N	−	1:100	0
BW5147	None	+	1:5	0
	None	+	1:100	0
	BW5147	+	1:5	0
	BW5147	+	1:100	0
	T101N	−	1:5	0
	T101N	−	1:100	0
Arthritis	None	+	1:5	0
thymocytes	None	+	1:100	0
	BW5417	+	1:5	0
	BW5417	+	1:100	2
	T101N	−	1:5	0
	T101N	−	1:100	0

[a]Cell line used as substrate in cytotoxicity assay employing a 30 minute incubation of cell line and sera dilution at 30°C followed by a 30 minute incubation of cells with a 1:8 dilution of rabbit complement. Cell viability was determined by trypan blue exclusion.

VI. CYTOKINES SECRETED BY A SUPPRESSOR INDUCER T CELL HYBRIDOMA T101N

The observation that CIA can be downregulated by inoculation of T cell hybridomas suggests two phases of activity are induced by inoculation: (1) Suppression of inflammation and (2) a remodeling of joint architecture to a form resembling normal joint structure. As noted earlier, both phases could be mediated by lymphokines. Initial studies were performed to characterize the soluble mediator(s) required for these two phases of activity (79). The studies showed that T101N cells secreted a mediator that inhibited IL-2-dependent proliferation of CTLL-20 cells in a dose-dependent fashion, that is, a contra-IL-2 cytokine. In addition, preincubation of CTLL-20 cells with the contra-IL-2 cytokine did not significantly alter the IL-2 responsiveness of the cells to recombinant IL-2.

The contra-IL-2 activity found in the T101N culture supernatant was purified and the physiochemical characteristics of the IL-2 inhibitor determined. Table 5

Table 5 Physiochemical Characteristics of Contra-IL-2 Activity

Physiochemical property	Contra-IL-2 activity range
pH	3–9
Temperature	20–60 °C
Molecular weight	> 30,000 daltons
Amicon filtration	
Agarose gel filtration	> 100,000 daltons

presents some of the characteristics that have been determined to date. In brief, the mediator loses activity after extended incubation at 4 °C, is resistant to freeze-thawing, has a molecular weight of greater than 30,000 daltons, and has peak activity in the neutral pH range (6–8) and at relatively physiologic temperatures. Contra-IL-2 activity can be lost upon incubation of the culture media with pepsin or pronase but is resistant to papain, keratinase, amylase, phospholipase, and chondroitinase. These results are consistent with the physiochemical characteristics of cytokines.

On A-1.5 M agarose chromatography, contra-IL-2 activity did not coelute with absorbing protein material. Contra-IL-2 activity eluted at the void volume of the column, indicative of a large aggregative suppressive molecule (79). Chromatographically purified contra-IL-2 was then concentrated and administered to naive mice before immunization with type II collagen. The data generated showed that animals that were administered chromatographically purified contra-IL-2 exhibited a reduced incidence of arthritis early in the time course of the disease when compared to control animals. Measurement of the edema of hind paws indicated that contra-IL-2–administered animals did not indicate the flaring incident at day 34 of the time course. Histochemical analysis of the hind paw joints of the mice indicated that mice administered contra-IL-2 developed a less severe form of CIA. These data show that a contra-IL-2 cytokine, when administered to mice before the induction of collagen-induced arthritis, can modulate the cartilage pathology associated with CIA. IL-2 is an important mediator of T cell activation. Therefore, an IL-2 inhibitor could represent a nonantigen-specific (driven) modulator of inflammation. A nonantigen-specific inhibitor of inflammation, such as a contra-IL-2 cytokine, may have relevance in the human disease. To this point, Smith et al. (80) reported on an inhibitor to interleukin-2 found in human serum and synovial fluid that inhibited the proliferation of normal peripheral blood lymphocytes in response to concanavalin A and phytohemagglutinin. This inhibitor, a 70 kD protein, was found to be present in decreased concentrations in the synovial fluid of patients with rheumatoid arthritis in comparison to patients with other types of arthritis. Analogous data have been generated in our laboratory. To this point, the IL-2 antagonist from the T101N cell line has also been found to inhibit the proliferation of mitogen-stimulated splenic lymphocytes (81). Lymphocytes cultured in the presence of T101N culture supernatant and concanavalin A exhibited a maximum of 77% inhibition of tritiated thymidine uptake compared to control cells incubated with concanavalin A, media, or BW5147 culture supernatant (81). A maximum of 52% reduction in tritiated thymidine uptake was observed in lipopolysaccharide-stimulated lymphocytes upon incubation with T101N culture supernatant (unpublished results). These data suggest an effect on IL-2-dependent B cell population as well. Lymphocytes incubated with mitogens for 2 days before the addition of culture supernatant containing contra-IL-2 activity showed a 65% reduction in tritiated thymidine uptake in comparison to the control cultures. These data, taken together, suggest that the contra-IL-2 activity contained in the T101N culture supernatant is able to interrupt the proliferation of activated lymphocytes, as well as inhibit an activation step of lymphocytes. Both these observations have implications for inhibition of pannus formation and lymphocyte infiltration into the joints.

Recent studies have investigated the molecular aspects of contra-IL-2 inhibition of lymphocyte activation (see Table 6). In situ hybridization studies have demonstrated that splenic lymphocytes incubated with concanavalin A and T101N contra-IL-2 contain reduced levels of messenger RNA coding for interleukin-2 (81). In splenic lymphocyte cultures incubated in the presence of 2.0 μg/ml concanavalin A, greater than 55% of the lymphocytes contained high levels of mRNA coding for interleukin-2. In comparison, only 20% of the cells from lymphocyte cultures that were incubated with concanavalin A and the culture supernatant from the T101N hybridoma cells contained high levels of mRNA coding for interleukin-2. These data indicate that the contra-IL-2 lymphokine produced by the T101N hybridoma can function in reducing endogenous mRNA levels for interleukin-2. The reduction of mRNA levels for IL-2 elucidates a further mechanism of T cell deactivation. T cells require IL-2 as both a paracrine and an autocrine signal for full differentiation and activation. A reduction in transcriptional and translational levels for IL-2 would limit the amount of soluble, secreted

Table 6   Contra-IL-2 Activity

Secretion:	Suppressor-inducer T cell hybridomas
Function	1. Inhibits [³H]thymidine uptake of CTLL-20 cells
	2. Inhibits [³H]thymidine uptake of ConA-stimulated lymphoid cells
	3. Reduces mRNA levels for IL-2 in ConA-stimulated lymphoid cells
	4. Chromatographically purified material modulates the induction and expression of CIA
	5. Reduces expression of MHC-encoded cell surface glycoproteins of lymphoid cells in vivo

IL-2 that could be utilized in T cell differentiation. In such a case, since both antigen and IL-2 are required for full T cell activation, contra-IL-2 cytokines could limit cartilage pathology through limiting T cell activation and differentiation regardless of the levels of arthritogenic antigen available to the cells.

VII. IMPLICATION FOR AMELIORATION OF DISEASE BY CYTOKINES AND CONTRA CYTOKINES

In recent years, many studies have focused on the involvement of the immune system in the articular inflammation occurring in rheumatoid arthritis. The pathology generated in this disease is believed to be, at least in part, the result of autoimmune reactivity, presumably to some component of the joint. The control of the inflammatory response, which involves both humoral and cellular immune responses, can be modulated by the production and secretion of cytokines. In 1984, it was reported that 100 molecules were known that could mediate some aspect of the inflammatory process, and about 50 of those molecules were cytokines (82). An understanding of the principal cytokines involved in the inflammatory process and joint remodeling would provide insight for the development of immunotherapies to downregulate the inflammatory process.

Interleukin-1 (IL-1) is a cytokine produced by many different cell types (83) and is thought to play an important role in the pathogenesis of rheumatoid arthritis. Injection of IL-1 into the joints of normal rabbits results in a dose-dependent increase in the inflammatory cells within the joint cavity (84). Concomitant with the appearance of this cellular infiltrate is a loss of proteoglycan from the matrix of the articular cartilage. These observations are similar to those that appear in antigen-induced arthritis but occur much more rapidly and are transient.

Many of the biologic activities of IL-1 are relevant to the pathology observed in rheumatoid arthritis. Purified IL-1 has been shown to (1) inhibit the synthesis of proteoglycans by articular cartilage (85); (2) stimulate the secretion of proteoglycan- and collagen-degrading proteases in rabbit chondrocytes (86); (3) stimulate bone resorption in culture (87); (4) stimulate fibroblast proliferation (88); (5) stimulate the production of collagen and fibronectin by chondrocyte cultures (89); (6) stimulate the release of lytic enzmyes and prostaglandin E_2 (90); (7) stimulate the synthesis of interleukin-2 (91) and interleukin-2 receptor (92) when a second activating signal (antigen or mitogen) is present; and (8) have chemotactic effects on T lymphocytes (93). These functions and the observation that interleukin-1 is present in the synovial fluid of patients with rheumatoid arthritis (94) suggest that IL-1 has a role in the initiation of the cellular infiltrate and in the erosion of cartilage and bone observed in the rheumatoid joint.

For the antigen-specific activation of T lymphocytes to occur, two distinct signals must occur. In addition to the presence of interleukin-1, antigen must be presented in conjunction with Ia antigen. The presence of these two signals stimulates interleukin-2 and interleukin-2 receptor production by the T lymphocyte. The principle action of IL-2 is to stimulate the proliferation and differentiation of T helper lymphocytes (95) and T suppressor cells (96). It can also function to promote the growth and differentiation of certain activated B cells (97–100) and stimulate T cell production of B cell growth factor (101) and interferon-γ (102).

The specific involvement of interleukin-2 in experimentally induced arthritis and rheumatoid arthritis is not clearly understood. Impaired IL-2 production and response have been observed in several animal models of autoimmune rheumatoid disease (103–106). Other studies have shown that the lymphocytes found in the synovial fluids of patients with rheumatoid arthritis are responsive to interleukin-2 (107) and IL-2 secretion is increased (108,109).

Other interleukins have been examined for possible involvement in the inflammatory response observed in rheumatoid arthritis. Interleukin-3 and the mRNA transcript encoding for IL-3 were not detected in the synovium and synovial cells of patients with rheumatoid arthritis (110). Interleukin-4 is a T cell cytokine that affects the activation and differentiation of lymphoid cells. Recent studies by Llorente et al. (111) suggest that IL-4 exhibits contra-IL-2 activity on B lymphocytes. It has recently been reported that IL-4 may also act as an autocrine signal in some murine T helper lymphocyte clones, independent of interleukin-2 production (112) and possibly acting synergistically with IL-2 (113).

Interleukin-6, a cytokine involved in the activation and differentiation of T and B lymphocytes (114–116), has been implicated in the induction of arthritic lesions. Human synoviocytes have been shown to produce high levels of interleukin 6 in vitro (117). The IL-6 produced by the synoviocytes is capable of stimulating the secretion of immunoglobulin, suggesting that IL-6 may play a role in the induction of hypergammaglobulinemia and rheumatoid factor production observed in rheumatoid arthritis. Lymph node cells from mice with collagen-induced arthritis produced high levels of interleukin-6 upon in vitro stimulation with collagen (118). Increased levels of interleukin-6 have also been observed in the serum of mice with CIA (118) and the serum and synovial fluids of patients with rheumatoid arthritis (117,119,120).

Several inhibitors to interleukins have been observed and may be important inflammatory mediators. Inhibitors to interleukin-1 function have been noted in several laboratories (121–124). Several studies have reported on inhibitors to interleukin-2 (45,60,61), particularly those found in the serum and synovial fluid of patients with rheumatoid arthritis (82,125,126). Interleukin-2 inhibitor was reported to be found in reduced concentrations in the synovial fluid of patients with rheumatoid arthritis compared to patients with other forms of arthritis (82,126). This suggests that the inflammatory response may be due to diminished inhibitory signals to the T lymphocytes within the joints. However, other studies show that the synovial fluid of rheumatoid patients is able to inhibit the proliferation of normal lymphocytes in response to mitogen (125).

In addition to the interleukins, other cytokines may mediate the inflammation of arthritis. Several hematopoietic growth factors have been reported to be present in the synovial fluid of rheumatoid arthritis patients. Granulocyte-macrophage colony stimulating factor (127), macrophage colony-stimulating factor (110), and a mast cell growth factor have been found to be present in increased amounts in the synovial fluids of patients with inflammatory arthritis. The role of these cytokines in rheumatoid arthritis is not understood at this time, but it is likely that they are involved in the modulation of the immune response. For example, granulocyte-macrophage colony stimulating factor increases Ia expression and the secretion of interleukin-1 in murine macrophages (128). The modulation of interleukin-1 secretion by this cytokine could be important in the modulation of the inflammatory response observed in arthritis.

Interferons are another class of proteins involved in the regulation of the immune response. For this reason, several laboratories have looked at the role of interferons in the immunoregulation of inflammatory arthritis. The presence of interferon-γ (IFN-γ) in the serum and synovial fluid of patients with rheumatoid arthritis has been somewhat controversial. Several investigators have detected IFN-γ in the serum and synovial fluids of rheumatoid arthritis (RA) patients (129–132); other laboratories have reported that IFN-γ is not present or is present only at very low levels (133) and that the synthesis of IFN-γ is impaired in RA patients (134,135).

Transforming growth factor β (TGF-β) is a multifunctional regulatory polypeptide synthesized by many different cell types (136) and found in relatively high concentrations in bone (137). This cytokine has regulatory effects on the immune system and could also be an important cytokine for joint remodeling in inflammatory arthritis. Both T and B lymphocytes synthesize TGF-β. The TGF-β acts to inhibit IL-2-dependent B lymphocyte proliferation, IL-2-dependent immunoglobulin production (138), and IL-2-dependent T lymphocyte proliferation (139). The synthesis of both IL-2 and TGF-β by activated T lymphocytes suggests that TGF-β acts as a feedback control for T cell proliferation. Chondrocyte proliferation (140) and the synthesis of fibronectin, collagen, and collagen-related proteins (69) can also be modulated by TGF-β. Recent studies from this laboratory have shown an in vivo role for TGF-β in the modulation of inflammation and joint reconstruction in vivo (141). Repeated injection of TGF-β into inflamed joints results in the amelioration of joint pathology based on the degree of CIA.

Tumor necrosis factor has been found to induce the production of collagenase and prostaglandin E_2 in synovial cells (142), stimulate bone resorption (143), and cause the adherence of neutrophils to endothelial cells (144), as well as prevent the resynthesis of bone matrix molecules (143). The action of tumor necrosis factor in other inflammatory processes and its action on synovial cells and bone imply that tumor necrosis factor may be involved in the modulation of inflammation observed in arthritis.

The use of lymphokines as a new and novel form of immunotherapy in the treatment of inflammatory arthritis may be useful as a way to downregulate the inflammation of the disease and to initiate the repair of the affected joints.

Interferon-γ has been reported to inhibit the bone resorptive properties of IL-1 (87) and to inhibit osteoclast formation (145). These observations suggest that IFN-γ may be useful as an immunotherapeutic agent in arthritis. Recent studies have shown the rheumatoid arthritis patients administered recombinant interferon-γ exhibited fewer swollen joints (146) and a decrease in joint tenderness (147).

The use of nonspecific immunoregulatory cytokines and drugs has resulted in suppression of the synovitis observed in inflammatory arthritis; the suppression of the immune response in these treatments can result in many side effects as a result of long-term treatment (148). The existence of a specific immunoregulatory cytokine antagonist could provide a method to regulate inflammatory synovitis without comprising the immune system or producing severe side effects. Alternatively, these molecules could be used in combination therapy, alternating drugs, cytokines, and cytokine antagonists based on the status of the inflamed joint. However, such novel therapeutic approaches would likely require additional methods detailing joint physiology.

The data summarized here detail the effects of a T cell hybridoma and a contra-IL-2 lymphokine that it produces. This T cell hybridoma is capable of suppressing the immune response to collagen, inhibiting the activation of T lymphocytes, delaying the onset of collagen-induced arthritis, and diminishing the joint pathology observed in collagen-induced arthritis.

There may be potential for the production of a similar hybridoma and lymphokine for use as an immunotherapeutic agent in the human disease. Recently, Ichikawa et al. (149) reported the spontaneous improvement of a patient with juvenile rheumatoid arthritis that occurred after a prominent increase in the number of activated T suppressor cells in the peripheral and bone marrow blood. If human suppressor T lymphocytes are involved in the downregulation of the flaring episodes observed in rheumatoid arthritis, these lymphocytes may act via the production of lymphokines that can modulate the inflammatory response. These lymphocytes could be used to produce a human T cell hybridoma with characteristics similar to those of the murine T101N hybridoma.

REFERENCES

1. Trentham, D.E. (1982). Collagen arthritis as a relevant model for rheumatoid arthritis. Evidence pro and con. Arthritis Rheum. 25:911–916.
2. Stuart, J.M., Townes, A.S., and Kang, A.H. (1982). The role of collagen autoimmunity in animal models and human diseases. J. Invest. Dermatol. 79 (Suppl. 1):121s–127s.
3. Trentham, D.E. (1985). Immune response to collagen. In: Immunology of Rheumatic Diseases, Gupta, S., and Talal, N., eds. Plenum Press, New York, pp. 301–323.
4. Stuart, J.M., Townes, A.S., and Kang, A.H. (1984). Collagen autoimmune arthritis. Annu. Rev. Immunol. 2:199–218.

5. Holmdahl, R., Klareskog, L., Rubin, K., Bjork, J., Smedegard, G., Jonsson, R., and Andersson, M. (1986). Role of T lymphocytes in murine collagen induced arthritis. Agents Actions 19:295–305.

6. Trentham, D.E., Townes, A.S., and Kang, A.H. (1977). Autoimmunity to type II collagen: An experimental model of arthritis. J. Exp. Med. 146:857–868.

7. Courtenay, J.S., Dallman, M.J., Dayan, A.D., Martin, A., and Mosedale, B. (1980). Immunisation against heterologous type II collagen induces arthritis in mice. Nature 283:666–668.

8. Holmdahl, R., Jansson, L., Larsson, E., Rubin, K., and Klareskog, L. (1986). Homologous type II collagen induces chronic and progressive arthritis in mice. Arthritis Rheum. 29:106–113.

9. Stuart, J.M., Cremer, M.A., Kang, A.H., and Townes A.S. (1979). Collagen-induced arthritis in rats. Evaluation of early immunologic events. Arthritis Rheum. 22:1344–1351.

10. Stuart, J.M., Townes, A.S., and Kang, A.H. (1982). Nature and specificity of the immune response to collagen in type II collagen-induced arthritis in mice. J. Clin. Invest. 69:673–683.

11. Trentham, D.E., Townes, A.S., Kang, A.H., and David, J.R. (1978). Humoral and cellular sensitivity to collagen in type II collagen-induced arthritis in rats. J. Clin. Invest. 61:89–96.

12. Trentham, D.E., Dynesius, R.A., and David, J.R. (1978). Passive transfer by cells of type II collagen-induced arthritis in rats. J. Clin. Invest. 62:359–366.

13. Stuart, J.M., Cremer, A.S. Townes, A.S., and Kang, A.H. (1982). Type II collagen-induced arthritis in rats. Passive transfer with serum and evidence that IgG anticollagen antibodies can cause arthritis. J. Exp. Med. 155:1–16.

14. Klareskog, L., Holmdahl, R., Larsson, E., and Wigzell, H. (1983). Role of T lymphocytes in collagen II induced arthritis in rats. Clin. Exp. Immunol. 51:117–125.

15. Holmdahl, R., Rubin, K., Klareskog, L., Dencker, L., Gustafson, G., and Larsson, E. (1985). Appearance of different lymphoid cells in synovial tissue and in peripheral blood during the course of collagen II-induced arthritis in rats. Scand. J. Immunol. 21:197–204.

16. Janossy, G., Panayi, G., Duke, O., Bofill, M., Poulter, L.W., and Goldstein, G. (1981). Rheumatoid arthritis: A disease of T lymphocytes/macrophages immunoregulation. Lancet 2:839–842.

17. Lindblad, S., Klareskog, L., Hedfors, E., Forsum, U., and Sundstrom, C. (1983). Phenotypic characterization of synovial tissue cells in situ in different types of synovitis. Arthritis Rheum. 26:1321–1332.

18. Poulter, L.W., Duke, O., Panayi, G.S., Hobbs, S., Raftery, M.J., and Janossy, G. (1985). Activated T lymphocytes of the synovial membrane in rheumatoid arthritis and other arthropathies. Scand. J. Immunol. 22:683–690.

19. Dallman, M., and Fathman, C.G. (1985). Type II collagen-reactive T cell clones from mice with collagen-induced arthritis. J. Immunol. 135:1113–1118.

20. Holmdahl, R., Klareskog, L., Rubin, K., Larsson, E., and Wigzell, H. (1985). T lymphocytes in collagen II-induced arthritis in mice: Characterization of arthritogenic collagen II-specific T cell lines and clones. Scand. J. Immunol. 22:295–306.

21. Hom, J.T., Stuart, J.M., and Chiller, J.M. (1986). Murine T cells reactive to type II collagen. I. Isolation of lines and clones and characterization of their antigen-induced proliferative response. J. Immunol. 136:769–775.

22. Hom, J.T., Stuart, J.M., Tovey, J., and Chiller, J.M. (1986). Murine T cells reactive to type II collagen. II. Functional characterization. J. Immunol. 136:776–782.

23. Helfgott, S.M., Dynesius-Trentham, R., Brahn, E., and Trentham, D.E. (1985). An arthritogenic lymphokine in the rat. J. Exp. Med. 162:1531–1545.

24. Staines, N.A., Hardingham, T., Smith, M., and Henderson, B. (1981). Collagen-induced arthritis in the rat: Modification of immune and arthritic responses by free collagen and immune anti-collagen antiserum. Immunology 44:737–744.

25. Schoen, R.T., Greene, M.I., and Trentham, D.E. (1982). Antigen-specific suppression of type II collagen-induced arthritis by collagen-coupled spleen cells. J. Immunol. 128:717–719.

26. Cremer, A.S., Hernandez, A.D., Townes, A.S., Stuart, J.M., and Kang, A.H. (1983). Collagen-induced arthritis in rats: Antigen specific suppression of arthritis and immunity by intravenously injected naive type II collagen. J. Immunol. 131:2995–3000.

27. Englert, M.E., Landes, M.J., Oronsky, A.L., and Kerwar, S.S. (1984). Suppression of type II collagen-induced arthritis by intravenous administration of type II collagen or its constituent peptide alpha-1 (II) CB_{10}. Cell. Immunol. 87:357–365.

28. Brahn, E., and Trentham, D.E. (1984). Antigen-specific suppression of collagen arthritis by adoptive transfer of spleen cells. Clin. Immunol. Immunopathol. 31:124–131.

29. Ranges, G.E., Sriram, S., and Cooper, S.M. (1985). Prevention of type II collagen-induced arthritis by in vivo treatment with anti-L3T4. J. Exp. Med. 162:1105–1110.

30. Thompson, H.S.G., and Staines, N.A. (1985). Gastric administration of type II collagen delays the onset and severity of collagen-induced arthritis in rats. Clin. Exp. Immunol. 64:581–586.

31. Thompson, H.S., and Staines, N.A. (1986). Suppresson of collagen-induced arthritis with pergastrically or intravenously administered type II collagen. Agents Actions 19:318–319.

32. Nagler-Anderson, C., Bober, L.A., Robinson, M.E., Siskind, G.W., and Thorbecke, G.J. (1986). Suppression of type II collagen-induced arthritis by intragastric administration of soluble type II collagen. Proc. Natl. Acad. Sci. USA 83:7443–7446.

33. Arai, K., Kaibara, N., Takagishi, K., Hotokebuchi, T., and Arita, C. (1987). Reversal of antigen-induced resistance to collagen arthritis by cyclophosphamide. Clin. Immunol. Immunopathol. 43:325–332.

34. Kresina, T.F., and Moskowitz, R.W. (1985). Adoptive transfer of suppression of arthritis in the mouse model of collagen-induced arthritis: Evidence for a type II collagen-specific suppressor T cell. J. Clin. Invest. 75:1990–1998.

35. Kresina, T.F., and Finegan, C.K. (1986). Restricted expression of anti-type II collagen antibody isotypes in mice suppressed for collagen-induced arthritis. Ann. Rheum. Dis. 45:60–66.

36. Grutzmann, R., and Hammerling, G.J. (1978). Characterization and functional analysis of T cell hybrids. Curr. Top. Microbiol. Immunol. 81:188–191.

37. Hagiwara, H., Yokota, T., Luh, J., Lee, F., Arai, K-I., Arai, N., and Zlotnik, A. (1988). The AKR thymoma BW5147 is able to produce lymphokines when stimulated with calcium ionophore and phorbol ester. J. Immunol. 140:1561–1565.

38. Okuda, K., Minami, M., Sherr, D.H., and Dorf, M.E. (1981). Hapten-specific T cell responses to 4-hydroxy-3-nitrophenyl acetyl. XI. Pseudogenetic restrictions of hybridoma suppressor factors. J. Exp. Med. 154:468–479.

39. Jones, C.M., Braatz, J.A., and Hebermaan, R.B. (1982). T lymphocyte hybridoma which generate MIF/MAF in phagocytosis, past and future. In: Phagocytosis: Past and Future. Karnovsky, M.L., and Bolis, L., eds. Academic Press, New York, p. 323.

40. Ruddle, N.H. (1978). T cell hybrids with specificity for individual antigens. Curr. Top. Microbiol. Immunol. 81:203–211.

41. Simpson, E., and Beverly, P.C.L. (1977). T cell subpopulations. Prog. Immunol. III:206.

42. Gershon, R.K., and Kondo, K. (1970). Cell interactions in the induction of tolerance: The role of thymic lymphocytes. Immunology 18:723–737.

43. Germain, R.N., and Benacerraf B. (1981). A single major pathway of T-lymphocyte interactions in antigen-specific immune suppression. Scand. J. Immunol. 13:1–10.

44. Dorf, M.E., and Benacerraf, B. (1984). Suppressor cells and immunoregulation. Annu. Rev. Immunol. 2:127–158.

45. Asherson, G.L., Colizzi, V., and Zembala, M. (1986). An overview of T suppressor cells circuits. Annu. Rev. Immunol. 4:37–68.

46. Claman, H.N., Miller, S.D., Sy, M.-S., and Moorhead, J.W. (1980). Suppressive mechanisms involving sensitization and tolerance in contact allergy. Immunol. Rev. 50:105–132.

47. Yamauchi, K., Murphy, D., Cantor, H., and Gershon, R.K. (1981). Analysis of antigen-specific Ig-restricted cell-free material made by I-J$^+$Ly-1 cells (Ly-1 TsiF) that induces Ly-2$^+$ cells to express suppressive activity. Eur. J. Immunol. 11:905–912.

48. Green, D.R., Flood, P.M., and Gershon, R.K. (1983). Immunoregulatory T cell pathways. Annu. Rev. Immunol. 1:439–463.

49. Tada, T. and Okumura, K., (1980). The role of antigen specific T cell factors in the immune response. Adv. Immunol. 28:1–87.

50. Kontiainen, S., and Feldmann, M., (1977). Suppressor cell induction in vitro. III. Antigen-specific suppression by supernatants of suppressor cells. Eur. J. Immunol. 7:310–314.

51. Minami, M., Okuda, K., Furusawa, S., Benacerraf, B., and Dorf, M.E. (1981). Analysis of T cell hybridomas. I. Characterization of H-2 and IgH-restricted monoclonal suppressor factors. J. Exp. Med. 154:1390–1402.

52. Bear, H.D. (1987) Production of tumor-specific suppressor T cell hybridomas. J. Surg. Res. 42:369–376.

53. Greene, W.C., Fleisher, T.A., Nelson, D.L., and Waldmann, T.A. (1982). Production of human suppressor T cell hybridomas. J. Immunol. 129:1986–1992.

54. Grillot-Courvalin, C., Brouet, J.-C., Berger, R., and Bernheim, A. (1981). Establishment of a human T-cell hybrid line with suppressive activity. Nature 292:844–845.

55. Murakami, M., and Cathcart, M.K. (1986). Suppression of polyclonal immunoglobulin production by a soluble factor produced by a human thymus hybridoma. Immunopharmacology 11:141–154.

56. Adorini, L., Doria, G., and Ricciardi-Castagnoli, P. (1982). Fine antigenic specificity and genetic restriction of lysozyme-specific suppressor T cell factor produced by radiation leukemia virus-transformed suppressor T cells. Eur. J. Immunol. 12:719–724.

57. Rich, R.R., El Masry, M.N., and Fox, E.J. (1986). Human suppressor T cells: Induction differentiation and regulatory functions. Hum. Immunol. 17:369–387.
58. Durham, J.C., Stephens, D.S., Rimland, D., Nassar, V.H., and Spira, T.J. (1987). Common variable hypogammaglobulinemia complicated by an unusual T-suppressor/cytotoxic cell lymphoma. Cancer 59:271–276.
59. Emara, M., and Battisto, J.R. (1987). A syngeneic splenic cell antigen induces a suppressor T cell in lymph nodes that controls cytotoxic T-cell and primary antibody responses. Cell. Immunol. 105:205–219.
60. Malkovsky, M., Asherson, G.L., Chandler, P., Colizzi, V., Watkins, M.C., and Zembala, M. (1983). Nonspecific inhibitor of DNA synthesis elaborated by T acceptor cells. I. Specific hapten- and I-J driven liberation of an inhibitor of cell proliferation by Lyt 1^-2^+ cyclophosphamide-sensitive T acceptor cells armed with a product of Lyt 1^+2^+ specific suppressor cells. J. Immunol. 130:785–790.
61. Malkovsky, M., Asherson, G.L., Stockinger, B. and Watkins, M.C. (1982). Nonspecific inhibitor released by T acceptor cells reduces the production of interleukin-2. Nature 300:652–655.
62. Postlethwaite, A.E., Snyderman, R., and Kang, A.H. (1976). The chemotactic attraction of human fibroblasts to a lymphocyte-derived factor. J. Exp. Med. 144:1188–1203.
63. Rola-Pleszczynski, M., Lieu, H., Hamel, J., and Lemaire, I. (1982). Stimulated human lymphocytes produce a soluble factor which inhibits fibroblast migration. Cell. Immunol. 74:104–110.
64. Wahl, S.M., and Gately, C.L. (1983). Modulation of fibroblast growth by a lymphokine of human T cell and continuous T cell line origin. J. Immunol. 130:1226–1230.
65. Johnson, R.L., and Ziff, M. (1976). Lymphokine stimulation of collagen accumulation. J. Clin. Invest. 58:240–252.
66. Wahl, S.M., Wahl, L.M., and McCarthy, J.B. (1978). Lymphocyte-mediated activation of fibroblast proliferation and collagen production. J. Immunol. 121:942–946.
67. Postlethwaite, A.E., Smith, G.N., Mainardi, C.L., Seyer, J.M., and Kang, A.H. (1984). Lymphocyte modulation of fibroblast function in vitro. Stimulation and inhibition of collagen production by different effector molecules. J. Immunol. 132:2470–2477.
68. Jimenez, S.A., Freundlich, B., and Rosenbloom, J. (1984). Selective inhibition of human diploid fibroblast collagen synthesis by interferons. J. Clin. Invest. 74:1112–1116.
69. Ignotz, R.A., and Massague, J. (1986). Transforming growth factor-beta stimulates the expression of fibronectin and collagen and their incorporation into the extracellular matrix. J. Biol. Chem. 261:4337–4345.
70. Roberts, A.B., Sporn, M.B., Assoian, R.K., Smith, J.M., Roche, N.S., Wakefield, L.M., Heine, U.I., Liotta, L.A., Falanga, V., Kehrl, J.H., and Fauci, A.S. (1986). Transforming growth factor type beta: Rapid induction of fibrosis and angiogenesis in vivo and stimulation of collagen formation in vitro. Proc. Natl. Acad. Sci. USA 83:4167–4171.
71. Raghow, R., Postlethwaite, A.E., Keski-Oja, J., Moses, H.L., and Kang, A.H. (1987). Transforming growth factor-beta increases steady state levels of type I

procollagen and fibronectin messenger RNAs posttranscriptionally in cultured human dermal fibroblasts. J. Clin. Invest. 79:1285-1288.

72. Wrana, J. L., Maeno, M., Hawrylyshyn, B., Yao, K.-L., Domenicucci, C., and Sodek, J. (1988). Differential effects of transforming growth factor-beta on the synthesis of extracellular matrix proteins by normal fetal rat calvarial bone cell populations. J. Cell. Biol. 106:915-924.

73. Varga, J., Rosenbloom, J., and Jimenez, S.A. (1987). Transforming growth factor beta (TGF β) causes a persistent increase in steady-state amounts of type I and type III collagen and fibronectin mRNAs in normal human dermal fibroblasts. J. Biochem. 247:597-604.

74. Kresina, T.F. (1987). Antigen specific T cell hybridomas inhibit the generation of murine collagen-induced arthritis. In: Clinical Immunology. Pruzanski, W., and Selligmann, M., eds. Elsevier Science, Amsterdam, pp. 113-118.

75. Kresina, T. F., Immunotherapy of experimental arthritis: Analysis of the articular cartilage of mice suppressed for collagen-induced arthritis by a T-cell hybridoma. Am. J. Pathol. 129:257-266.

76. Kresina, T. F. (1988). Down-regulation of murine collagen-induced arthritis by a T cell hybridoma. Exp. Cell. Biol. 56:86-102.

77. Kresina, T.F. (1988). Antigen specific down regulation of murine collagen induced arthritis: T suppressor cell circuits in arthritis immunotherapy. Int. Rev. Immunol. 4:91-106.

78. Wooley, P.H., Luthra, H.S., Stuart, J.M., and David, C.S. (1981). Type II collagen-induced arthritis in mice. I. Major histocompatibility complex (I region) linkage and antibody correlates. J. Exp. Med. 154:688-700.

79. Kresina, T.F. (1990). Contra-IL-2 derived from mice suppressed for collagen-induced arthritis. Cell. Immunol. 125:171-182.

80. Smith, M.D., Haynes, D.R., and Roberts-Thomson, P.J. (1989). Interleukin 2 and interleukin 2 inhibitors in human serum and synovial fluid. I. Characterization of the inhibitor and its mechanism of action. J. Rheumatol. 16:149-157.

81. Spannaus-Martin, D.J., and Kresina, T.F. (1989). Mediators of immunotherapy of experimental arthritis I. Identification of contra-IL-2 activity derived from a cloned population of suppressor-inducer T cells. Las Vegas: Orthopedic Research Society, Paper 533.

82. Billingham, M.E.J. (1987). Cytokines as mediators. Br. Med. Bull. 43:350-370.

83. Oppenheim, J.J., Kovacs, E.J., Matsushima, K., and Durum, S.K. (1986). There is more than one interleukin 1. Immunol. Today 7:45-56.

84. Pettipher, E.R., Higgs, G.A., and Henderson, B. (1986). Interleukin 1 induces leukocyte infiltration and cartilage proteoglycan degradation in the synovial joint. Proc. Natl. Acad. Sci. USA 83:8749-8753.

85. Tyler, J.A. (1985). Chondrocyte-mediated depletion of articular cartilage proteoglycans in vitro. Biochem. J. 225:493-507.

86. Pasternak, R.D., Hubbs, S.J., Caccese, R.G., Marks, R.L., Conaty, J.M., and DiPasquale, G. (1986). Interleukin-1 stimulates the secretion of proteoglycan- and collagen-degrading proteases by rabbit articular chondrocytes. Clin. Immunol. Immunopathol. 41:351-367.

87. Gowan, M., Wood, D.D., Ihrie, E.J., McGuire, M.K.B., and Russell, R.G.G. (1983). An interleukin 1 like factor stimulates bone resorption in vitro. Nature 306:378-380.

88. Schmidt, J.A., Mizel, S.B., Cohen, D., and Green, I. (1982). Interleukin 1, a potential regulator of fibroblast proliferation. J. Immunol. 128:2177–2182.
89. Krane, S.M., Dayer, J.-M., Simon, L.S., and Byrne, M.S. (1985). Mononuclear cell-conditioned medium containing mononuclear cell factor (MCF), homologous with interleukin-1, stimulates collagen and fibronectin synthesis by adherent rheumatoid synovial cells: Effects of prostaglandin E_2 and indomethacin. Collagen Relat. Res. 5:99–117.
90. Schnyder, J., and Payne, T. (1985). Effect of interleukin-1 and 2 on enzyme secretion and prostaglandin formation by chondrocytes. Br. J. Rheumatol. (Suppl. 1) 24:128–132.
91. Smith, K.A. (1980). T-cell growth factor. Immunol. Rev. 51:337–357.
92. Kaye, J., Gillis, S., Mizel, S.B., Shevach, E.M., Malek, T.R. Dinarello, C.A. Lachman, L.B., and Janeway, C.A. (1984). Growth of a cloned helper T cell line induced by a monoclonal antibody specific for the antigen receptor: Interleukin-1 is required for the expression of receptors for interleukin-2. J. Immunol. 133:1339–1345.
93. Sauder, D.H. (1984). Epidermal cytokines: Properties of epidermal cell thymocyte-activating factor (ETAF). Lymph. Res. 4:145–152.
94. Nouri, A.M.E., Panayi, G.S., and Goodman, S.M. (1984). Cytokines and the chronic inflammation of rheumatic disease. I. The presence of interleukin-1 in synovial fluids. Clin. Exp. Immunol. 55:295–302.
95. Smith, K.A. (1988). Interleukin-2: Inception, impact and implications. Science 240:1169–1176.
96. Ting, C.-C., Yang, S.S., and Hargrove, M.E. (1984). Induction of suppressor T cells by interleukin-2. J. Immunol. 133:261–266.
97. Efrat, S., and Kaempfer, R. (1984). Control of biologically active interleukin 2 messenger RNA formation in induced human lymphocytes. Proc. Natl. Acad. Sci. USA 81:2601–2605.
98. Nakanishi, K., Malek, T.R., Smith, K.A., Hamaoka, T., Shevach, E.M., and Paul, W.E. (1984). Both interleukin 2 and a second T cell-derived factor in EL-4 supernatant have activity as differentiation factors in IgM synthesis. J. Exp. Med. 160:1605–1621.
99. Mittler, R., Rao, P., Olini, G., Westberg, E., Newman, W., Hoffman, M., and Goldstein, G. (1985). Activated human B cells display a functional IL 2 receptor. J. Immunol. 134:2393–2399.
100. Ralph, P., Jeong, G., Welte, K., Mertelsmann, R., Rabin, H., Henderson, L.E., Souza, L.M., Boone, T.C., and Robb, R. J. (1984). Stimulation of immunoglobulin secretion in human B lymphocytes as a direct effect of high concentrations of IL 2. J. Immunol. 133:2442–2445.
101. Howard, M., Matis, L., Malek, T.R., Shevach, E., Kell, W., Cohen, D., Nakanishi, K., and Paul, W.E. (1983). Interleukin 2 induces antigen-reactive T cell lines to secrete BCGF-I. J. Exp. Med. 158:2024–2039.
102. Farrar, J.J., Benjamin, W.R., Hilfiker, M.L., Howard, M., Farrar, W.L., and Fuller-Farrar, J. (1982). The biochemistry, biology, and role of interleukin 2 in

the induction of cytotoxic T cell and antibody-forming B cell responses. Immunol. Rev. 63:129–166.

103. Davidson, W.F., Roths, J.B., Holmes, K.L., Rudikoft, E., and Morse, H.C., III (1984). Dissociation of severe lupus-like disease from polyclonal B cell activation and IL 2 deficiency in C3H-1pr/1pr mice. J. Immunol. 133:1048–1056.

104. Dauphinee, M.J., Kipper, S.B. Wofsy, D., and Talal, N. (1981). Interleukin 2 deficiency is a common feature of autoimmune mice. J. Immunol. 127:2483–2487.

105. Talal, N., Dauphinee, M.J., and Wofsy, D. (1982). Interleukin-2 deficiency, genes, and systemic lupus erythematosus. Arthritis Rheum. 25:838–842.

106. Santoro, T.J., Luger, T.A., Ravache, E.S., Smolen, J.S., Oppenheim, J.J., and Steinberg, A.D. (1983). In vitro correction of the interleukin 2 defect of autoimmune mice. Eur. J. Immunol. 13:601–604.

107. Stamenkovic, I., Stegagno, M., Wright, K.A., Krane, S.M., Amento, E.P. Colvin, R.B., Duquesnoy, R.J., and Kurnick, J.T. (1988). Clonal dominance among T-lymphocyte infiltrates in arthritis. Proc. Natl. Acad. Sci. USA 85:1179–1183.

108. Lemm, G., and Warnatz, H. (1986). Evidence for enhanced interleukin-2 (IL-2) secretion and IL-2 receptor presentation by synovial fluid lymphocytes in rheumatoid arthritis. Clin. Exp. Immunol. 64:71–79.

109. Nouri, A.M.E., Panayi, G.S., and Goodman, S.M. (1984). Cytokines and the chronic inflammation of rheumatic disease. II. The presence of interleukin-2 in synovial fluids. Clin. Exp. Immunol. 58:402–409.

110. Firestein, G.S., Xu, W.D., Townsend, K., Broide, D., Alvaro-Garcia, J., Glasebrook, A., and Zvaifler, N.J. (1988). Cytokines in chronic inflammatory arthritis. I. Failure to detect T cell lymphokines (IL-2 and IL-3) and the presence of CSF-1 and a novel mast cell growth factor in rheumatoid arthritis. J. Exp. Med. 168:1573–1586.

111. Llorente, L., Crevon, M.-C., Karray, S., Defrance, T., Banchereau, J., and Galanaud, P. (1989). Interleukin (IL) 4 counteracts the helper effect of IL-2 on antigen-activated human B cells. Eur. J. Immunol. 19:765–769.

112. Lichtman, A.H., Kurt-Jones, E.A., and Abbas, A.K. (1987). B-cell stimulatory factor 1 and not interleukin 2 is the autocrine growth factor for some helper T lymphocytes. Proc. Natl. Acad. Sci. USA 84:824–827.

113. Carding, S. R., and Bottomly, K. (1988). IL-4 (B cell stimulatory factor 1) exhibits thymocyte growth factor activity in the presence of IL-2 J. Immunol. 140:1519–1526.

114. Takai, Y., Wong, G.G., Clark, S.C., Burakoff, S.J., and Herrmann, S.H. (1988). B cell stimulatory factor-2 is involved in the differentiation of cytotoxic T lymphocytes. J. Immunol. 140:508–512.

115. Garman, R.D., Jacobs, K.A., Clark, S.C., and Raulet, D.H. (1987). B-cell stimulatory factor 2 (beta 2 interferon) funtions as a second signal for interleukin-2 production by mature murine T cells. Proc. Natl. Acad. Sci. USA 84:7629–7633.

116. Kishimoto, T. (1985). Factors affecting B-cell growth and differentiation. Annu. Rev. Immunol. 3:133–157.

117. Guerne, P.-A., Zuraw, B.L., Vaughan, J.H., Carson, D.A. and Lotz, M. (1989). Synovium as a source of interleukin-6 in vitro. Contribution to local and systemic manifestations of arthritis. J. Clin Invest. 83:585–592.

118. Takai, Y., Seki, N., Senoh, H., Yokota, T., Lee, F., Hamaoka, T., and Fujiwara, H. (1989). Enhanced production of interleukin-6 in mice with type II collagen-induced arthritis. Arthritis Rheum. 32:594–600.

119. Waage, A., Kaufmann, C., Espevik, T., and Husby, G. (1989). Interleukin-6 in synovial fluid from patients with arthritis. Clin. Immunol. Immunopathol. 50:394–398.

120. Houssiau, F., Devogelaer, J.-P., Van Damme, J., de Deuxchaisnes, C.N., and Van Snick, J. (1988). Interleukin-6 in synovial fluid and serum of patients with rheumatoid arthritis and other inflammatory arthritides. Arthritis Rheum. 31:784–788.

121. Balavoine, J.-F., deRochemonteix, B., Williamson, K., Seckinger, P., Cruchaud, A., and Dayer, J.-M. (1986). Prostaglandin E_2 and collagenase production by fibroblasts and synovial cells is regulated by urine-derived human interleukin 1 and inhibitor(s). J. Clin. Invest. 78:1120–1124.

122. Seckinger, P., and Dayer, J.-M. (1987). Interleukin-1 inhibitors. Ann. Inst. Pasteur Immunol. 138:486–488.

123. Prieur, A.-M., Kaufmann, M.-T., Griscelli, C., and Dayer, J.-M. (1987). Specific interleukin-1 inhibitor in serum and urine of children with systemic juvenile chronic arthritis. Lancet 2:1240–1242.

124. Westacott, C.I., Whicher, J.T., Hutton, C.W., and Dieppe, P.A. (1988). Increased spontaneous production of interleukin-1 together with inhibitory activity in systemic sclerosis. Clin. Sci. 75:561–567.

125. Miossec, P., Kashiwado, T., and Ziff, M., (1987). Inhibitor of interleukin-2 in rheumatoid synovial fluid. Arthritis Rheum. 30:121–129.

126. Yamagata, N., Kobayashi, K., Kasama, T., Fukushima, T., Tabata M., Yoneya, I., Shikama, Y., Kaga, S., Hashimoto, M., Yoshida, K., Sekine, F., Negishi, M., Ide, H., Mori, Y., and Takahashi, T. (1988). Multiple cytokine activities and loss of interleukin 2 inhibitor in synovial fluids of patients with rheumatoid arthritis. J. Rheum. 15:1623–1627.

127. Xu, W.D., Firestein, G.S., Taetle, R., Kaushansky, K., and Zvaifler, N.J. (1989). Cytokines in chronic inflammatory arthritis.II. Granulocyte-macrophage colony stimulating factor in rheumatoid synovial effusions.J. Clin. Invest. 83::876–882.

128. Morrissey, P.J., Bressler, L., Park, L.S., Alpert, A., and Gillis, S. (1987). Granulocyte-macrophage colony-stimulating factor augments the primary antibody response by enhancing the function of antigen-presenting cells. J. Immunol. 139:1113–1119.

129. Buchan, G., Barrett, K., Fujita, T., Taniguchi, T., Maini, R., and Feldmann, M. (1988). Detection of activated T cell products in the rheumatoid joint using cDNA probes to interleukin-2 (IL-2), IL-2 receptor, and IFN-gamma. Clin. Exp. Immunol. 71:295–301.

130. Husby, G., and Williams, R.C. (1985). Immunohistochemical studies of interleukin-2 and gamma-interferon in rheumatoid arthritis. Arthritis Rheum. 28:174–181.

131. Degre, M., Mellbye, D.J., and Clarke-Jenssen, O. (1983). Immune interferon in the serum and synovial fluid in rheumatoid arthritis and related disorders. Ann. Rheum. Dis. 42:672–676.

132. Cesario, T.C., Andrews, B.S., Martin, D.A., Jason, M., Treadwell, T., Friou, G., and Tilles, J.A. (1983). Interferon in synovial fluid and serum of patients with rheumatic disease. J. Rheumatol. 10:647–650.

133. Firestein, G.S., and Zvaifler, N.J. (1987). Peripheral blood and synovial fluid monocyte activation in inflammatory arthritis. II. Low levels of synovial fluid and synovial tissue interferon suggest that gamma-interferon is not the primary macrophage activating factor. Arthritis Rheum. 30:864–871.

134. Stolzenburg, T., Binz, R., Fontana, A., Felder, N.A., and Wagenhauser, F.J. (1988). Impaired mitogen-induced interferon gamma production in rheumatoid arthritis and related diseases. Scand. J. Immunol. 27:73–82.

135. Combe, B., Pope, R.M., Fischbach, M., Darnell, B., Baron, S., and Talal, N. (1985). Interleukin-2 in rheumatoid arthritis: Production of and response to interleukin-2 in rheumatoid synovial fluid, synovial tissue and peripheral blood. Clin. Exp. Immunol. 59:520–528.

136. Sporn, M.B., Roberts, A.B., Wakefield, L.M., and Assoian, R. K. (1986). Transforming growth factor-beta: Biological function and chemical structure. Science 233:532–534.

137. Seyedin, S.M., Thompson, A.Y., Bentz, H., Rosen, D.M., McPherson, J.M., Conti, A., Sigel, N.R., Gallupi, G.R., and Piez, K.A. (1986). Cartilage-inducing factor-A. Apparent identity to transforming growth factor-beta. J. Biol. Chem. 261:5693–5695.

138. Kehrl, J.H., Roberts, A.B., Wakefield, L.M., Jakowlew, S., Sporn, M.B., and Fauci, A.S. (1986). Transforming growth factor beta is an important immuno-modulatory protein human B lymphocytes. J. Immunol. 137:3855–3860.

139. Kehrl, J.H., Wakefield, L.M., Roberts, A.B., Jakowlew, S., Alvarez-Mon, M., Derynck, R., Sporn, M.B., and Fauci, A.S. (1986). Production of transforming growth factor beta by human T lymphocytes and its potential role in the reduction of T cell growth. J. Exp. Med. 163:1037–1050.

140. O'Keefe, R.J., Puzas, J.E., Brand, J.S., and Rosier, R.N. (1988). Effects of transforming growth factor-beta on matrix synthesis by growth plate chondrocytes. Endocrinology 122:2953–2960.

141. Kresina, T.F., and Newman, W. Amelioration of CIA by in vivo administration of TGF-β. (Submitted).

142. Dayer, J.-M., Beutler, B., and Cerami, A. (1985). Cachectin/tumor necrosis factor stimulates collagenase and prostaglandin E_2 production by human synovial cells and dermal fibroblasts. J. Exp. Med. 162:2163–2168.

143. Bertolini, D.R., Nedwin, G.E., Bringman, T.S., Smith, D.D., and Mundy, G.R. (1986). Stimulation of bone resorption and inhibition of bone formation in vitro by human tumour necrosis factors. Nature 319:516–518.

144. Gamble, J.R., Harlan, J.M., Klebanoff, S.J., and Vadas, M.A. (1985). Stimulation of the adherence of neutrophils to umbilical vein endothelium by human recombinant tumor necrosis factor. Proc. Natl. Acad. Sci. USA 82:8667–8671.

145. Takahashi, N., Mundy, G.R., and Roodman, G.D. (1986). Recombinant human interferon-gamma inhibits formation of human osteoclast-like cells. J. Immunol. 137:3544–3549.

146. Wolfe, F., Cathey, M.A., Hawley, D.J., Balser, J.P., and Schindler, J.D. (1986). Clinical trial with rIFN-G in rheumatoid arthritis. In: Biologically Based Immunomodulators in the Therapy of Rheumatic Diseases. Pincus, S.H., Pisetsky, D.S., and Rosenwasser, L.J., Eds. Elsevier, Amsterdam, pp. 379–396.

147. Veys, E.M., Mielants, H., Verbruggen, G., Grosclaude, J.-P., Meyer, W., Galazka, A., and Schindler, J. (1988). Interferon gamma in rheumatoid arthritis—a double blind study comparing human recombinant interferon gamma with placebo. J. Rheumatol. 15:570–574.

148. Weinstein, A., and Utsinger, P.D. (1985). Immunoregulatory drugs. In: Rheumatoid Arthritis. Utsinger, P.D., Zvaifler, N.J., and Ehrlich, G.E., eds. J.B. Lippincott, Philadelphia, pp. 635–644.

149. Ichikawa, M., Yanagisawa, M., Kawai, H., Kamijo, T., Komiyama, A., and Akabane, T. (1988). Spontaneous improvement of juvenile rheumatoid arthritis after T lymphocytosis with suppressor phenotype and function. J. Clin. Lab. Immunol. 27:197–201.

10

Induction and Regulation of Arthritis by T Cell-Derived Collagen Binding Proteins

David E. Trentham
Harvard Medical School and Beth Israel Hospital, Boston, Massachusetts

I. INTRODUCTION

This chapter describes the present knowledge and therapeutic potential for inflammatory arthritis of a unique set of proteins designated T cell-derived antigen binding molecules (TABM) or antigen-specific lymphokines or factors. The term TABM is used to assist in distinguishing these antigen binding proteins from conventional lymphokines or interleukins, which have no antigen uniqueness with regard to their generation or effector functions. Much of the content of this chapter deals with proteins that bind to type II collagen, as does collagenase. However, the T cell origin and lack of degradative activity clearly distinguish these collagen binding factors from members of the collagenase family of enzymes. To adequately discuss the potential therapeutic usefulness of collagen binding TABM, the review also provides an update on the increasing evidence that autoimmunity to type II collagen is pivotal for the expression of joint and eye inflammation in certain human connective tissue diseases. Because it could be critical for the understanding of inflammatory arthritis, the primary pathogenesis of collagen arthritis is also covered.

The intent of this chapter is not simply to provide coverage of totally accepted areas but to delineate recent information, much of which is preliminary and require further scientific scrutiny. Thus, the goal of this review is to pinpoint promising new insights for which additional investigative work could lead to major therapeutic breakthroughs for patients with inflammatory arthritis. Only a highly condensed reference list is included since reviews of TABM (1,2) and autoimmunity to collagen (3–6) have recently appeared.

II. TABM

One of the major contributors to the field of TABM, Robert Cone, has convincingly traced the origin of awareness of the functional profile of TABM to work that suggested the presence of antibodylike but clearly nonimmunoglobulin activities in states of tuberculin hypersensitivity (2). Even today, TABM can be succinctly considered highly potent effector molecules, uniquely programmed by antigen and both displayed on their surface and released in a soluble form by certain T cells. These aspects are extremely analogous to B cells and their production of antibodies. In fact, TABM can accurately be described as antibodylike proteins released by T cells. The ability of T cells that produce TABM to recognize conformational or native epitopes on at least certain antigens and to interact with antigen without constraints imposed by contiguous structures designed by the major histocompatibility complex (MHC) are also strikingly parallel to that of B cells and antibodies.

The conformational but not MHC-restricted properties of TABM have been features consistently uncovered by laboratories investigating a number of such factors (7–25). Despite clear-cut experimental outcomes, these two attributes have provoked prolonged controversy, largely among those outside of the field. Although workers described the findings that appeared "under their noses,"TABM appeared to be heretical "beasts" to the proponents of classic cellular immunology, who knew that T cells experience sequential epitopes passed to them in a processed fashion by antigen-presenting cells and that MHC governance operated in the helper, suppressor, and cytotoxic T cell limbs.

Fortunately, Askenase and associates appear to have recently provided data that coherently explain, even for TABM agnostics, the peculiarities of TABM (25). If their findings with one TABM system turn out to be universally applicable, the following scenario for TABM will be established. TABM are not the offspring of fully mature CD4 or CD8 cells but exist on the surface and are shed from cells that have received relatively scant programming by the thymus. Although the absence of B cell and macrophage markers and the presence of Thy-1, at least in the mouse, enable the TABM-generating cells to be included within the T cell repertoire, they are phenotypically, "triple negative"; that is, they fail to stain with antisera to CD3, CD4, and CD8, as well as to MHC class I and II molecules. Askenase's TABM-producing cell is even more intriguing in that it is described as interleukin-2 receptor negative, capable of recognizing conformational epitopes, and exhibiting an ability to proliferate when exposed to interleukin-3. The presence of these TABM-producing cells in nude mice, in which mature T cells do not exist (25), has made these discoveries particularly convincing. Perusal of much of the TABM literature yields information consistent with the revelation of Askenase et al. that TABM are immunoglobulinlike products of cells that are somewhere between classic mature T cells and B cells. This startlingly simple explanation completely explains the unusual properties of TABM, which were previously judged to be maverick. Even the site of tissue residence of Askenase's TABM- producing cell is unusual—rather than being largely blood or lymph borne or remaining within splenic or lymph node structures, the cell seems to exist in at least sizable quantities in the skin.

This dermal residence ties in nicely with a two-tier demarcation to delayed-type hypersensitivity (DTH) recently proposed by the group at Yale (25). In a sensitized host, relevant antigen injected into the skin quickly interacts, not with intermediary antigen-presenting cells, but with Thy-1$^+$, triple negative TABM-producing cells via antigen binding surface molecules. The cell is devoid of MHC determinants and, when required, the antigen binding molecule interdigitates with quarternary epitopes, just as antibodies are capable of doing.

The TABM-producing cell then releases the TABM, and these highly soluble proteins recruit additional elements of the inflammatory and immune system. Non-antigen binding regions of the TABM, possibly analogous to the Fc portion of immunoglobulin, bind to specific TABM receptors on mast cells and trigger degranulation and release of a variety of vasoactive materials, such as histamine and bradykinin. This process enables an early stage of DTH to be recognized as a "wheal-and-flare" by 2 h after antigen challenge. Although the precise pathways have not been elucidated, TABM also probably influence antigen presenting cells to relinquish a dormant state, engulf antigen, and present it in a partially degraded state to antigen-relevant CD4$^+$ helper T cells. By this mechanism, the classic stage, which is actually a second phase of DTH, begins and culminates in the full-blown expression of DTH 24–48 h later.

The two-stage pathway of DTH, that is, initiation by TABM and magnification by CD4$^+$ cells, may have biologic relevance far beyond the purpose of eliciting positive skin tests to recall antigens. Autoimmunity has previously been considered a response provided by disease-specific autoantibodies or interleukins generated vicariously as a byproduct of disease-specific CD4$^+$ cells. Additional possibilities can now be formulated. Autoimmunity can be at least partially subserved by disease-specific TABM. A look at the biochemical and functional properties of previously described TABM is thus in order.

Similarities of TABM with antibodies continue to be evident when the physico-chemical and functional properties of TABM are analyzed. Although no TABM has been sequenced at present, large-scale manufacture by T cell lines or hybridomas and purification by antigen or antibody affinity techniques have enabled considerable progress to be achieved in terms of understanding the structure and composition of TABM. TABM are smaller than immunoglobulins and frequently display a tendency to aggregate into various sizes. Molecular weights of approximately 45, 60, or even 120 kD have been frequently identified (1,2). Perhaps quite importantly, TABM isotypes (or classes) have been detected in several systems (1,2). It appears likely that additional work will enable classification of TABM, based on shared major framework regions, into IgG, IgM, and IgA equivalents, for example. Currently, a cartoon mimicking the structure of an IgG molecule appears to reflect reasonably well the conceived appearance of a TABM, although the valency of TABM with respect to antigen is far from worked out.

Several physicochemical properties of TABM have unfortunately impeded analysis of these effector proteins. Such drawbacks include their size similarity to albumin, resulting in albumin-attributable contamination of TABM preparations and incorrectness of antisera, their propensity to adhere avidly to plastic, and their lability during attempted prolonged storage, particularly in a highly purified state (1,2). The initial sequencing or production of a TABM by recombinant means will therefore represent a substantial breakthrough in this field.

Mainly immunoregulatory functions have been described for TABM. It is probable that many of the so-called antigen-specific T suppressor factors described in a biochemically elegant fashion close to a decade ago were actually TABM (26). Although the initial reports were enthusiastically received, the scant amount of material available and the functional ambiguities in the systems dampened interest in the area of antigen-specific suppressor factors. Over the next few years the area received more inattention or criticism than additional work. Recently, however, hapten-or antigen-specific TABM have been described in the mouse with T helper, T suppressor-inducer, and even T contrasuppressor capabilities (2). Additional TABM able to influence atopic states have been detected (2). Finally, TABM capable of monitoring tissue inflammation have been reported in the rat (19–21); these TABM are type II collagen binding and are the dominant subject of the remainder of this chapter.

III. AUTOIMMUNITY TO COLLAGEN AS A RELEVANT EFFECTOR MECHANISM IN INFLAMMATORY ARTHRITIS

Collagen-binding TABM are unlikely to have relevance for inflammatory arthritis unless autoimmunity to type II collagen at least partly contributes to the fundamental pathogenesis of these diseases. The designation inflammatory arthritis is used because of the demonstrated presence of autoimmunity of collagen in patients with rheumatoid arthritis, psoriatic arthritis, juvenile rheumatoid arthritis, and relapsing polychondritis (reviewed in Ref. 4). The most compelling evidence that autoimmunity to collagen actually provokes human disease is the ability of sensitization to native, but not denatured, type II collagen to initiate in rats (27), mice (28,29), and monkeys (30–33) a morphologic counterpart to chronic inflammatory arthritis. The recent work with primates (3,30–33) has kindled further interest in this possibility, as has the recognition that rats with collagen arthritis frequently exhibit anterior uveitis, a composite that recapitulates the damage encountered in many patients with juvenile rheumatoid arthritis (O'Brien, Albert, and Trentham, unpublished data).

Not only has the recent work in collagen arthritis become more compelling, but the use of more sophisticated T cell (34) and autoantibody techniques has substantiated earlier reports that a substantial proportion of patients with inflammatory arthritis exhibit autoimmunity to type II collagen. This knowledge has more firmly wedded the animal model work with human disease.

Studies in animals and humans have reached a point at which probably the only way that the collagen autoimmunity theory can be more substantially tested is by ascertaining the effect of collagen-specific immunosuppression on inflammatory arthritis in humans. Attempts by the author to induce tolerance to type II collagen by peroral antigen administration, as has been done in collagen arthritis (35), will start in patients with inflammatory arthritis in the very near future. If efficient and antigen-specific immunosuppression is achieved, a judgment regarding the validity of the collagen hypothesis could be reached by observing the effect on disease expression. Additional avenues, such as the use of T cell vaccination (36), could also be tried to solidify or refute the collagen hypothesis.

IV. ARTHRITOGENIC FACTOR

Efforts to determine whether lymphokines were the major inciting factor in collagen arthritis were upscaled when it became apparent that antibodies to collagen lacked the capacity to induce proliferative synovitis in passive transfer experiments in the rat (19). To quantify any effect that antibody had on the synovium, a bioassay was developed in which the synovium of the knee was analyzed by light microscopy after intra-articular injection of test material in an immunologically naive animal (19). In contrast to antibody, alliquots of type II collagen-specific T cells, obtained from T cell lines expanded by periodic exposure to type II collagen in vitro, proved to be highly efficient at creating a prolonged proliferative synovitis that closely simulated the lesion in the primary model (37). Marked joint inflammation was apparent even when as few as 1000 T cells were injected (37). The highly cellular nature of the experimental synovitis induced by collagen-reactive T line cells strongly suggested that the process involved lymphokine release, and additional experiments showed that the line cell lesion could be recreated by injection of supernatant material derived from cultures containing collagen-specific T cells (19).

Initial estimates of molecular size used gel filtration and isolated the active principle to a 60–70 kD range (19). A paradox arose when attempts to upgrade production of the lymphokine(s) of interest by mitogen stimulation of cells were totally unsuccessful. The possibility that the arthritogenic protein was not a conventional interleukin, and thus would not be efficiently generated by mitogen exposure, was then considered. Because the cell line-induced synovitis depended specifically on type II collagen-sensitized T cells, it was hypothesized that the 60–70 kD protein was also collagen specific and, thereby, a newly discovered TABM. Because TABM can be purified by antigen affinity chromatography, columns of type II collagen were constructed as a test ligand. Experiments predicated on this notion yielded an approximately 65 kD protein that bound to type II collagen. When instilled into the knee, the factor created the same magnitude of joint inflammation as did the use of line cells (19,37). As little as 10 μg of protein, which was designated arthritogenic factor (AF), produced substantial inflammation and even cartilage erosion in the knee joint bioassay. To determine whether AF was an exclusive attribute of the collagen model, analogous studies were conducted in rats with adjuvant arthritis, resulting in a biochemically and functionally identical AF species being identified (20).

All the properties of other TABM seem to apply to AF. These include (1) production by T cells; (2) ability to bind conformational determinants on the inducing antigen; (3) existence on the surface of T cells, as determined by a monospecific antibody and flow cytometry; (4) non-MHC restriction, demonstrated by an ability of rat AF to induce synovitis across strains and in the mouse; (5) the ability to interact with mast cells (see later); and (6) isoelectric point similarities and recognition by certain other TABM antisera, suggesting isotypic identities of AF with murine TABM (performed in collaboration with Cone). Although the parental cell for AF was initially assumed to be CD4$^+$ because greater than 90% of the line cells routinely used to generate AF displayed CD4 (19–21), the findings of Askenase et al. (25) are currently stimulating a reappraisal to determine whether a minority population within the lines is the actual generator of AF.

The way in which AF triggers sustained synovial inflammation is a major unanswered question. Additional pathways, recruited by AF, are likely to operate. Within 2 h of instillation of AF, mast cells in the subsynovial region of the knee start to undergo degranulation (21). In addition, polymorphonuclear leukocytes are transversing through nascent openings in the subsynovial capillaries into extraluminal sites by this time.

Although much of the inflammation in the initial stage appears to be quite nonspecific, some attribute(s) of AF must enable the protein to incite synoviocyte proliferation, which is recognizable by 24–48 h after injection and persists for weeks thereafter. One way the process would become better defined is to ascertain whether synoviocytes possess receptors for AF. Alternatively, communications between AF and chondrocytes could be involved.

The recognition of AF, coupled with the outcome of passive transfer experiments (19), now allow a fairly coherent understanding of the pathogenesis of collagen arthritis. The primary pathway is surprisingly simple. Immunogenetic governance is critical (29). In a susceptible animal, injection of type II collagen possessing unaltered quarternary epitopes in a vehicle that promotes interactions with immunocompetent cells (adjuvant oil) leads to clonal expansion of collagen autoreactive T cells that produce the TABM, AF. Homing of AF to joint tissues both initiates and helps to propagate collagen arthritis. Although antibodies to collagen could accelerate the magnitude of synovial inflammation when disease is established, immunoglobulin is not the inciting factor. Evidence for this statement includes the clear presence of synovial changes on day 3 postimmunization (38), which is well before the onset of collagen antibody production, as well as the inability of passively administered antibody to provoke a hypertrophic synovial lesion (19). Whether a similar process contributes to the onset of inflammatory arthritis in humans is a speculation deserving scrutiny.

V. ANTIARTHRITIC FACTOR

During recent studies, a second collagen-binding TABM has been identified. Because the work is unpublished, only a very preliminary description of the new TABM is included in this review. The protein has a molecular weight of approximately 55 kD, is antigenically distinct from AF, suggesting that it is not merely a fragment of the larger protein AF, and has the ability to suppress the induction of collagen arthritis and modify the immune response to collagen in a non-MHC–restricted manner when administered intravenously to collagen-immunized rats. Because its cell of origin does not bear the CD8 phenotype, it is likely that the collagen-specific antiarthritic factor belongs to the TABM family of T suppressor-inducer factors (TsiF). It is possible that collagen-binding TsiF regulate, endogenously, collagen arthritis. The maximum disease severity in the primary model is exhibited in the rat 15–30 days postimmunization; a gradual subsidence in joint inflammation occurs thereafter, with exacerbations promptly achievable with booster doses of collagen. Within the complex T cell circuitry, TABM-producing cells could activate suppressor T cell elements and thereby attenuate disease manifestations in the collagen model. By extrapolation, TABM—TsiF appear to have considerable potential as novel future therapies for autoimmune disease.

VI. POTENTIAL FOR TABM IN THE TREATMENT OF AUTOIMMUNE DISEASE

The existing knowledge of TABM strongly suggests that they possess almost ideal properties for the treatment of autoimmune disease. The attractive features include (1) the prospect that each autoimmune disease is uniquely driven by a central self antigen response and is thereby capable of being palliated by an autoantigen-specific intervention; (2) TABM being both antigen-specific and potent immunoregulatory molecules; (3) TABM being at their effector stage, non-MHC–restricted and even active across species, thus heterologous TABM might be fully sufficient and emanently safe for use in unrelated humans with an autoimmune disease; (4) TABM being fairly small proteins and, theoretically, synthesizable by recombinant DNA technology—active peptide fragments are also a possibility; (5) the cell surface expression of TABM, enabling efficient immunotoxin destruction of disease producing TABM-bearing T cells; (6) the prospect the subcutaneous administration would be sufficient for TABM therapy; (7) the possibility of co-TABM directed therapy, all targeted at an antigen-specific response, for example, elimination of AF-producing T cells by immunotoxin and simultaneous administration of collagen-binding TsiF.

Autoimmune disease other than inflammatory arthritis could be susceptible to TABM therapy. If native DNA is the antiself reactivity pivotal for the expression of systemic lupus erythematosus, DNA-binding TABM might be therapeutically useful. Allograft survival, allergic states, and cancer immunotherapy represent additional areas that might be approached by TABM.

Coexistent with the attractive but speculative status of TABM are theoretical concerns. An immunogenic potential exists, particularly since TABM would probably need to be administered parenterally. An anti-TABM response could nullify or limit the intended effect of TABM. Moreover, a contra-TABM response, similar to an anti-idiotypic cascade, could be generated by the immune system and abort the intended therapeutic effect. Regardless of these reservations, TABM appear to represent almost a singular new opportunity for the disciplines of cellular immunology and molecular biology to formulate effective therapeutic measures for autoimmune disease. Full utilization of the TABM approach in the upcoming decade could lead to better control of autoimmune disease.

REFERENCES

1. Cone, R.E. (1987). Non-MHC-restricted T cell antigen-binding proteins. Methods Enzymol. 150:666–681.
2. Cone, R.E., Zheng, H., Chue, B., Beaman, K., Ferguson, T., and Green, D.R. (1988). T cell-derived antigen binding molecules (TABM): Molecular and functional properties. Int. Rev. Immunol. 3:205–228.
3. Stuart, J.M., and Kang, A.H. (1986). Monkeying around with collagen autoimmunity and arthritis. Lab. Invest. 54:1–3.
4. Trentham, D.E. (1987). Clues provided by animal models of arthritis. Rheum. Dis. Clin. North Am. 13:307–318.
5. Breedveld, F.C., and Trentham, D.E. (1987). Progress in the understanding of inducible models of chronic arthritis. Rheum. Dis. Clin. North Am. 13:531–544.
6. Trentham, D.E. (1988). Collagen arthritis in rats, arthritogenic lymphokines and other aspects. Int. Rev. Immunol. 4:25–33.

7. Van Loveren, H., Meade, R., and Askenase, P.W. (1983). An early component of delayed-type hypersensitivity mediated by T cells and mast cells. J. Exp. Med. 157:1604–1617.

8. Kops, S.K., Van Loveren, H., Rosenstein R.W., Ptak, W., and Askenase, P.W. (1984). Mast cell activation and vascular alterations in immediate hypersensitivity-like reactions induced by a T cell-derived antigen-binding factor. Lab. Invest. 50:421–434.

9. Van Loveren, H., Kraeuter-Kops, S., and Askenase, P.W. (1984). Different mechanisms of release of vasoactive amines by mast cells occur in T cell-dependent compared to IgE-dependent cutaneous hypersensitivity responses. Eur. J. Immunol. 14:40–47.

10. Van Loveren, H., Kato, K., Meade, R., Green, D.R., Horowitz, M., Ptak, W., and Askenase, P.W. (1984). Characterization of two different Ly-1 + T cell populations that mediate delayed-type hypersensitivity. J. Immunol. 133:2402–2411.

11. Van Loveren, H., and Askenase, P.W. (1984). Delayed-type hypersensitivity is mediated by a sequence of two different T cell activities. J. Immunol. 133:2397–2401.

12. Van Loveren, H., Den Otter, W., Meade, R., Terheggen, P.M.A.B., and Askenase P.W. (1985). A role for mast cells and the vasoactive amine serotonin in T cell-dependent immunity to tumors. J. Immunol. 134:1292–1299.

13. Kops, S.K., Ratzlaff, R.E., Meade, R., Iverson, G.M., and Askenase, P.W. (1986). Interaction of antigen-specific T cell factors with unique "receptors" on the surface of mast cells: Demonstration in vitro by an indirect rosetting technique. J. Immunol. 136:4515–4524.

14. Ptak, W., Bereta, M., Ptak, M., and Askenase, P.W. (1986). Isotype-like suppression of T cell-mediated immunity in vivo I. Delayed-type hypersensitivity specificity of T cell suppression induced by antigen-binding T cell factors that initiate contact sensitivity. J. Immunol. 136:1554–1563.

15. Van Loveren, H., Ratzlaff, R.E., Kato, K., Meade, R., Ferguson, T.A., Iverson, G.M., Janeway, G.A., and Askenase, P.W. (1986). Immune serum from mice contact-sensitized with picryl chloride contains an antigen-specific T cell factor that transfers immediate cutaneous reactivity. Eur. J. Immunol. 16:1203–1208.

16. Ptak, W., Bereta, M., Ptak, M., and Askenase, P.W. (1986). Isotype-like suppression of T cell-mediated immunity in vivo. II. Suppression of the early component of contact sensitivity by a Ly-2 + T cell-derived suppressor fator that binds to contact sensitivity-initiating, antigen-specific, Ly-1+ T cell-derived factors that are of different antigen specificities. J. Immunol. 136:1564–1570.

17. Ferguson, T.A., and Iverson, G.M. (1986). Isolation and characterization of an antigen-specific suppressor inducer molecule from serum of hyperimmune mice by using a monoclonal antibody. J. Immunol. 136:2896–2903.

18. Cone, R.E., Gerardi, D.A., Davidoff, J., Petty, J., Kobayashi, K., and Cohen, S. (1987). Quantitation of T cell antigen-binding molecules (TABM) in the sera of nonimmunized, immunized, and desensitized mice. J. Immunol. 138:234–239.

19. Helfgott, S.M., Dynesius-Trentham, R., Brahn, E., and Trentham, D.E. (1985). An arthritogenic lymphokine in the rat. J. Exp. Med. 162:1531–1545.

20. Helfgott, S.M., Kieval, R.I., Breedveld, F.C., Brahn, E., Young, C.T., Dynesius-Trentham, R., and Trentham, D.E. (1988). Detection of arthritogenic factor in adjuvant arthritis. J. Immunol 140:1838-1843.

21. Caulfield, J.P., Hein, A., Helfgott, S.M., Brahn, E., Dynesius-Trentham, R.A., and Trentham, D.E. (1988). Intraarticular injection of arthritogenic factor causes mast cell degranulation, inflammation, fat necrosis, and synovial hyperplasia. Lab. Invest. 59:82-95.

22. Meade, R., Van Loveren, H., Parmentier, H., Iverson, G.M., and Askenase, P.W. (1988). The antigen-binding T cell factor PCl-F sensitizes mast cells for in vitro release of serotonin: Comparison with monoclonal antibody. J. Immunol. 141:2704-2713.

23. Chue, B., Ferguson, T.A., Beaman, K.D., Rosenman, S.J., Cone, R.E., Flood, P.M., and Green, D.R. (1989). An approach to the unification of suppressor T cell circuits: A simplified assay for the induction of suppression by T cell-derived, antigen-binding molecules (T-ABM). Cell. Immunol. 118:30-40.

24. Dietsch, G.N., and Hinricks, D.J. (1989). The role of mast cells in the elicitation of experimental allergic encephalomyelitis. J. Immunol. 142:1476-1481.

25. Herzog, W.R., Meade, R., Pettinicchi, A., Ptak, W., and Askenase, P.W. (1989). Nude mice produce a T cell-derived antigen-binding factor that mediates the early component of delayed-type hypersensitivity. J. Immunol. 142:1803-1812.

26. Fresno, M., McVay-Boudreau, L., Nabel, G., and Cantor, H. (1981). Antigen-specific T lymphocyte clones. II. Purification and biological characterization of an antigen-specific suppressive protein synthesized by cloned T cells. J. Exp. Med. 153:1260-1273.

27. Trentham, D.E., Townes, A.S., and Kang, A.H. (1977). Autoimmunity to type II collagen: An experimental model of arthritis. J. Exp. Med. 146:857-868.

28. Courtenay, J.S., Dallman, M.J., Dayan, A.D., Martin, A., and Mosedale, B. (1980). Immunisation against heterologous type II collagen induces arthritis in mice. Nature 283:666-668.

29. Wooley, P.H., Luthra, H.S., Stuart, J.M., and David, C.S. (1981). Type II collagen-induced arthritis in mice. I. Major histocompatibility complex (I region) linkage and antibody correlates. J. Exp. Med. 154:688-701.

30. Cathcart, E.S., Hayes, K.C., Gonnerman, W.A., Lazzari, A.A., and Franzblau, C. (1986). Experimental arthritis in a nonhuman primate. I. Induction by bovine type II collagen. Lab. Invest. 54:26-31.

31. Rubin, A.S., Healy, C.T., Martin, L.N., Baskin, G.B., and Roberts, E.D. (1987). Experimental arthropathy induced in rhesus monkeys (Macaca mulatta) by intradermal immunization with native bovine type II collagen. Lab. Invest. 57:524-534.

32. Yoo, T.J., Kim, S.-Y., Stuart, J.M., Floyd, R.A., Olson, G.A., Cremer, M.A., and Kang, A.H. (1988). Induction of arthritis in monkeys by immunization with type II collagen. J. Exp. Med. 168:777-782.

33. Terato, K., Arai, H., Shimozura, Y., Fukuda, T., Tanaka, H., Watanabe, H., Nagai, Y., Fujimoto, K., Okubo, F., Cho, F., Honjo, S., and Cremer, M.A. (1989). Sex-linked differences in susceptibility of cynomologus monkeys to type II collagen induced arthritis: Evidence that epitope-specific immune suppression is involved in the regulation of type II collagen autoantibody formation. Arthritis Rheum. 32:748-758.

34. Londei, M., Savill, C.M., Verhoef, A., Brennan, F., Leech, Z.A., Duance, V., Maini, R.N., and Feldmann, M. (1989). Persistence of collagen type II-specific T-cell clones in the synovial membrane of a patient with rheumatoid arthritis. Proc. Natl. Acad. Sci. USA 86:636–640.

35. Nagler-Anderson, C., Bober, L.A., Robinson, M.E., Siskind, G.W., and Thorbecke, G.J. (1986). Suppression of collagen arthritis by the peroral administration of type II collagen. Proc. Natl. Acad. Sci. USA 83:7443–7446.

36. Brahn, E., and Trentham, D.E. (1987). Attenuation of collagen arthritis and modulation of delayed-type hypersensitivity by type II collagen reactive T-cell lines. Cell Immunol. 109:139–147.

37. Brahn, E., and Trentham, D.E. (1989). Experimental synovitis induced by collagen-specific T cell lines. Cell. Immunol. 118:491–503.

38. Breedveld, F.C., Dynesius-Trentham, R., De Sousa, M., and Trentham, D.E. (1989). Collagen arthritis in the rat is initiated by CD4 + T cells and can be amplified by iron. Cell. Immunol. 121:1–12.

11

Experimental Arthritis: Importance of T Cells and Antigen Mimicry in Chronicity and Treatment

Wim B. van den Berg, Maries F. van den Broek,
Levinus B. A. van de Putte, Mieke C. J. van Bruggen,
and Peter L. E. M. van Lent
University Hospital St. Radboud, Nijmegen, The Netherlands

I. INTRODUCTION

Rheumatoid arthritis is a systemic disease of unknown etiology, with as main manifestation a chronic inflammation in multiple joints. In many patients the arthritis is characterized by exacerbations and remissions. Current theories of the pathogenesis include a genetically regulated immunologic reaction directed at an exogenous agent that localizes to the joints or an articular autoantigen. These two concepts originate from studies in experimental arthritis models, and an important breakthrough is that they are not mutually exclusive.

Considerable evidence has recently emerged that immunologic reactions directed at exogenous or host antigen may overlap. This may provide new insights not only in the pathogenetic mechanisms but also in possibilities for therapy. We summarize our current understanding of the major experimental arthritis models, with particular emphasis on T cells and aspects of antigen mimicry. Other details can be found in a recent review (1). The spontaneously developing MRL-1pr/1pr mouse model (2), proteoglycan arthritis (3), pristane arthritis (4), and a number of nonimmune arthritis models are not covered here.

In theory, chronic joint inflammation must result from a continuous stimulus, which can be the perpetual supply of antigen from the circulation of persisting antigen in the joint. The potential relevance of these mechanisms is illustrated in both antigen-induced arthritis (AIA) and streptococcal cell wall (SCW)-induced arthritis. In addition, structures of the joint itself, like collagen type II or proteoglycan, may function as persisting antigen, the arthritis thus being the result of an autoimmune response. That tolerance against these structures can be broken has been demonstrated in the collagen-induced arthritis (CIA) and the proteoglycan arthritis models. In essence, heterologous collagen type II or enzymatically modified proteoglycan are used to induce cross-reactive autoimmunity. This principle becomes of more physiologic relevance when autoimmune responses to joint structures are initiated by exogenous stimuli. In this light the recent recognition of mimicry between bacteria and cartilage proteoglycans seems of utmost importance.

II. COMMON PATHOGENETIC MECHANISMS IN EXPERIMENTAL ARTHRITIDES

A. Collagen-Induced Arthritis

Collagen-induced arthritis (CIA) is an experimentally induced autoimmune model of chronic erosive arthritis in both rats and mice. It is produced by sensitization to native type II collagen, a major component of articular cartilage. Denatured type II collagen or other collagen types are not arthritogenic. In the active model, binding of anti-collagen II antibodies to the articular cartilage surface probably plays an important initiating role (5). Although passive transfer of the disease has been achieved with antibodies, the arthritis seems rather transient and a major role must be attributed to T cells. Arthritis does not develop in nude or cyclosporin A-treated rats, the joint inflammation can be convincingly transferred with T cell lines or clones (6,7), and disease seems to be regulated by suppressor T cells ((8,9). Recent work demonstrated that arthritogenicity of T cell lines correlated with the capacity to generate a collagen II binding lymphokine (10). Details of this model are discussed in a separate chapter of this book.

B. Adjuvant Arthritis

Adjuvant arthritis (AA) is induced by intradermal administration of Freund's complete adjuvant containing heat-killed mycobacteria. The volume, type of oil, and composition of the emulsion are important variables that determine the incidence of arthritis in susceptible rats. The active component in the bacteria is the cell wall peptidoglycan, and it seems clear that the disease can be induced with various bacteria (11). Recent data suggest that the joint inflammation is in fact an autoimmune process triggered by structural mimicry between bacteria and cartilage proteoglycans (see later). A complicating aspect of current understanding is that not all adjuvant active materials are derived from bacteria. At least one oil, CP20961, is adjuvant active itself and can induce an arthritis indistinguishable from the classic adjuvant disease (12). Perhaps there are two potential mechanisms underlying chronic joint inflammation in adjuvant disease: one related to a cross-reactive autoimmune T cell reaction triggered by a response to bacterial cell wall antigens, and a second mechanism based on nonspecific immunomodulation, resulting in expression of normally suppressed autoimmunity.

There is no doubt that adjuvant arthritis is T cell dependent. The strongest argument for an autoimmune process is the induction of arthritis by passive transfer of T cells from diseased animals (13). The pathogenetic mechanism has been further explored using T cell lines and clones reactive to Mycobacterium tuberculosis (Mt). Holoshitz et al. (14–16) showed that a T cell line, called A2, isolated from AA Lewis rats and further selected in vitro with Mt, could induce arthritis in irradiated syngeneic recipients. Subsequent cellular cloning yielded the arthritogenic T cell clone A2b. This clone did not show reactivity with collagen type II, which underscores the claim of different pathogenetic pathways in AA and CIA (17). Further characterization of reactivity revealed distinct responsiveness to cartilage proteoglycans (18). That the clone could induce arthritis only in irradiated recipients suggests that tolerance exists in normal animals against such threatening autoimmune responses. Further suggestive evidence for the existence of tolerance against proteoglycans, which is regulated by cross-reactive responses to bacteria, comes from the observations in germ-free animals. Pathogen-free or coventionally bred F344 are generally resistant to adjuvant arthritis, whereas germ-free F344 rats are highly susceptible. Colonization of the germ-free rats with gram-negative bacteria again suppressed the disease susceptibility (19,20). This issue is addressed later in the discussion of SCW arthritis.

C. Streptococcal Cell Wall Arthritis

Streptococcal cell wall-induced arthritis is elicited in susceptible rats by systemic administration of cell wall fragments, which are highly resistant to biodegradation (21). Normally, cell wall fragments of group A streptococci are used, but a similar disease can be induced with cell wall fragments from other bacteria, such as *Lactobacillus casei* or *Eubacterium aerofaciens* (22,23). The latter models are of particular interest with respect to human disease, since these bacteria are components of the normal gastrointestinal flora. This implies that an enormous load of potential arthritogenic stimuli is continuously present in the normal gastrointestinal tract.

Within 24 h of administration of cell wall fragments acute inflammation develops in peripheral joints coincident with the localization of cell wall fragments in the blood vessels of the synovium and in the subchondral bone marrow. This acute inflammation subsides over the next week. Acute disease is inducible in all rat strains tested and also occurs in nude or thymectomized rats, indicating in-dependence of T cells.

The acute phase is followed within 2 weeks by a chronic erosive polyarthritis, which involves mainly peripheral joints. In contrast with the acute phase, the chronic joint inflammation develops in only a limited number of rat strains, with the highest incidence in Lewis rats (24,25).

Early studies on the SCW arthritis model demonstrated that the poorly degradable fragments persisted in the joint tissues for months. Arthritogenicity is associated with lysozyme resistance. Evidence that the persistence of fragments in the joints is of utmost importance for chronicity of the arthritis emerged from elegant studies with the enzyme mutanolysin. Degradation of the cell walls with this enzyme, either in vitro or even in vivo, clearly inhibited the development of chronic arthritis (26). Similar results were obtained when the cell walls were rendered susceptible to lysozyme cleavage by acetylation (27).

Although macrophages become stimulated by the persistent bacterial fragment, cogent evidence now exists that the chronic phase of SCW arthritis is dependent on T cells. The chronic phase was not inducible in nude Lewis rats, and cyclosporin A effectively inhibited this phase (28–30). In line with observations in other arthritis models it seemed reasonable to suggest that SCW-specific immunity played an important role in the chronic phase. We therefore explored SCW-specific T cell responses in both SCW arthritis-resistant (F344) and arthritis-susceptible (Lewis) rat strains. The data were striking: susceptible Lewis rats mounted distinct SCW-specific T cell immunity after various immunization protocols, whereas the resistant F344 rats were totally unable to mount a T cell response against the SCW (31). Control studies with other antigens demonstrated that F344 rats are fully capable of mounting distinct T cell responses. Tolerance against SCW material is probably a highly protective mechanism in view of the discussion raised earlier about threatening cross-reactive autoimmune responses. Immunity to car-tilage proteoglycans could be induced with bacteria. Along this line, we assumed that F344 rats became tolerized against bacteria early in life through contact with gut flora. The next step was to see whether germ-free F344 rats were able to mount SCW-specific T cell responses and, as a consequence, to develop SCW arthritis. The data were clear-cut: germ-free animals develop SCW—specific T cell immunity and show chronic SCW arthritis, indistinguishable from that observ-ed in conventional Lewis rats (manuscript in preparation).

Although there is no doubt that persistent SCW play a pivotal role in the pathogenesis of SCW arthritis, it remains to be explored whether cross-reactive autoimmune responses, like those in adjuvant arthritis, play an active part in this model. SCW contain peptidoglycan, the active moiety in adjuvants, and when properly mixed with oil, SCW can induce classic adjuvant arthritis (unpublished observations). On the other hand, passive transfer of the disease with T cells from SCW arthritic animals has not, to our knowledge, been described so far. The recent finding that a line selected with SCW could transfer arthritis to naive recipients (32) indicates the potential of SCW-primed T cells but in our opinion does not provide ultimate proof that these T cells are of utmost importance in the active SCW arthritis model. This field certainly deserves further attention.

D. Antigen-Induced Arthritis

Antigen-induced arthritis is, in contrast to those described earlier, a model of unilateral arthritis. It is induced by intra-articular injection of antigen into the knee joint of animals previously immunized with the same antigen. The arthritis remains confined to the injected joint, and it provides the opportunity to study the behavior of an arthritic joint compared to the contralateral naive joint within the same animal. Immunization is performed with antigen in complete Freund's adjuvant to induce strong humoral and cell-mediated immunity. Upon intra-articular injection of a large amount of antigen, an Arthus type of reaction develops, followed by a T cell-mediated chronic inflammation. Two determinants appeared of utmost importance for chronicity: sufficient antigen retention in the joint tissues, combined with proper T cell-mediated delayed hypersensitivity (33–35). Antigen can be retained in two ways: by antibody-mediated trapping (34) and by charge-charge interactions. Of interest is that electrical charge of the antigen determines both the site and the amount of antigen retained in the joint (36–38). Negatively charged antigen has no affinity for cartilage, and large amounts of antibody are required for its retention, primarily in loose collagenous connective tissue but not in hyaline cartilage. In contrast, positively charged antigen (pI above 8.5) is retained in substantially greater amounts and is found in both collagenous connective tissues and hyaline cartilage. Free cationic antigen can deeply penetrate dense hyaline articular cartilage, but immune complexes are found only in the superficial layers (37). Retention in collagenous tissues is of critical importance, since leukocytes cannot easily penetrate those tissues and antigen escapes clearance by the phagocytic system.

Chronicity of the arthritis in this model is probably related to the generation of local hyperreactivity. Antigen is trapped in the collagenous tissues of the joint, and tiny amounts of antigen are continuously released from these depots to sustain low-grade chronic arthritis. Under those conditions it is expected that the T cell infiltrate gains specificity. It has been shown that T cell clones are better retained in the synovial tissue in the presence of the homologous antigen (39). Moreover, it was found that approximately 50% of the local plasma cells produce antibodies specific to the retained antigen (33). Ultimate proof for a state of antigen-specific local hyperreactivity emerged from studies in the murine AIA model using cationic bovine serum albumin (BSA) as the antigen. Local challenge with nanogram amounts of antigen appeared sufficient to induce a measurable exacerbation of the smouldering inflammatory process, whereas these tiny doses did not induce arthritis in the contralateral naive joint (40).

E. General Conclusions

None of the models discussed earlier should be equated with specific forms of human arthritis, but the data may provide general insights to the immunopathogenesis. An important concept from the various models is that joint pathology can be induced by a variety of stimuli. It may suggest that the condition of rheumatoid arthritis is a collection of common end points induced by different stimuli. In addition, it could indicate that the various stimuli play a role in just one patient, in concert, or separately in various stages of the disease. This would of course complicate therapeutic intervention.

To get an impression of common concepts within the various models, we have summarized important details in Table 1. It is clear that T cell responses play a dominant role in *chronic* arthritis. This is also true in the human situation. Therapies like immunosuppression, lymphapheresis, or total lymphoid irradiation all are of benefit to the rheumatoid arthritis (RA) patient. The second important lesson from the models is that there are two forms of continuous stimuli in the joint: either the local persistence of exogenous antigens, like the nondegradable cell walls or antigen trapped in collagenous reservoirs, or articular cartilage autoantigens, like collagen type II and proteoglycans. Apart from the SCW, which are trapped in the synovium, all other stimuli focus on the cartilage as the main source of potential antigens. In the case of SCW, the cartilage could as well function as the antigenic reservoir because of cross-reactivity between SCW and cartilage proteoglycan (PG). Of interest is that destructive forms of rheumatoid arthritis tend to decline at the moment the cartilage is fully destroyed. Moreover, total joint replacement often results in a complete remission of the arthritis in

Table 1 Pathogenetic Mechanisms in Experimental Models of Chronic Arthritis[a]

Model	Immunization	Induction	Persistent antigen	Autoimmunity	T cells
CIA	CII/CFA	—	—	CII	+
AA	CFA	—	—	PG	+
SCW	—	IP SCW	SCW	PG?	+
AIA	Ag/CFA	IA Ag	Ag	—	+

The table has a spanning header "Chronic stimulus" over the Persistent antigen, Autoimmunity, and T cells columns.

[a]Persistent antigen relates to local retention in the joint.
CII, collagen type II; PG, proteoglycan; CFA, complete Freund's adjuvant; SCW, streptococcal cell walls.

that joint, without the need for concomitant synovectomy. These are strong arguments for a direct role of cartilage in the pathogenesis of RA.

The third important lesson from the models is that microbial components, particularly cell wall fragments derived from enteric organisms, are potential etiologic agents in humans. Apart from their ability to induce arthritis by direct localization to the joint tissue, they may induce arthritis remotely as a result of structural mimicry with joint structures. There is ample evidence from clinical observations that bacterial infections and development of arthritis may somehow be related. Arthritis is associated with streptococcal infections of the throat; infections of the gastrointestinal or urinary tract (Reiter's syndrome and reactive arthritis); jejunal bypass surgery for obesity, often resulting in bacterial overgrowth; and inflammatory bowel diseases, like Crohn's disease.

III. CONTRIBUTION OF FLARE REACTIONS TO CHRONICITY

Chronicity of arthritis may result from a perpetual supply of antigen leading to repeated reactivation of joint inflammation. Clearly, such a mechanism makes sense when a relevant stimulus is continuously, or at least intermittently, present in the circulation. An obvious source of such antigens may be the bacterial load in the gastrointestinal tract. We first studied the potential relevance of flare reactions in a well-characterized arthritis model, the murine AIA using mBSA as the antigen. As stated earlier, an arthritic joint bearing a chronic T cell infiltrate displays distinct local hyperreactivity against the retained antigen. However, this is not restricted to the retained antigen but also applies to antigen coming from the circulation. Flare reactions could be induced after intravenous or even oral antigen challenge, and doses of 10 ng of the antigen appeared sufficient to reactivate the arthritic joint (40,41). The state of hypersensitivity is antigen specific, that is, confined to the retained antigen, but may of course also hold for cross-reactive antigens (see later). The flare is T cell dependent: it could be blocked with anti-lymphocyte serum or anti-Ia treatment, whereas cobra venom factor treatment, to lower complement, was ineffective (42,43). A further determinant of the flare is the amount of systemic antigen reaching the joint tissue, and this is dependent upon systemic antibodies and physicochemical properties of the antigen (44,45).

In addition, flare reactions were studied using bacterial cell wall fragments. Since cell wall fragments are irritants in their own right, some of the flares induced with such stimuli may be nonspecific (46,47). However, cogent evidence now exists that specific T cell immunity plays a major role in bacterial reactivations as well (48,49). We compared the induction of flare reactions with SCW in both Lewis and F344 rats, the latter being unable to mount adequate T cell immunity against SCW. Injection of SCW into the knee joint induced a transient monoarthritis in both strains, but reactivation of the subsided arthritis by intravenous challenge with SCW could be evoked in the Lewis rat only. Even repeated IV challenges with SCW failed to induce a flare in the F344 rat, but the Lewis rat went through an exacerbation after every challenge. Moreover, removal of T helper cells by monoclonal antibodies, shortly before induction of an exacerbation, rendered Lewis rats refractory to these flares (49). Further proof of an important role of SCW- specific T cells emerged from a comparison of a series of heterologous cell wall fragments for their potential to induce exacerbations and to elicit proliferation of SCW—specific T cells in vitro. A strong correlation was found between these features (Table 2). Apart from pointing to a role for SCW-specific T cells in exacerbations, this experiment nicely illustrates that cross-reactive antigens may be involved in exacerbations and therefore in chronicity. Once a state of local hyperreactivity has been reached, every stimulus showing cross-reactivity at the T cell level could propagate the inflammatory process (Fig. 1). In terms of human arthritis, it is easy to see that a primary arthritis may be caused by a reaction to a certain bacterial species, but that once a state of local hyperreactivity has been induced the arthritis may be sustained by other bacteria displaying structural mimicry. Along the same line, cross-reactive autoantigens could function as second antigens as well.

Therapy should be focused on abrogation of local hyperreactivity. One approach is to specifically downregulate local T cell immunity, either by specific antigen treatment or T cell vaccination (50), in the hope of achieving tolerance. Experiments to modulate immunity were successful when treatment was started either before or in the active phase of generation of immunity. The present experiments illustrate that late treatment could cause exacerbations as well. Other promising approaches are to block T cell influx. Detailed knowledge of homing receptors

Table 2 Correlation Between the Capacity of Heterologous Cell Walls to Induce a Flare of SCW Arthritis and to Stimulate SCW-Primed T Cells In Vitro[a]

Cell walls (10 μg/ml)	Severity of flare	Proliferative response		
		Experiment 1	Experiment 2	Experiment 3
S. pyogenes	Severe	100	100	100
S. faecium	Severe	63	64	69
P. productus	Moderate	30	20	23
L. casei	None	9	7	3
P. acnes	None	7	11	3
M. formicicum	None	7	3	6

[a]Arthritis is induced by IA injection of SCW. A flare is induced by IV injction of 300 μg cell walls of various bacteria 17–25 days after arthritis induction. Details of the flare reactions can be found in Refs. 46–49. The proliferative responses are expressed as a percentage of the response to the priming antigen (SCW).

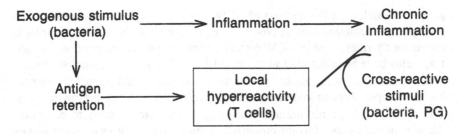

Fig. 1 Factors determining chronicity of joint inflammation.

would probably provide new tools. Moreover, elegant studies have demonstrated that various heparine derivatives, lacking anticlotting activity, could suppress adjuvant arthritis, probably also by interference with T cell influx (51).

IV. CONTRIBUTION OF CROSS-REACTIVE CARTILAGE RESPONSES

There is no doubt that bacteria can induce T cell responses against cartilage proteoglycans on account of structural mimicry (9,52). However, the contribution of those responses in chronicity of the various arthritis models is still a moot point. When Lewis rats were immunized with SCW in IFA emulsion, the lymph node cells clearly responded to SCW. In addition, the response was monitored against a variety of cartilage constituents. No response was found against collagen type II. The proteoglycan fraction was separated by density centrifugation in a protein-rich and proteoglycan-rich fraction. The response of SCW-primed cells was highest against the protein-rich fraction, suggesting that the cross-reactive epitope lies on a protein or on a small proteoglycan associated with protein. To investigate the relevance of cross-reactive responses we looked for joint pathology in SCW-IFA–primed animals. Mere immunization did not induce arthritis. Because it might be possible that cross-reactive epitopes are not accessible in intact cartilage in we then exposed epitopes by intra-articular injection with papaine. Such a treatment results in a short-lasting arthritis in OVA-primed Lewis rats, but the arthritis was significantly prolonged in SCW-primed animals (van den Broek, in preparation). However, this arthritis is not chronic at all: after 14 days no inflammation could be detected indicating that this combination does not create a self-perpetuating system. These findings are in line with the transient monoarthritis induced by intra-articular injection of SCW fragments in Lewis rats. Shortly after injection the fragments induce arthritis, with concomitant joint damage. After 4 weeks the arthritis has waned. This despite that SCW-specific immunity and therefore cross-reactive anticartilage responses have been mounted, as reflected by the potential to induce flare reactions in such joints with tiny amounts of SCW (see earlier). It further indicates that in the chronicity of the standard SCW arthritis model, after IP injection of SCW, the depot of SCW remote from the joint plays a dominant role. A possible mechanism could be that the arthritis is continuously reactivated by SCW material coming from the circulation. In fact, fragments have been detected in the blood long after IP administration (Stimpson, personal communication). A second mechanism could be that the remote bacterial depot plays an immunomodulatory role, either to prevent downregulation of the SCW-specific immunity or to stimulate autoimmunity to other cartilage epitopes by its adjuvant property. Studies are now in progress to isolate T cell lines from different phases of SCW arthritis, to select with various SCW and cartilage epitopes, and subsequently to investigate the in vivo potential of the various lines or clones, with slightly different antigen specificities, to induce arthritis.

It seemed clear from the impressive work with T cell clones that at least in adjuvant arthritis the joint inflammation is caused by a cross-reactive response to cartilage proteoglycan. However, conflicting data also exists in this model. Recipient rats must be irradiated when the arthritis is transferred with the A2 line or subclone to eliminate existing suppression (14,15). In contrast, arthritis can easily be transferred to nonirradiated recipients with total T cells isolated from adjuvant arthritic rats (19,53). This may implicate additional pathogenetic mechanisms underlying active adjuvant disease.

Finally, it is still unclear why IP injection of SCW or *Lactobacillus* induces arthritis in Lewis rats but induces a form of carditis or coronary arteritis in mice (54). It is tempting to speculate that cross-reactivity somehow directs responses to one or the other organ. Small differences exist between proteoglycans from endocardiac and articular cartilage, on the one hand, and proteoglycans from rat and mouse, on the other hand. Detailed mimicry studies at the (T cell) epitope level may yield important information regarding the pathogenesis of both arteritis and arthritis.

V. REGULATION OF ANTIBACTERIAL RESPONSES

Nonresponsiveness to SCW appeared the underlying mechanism of the resistance of F344 rats to SCW arthritis (31). This was not caused by a defect in the T cell receptor (hole in the repertoire) but was apparently due to active suppression. F344 rats can recognize SCW, as shown by the distinct SCW responses in germ-free animals, but became tolerized early in life, probably by environmental or gut flora bacteria. It is unclear so far whether this persistent bacterial load plays a role only in the induction or also in maintenance of immunologic tolerance to bacterial antigens. Lewis rat are defective in this tolerance, resulting in a high susceptibility for bacterium-induced arthritis. In fact, Lewis rats are the preferred strain in quite a number of autoimmune models and may be proper representatives for people in whom tolerance is easily broken and who therefore suffer from autoimmune diseases. The reason for susceptibility to SCW arthritis does not merely reside in the MHC genes, since susceptible Lewis and resistant F344 rats are identical on the RT1.A and RT1.B loci (MHC class I and II, respectively).

It is known from the adjuvant arthritis model that animals that have experienced AA are resistant to subsequent induction of AA. Recently, studies by van Eden et al. (55) characterized the immunodominant protein of Mt, the 65 kD heat-shock protein, and demonstrated that pretreatment with this protein protected Lewis rats against adjuvant arthritis. This 65 kD protein is immunologically related to a similarly sized ubiquitous bacterial common antigen and a 65 kD-like protein has been demonstrated in streptococci as well (56). We studied the potential of this antigen to protect Lewis rats against SCW arthritis. Pretreatment with 50 μg 65 kD in oil until as short as 5 days before SCW challenge fully protected against the development of SCW arthritis, and the protection appeared to be transferable by splenic T cells (57).

Interestingly, SCW-specific T cell responses normally found in SCW-challenged Lewis rats were significantly diminished. Moreover, concanavalin A (ConA) responses were suppressed, too. Further experiments were done to reveal the nature of the 65 kD-induced suppression. When OVA-preimmunized 65 kD-pretreated animals were rechallenged with OVA + SCW, the rats showed a significantly suppressed DTH. This suggest the following mechanism for 65 kD-induced protection. Treatment with 65 kD induces a state of latent immunosuppression, which is activated only when the immune system encounters bacterial stimuli containing the 65 kD-like epitope. At that moment, the activated immunosuppression downregulates bacterium-specific responses but, at the same time, also responses to nonrelated proteins (Fig. 2). This nonspecific feature is not uncommon at certain stages of immunosuppression.

A point of considerable concern is that treatment with 65 kD in an established phase of SCW arthritis clearly induced an exacerbation of the joint inflammation. This is not surprising in view of the phenomenon of flare reactions of arthritis discussed earlier. However, it stresses the need of modulatory antigens lacking this property. Tolerance induction has been convincingly achieved with

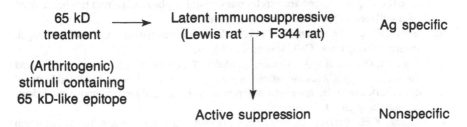

Figure 2 Schematic presentation of 65 kD-mediated suppression.

antigen pretreatment in a number of other models, like collagen type II-induced arthritis (58) or allergic encephalomyelitis (59,60). Using fragments of myelin basic protein it has been nicely demonstrated that the protein contains disease-inducing as well as nonencephalitogenic, tolerogenic epitopes (59). Suppression could be induced with both fragments, but suppression was more complete with the latter. It is our hope that bacterial or cross-reactive cartilage epitopes can be defined that can be used to induce suppression even at later stages of arthritis, without the threat of exacerbations. Epitopes lacking arthritogenicity seem the ideal candidates to look for.

REFERENCES

1. Wilder, R.L. (1988). Experimental animal models of chronic arthritis: In: Immunopathogenetic Mechanisms of Arthritis. Goodacre, J., and Carson Dick, W., eds. MTP Press, Lancaster, p. 157.
2. Hang, L., Theofilopoulos A.N., and Dixon, F.J. (1982). A spontaneous rheumatoid arthritis-like disease in MRL/1 mice. J. Exp. Med. 155:1690.
3. Glant, T.T., Mikecz, K., Arzoumanian, A., and Poole, A.R. (1987). Proteoglycan induced arthritis in BALB/c mice. Arthritis Rheum. 30:201.
4. Hopkins, S.J., Freemont, A.J., and Jayson, M.I.V. (1984). Pristane induced arthritis in BALB/c mice. Rheumatol. Int. 5:21.
5. Stuart, J., Townes, A., and Kang, A. (1984). Collagen autoimmune arthritis. Annu. Rev. Immunol. 2:199.
6. Trentham, D.E. (1982). Collagen arthritis as relevant model for rheumatoid arthritis. Evidence pro and con. Arthritis Rheum. 25:911.
7. Holmdal, R., Klareskog, L., Rubin, K., Larsson, E., and Wigzell, H. (1985). T lymphocytes in collagen II-induced arthritis in mice. Characterization of arthritogenic collagen II-specific T-cell lines and clones. Scand. J. Immunol. 22:295.
8. Kresina, T.F., and Moskowitz, R.W. (1985). Adoptive transfer of suppression of arthritis in the mouse model of collagen induced arthritis. Evidence for a type II collagen-specific suppressor T cell. J. Clin. Invest. 75:1990.
9. Burrai, I., Henderson, B., Knight, S.C., and Staines, N.A. (1985). Suppression of type II collagen-induced arthritis by transfer of lymphoid cells from rats immunized with collagen. Clin. Exp. Immunol. 61:368.
10. Brahn, E., and Trentham, D.E. (1989). Experimental synovitis induced by collagen specific T cell lines. Cell. Immunol. 118:491.
11. Kohashi, O., Tanaka, A., Kotani, S., Shiba, T., Kusumoto, K., Ykogawa, K., and Ozawa, A. (1980). Arthritis inducing ability of a synthetic adjuvant, MDP and bacterial dissacharide peptides related to different oil vehicles and their composition. Infect. Immunology 29:70.
12. Chang, Y.H., Pearson, C., and Abe, C. (1980). Adjuvant polyarthritis IV. Induction by a synthetic adjuvant. Arthritis Rheum. 23:62.
13. Taurog, J., Sandberg, G., and Mahowald, M. (1983). The cellular basis of adjuvant

arthritis. I. Enhancement of cell mediated passive transfer by ConA and immunosuppressive treatment of the recipient. Cell. Immunol. 75:271.

14. Holoshitz, J., Naparstek, Y., Ben-Nun, A., and Cohen, I.R. (1983). Lines of T lymphocytes induce or vaccinate against autoimmune arthritis. Science 219:56.

15. Holoshitz, J., Matitiau, A., and Cohen, I.R. (1984). Arthritis induced in rats by clones of T lymphocytes responsive to mycobacteria but not to collagen type II. J. Clin. Invest. 73:211.

16. Cohen, I.R., Holoshitz, J., van Eden, W., and Frenkel, A. (1985). Lines of T lymphocytes illuminate pathogenesis and affect therapy of experimental arthritis. Arthritis Rheum. 28:841.

17. Taurog, J.D., Kerwar, S.S., McReynolds, R.A., Sandberg, G.P., Leary, S.L., and Mahowald, M.L. (1985). Synergy between adjuvant arthritis and collagen induced arthritis in rats. J. Exp. Med. 162:962.

18. van Eden, W., Holoshitz, J., Nevo, Z., Frenkel, A., Klajman, A., and Cohen, I.R. (1985). Arthritis induced by a T lymphocyte clone that responds to Mycobacterium tuberculosis and to cartilage proteoglycans. Proc. Natl. Acad. Sci. USA 82:5064.

19. Kohashi, O., Kohashi, Y., Takahashi, T., Ozawa, A., and Shigematsu, N. (1985). Reverse effect of gram positive bacteria vs gram negative bacteria on adjuvant induced arthritis in germ free rats. Microbiol. Immunol. 29:487.

20. Kohashi, O., Kohashi, Y., Takahashi, T., Ozawa, A., and Shigematsu, N. (1986). Suppressive effect of *Escherichia coli* on adjuvant induced arthritis in germ free rats. Arthritis Rheum. 29:547.

21. Cromartie, W.J., Craddock, J.C., Schwab, J.H., Anderle, S.K., and Yang, C.H. (1977). Arthritis in rats after systemic injection of streptococcal cells or cell walls. J. Exp. Med. 146:1585.

22. Lehman, T.J.A., Allen, J.B., Plotz, P.H., and Wilder, R.L.(1984). *Lactobacillus casei* cell wall induced arthritis in rats: cell wall fragment distribution and persistence in chronic arthritis-susceptible LEW/N and resistant F344/N rats. Arthritis Rheum. 27:939.

23. Severijnen, A.J., van Kleef, R., Hazenberg, M.P., and van de Merwe, J.P. (1989) Cell wall fragments from major residents of the human intestinal flora induce chronic arthritis in rats. J. Rheumatol. in press.

24. Wilder, R.L., Calandera, G.B., Garvin, A.J., Wright, K.D., and Hansen, C.T. (1982). Strain and sex variation in the susceptibility of streptococcal cell wall induced polyarthritis in the rat. Arthritis Rheum. 25:1064.

25. Wilder, R.L., Allen, J.B., Wahl, L.M., Calandra, G.B. ,and Wahl, S.M. (1983). The pathogenesis of group A streptococcal cell wall induced polyarthritis in the rat. Comparative studies in arthritis resistant and susceptible inbred rat strains. Arthritis Rheum. 26:1442.

26. Janusz, M.J., Chetty, C.C., Eisenberg, R.A., Cromartie, W.J., and Schwab, J.H. (1984). Treatment of experimental erosive arthritis in rats by injection of the muralytic enzyme mutanolysin. J. Exp. Med. 160:1360.

27. Stimpson, S.A., Lerch, R.A., Cleland, D.R., Yarnall, D.P., Clark, R.L., Cromartie, W.J., and Schwab, J.H. (1986). Effect of acteylation on arthropatic activity of group A streptococcal cell walls. Arthritis Rheum. 29:S101.

28. Allen, J.B., Malone, D.G., Wahl, S.M., Calandra, G.B., and Wilder, R.L. (1985).

The role of the thymus in streptococcal cell wall induced arthritis and hepatic granuloma formation. J. Clin. Invest. 76:1042.

29. Yocum, D.E., Allen, J.B., Wahl, S.M., Calandra, G.B., and Wilder, R.L. (1986). Inhibition by cyclosporin A of streptococcal cell wall induced arthritis and hepatic granulomas in rats. Arthritis Rheum. 29:262.

30. Wilder, R.L., Allen, J.B., and Hansen, C.T. (1987). Thymus dependent and independent regulation of Ia antigen expression in situ by cells in the synovium with streptococcal cell wall induced arthritis. Differences in site and intensity of expression in euthymic, athymic and cyclosporin A treated LEW and F344 rats. J. Clin. Invest. 79:1160.

31. van den Broek, M.F., van Bruggen, M.C.J., van de Putte, L.B.A., and van den Berg, W.B. (1988). T cell responses to streptococcal antigens in rats: Relation to susceptibility to streptococcal cell wall induced arthritis in rats. Cell. Immunol. 116:216.

32. Quinn DeJoy, S., Ferguson, K.M., Sapp, T.M., Zabriskie, J.B., Oronsky, A.R., and Kerwar, S.S. (1989). Streptococcal cell wall arthritis. Passive transfer of disease with a T cell line and crossreactivity of streptococal cell wall antigens with *Mycobacterium tuberculosis*. J. Exp. Med. 170:369.

33. Cooke, T.D., and Jasin, H.E. (1972). The pathogenesis of chronic inflammation in experimental antigen induced arthritis. I. The role of antigen on the local immune response. Arthritis Rheum. 15:327.

34. Cooke, T.D., Hurd, E.R., Ziff, M., and Jasin, H.J. (1972). The pathogenesis of chronic inflammation in experimental antigen induced arthritis. II. Preferential localization of antigen antibody complexes to collagenous tissues. J. Exp.Med. 135:323.

35. Brackertz, D., Mitchell, G.F., Vadas, M.A., and Mackay, I.R. (1977). Studies on antigen induced arthritis in mice. III. Cell and serum transfer experiments. J. Immunol. 118:1645.

36. van den Berg, W.B., van de Putte, L.B.A., Zwarts, W.A., and Joosten, L.A.B. (1984). Electrical charge of the antigen determines intraarticular antigen handling and chronicity of arthritis in mice. J. Clin. Invest. 74:1850.

37. van den Berg, W.B., and van de Putte, L.B.A. (1985). Electrical charge of the antigen determines its localization in the mouse knee joint: Deep penetration of cationic BSA in hyaline articular cartilage. Am. J. Pathol. 121:224.

38. van Lent, P.L.E.M., Dekker, C., Mosterd, J., van den Bersselaar, L., and van den Berg, W.B. (1989). Allergic arthritis by cationic proteins: role of molecular weight. Immunology.

39. Klasen, I.S., Ladestein, R.M.T., van den Berg, W.B., and Benner, R. (1989). Requirements for flare reactions of joint inflammation induced in mice by cloned MT4+,Lyt2- T cells. Arthritis Rheum. 32:330.

40. Lens, J.W., van den Berg, W.B., and van de Putte, L.B.A. (1984). Flare up of antigen induced arthritis in mice after challenge with intravenous antigen. Studies on the characteristics of and mechanisms involved in the reaction. Clin. Exp. Immunol. 55:287.

41. Lens, J.W., van den Berg, W.B., and van de Putte, L.B.A. (1984). Flare up of

antigen induced arthritis in mice after challenge with oral antigen. Clin. Exp. Immunol. 58:364.

42. Lens, J.W., van den Berg, W.B., van de Putte, L.B.A., Berden, J.H.M., and Lems, S.P.M. (1984). Flare up of antigen induced arthritis in mice after challenge with intravenous antigen: Effects of pretreatment with cobra venom factor and anti lymphocyte serum. Clin. Exp. Immunol. 57:520.

43. van den Broek, M.F., van den Berg, W.B., and van de Putte, L.B.A. (1986). Monoclonal anti-Ia antibodies suppress the flare up reaction of antigen induced arthritis in mice. Clin. Exp. Immunol. 66:320.

44. Lens, J.W., van den Berg, W.B., van de Putte, L.B.A., and Zwarts W.A. (1986). Flare up of antigens induced arthritis in mice after challenge with intravenous antigen: Kinetic of antigen in the circulation and localization of antigen in the arthritic and noninflamed joint. Arthritis Rheum. 29:665.

45. van Lent, P.L.E.M., van den Bersselaar, L., Grutters, G.J.F., and van den Berg, W.B. (1989). Fate of antigen after intravenous and intrarticular injection into mice: Role of molecular weight and charge. J. Rheumatol. in press.

46. Esser, R.E., Stimpson, S.A., Cromartie, W.J., and Schwab, J.H. (1985). Reactivation of streptococcal cell wall induced arthritis by homologous and heterologous cell wall polymers. Arthritis Rheum. 28:1402.

47. Stimpson, S.A., Esser, R.E., Carter, B.P., Sartor, R.B., Cromartie, W.J., and Schwab, J.H. (1987). Lipopolysacharide induces recurrence of arthritis in rat joints previously injured by polysaccharide-peptidoglycan. J. Exp.Med. 165:1688.

48. van den Broek, M.F., van den Berg, W.B., Severijnen, A.J., and van de Putte, L.B.A. (1988). Streptococcal cell wall induced arthritis and flare up reactions in mice induced by homologous and heterologus cell walls. Am. J. Pathol. 133:125.

49. van den Broek, M.F., van Bruggen, M.C.J., Stimpson, S.A., Severijnen, A.J., van de Putte, L.B.A., and van den Berg, W.B. (1989). Flare up of streptococcal cell wall induced arthritis in Lewis and F344 rats: The role of T lymphocytes. Clin. Exp. Immunol. in press.

50. Cohen, I.R., and Weiner, H.L. (1988). T cell vaccination. Immunol. Today 9:332.

51. Lider, O., Baharav, E., Mekori, Y.A., Miller, T., Naparstek, Y., Vlodavsky, I., and Cohen, I.R. (1989). Suppression of experimental autoimmune diseases and prolongation of allograft survival by treatment of animals with low doses of heparins. J. Clin. Invest. 83:752.

52. van den Broek, M.F., van den Berg, W.B., Arntz, O.J., and van de Putte, L.B.A. (1988). Reaction of bacterium primed murine T cells to cartilage components: A clue for the pathogenesis of arthritis. Clin. Exp. Immunol. 72:9.

53. Billingham, M.E.J., Fairchild, S., Griffin, E., Drayer, L., and Hicks, C. (1989). Monoclonal antibody therapy for arthritis. In: Therapeutic Control of Inflammatory Disease. Lewis, A.J., and Otterness, I. eds. Elsevier, New York, in press.

54. Lehman, T.J.A., Walker, S.M., Mahnovski, V., and McCurdy, D. (1985). Coronary arteritis in mice following the systemic injection of group B *Lactobacillus casei* cell walls in aqueous suspension. Arthritis Rheum. 28:652.

55. van Eden, W., Thole, J.E.R., van der Zee, R., Noordzij, A., van Embden, J.D.A., Hensen, E.J., and Cohen, I.R. (1988). Cloning of the mycobacterial epitope recognized by T lymphocytes in adjuvant arthritis. Nature 331:171.

56. Thole, J.E.R., Hinderson, P., de Bruyn, J., Cremers, F., van der Zee, R., de Cock, H., Tomassen, J., van Eden, W., and van Embden, J.D.A. (1988). Antigenic relatedness of a strongly immunogenic 64 kDa mycobacterial protein antigen with a similarly sized ubiquitous bacterial common antigen. icrob. Pathogenesis 4:71.

57. van den Broek, M.F., Hogervorst, E.J.M., van Bruggen, M.J.C., van Eden, W., van der Zee, R., and van den Berg, W.B. (1989). Protection against streptococcal cell wall induced arthritis by pretreatment with the 65-kD mycobacterial heat shock protein. J. Exp. Med. 170:449.

58. Thompson, H.S.G., Henderson, B., Spencer, J.M., Peppard, J.V., and Staines, N.A. (1988). Tolerogenic activity of polymerized type II collagen in preventing collagen induced arthritis in rats. Clin. Exp. Immunol. 72:20.

59. Higgins, P.J., and Weiner, H.L. (1988). Suppression of experimental autoimmune encephalomyelitis by oral administration of myelin basic protein and its fragments. J. Immunol. 140:440.

60. Bitter, D.M., and Whitacre, C.C. (1988). Suppression of experimental autoimmune encephalomyelitis by the oral administration of myelin basic protein. Cell. Immunol. 112:364.

12

A Mycobacterial 65 kD Heat-Shock Protein and T Cells in Experimental Arthritis: Possibilities for Immunotherapy

Willem van Eden, Claire J. P. Boog, Els J. M. Hogervorst, and Marca H. M. Wauben
University of Utrecht, Utrecht, The Netherlands

Ruurd van der Zee and Jan D. A. van Embden
National Institute of Public Health and Environmental Hygiene, Bilthoven, The Netherlands

I. AUTOIMMUNE ARTHRITIS: A T CELL DISEASE

As a common characteristic, autoimmune disorders show a loss of self integrity due to a pernicious reactivity of the immune system directed against self structures. It is generally assumed that this reactivity of the immune system is due to a specific recognition of endogenous self target antigens. That this may be correct is indicated by the possibilities of experimentally inducing autoimmune disease by immunization of the animal with a self constituent, such as basic protein of myelin and thyroglobulin. In such cases disease is specifically targeted at those organs that contained the self constituent used for the immunization. In most of these experimental models T cells were found to be responsible for the immunopathology that evolved (1).

Whether human autoimmune disease may be caused by a similar T cell-mediated reactivity directed at certain self target molecules is unknown at present. So far, no target structures have been defined with certainty in such clinical syndromes as Hashimoto's thyroiditis, multiple sclerosis, diabetes mellitus, or rheumatoid arthritis.

A constant finding in these diseases, however, is their occurrence in association with certain HLA phenotypes. Being aware of the biologic function of HLA molecules in general as antigen presenting structures in T cell recognition

253

processes, the contribution of HLA to these diseases is probably in controlling antigen-specific T cell responses. In the experimental models a similar contribution of the major histocompatibility complex (MHC) has been documented. So, the presence of HLA associations in these diseases is compatible with the possibility that human autoimmune diseases are under the control of specific T cell recognition of antigens, which may be either the endogenous self target antigens or exogenous triggering antigens. Moreover, in trying to explain in a teleologic way the unique polymorphism of the MHC, the HLA associations may give support to certain theories concerning the origin of these diseases.

The most probable explanation for the extreme polymorphism of the MHC is that it evolved during evolution under the selective pressure exerted by virulent infectious organisms. Polymorphism at the population level secured the population against extermination due to a certain lethal infectious organism. During such an evolutionary process, selection must have been weeding out the unsuitable genotypes. We are now left with those genes that provide us with a strong and mostly effective immune response to exogenous microbial antigens. What we face now, however, with autoimmune diseases may be the other side of the coin. An effective response to microbial antigens may overshoot its goal and strike the host by attacking endogenous self antigens. Selection has not been operative against such diseases, since they usually develop late in life, mostly after the age of reproduction. If this reasoning is correct, one may conclude that in individuals with certain predisposing MHC types autoimmune disease may be evoked by the exposure to certain microbial antigens. Autoimmune arthritis is an obvious candidate disease for such a situation (see Table 1) (2). Reactive arthritis is by definition the result of an exposure to such bacteria as *Yersinia*, *Shigella*, gonococci, and *Campylobacter*. Furthermore, *Borrelia* spirochetes induce Lyme arthritis, a clinical syndrome that has an immunopathologic picture indistinguishable from that of rheumatoid arthritis. Streptococci cause acute rheumatic fever and many infectious diseases, varying from mycobacterioses to histoplasmosis, feature, at least transiently, episodes of arthritic disease.

The evidence in humans that autoimmune arthritis could be triggered by microbial antigens is supported by a number of experimental models. One of these models is the well-known model of adjuvant arthritis (AA). AA can be induced in susceptible rats by immunization with mycobacterial antigens, suspended in mineral oil, a preparation known as Freund's complete adjuvant. The model, developed by Pearson in the late 1950s, has been studied intensively because of the well-described striking resemblance of its pathology to human rheumatoid arthritis (3). That T cells could play a central role in AA was indicated by the findings that disease could be transferred to naive animals with lymphocytes taken from AA rats (4) and, furthermore, that pretreatment of rats with antithymocyte antibodies inhibited development of disease (5). A more definite claim for the essential role of T cells in the disease came from the experiments of Holoshitz

Table 1 Bacterial Species and Arthritic Disease in Humans

Bacterium	Nature of arthritis	Clinical situation
Streptococcus gr. A	Migratory polyarthritis	Acute rheumatic fever
Yersinia	Limited polyarthritis	Enteritis, HLA-B27
Shigella	Limited polyarthritis	Enteritis, HLA-B27
Salmonella	Limited polyarthritis	Enteritis, HLA-B27
Campylobacter	Limited polyarthritis	Enteritis, HLA-B27
Klebsiella?	Ankylosing spondylitis	?, HLA B-27
Borrelia burgdorferi	Migratory polyarthritis	Lyme disease
M. bovis BCG	Polyarthritis, small joints	Cancer immunotherapy
Chlamydia	Relapsing polyarthritis	Reiter's disease, HLA-B27

et al. It was shown that a T lymphocyte line, called A2, obtained from Lewis rats after Mt (*Mycobacterium tuberculosis*) immunization, and propagated by further in vitro selection with Mt, could induce AA disease in irradiated syngeneic recipients (6). Thus, under conditions of hyperimmunization with crude mycobacterial antigens, Lewis rats were found capable of generating a T cell response with autoimmune potential. Subsequent cellular cloning of the A2 cell line revealed the presence of a virulently arthritogenic T cell clone, called A2b (7). This A2b clone demonstrated that T cells with a single antigenic specificity could elicit in vivo a fulminant form of autoimmune arthritis. Inoculation of A2 into non irradiated recipient rats did not cause arthritis but resistance against AA instead. Similar resistance was also found to result from inoculation with another A2-derived nonarthritogenic subclone, called A2c. Moreover, inoculation of A2c in rats with AA resulted in early remission of disease (8). Besides responding to mycobacteria, the selecting antigen, A2 was found to be weakly reactive with collagen type II. For the arthritogenic subclone A2b, no reactivity with purified collagen type II preparations was ever found (7). This A2b clone, however, did show reactivity with crude cartilage preparations, especially with preparations enriched for proteoglycan molecules (9). Similar findings were obtained with the original A2 cell line and the protective subclone, A2c. Furthermore, both A2b-immunized rats and rats with actively induced AA were found to exhibit delayed-type hypersensitivity (DTH) reactivity to the proteoglycan-containing preparations. From these observations it was concluded that the phenomenon of AA was probably due to the presence within mycobacteria of a molecule having a structural resemblance to a cartilage proteoglycan molecule, possibly the core protein (10). Since this resemblance was defined by the reactivity of an arthritogenic effector cell itself, it is likely that the immunization with such a mimicking mycobacterial antigen is enough for triggering AA. That A2c, a protective clone, showed a similar cross-specificity indicated that T cell recognition of such a mimic antigen could potentially have complex consequences. The outcome of in vivo exposure to a potentially arthritogenic antigen could so depend on the balance of functionally distinct, but related, T cell clones. Further characterization of the arthritogenic antigen could therefore possibly turn out to be meaningful, not only for further understanding the basis of AA, but in addition to generate the tools to analyze mechanisms of protection.

II. ARTHRITIS T CELL CLONES IDENTIFY THE 65 kD HEAT-SHOCK PROTEIN IN MYCOBACTERIA

Since mycobacterial species are notoriously difficult to grow in vitro, molecular cloning of their antigens seemed the solution for the development of diagnostics and vaccines. Thole et al. have been involved in cloning antigens of *Mycobacterium bovis* BCG, the strain used for tuberculosis vaccines, in *Escherichia coli* K12. A total of six different antigens were expressed as 30, 65, 70, 90, 95, and more than 100 kD molecular weights (11). From serology in mycobacterial diseases one antigen, the 65 kD protein, was already identified as a potent immunogen. By further subcloning of the latter coding gene an overproducing strain was obtained. From this strain the 65 kD could easily be purified and subsequently further characterized (12). By testing this particular protein in proliferation assays, the protein was found to stimulate A2, A2b, and A2c to an extent that exceeded even the stimulation obtained with the original selecting antigen, whole *M. tuberculosis* (13). All other mycobacterial recombinant proteins available to us at that time were found negative. Sequencing of the *M. bovis* BCG 65 kD protein coding gene revealed that it was composed of 540 amino acids and that it was identical with the *M. tuberculosis* 65 kD protein. Furthermore, the protein turned out to have a homology of more than 95% with its *Mycobacterium leprae*-derived counterpart. Thus, the antigen found responsible for triggering our arthritis T cells turned out to be a protein molecule conserved between various mycobacterial species. Furthermore, a panel of both polyclonal and monoclonal antibodies with specificity for this 65 kD mycobacterial protein was found to recognize, in Western blots, antigens of similar molecular weights in many other bacterial species. These species included arthritis-associated species, such as streptococci, *Klebsiella*, *Shigella*, *Yersinia*, gonococci, and *Campylobacter*. From these observations it was concluded that the 65 kD protein was a member of a family of proteins called "common antigen" (14). Further analysis revealed extensive sequence homology with the GroEL protein of *E. coli*, which is a so-called heat-shock or stress protein (15,16). The latter GroEL protein is a major essential protein present in virtually all bacterial cells. The expression of the GroEL gene(s) is upregulated under conditions that are stressful for the organism. The GroEL was also found to be a major protein present in mitochondria of eukaryotic cells, and also in plant chloroplasts. The reason for the evolutionary conservation of these molecules is probably related to their function as so-called molecular chaperones, which are essential to cell integrity, being involved in the assembly and possibly intracellular translocation of other multisubunit proteins.

From a number of bacterial and parasitic infections it has become apparent that members of the heat-shock protein (HSP) families are frequent and efficient inducers of immune reactivity (17). This may be related to their enhanced expression during the stress that bacteria undergo being within the hostile environment of the host. Be that as it may, the T cells of the AA model now have also shown that when part of a dead complex antigen, T cells may select the 65 kD protein to respond to, resulting in a pernicious form of autoimmune arthritis. It is tempting to speculate that this responsiveness to these conserved molecules may be similarly responsible for other forms of bacteria-induced autoimmune arthritides. Moreover, it seems attractive to assume that, in such cases, there is an additional role for the homologous endogenous counterpart expressed by the host tissues themselves in the disease. Such a role could be in serving as a target structure for the autoimmune reactivity triggered by the bacterial counterpart. Alternatively, responses directed at such endogenous HSPs could theoretically have an influence on their functioning as chaperone molecules. which could indirectly change processing or presentation, for instance in antigen presenting cells. This could, of course, indirectly contribute to inflammatory responses or cause additional immunologic epiphenomena in the disease process.

III. T CELL EPITOPE DEFINITION IN ADJUVANT ARTHRITIS

To further characterize both the nature of the structural mimicry between mycobacteria and cartilage and the nature of the differences between the functionally distinct clones A2b and A2c, a mapping of the T cell epitopes on the 65 kD protein was undertaken (13). By the construction of deletion mutants of the 65 kD gene, and deletion mutants of this gene fused with the β-galactosidase gene, parts of the protein were expressed. From an analysis of the responses of A2b and A2c to the expressed molecular fragments, it was deduced that both A2b and A2c recognized an area in the molecule located between amino acids at position 171–234. This area was short enough to cover subsequently by peptide synthesis. From the peptides synthesized, those peptides that included the area from positions 180 to 188 were found to stimulate A2b and A2c. The synthetic nonapeptide 180–188 was also found to be fully stimulatory by itself to both clones. The inevitable conclusion from this was that A2b and A2c had identical fine specificity for the 180–188 epitope located within the 65 kD molecule of mycobacteria. Therefore A2b and A2c are most likely to be clones with identical T cell receptors and therefore idiotypes or better clonotypes, but with different intrinsic functional characteristics. Apparently, the 180–188 T cell epitope itself was capable of activating arthritis-related regulatory T cells, no matter whether the cells were virulently arthritogenic or merely protective. The relevance for arthritis of this epitope was most probably defined by its unique structural resemblance to a cartilage-associated antigen, giving this epitope the capacity to direct responses to cartilage-containing target organs, such as joint tissues.

A search for sequence homologies of the epitope with known sequences of link and core proteins of proteoglycans revealed an incomplete homology with a link protein sequence derived from rat chondrosarcomas (18,19). Whether this sequence homology sufficiently explains the phenomenon of adjuvant arthritis remains to be seen. Positive responses of A2b to synthetic peptides based on sequence homologies have been found, but they were sometimes very weak and therefore inconclusive. To fully characterize the boundaries of recognition by such clones as A2b, we wished to have the disposal of a virtually unlimited source of variant peptides. This was achieved by a modification of the well-known PEPSCAN method of peptide synthesis, originally designed to synthesize sequentially overlapping sets of nested peptides for B cell epitope mapping (20). In the PEPSCAN method, automated synthesis is performed on polyethylene pins. The scanning procedure for B cell epitopes is done by direct incubation of the pins with antibodies. Specific binding of antibodies is then assayed in an enzyme-linked immunosorbent assay (ELISA) system directly on these pins. To use this same very efficient synthesis method for T cell epitope mapping a modification of the method was introduced by van der Zee et al., which enabled us to recover the peptides from their solid supports (21). In the modified procedure a cleavable tripeptide is introduced as a spacer between the solid support and the peptide. After cleavage with formic acid under mild conditions sufficient amounts of peptide were obtained for performing a small series of proliferation assays in the standard way, in the presence of added antigen presenting cells. All overlapping peptides comprising the minimal sequence 180–186 were found to stimulate clones A2b and A2c. Moreover, variant peptides with substitutions at positions 187 and 188 of the original 180–188 peptide were fully stimulatory. So, the critical sequence for recognition was found to be only seven amino acids long. Some substitutions were permitted within this critical sequence, although the stimulatory capacities of such substituted peptides have so far been significantly below the original nonsubstituted sequence. Recently, using this modified PEPSCAN procedure, substituted peptides have been obtained that were efficiently inhibitory to responses of A2b in the presence of the nonsubstituted 180–188 peptide (Wauben et al., in preparation). We are currently testing whether such inhibitory peptides, which probably exert competition at the level of binding in the antigen presenting MHC molecule, can be used for in vivo modulation of the disease process. Such an approach has already been found to be successful in myelin basic protein-triggered experimental allergic encephalomyelitis (EAE) in mice (22). It will be interesting to test whether this approach is equally effective in AA, in which there probably is a mimicry, not an identity relationship between triggering antigen and target antigen. Furthermore, by blocking T cell responses directed at 180–188, both the arthritogenic A2b(-like) cells and the protective A2c(-like) cells may be equally inhibited. Whatever the outcome of the in vivo experiments, it is clear from the EAE experience that molecular information on the nature of disease-triggering T cell epitopes may give attractive possibilities to specific immunologic intervention to the benefit of the host. One of the questions to be dealt with in such complex models as AA in rats, is whether such diseases can be controlled by the manipulation of responses directed against just a single antigenic epitope. The experience with our protective clone A2c, however, is promising in this particular respect.

IV. IMMUNOTHERAPEUTIC ASPECTS OF THE 65 kD PROTEIN

Arthritogenic clone A2b and protective clone A2c both recognized a single epitope of the 65 kD protein of mycobacteria. It was therefore obviously important to investigate whether active immunization with the 65 kD protein would activate A2b(-like) T cells and induce AA, or whether it would activate A2c-like T suppressor-inducers and induce resistance to AA. Unlike immunization with whole mycobacteria, the administration of the 65 kD antigen emulsified in oil did not induce AA. So, it had to be concluded that in vivo the consequences of immunization to 65 kD either were dependent on the mycobacterial context surrounding the 65 kD molecule or that additional arthritogenic epitopes were present in Mt. However, the crucial importance of the 65 kD molecule in AA has now become apparent in various ways.

When animals, after immunization with the 65 kD protein, are subsequently challenged with whole Mt in oil to induce AA, animals may either fail to develop disease at all or develop only mild disease (13). Recently, the protective effects of 65 kD preimmunization were found to be more dramatic in the distinct model of streptococcal cell wall-induced arthritis (SCW arthritis) by van den Broek et al. (23). Immunization with 50 µg of 65 kD protein in oil until only 5 days before SCW immunization was found to protect fully against the development of SCW arthritis. This protection was found to be transferable with splenic T cells to naive recipients. From in vivo cross-priming experiments, evidence was obtained for the immunologic relationship between the mycobacterial 65 kD and an antigen present in the streptococcal cell wall, presumably the streptococcal 65 kD homolog. The findings in the SCW model further support the possibility that the 65 kD HSP is a common denominator in models of bacterially induced arthritis. Further experimentation will be done to see whether 65 kD preimmunization also induces protection in nonbacterial arthritis models. Although no protection has been seen in experimentally induced nonspecific forms of joint inflammation, such as those caused by intra-articular zymosan inoculation, in the model of pristane-induced arthritis in mice 65 kD preimmunization was found to be protective (Thompson, personal communication). This indicates that the development of autoimmune arthritic processes can be prevented by 65 kD preimmunization or, perhaps even better, vaccination, irrespective of their triggering immunogen.

Exposure to the 65 kD protein during arthritis, however, may lead to exacerbations of the disease process. This has been noted both in the AA and in the SCW experimental models. In itself, this can be taken as supporting the pivotal role of 65 kD in these forms of arthritis. However, if we are interested in defining agents that can be used to enforce an immunotherapeutic effect in arthritis, the conditions of 65 kD administration must apparently be determined carefully. Experiments have already shown that the dosage and the manner of administration are of critical importance in this respect. It is becoming evident now that, depending on the circumstances, existing disease can also be successfully mitigated by the administration of the 65 kD protein of mycobacteria, at least in the experimental situation.

V. ANTIGEN-SPECIFIC IMMUNE REGULATION IN ADJUVANT ARTHRITIS

Lewis rats are particularly susceptible to developing AA after mycobacterial immunization. From such in vivo immunized rats T cell line A2 was selected, because of its arthritogenic potential. The selection was done in vitro with whole heat-killed mycobacteria (Mt). Recently, we have been selecting an additional T cell line, B1, from Lewis rats, also after Mt immunization in vivo, but in vitro selection was done with the 65 kD protein. Mapping the T cell epitopes seen by this new B1 T cell line again showed specificity for the 180–188 epitope that was also recognized by A2 and its subclones. Thus in Lewis rats the response directed at the arthritis epitope 180–188 seems to dominate the T cell reactivity after Mt immunization. That this is probably true was further indicated by the finding that after Mt immunization draining lymphode lymphocytes can be obtained that show in vitro a proliferation in the presence of the 180–188 synthetic peptide (Hogervorst et al., in preparation). So, also at the level of polyclonal T lymphocytes, responses to 180–188 can be obtained.

Observations made in other rat strains, which are less susceptible to AA, have now shown that responsiveness to the 180–188 epitope and arthritis susceptibility are probably positively correlated. BN rats, carrying an MHC haplotype that differs from that in the Lewis, were found low responders to 65 kD and also 180–188. Fisher rats, carrying an MHC haplotype identical to that of Lewis rats were found to be responders to 65 kD, but they failed to respond to 180–188 after Mt immunization. Although MHC identical with Lewis rats, Fisher rats are known to be notoriously resistant to induction of AA. One exceptional case of severe AA in a Fischer rat, however, turned out to be exquisitely informative. This single rat showed a strong 180–188 response. Thus, at least in the context of Lewis MHC, responses directed at 180–188 of the 65 kD protein seem to go along with the development of AA.

VI. RESPONSES TO THE 65 kD HSP IN HUMAN RHEUMATOID ARTHRITIS

Bacterial antigens have been shown to trigger arthritis in the experimental situation. The 65 kD molecule of mycobacteria is such an antigen and may even be a common denominator in different experimental models (see Table 2). It is a conserved molecule and obviously also human individuals are constantly exposed to exogenous organisms that express this 65 kD protein. Because it is a member of the HSP families of proteins, immune responses seem to be elicited frequently by this particular 65 kD protein. In other words, the 65 kD molecule is also known to behave as a so-called dominant immunogen for human beings (17).

In the model of AA the HSP seems to trigger arthritis on the basis of structural mimicry of its 180–188 epitope with a proteoglycan protein. The latter core protein is also of a conserved nature among mammalian species, and we were not surprised to see that A2b was found capable of recognizing proteoglycan-containing preparations of rat and human origin equally well (9). Thus, the potential to dangerous mimicry as seen in the rat disease seems to exist in humans as well. An alternative possibility is that the endogenous host HSPs actually serve as a target structure in arthritis, and rat and humans are likely to behave similarly. Preliminary sequencing data obtained by PCR have already indicated the identities between human and rat 65 kD HSPs (van der Zee et al., in preparation). It thus seems that we must accept the possibility that the potential for breaking self tolerance present in bacterial HSP 65 is equally present in both rats and

Table 2   Mycobacterial 65 kD Heat-Shock Protein in Experimental Arthritis

Feature	References
Dominant mycobacterial antigen in susceptible Lewis rats	Hogervorst et al., in preparation
Structural resemblance to a cartilage-associated molecule	9, 18
Recognized by arthritis-regulatory T cells	13
Immunization induces resistance against AA, SCW arthritis, and pristane-induced arthritis	13, 23, Thompson, personal communication

humans. A summary of all sequences known thus far of the critical area 180–186 of 65 kD heat-shock proteins present in various organisms is given in Table 3.

Although the substitutions found between the prokaryotic and eukaryotic sequences are of a conserved nature (28), in comparison to the overall sequence conservation of this protein the 180–186 turns out to be a relatively nonconserved area of the molecule. This obviously makes sense and may well explain that the rat after immunization with the whole protein selects this area of the molecule for recognition. It may be of further interest to note that in the screening of a large number of substituted peptides synthesized by the PEPSCAN method for stimulating the arthritogenic clone A2b, those substitutions that were permitted within the mycobacterial 180–186 were without exception found to be present within the sequences given in Table 3 (Wauben et al., in preparation). Despite this suggestive evidence, so far no conclusive answer can be given to the question of whether the mammalian 180–186 structure can serve in itself as a target in autoimmune arthritis. Be that as it may, the more important questions are, first, whether human individuals encounter these bacterial antigens in such a manner that arthritis may be triggered, and second, whether human individuals are capable of selecting an arthritogenic epitope, such as 180–188, to respond to.

It has been reported that hyperimmunization with mycobacteria in the human may also lead to the development of arthritis. This was seen in about 10% of the cases in a series of patients treated with BCG immunotherapy for cancer (29). This may well represent the human equivalent of AA. Although convincing in itself—the potential to develop arthritis after bacterial immunization seems to be present in humans—the question whether chronic rheumatoid arthritis may also be triggered by bacterial antigens remains more difficult to answer. However, responses against mycobacterial antigens in RA patients have now been shown

Table 3 Summary of Known 180–186 Sequences

Organism	Protein	Positions 180–186	Reference
Mycobacterium tuberculosis	65 kD protein	T F G L Q L E	16
M. bovis BCG	65 kD protein	T F G L Q L E	12
M. leprae	65 kD protein	T F G L Q L E	24
Escherichia coli	GroEL	G L Q D E L D	25
Coxiella burnetii	62 kD protein	G L E N A L E	26
Saccharomyces cerevisiae	HSP 60	T L E D E L E	27
Human	P1	T L N D E L E	28
Ricinus communis	Rubisco binding protein	S F E T T V D	25
Triticum aestivum	Rubisco binding protein	S F E T T V E	25

in a number of studies. Antigens tested included an acetone-precipitable fraction of mycobacteria, originally developed as a preparation enriched for the antigen recognized by A2, A2b, and A2c in the rat AA model (30) and also, more recently, the recombinant 65 kD HSP of mycobacteria (31). In these studies, the responses were more easily obtained in lymphocytes obtained from patients with a recent onset of disease than in patients with more advanced disease. This could well indicate that these responses were related to the cause of arthritis. Furthermore, responses were found to be more prominent in synovial fluid lymphocytes than in peripheral blood lymphocytes. Moreover, similar findings of responses obtained with the 65 kD protein have been made in patients with reactive forms of arthritis (32). In addition to T cell proliferation data, some studies have now shown a rise in 65 kD antibodies in sera obtained from both adult RA patients (33) and children with juvenile chronic arthritis (Cohen, personal communication).

In summary, it seems that arthritis patients tend to exhibit the signs of an immunologic experience with the mycobacterial 65 kD protein. The question remains of whether this results from bacterial priming at the start of disease or whether this sensitization to the mycobacterial antigen is instead the result of the disease process. Genetic data, however, can be taken as arguing in favor of the first possibility. Ottenhoff et al. have shown that in leprosy patients, individuals who have been chronically exposed to mycobacterial antigens, the HLA-DR4-positive individuals exhibited without exception strong hypersensitivity reactions in the skin after intracutaneous inoculation with *M. tuberculosis* tuberculin (34). In constrast, individuals without HLA-DR4 were found either not to respond at all or to respond weakly upon tuberculin skin testing. Thus the presence of HLA-DR4, which has no known association with leprosy or any other mycobacteriosis, seems to control the capacity to develop strong mycobacteria-specific T cell responses. Similar findings were made by Palacios-Boix et al. in vitro (35). By performing proliferation assays they showed that lymphocytes taken from HLA-DR4-positive donors responded more vigorously to the acetone-precipitable fraction (AP) of MT than lymphocytes from HLA-DR4-negative donors. This observation was made both in healthy donors and in RA patients. In other words, HLA-DR4 seems to be an immune response gene with specificity for some mycobacterial antigen. The consequence is that the association of HLA-DR4 with human RA is in fact due to the HLA-DR4-mediated control of the specific immune response to mycobacteria.

If such reasoning is correct, it is difficult to argue that the antimycobacterial reactivity in RA is the result of the disease process, not a causal relationship to the disease (see Table 4).

From this discussion it is clear that more data must be collected, preferably on responses to the 65 kD HSP using T cells obtained directly from the sites of the autoimmune inflammatory lesions in human arthritic disease. In doing so, attention should be given to determining the precise epitopes recognized by

Table 4 Mycobacteria and RA in Humans

T cells from synovium respond to mycobacterial antigens (30–32)

Patient sera contain antibodies with specificity for
mycobacterial antigen (33; Cohen, personal
communication)

HLA-DR4 associated with RA and tuberculin skin
hypersensitivity (34)

HLA-DR4 associated with in vitro proliferative
responses to mycobacterial antigens (35)

individuals in relation to their HLA phenotypes. Such an approach may be expected to provide the information that we need to make the proper comparisons
between rat AA and human arthritis (36).

Once we have identified the relevant T cell epitopes in the disease process,
tangible benefits to patients are expected to emerge in the future. As has now
been shown in the experimental rat model, antigens identified by the specific
recognition of the relevant T cell populations can be used to modulate the disease
process in vivo. The conditions for doing so are at present being defined in the
experimental disease. Since no specific therapy is available for the treatment of
chronic arthritis, obviously we are obliged to further explore any procedure so
effective in animal models (Table 5).

Table 5 Lessons of the AA Model

Autoimmune arthritis can be the consequence of a
"physiologic" exogenous trigger.

T cells of a single epitope specificity may evoke
autoimmune arthritis.

Specific immunotherapy in autoimmune arthritis is
possible and can be achieved through the manipulation with a single T cell specificity.

Specific vaccination with immunogens containing (a)
defined T cell epitope(s) can prevent autoimmune
arthritis.

REFERENCES

1. Cohen, I.R. (1986). Regulation of autoimmune disease: Physiological and therapeutic. Immunol Rev. 94:5–21.
2. Klein, J. (1986). The Natural History of the MHC. John Wiley & Sons, New York, p. 656.
3. Pearson, C.M. (1956). Development of arthritis, periarthritis and periostitis in rats given adjuvant. Proc. Soc. Exp. Biol. Med. 91:95–101.
4. Whitehouse, D.J., Whitehouse, M.W., and Pearson, C.M. (1969). Passive transfer of adjuvant-induced arthritis and allergic encephalomyelitis in rats using thoracic duct lymphocytes.Nature 224:1322.
5. Kayashima, K., Koga, T., and Onone, K. (1978). Role of T lymphocytes in adjuvant arthritis. II. Different subpopulations of T lymphocytes functioning in the development of the disease. J. Immunol. 120:1127.
6. Holoshitz, J., Naparstek, Y., Ben-Nun, A., and Cohen, I.R. (1983). Lines of T lymphocytes induce or vaccinate against autoimmune arthritis. Science 219:56–58.
7. Holoshitz, J., Matitiau, A., and Cohen, I.R. (1984). Arthritis induced in rats by clones of T lymphocytes responsive to mycobacteria but not to collagen type II. J. Clin. Invest. 73:211–215.
8. Cohen, I.R., Holoshitz, J., van Eden, W., and Frenkel, A. (1985). Lines of T lymphocytes illuminate pathogenesis and affect therapy of experimental arthritis. Arthritis Rheum. 28:841–845.
9. van Eden, W., Holoshitz, J., Nevo, Z., Frenkel, A., Klajman, A., and Cohen, I.R. (1985). Arthritis induced by a T lymphocyte clone that responds to *Mycobacterium tuberculosis* and to cartilage proteoglycans. Proc. Natl. Acad. Sci. USA 82:5064–5067.
10. van Eden, W., Holoshitz, J., and Cohen, I.R. (1987). Antigenic mimicry between mycobacteria and cartilage proteoglycans: The model of adjuvant arthritis. Concepts Immunopathol. 4:144–170.
11. Thole, J.E.R., Dauwerse, H.G., Das, P.K., Groothuis, D.G., Schouls, L.M., and van Embden, J.D.A. (1985). Cloning of the *Mycobacterium bovis* BCG DNA and expression of antigens in *Escherichia coli*. Infect. Immun. 50:800–806.
12. Thole, J.E.R., Keulen, W., Kolk, A., Groothuis, D., Berwald, L., Tiesjema, R., and van Embden, J.D.A. (1987). Characterisation, sequence determination and immunogenicity of a 64-kilodalton protein of *Mycobacterium bovis* BCG, expressed in *Escherichia coli* K-12. Infect. Immun. 55:1466–1475.
13. van Eden, W., Thole, J.E.R., van der Zee, R., Noordzij, A., van Embden, J.D.A., Hensen, E.J., and Cohen, I.R. (1988). Cloning of the mycobacterial epitope recognized by T lymphocytes in adjuvant arthritis. Nature 331:171–173.
14. Thole, J.E.R., Hindersson, P., De Bruyn, J., Cremers, F., van der Zee, R., De Cock, H., Tommassen, J., van Eden, W., and van Embden, J.D.A. (1988). Antigenic relatedness of a strongly immunogenic 65 kD mycobacterial protein antigen with a similarly sized ubiquitous bacterial common antigen. Microb. Pathogenesis 4:71–83.
15. Young, D.B., Ivanyi, J., Cox, J.H., and Lamb, J.R. (1987). The 65 kDa antigen of mycobacteria—a common bacterial protein? Immunol. Today 8:215–219.

16. Shinnick, T.M., Vodkin, M.H., and Williams, J.C. (1988). The *Mycobacterium tuberculosis* 65 kD antigen is a heat-shock protein which corresponds to common antigen and to the *Escherichia coli* GroEL protein. Infect Immun. 56:446–451.

17. Young, D.R., Lathigra, R., Hendrix, R., Sweetser, D., and Young, R.A. (1988). Stress proteins are immune targets in leprosy and tuberculosis. Proc. Natl. Acad. Sci. USA 85:4267.

18. van Eden, W., Hogervorst, E.J.M., Hensen, E.J., van der Zee, R., van Embden, J.D.A., and Cohen, I.R. (1989). A cartilage mimicking T cell epitope on a 65 kD mycobacterial heat-shock protein: Adjuvant arthritis as a model for human rheumatoid arthritis. In: Molecular Mimicry: Chemical Similarity Between Microbe and Host Protein as a Source of Autoimmunity. Oldstone, ed. Curr. Top. Microbiol. Immunol. 145:27–43.

19. Cohen, I.R. (1988). The self, the world and autoimmunity. Sci. Am. 255:34–42 (April).

20. GeEysen, H.M., Meloen, R.H., and Barteling, S.J. (1984). Use of peptide synthesis to probe viral antigens for epitopes to a resolution of a single amino acid. Proc. Natl. Acad. Sci. USA 81:3998.

21. van der Zee, R., van Eden, W., Meloen, R.H., Noordzij, A., and van Embden, J.D.A. (1989). Efficient mapping and characterization of a T cell epitope by the simultaneous synthesis of multiple peptides. Eur. J. Immunol. 19:43–49.

22. Sakai, K., Mitchell, D.J., Hodgkinson, S.J., Zamvil, S.S., Rothbard, J.B., and Steinman, L. Allele-specific therapy of autoimmune disease with peptides blocking T cell-MHC interaction: Prevention of EAE with nonencephalitogenic peptides. Cold Spring Harbor Laboratory, in press.

23. van den Broek, M.F., Hogervorst, E.J.M., van Bruggen, M.C.J., van Eden, W., van der Zee, R., and van den Berg, W. (1989). Protection against streptococcal cell-wall induced arthritis by pretreatment with the 65 kD mycobacterial heat-shock protein. J. Exp. Med. 170:449.

24. Mehra, V., Sweetser, D., and Young, A. (1986). Efficient mapping of protein antigenic determinants. Proc. Natl. Acad. Sci. USA 83:7013–7017.

25. Hemmingsen, S.M., Woolford, C., van der Views, S.M., Tilly, K., Dennis, D.T., Georgopoulos, C.P., Hendrix, R.W., and Ellis, R.J. (1988). Homologous plant and bacterial proteins chaperone oligomeric protein assembly. Nature 333:330–334.

26. Vodkin, M.H., and Williams, J.C. (1988). A heat shock operon in *Coxiella burnetii* produces a major antigen homologous to a protein in both mycobacteria and *Escherichia coli*. J. Bacteriol. 170(3):1227–1234.

27. Reading, D.S., Hallberg, R.L., and Myers, A.M. (1989). Characterization of the yeast HSP60 gene coding for a mitochondrial assembly factor. Nature 337:655–659.

28. Jindal, S., Dudani, A.K., Singh, B., Harley, C.B., and Gupta, R.S. (1989). Primary structure of a human mitochondrial protein homologous to the bacterial and plant chaperonins and to the 65 kD mycobacterial antigen. Mol. Cell. Biol. 9:2279–2283.

29. Torisu, M., Miyahara, T., Shinohara, N., Ohsato, K., and Sonozaki, H. (1978). A new side effect of BCG immunotherapy: BCG-induced arthritis in man. Cancer Immunother. 5:77–83.

30. Holoshitz, J., Klajman, A., Drucker, I., Lapidot, Z., Yaretzky, A., Frenkel, A., van Eden, W., and Cohen, I.R. (1986). T-lymphocytes of rheumatoid arthritis patients show augmented reactivity to a fraction of mycobacteria cross-reactive with cartilage. Lancet 2:305–309.

31. Res, P.C.M., Schaar, C.G., Breedveld, F.C., van Eden, W., van Embden, J.D.A., Cohen, I.R., and De Vries, R.R.P. (1988). Fluid T cell reactivity against the 65 kD heat-shock protein of mycobacteria in early onset of chronic arthritis. Lancet 2:478–480.

32. Gaston, J.H.S., Life, P.F., Bailey, L., and Bacon, P.A. (198). Synovial fluid T cells and 65 kD heat-shock protein (letter). Lancet 2:856.

33. Bahr, G.M., Rook, G.A.W., Al-Safar, M., van Embden, J., Stanford, J.L., and Behbehani, K. (1988). Antibody levels to mycobacteria in relation to HLA type: Evidence for non-HLA-linked high levels of antibody to the 65 kD heat-shock proein of *M. bovis* in rheumaoid arthritis. Clin. Exp. Immunol. 74:211–215.

34. Ottenhoff, T.H.M., Torres, P., De Las Aguas, J.T., Fernandez, R., van Eden, W., De Vries, R.R.P., and Stanford, J.L. (1986). Evidence for an HLA-DR4-associated immune response gene for *Mycobacterium tuberculosis*: A clue to the pathogenesis of rheumatoid arthritis. Lancet 2:310–313.

35. Palacios-Boix, A.A., Estrad, G.I., Colston, M.J., and Panayi, G.S. (1988). HLA-DR4 restricted lymphocyte proliferation to a *M. tuberculosis* extract in rheumatoid arthritis and healthy subjects. J. Immunol. 140:2–13.

36. Rook, G.A.W. (1988). Rheumatoid arthritis, mycobacterial antigens and agalactosyl IgG (meeting review). Scand. J. Immunol. 28:487.

13

Immunotherapy of Collagen-Induced Arthritis with Anti-Ia and Anti-IL-2R Antibodies

Paul H. Wooley
Wayne State University Medical School, Detroit, Michigan

Subhashis Banerjee
McGill University and Shriners Hospital for Crippled Children, Montreal, Quebec, Canada

I. INTRODUCTION

Type II collagen-induced arthritis (CIA) is an experimental disease induced in rats (1) and mice (2) by intradermal injection of native type II collagen, the major component of hyaline cartilage. CIA in mice exhibits a number of pathologic features in common with rheumatoid arthritis (RA) (3), including the clinical features of erythema and edema and the histologic appearance of synovial hypertrophy and hyperplasia, pannus formation, and the subsequent erosion of cartilage and bone.

A. MHC in CIA

The development of CIA is associated with genes of the major histocompatibility complex (MHC) in mice (4) and rats (5), which mimics the association of RA with HLA-DR4 (6). In mice, the association of susceptibility to arthritis induced by chick type II collagen has been specifically associated with the 1-A^q phenotype, based on the pattern of disease development in recombinant haplotype mice congenic to the C57/BL10 background (Table 1). In addition, the H-2^q haplotype does not express a functional I-E molecule on class II antigen-expressing cells (7). Since H-2^p haplotype mice (B10.P) are resistant to the induction of

Table 1 Incidence of CIA in Recombinant Haplotype Strains Immunized with Chick Type II Collagen

Strain		H-2			Arthritis (%)
B10.BYR	K^q	I-A^k	I-E^k	D^b	0
B10.AQR	K^q	I-A^k	I-E^k	D^d	0
B10.T(6R)	K^q	I-A^q	I-E^q	D^d	56
B10.DA	K^q	I-A^q	I-E^q	D^s	64
B10.RQF-1	K^q	I-A^q	I-E^q	D^f	85
B10.RQB-1	K^q	I-A^q	I-E^q	D^b	69
B10.RBQ-1	K^q	I-A^b	I-E^b	D^q	0
B10.RKQ-1	K^k	I-A^k	I-E^k	D^q	0
B10.RKQ-2	K^k	I-A^k	I-E^q	D^b	0
B10.AKM	K^k	I-A^k	I-E^k	D^q	0
B10.MBR	K^b	I-A^k	I-E^k	D^q	0

arthritis and B10.Q and B10.P mice express identical I-A α chains, Holmdahl et al. (8) have postulated that susceptibility may be associated with the limited variations seen between the 1-A$_\beta^q$ and I-A$_\beta^p$. However, the assignation of this association is complicated by the existence of multiple arthritogenic epitopes on the type II collagen molecule (9), demonstrated by the varied immunogenetic regulation of CIA susceptibility using different species sources of type II collagen (Table 2). Notably, B10.RIII mice (H-2^r) develop a high incidence of disease when immunized with bovine, porcine, or deer type II collagen, despite complete resistance to chick collagen. In contrast, B10.Q animals are resistant to arthritis induced with porcine collagen. Insufficient recombinant haplotypes

Table 2 Incidence of Arthritis (%) in Independent Haplotype Strains Immunized with Various Species of Type II Collagen

Strain	H-2	CII	BII	DII	RII	PII
B10.Q	q	84	63	54	26	8
B10.G	q	41	15	18	18	17
DBA/1	q	71	62	ND	ND	70
DBA/1LacJ	q	89	65	85	ND	90
BUB/J	q	77	ND	18	ND	17
SWR/J	q	0	0	0	0	0
B10.RIII	r	0	78	75	3	95
RIII/J	r	0	0	0	ND	0
LP.RIII/J	r	0	40	ND	ND	50

are available to accurately determine the major histocompatibility complex (MHC) association, and since B10.RIII mice express a functional I-E molecule on the cell surface, it is not known at present whether susceptibility to bovine type II collagen is associated with the I-A^r.

B. Arthritogenic Epitopes

Since the development of arthritis is invariably accompanied by a vigorous immune response to collagen, current hypotheses suggest that the presentation of certain "arthritogenic" epitopes on the collagen molecule in association with class II antigens of the H-q^q or H-2^r haplotypes results in an autoimmune response to type II collagen that results in a disease state. Evidence for reactivity against autologous collagen has been demonstrated for the DBA/1 strain, indicating the genetic capacity for autoreactivity (10,11). In addition to the presentation of collagen in an autoimmune manner, the strain must also possess a T cell repertoire with the capacity to recognize and respond to collagen in an autoimmune manner (12). Several mouse strains develop high antibody responses to type II collagen but remain resistant to the disease (4), which may be due to the recognition of nonautologous collagen epitopes. The successful transfer of disease with anti-type II collagen immunoglobulin from both murine arthritis (13,14) and rheumatoid disease (15) has provided evidence for an important and perhaps obligatory role of anticollagen antibodies in collagen arthritis. However, the T cell requirement has been demonstrated using congenitally athymic (*rnu/rnu*) nude rtas, which are resistant to disease induction by collagen immunization (16) but are more susceptible to arthritis caused by passive transfer of anticollagen immunoglobulin than *rnu/* + heterozygous rats (17).

II. IMMUNOTHERAPY WITH ANTI-Ia ANTIBODIES

Since antibodies directed against the class II MHC determinants have been successfully used in the prevention and therapy of experimental allergic encephalomyelitis (EAE) (18), the autoimmune disease of (NZB × NZW)F$_1$ (B/W) mice (19) and experimental allergic thyroiditis (20) in a series of studies by Steinman and McDevitt, we examined this immunotherapy in collagen arthritis (21). Monoclonal antibodies specifically raised against 1-A^q determinants were not available; therefore, both cross-reactive monoclonal antibodies and specific polyclonal antisera reactive against I-A^q, I-A^r, and I-E^r were investigated (Table 3).

Although the time course of the development of collagen arthritis is substantially different from that for the induction of EAE, the method of Steinman et al. (18) was employed for the administration of the immunotherapy. B10.Q mice were immunized on day 0 with 25 μg of chick type II collagen, solubilized in 0.1M acetic acid and emulsified in Freund's complete adjuvant (FCA) in a manner

Table 3 Antibodies Used in Collagen Arthritis Immunotherapy

Antisera	Source	Type	Specificity
MI 11	B10.AQR anti-B10.T (6R)	Polyclonal	Ia.10
MW 1	B10.BYR anti-B10.RQB-1	Polyclonal	Ia.16
MI 112	A.TH anti-A.TL	Polyclonal	Ia.1, 2, 3, 7
RT	Rabbit anti-B10.T(6R)	Polyclonal	I^q
25-9-17	C3H anti-C3H.SW	Monoclonal	I^b
MK D6	(B6 × A/J) anti-B10.D2	Monoclonal	I^d
H39-459	A.TH anti-A.TL	Monoclonal	Ia.7 (III)
H1093.2	A.TH anti-A.TL	Monoclonal	Ia.7 (I)
14-4-4	A.TH anti-A.TL	Monoclonal	Ia.7 (I)
13-4	A.TH anti-A.TL	Monoclonal	Ia.7 (I)
H7-86.2	A.TH anti-A.TL	Monoclonal	Ia.7 (II)
H9-15.4	A.TH anti-A.TL	Monoclonal	Ia.7 (III)
17-3-3	C3H.SW anti-C3H	Monoclonal	Ia.22
17-227	C3H.anti-C3H.SW	Monoclonal	Ia.25

previously shown to induce arthritis in 65–75% of mice (4). Groups of 10–15 mice were injected IP with 250 μl of polyclonal antisera on day −1 and day 0 and 500 μl antisera on day +1. Groups of 12–31 mice were injected with similar volumes of saline containing purified monoclonal antibodies at 1–3 mg/ml concentrations. No further antibody treatment was given to these animals. Using the same protocol, B10.RIII mice were injected IP with either polyclonal antisera or purified monoclonal antibodies in saline and immunized with 25 μg of bovine type II collagen.

The incidence of arthritis in control (saline-injected) B10.Q mice was 65%. Treatment of mice with the polyclonal antisera directed against I-A^q had a significant influence on the incidence of CIA. Irrespective of the specificity of the antisera (Ia.10, Ia.16, and Ia.3), the disease incidence was reduced to approximately 30%. However, the specificity of the monoclonals had a marked effect on the incidence of arthritis. The control monoclonal antibody (H10-93.2), directed against the Ia.7 antigen (not expressed on H-2^q cells), did not significantly influence the CIA incidence. Although the monoclonal antibodies MK D6 and H39-459 reacted in vitro with H-2^q lymphocytes, as assessed by cell surface antigen precipitation tests, their influence on the incidence of collagen arthritis was not significant. However, a substantial delay in the onset of arthritis was seen in mice treated with MK D6. The monoclonal 25-9-17 caused both a significant reduction in CIA incidence (30%) and a delay in the onset of disease.

The incidence of bovine CIA in B10.RIII was significantly reduced by the polyclonal sera (MI 112), from 88% in the saline-injected control to 28%. MI 112 reacts with I-A and I-E antigens expressed by H-2^r (Ia.1, 3, and 7).

A marked reduction in disease was seen in mice injected with the monoclonal antibodies H10-93.2, 14-4-4, and 13-4. These antibodies are specific for epitope I of the Ia.7 (I-E) molecule. Monoclonals reactive with either epitope II or epitope III did not suppress the disease incidence. However, mice treated with the monoclonal antibody 17-3-3 (anti-Ia.22) were seen to develop 100% disease incidence.

The development of the antibody response to type II collagen was found to be influenced by the anti-Ia antibody therapy. Although the final antibody titer was not significantly affected, the rate of anticollagen antibody production was reduced, judged by the titers measured 14 days after immunization. With the exception of the control monoclonal antibody (H10.93.2) and H39-459, IgG antibodies reactive with chick collagen were significantly lower in B10.Q mice. This effect was not as pronounced in B10.RIII mice, in which anti-bovine IgG antibodies were reduced only in mice treated with MI 112 or the monoclonal H10-93.2. Interestingly, the mice injected with monoclonal 17-3-3 developed significantly higher antibody responses, assessed at both 14 and 28 days after immunization. This correlated well with the observation of increased arthritis incidence and severity.

The peak delayed-type hypersensitivity response to type II collagen was not significantly influenced by anti-Ia therapy in either mouse strain. However, the DTH response to collagen in mice does not correlate well with the arthritogenic reaction and is typically early and transitory in most CIA—susceptible strains (9).

The mechanism by which anti-Ia antibody therapy suppresses the arthritogenic response to type II collagen is at present unclear. Anti-Ia antisera may delete a cell population bearing this marker (22), and candidates include the antigen presenting cell population, the B cell pool essential for the autoimmune response, or an activated T cell subset bearing Ia (23). However, evidence that the effect may not be exerted via the deletion of Ia-bearing cells is indicated by experiments carried out in F_1 hybrid animals. (B10.Q × B10)F_1 mice were obtained and injected with either a monoclonal antibody reactive with I-A^q (25-9-17) or a monoclonal specific for I-A^b (17-227). $F_1{}^{q/b}$ mice were susceptible to the induction of arthritis with chick type II collagen, and the 75% incidence of disease was reduced to 25% using monoclonal 25-9-17. These data correlated well with the effects of 25-9-17 on B10.Q immunized in a similar manner. In contrast, $F_1{}^{q/b}$ mice treated with monoclonal 17-227 did not show a significant reduction in disease incidence. The results are in concordance with the reports from studies in H-2$^{k/b}$ mice, in which a monoclonal antibody reactive to I-A^k markedly reduced the response to HGAL, but not TGAL (24). This observation favors the hypothesis of interference at the molecular level between the association of certain autoimmune epitopes with the class II antigen molecules.

Studies in EAE have indicated that anti-Ia therapy may be effective after the development of disease signs (25) and the concomitant development of autoreactive T cells. A similar effect has not been demonstrated to date for collagen arthritis after the onset of disease. This may be due to the delayed onset of the disease postimmunization, the pathologic mechanism that results in CIA, or the specificities of the anti-Ia antibodies tested at present.

Anti-Ia antibodies in vivo have also been shown to induce a T suppressor cell population capable of abrogating the DTH response to syngeneic tumor antigens, via interaction with the Ly-1$^+$ T responder cells (26). In a similar manner, T suppressor cells, which downregulate the response to myelin basic protein, may be induced by the use of anti-Ia in EAE (27). Alternatively, anti-Ia antibodies may block the induction of T helper cells in the absence of the induction of suppression (28). However, corresponding mechanisms have not been reported for the use of anti-Ia in CIA.

The overall success of anti-Ia therapy in suppressing collagen arthritis lends support to the use of anti-class II antigen therapy in rheumatoid arthritis, in which susceptibility to disease is associated with HLA-DR4. Although polyclonal or monoclonal antibodies of DR4 have not been formally studied in a clinical setting, Sany et al. (29,30) have used placenta-eluted gammaglobulin (PEGG) in the treatment of RA. In a trial of 31 patients, significant improvement was seen in 60% of individuals receiving high doses of PEGG over a 6 month period. Interestingly, a concomitant increase in mitogen responsiveness was seen during the gamma globulin therapy. These results must be treated with caution, since the PEGG preparation contains antibody reactivity directed against class I antigens, plus antiviral and antibacterial activity. PEGG was demonstrated to block stimulation in the mixed lymphocyte reaction, an activity consistent with anti-DR activity. However, formal evidence for the activity of anti-class II antibody in the immunotherapy of RA remains to be demonstrated. Moreover, the demonstration in mice that certain anti-Ia treatments can aggravate both the arthritis incidence and the immune response to type II collagen suggests that caution must be used until a full understanding of the mechanisms involved has been elucidated.

III. IMMUNOTHERAPY OF ARTHRITIS WITH AGENTS REACTIVE WITH IL-2R

A. Role of T Cells in Collagen-Induced Arthritis

Type II collagen-reactive T cells play a central role in the pathogenesis of CIA in rodents (16,31). After immunization in vivo, type II collagen is processed and presented by antigen presenting cells to CD_4^+ T "helper" (T_H) cells specific for type II collagen. These T cells are then activated and initiate the production of pathogenic anticollagen antibodies [which are known to be T cell dependent (32)] by type II collagen-reactive B cells. The disease is considered induced by the deposition of anti-type II collagen on surfaces of joint cartilage with subsequent activation of complement (32,33). This is followed by infiltration of polymorphonuclear and mononuclear cells into the joint. Numerous CD4$^+$ T cells are found in the synovium (16,32,34) in the acute phase of the disease. These cells may release a collagen-specific arthritogenic lymphokine (35) that has been shown to cause joint destruction. Type II collagen-specific T_H cell lines have been shown to be arthritogenic on adoptive transfer to naive animals (36,37). Hence T cells are important both in the "affector" phase of the disease in initating production of pathogenic anticollagen antibodies, as well as in the "effector" phase of the disease in causing joint destruction.

A suitable target for immunotherapy in this disease would thus be the T_H cells. In fact anti-CD4 antibodies, acting on the CD4 molecule expressed on all T_H cells, have been shown to prevent CIA on in vivo administration (38). In addition, anti-Ia antibodies blocking activation of the T_H cells by MHC class II expressing antigen presenting cells have also been shown to be useful in the prevention of CIA (Ref. 21 and see earlier discussion). However, the constitutive nature of expression of these targeted molecules on the surfaces of all T_H cells and antigen presenting cells, respectively, could lead to a broad immunosuppression. This could be detrimental to the animal.

B. IL-2 Receptor

Another potential target for immunosuppression could be a surface molecule expressed only on activated T_H cells. Treatment aimed at this molecule would spare resting and memory cells, which would not express this molecule. Such a target molecule is the interleukin-2 receptor (IL-2R, CD25). IL-2R are expressed on T cells (and to a lower extent on B cells and monocytes) only when the cells are activated (39–41). Stimulation of T cells with interleukin-2 leads to the growth and proliferation of these cells. The IL-2R on activated T cells is a noncovalently linked heterodimer of a 55 kD (p55) and a 75 kD (p75) chain (41). Each chain has a distinct IL-2 binding site. The coexpression of both the chains is necessary for the development of a high-affinity IL-2R on activated T cells. The p55 chain individually binds IL-2 with a kD of 10 nm, whereas the p75 chain individually binds IL-2 with a kD of 1 nm (42). Only when both the chains are expressed is the typical kD of 10 pM of the high-affinity IL-2R obtained by the synergistic action of the two chains. The majority of the IL-2R antibodies described so far are reactive to the p55 chain in mice (e.g., 7D$_4$, 3C7, and M7/20), rats (e.g., ART-18 and ART-65), and humans (e.g., anti-Tac). Recently, monoclonal antibodies reactive to the p75 chain of IL-2R in humans have been described (43). The anti-IL-2R antibodies are of two types: those that act on the IL-2 binding site on the IL-2R and those that bind to a site distinct from the IL-2 binding site (44). Examples of the former are anti-Tac (45), ART-18 (46), and M7/20 (47).

Examples of the latter are 7D4 (48) and ART-65 (49). The former type of antibodies can block IL-2-dependent T cell proliferation in vitro. Some of the latter type of antibodies, such as 7D4, can also do so, albeit less efficiently (50).

C. Use of Anti-IL-2R Antibodies in the Prevention of Graft Rejection

With selective immunosuppression of activated allogressive T cells in mind (41,44), the use of anti-IL-2R antibodies in vivo for the prevention of allograft rejection was studied. Anti-IL-2R treatment was shown to be effective in prolonging the survival of cardiac (51) and skin (52) allografts. An anti-IL-2R antibody has also been used successfully in the prevention of kidney allograft rejection in humans (53). There did not seem to be any side effects or complications with this treatment in any of these instances. This demonstrated not only that IL-2R$^+$ T cells are important in the graft rejection process but also that hyperactive aggressive immune cells could be specifically targeted to achieve a selective form of immunosuppression.

D. Use of an Anti-IL-2R Antibody in Arthritis

Since anti-IL-2R antibodies had been shown to be effective in suppressing the alloreactive cells involved in graft rejection, the use of anti-IL-2R antibodies in suppressing autoreactive cells in autoimmune diseases was the next step. We decided to investigate whether anti-IL-2R antibodies could, in fact, suppress CIA by targeting pathogenic type II collagen-reactive cells. We selected for our studies an anti-IL-2R antibody, 7D4 (48), which is a rat IgM antimouse IL-2R monoclonal antibody. It binds to a site on the p55 subunit of IL-2R distinct from the IL-2 binding site (54) but causes suppression of IL-2-dependent T cell proliferation in vitro (50,54). 7D4 could thus bind to the IL-2R regardless of IL-2 already bound to the IL-2R (50) and, having an IgM isotype, would efficiently bind complement in vivo.

Table 4 summarizes the results of our preliminary trial of 7D4 in the suppression of CIA (55). One group of DBA/1 Lac mice received 40 μg of 7D4, purified from ascites and culture supernatants over a goat anti-rat IgM column, IP for

Table 4 Effects of "Low-Dose" 7D4 in CIA

Agent	Incidence of arthritis	Day of onset of arthritis[a]	Mean severity
7D4	6/7	34 ± 2[b]	1.9[b]
Control	5/10	25 ± 3	3.6

[a]Mean ± SEM.
[b]$p < 0.05$.

7 days. Another group received buffer alone as a control. Both groups of mice immunized with 100 μg of native bovine type II collagen in complete Freund's adjuvant intradermally on the second day of the 7D4 or buffer injections. As shown in Table 4, 7D4 significantly delayed the onset and reduced the severity of arthritis compared to the control group.

Since 7D4 at the dose used did not seem to affect the incidence of arthritis, we next decided to use a higher dose of the antibody for improved efficacy. We used a rat IgM anti-Forsmann antigen antibody as control, similar to earlier studies (52). Two groups of DBA/1 mice were immunized interdermally with 100 μg native bovine type II collagen in complete Freund's adjuvant. One group was administered 200 μg of purified 7D4 IP for 6 days, and the other group was given 200 μg of the control antibody for 6 days, both starting 1 day before collagen immunization. As shown in Table 5, 7D4 with this increased dose not only decreased the severity of arthritis, as earlier, but also suppressed the incidence of arthritis (56). Since arthritis was earlier shown to correlate with complement-fixing IgG_{2a} isotype anticollagen antibodies in DBA/1 mice (57), we analyzed the anticollagen isotypes in these mice. There was a significantly reduced level of anticollagen antibodies of the IgG_{2a} and IgG_{2b} isotypes in the 7D4 group at 14 days (56) after immunization with collagen (Table 6). However, by 28 days after collagen immunization these differences in anticollagen antibody levels were much less. We also investigated whether 7D4 could downregulate delayed-type hypersensitivity (DTH) responses to type II collagen measured in the ears 10 days following collagen immunization. This is the time of peak DTH responses to type II collagen (21). Although the mean DTH responses were in fact lower in the 7D4-treated group (3×10^{-2} mm) than in the control group (6.8×10^{-2} mm), the variability of responses in the two groups was too great to be statistically significant. Since 7D4 did not cause a more complete suppression of CIA, and anticollagen antibodies did not seem to differ between the 7D4 and control groups 28 days after collagen immunization, we investigated the possibility of antirat antibodies being induced in these mice. Such antixenogeneic antibodies had been earlier shown to partially negate the beneficial effects of administration of anti-IL-2R antibodies in vivo (52). Indeed, both the 7D4 and the control groups showed

Table 5 Effects of "High-Dose" 7D4 in CIA

Agent	Incidence of arthritis	Day of onset of arthritis[a]	Mean severity
7D4	8/16[b]	36 ± 4	1.9[b]
Control	16/19	34 ± 2	3.4

[a]Mean ± SEM.
[b]$p < 0.05$.

Table 6 Anti-Type II Collagen Antibodies in "High-Dose" 7D4 Treatment of CIA[a]

Agent	Day 14					Day 28				
	Total Ig	IgG$_{2a}$ Subclass	IgG$_{2b}$ Subclass	IgG$_1$ Subclass	IgG$_3$ Subclass	Total Ig	IgG$_{2a}$ Subclass	IgG$_{2b}$ Subclass	IgG$_1$ Subclass	IgG$_3$ Subclass
7D4	52 ± 8[b]	10 ± 2[b]	15 ± 3[c]	9 ± 1	1 ± 0.2[d]	92 ± 15	32 ± 10	27 ± 6	20 ± 4	1 ± 0.3
Control	80 ± 8	23 ± 5	33 ± 5	13 ± 2	2 ± 0.3	102 ± 9	57 ± 3	45 ± 7	27 ± 4	1 ± 0.2

[a]All results are mean μg/ml ± SEM.
[b]$p < 0.02$.
[c]$p < 0.01$.
[d]$p < 0.05$.

the development of antirat antibodies. The development of antirat antibodies could probably account for lack of a better efficacy of 7D4 in vivo. It is also possible that coadministration of another anti-IL-2R antibody that binds to the IL-2 binding site, such as M7/20, could have a synergistic effect leading to a better response in vivo. This latter antibody has recently been shown to be effective in suppressing two spontaneously induced autoimmune diseases in mice, diabetes mellitus and lupus nephritis (58).

Remarkably enough, following our report on the effective use of an anti-IL-2R antibody in an animal model of arthritis, an antihuman IL-2R antibody has been shown to be beneficial in the treatment of patients with rheumatoid arthritis (59). Three patients with active erosive rheumatoid arthritis who were unresponsive to conventional treatment, including disease-modifying drugs, were administered a rat anti-human IL-2R antibody. All three patients showed a remarkable improvement with this antibody. In two of the three patients the benefit lasted up to 3 months. Further administration was not done to avoid the risk of antixenogeneic sensitization. This report has demonstrated the potential for the use of anti-IL-2R antibodies in the selective immunosuppression of human autoimmune diseases. This has also borne out the importance of the use of animal models of arthritis in the investigation of newer forms of immunotherapy and the possibility of extrapolating the findings in animal models to clinically relevant human situations.

E. Mode of Action of Anti-IL-2R Antibodies In Vivo

The exact mode of action of anti-IL-2R antibodies in vivo is not clear. They could act by directly blocking IL-2 binding to the IL-2R (60), opsonization of IL-2R$^+$ cells coated with the antibodies (49), antibody-dependent cell cytotoxicity (ADCC) (49), or complement-dependent target cell destruction (60). Target cell depletion in vivo may be the major mode of action of anti-IL-2R antibodies in vivo (49,61). An anti-rat IL-2R antibody, ART-65, which does not inhibit the binding of IL-2 to activated T cells nor have any inhibitory effect on IL-2-stimulated proliferation of T cells in vitro nevertheless is effective in vivo. It is as effective in inhibiting a graft-versus-host reaction in vivo as another anti-IL-2R antibody, ART-18, which binds to the IL-2 binding site on the IL-2R (49). Thus, anti-IL-2R antibodies do not necessarily have to bind to the IL-2 binding site on the IL-2R for efficacy in vivo. ART-65 presumably binds to the IL-2R on activated cells in vivo and eliminates them by ADCC and/or complement depletion. The same group of workers has recently reported an increase in circulatory levels of soluble IL-2R in situations in which administered anti-IL-2R antibodies were effective in vivo (61). This suggests the destruction of IL-2R$^+$ cells is necessary for the in vivo efficacy of anti-IL-2R antibodies. Furthermore, the observation that only intact anti-IL-2R antibodies, but not Fab fragments, were effective in suppressing allograft rejection in vivo supported their findings (61).

There is yet another mechanism of action of anti-IL-2R antibodies in vivo to explain their beneficial effects. It has been shown that T "suppressor" cells (T_s) are relatively spared by the anti-II-2R antibodies both in vitro as well as in vivo compared to other activated cells (62–64). The T_s cells are thus left free to exert their suppressive actions in vivo. In fact, different anti-IL-2R antibodies act on distinct T_s subsets in vivo and can exert synergistic beneficial effects on coadministration in vivo (65).

Anti-IL-2R antibody administration causes suppression of clinical manifestations of CIA, possibly by different mechanisms acting synergistically. The anti-IL-2R antibody probably blocks the "afferent" pathway of pathogenesis by suppressing the production of pathogenic anticollagen antibodies. It also possibly suppresses the "efferent" pathway by suppressing activated effector cells. This probably explains the reduction in severity of the disease. In addition, the anti-IL-2R antibody may spare collagen-reactive T_s cells (66), leading to suppression of the disease.

F. Use of IL-2 Toxins to Deplete IL-2R$^+$ Cells In Vivo

Although anti-IL-2R antibodies have proven to be effective in the suppression of allograft rejection and autoimmune diseases, they have a few drawbacks. Since the IL-2R described so far are nonpolymorphic in a species, anti-IL-2R antibodies must be generated across species. This has the potential of inducing the production of antixenogeneic antibodies, which could negate the beneficial effects of the administered anti-IL-2R antibody. This was observed in the immunosuppression of CIA. In addition, most currently available antibodies are directed against the p55 subunit of the IL-2R, which can exist alone or as part of the high-affinity IL-2R heterodimer (41). These antibodies may thus lack the specificity of action toward the high-affinity IL-2R uniquely expressed on activated T cells. IL-2 itself has a 100–1000 times higher affinity for the high-affinity IL-2R than the anti-IL-2R antibodies. This principle has been employed by various groups of investigators in devising a novel molecule to delete IL-2R$^+$ cells in vitro and in vivo. Recombinant chimeric fusion proteins of IL-2 with bacterial exotoxin products—IL2–PE40 (67) and IL-2–diphtheria toxin (68)—have been constructed for this purpose. IL-2–PE40 is a chimeric immunotoxin combining human IL-2 with the membrane penetration and ADP ribosylation regions of *Pseudomonas* exotoxin A. The IL-2 portion replaces the native membrane binding region of the exotoxin. Similarly, IL-2–diphtheria toxin is a fusion protein of the human IL-2 molecule and diphtheria toxin A in which IL-2 replaces the membrane binding region of the diphtheria toxin. Both toxins bind to the high-affinity IL-2R on T cells, are endocytosed via acid vesicles, and release the toxophore portion of the molecules intracellularly. The toxophore portions enzymatically inactivate the elongation factor 2 by ADP ribosylation (67,69). This causes blockage of cellular protein synthesis, leading to cell death. The IL-2–PE40 fusion immuno-toxin has been recently demonstrated to be effective in the treatment of yet another animal model of arthritis, adjuvant arthritis in rats (70). Activated T cells are important in the pathogenesis of this disease (70). As in the treatment of CIA with an anti-IL-2R antibody shown by us earlier, IL-2–PE40 administered IP reduced the severity of adjuvant arthritis with a delay in the onset of clinical symp-toms. Some of the rats treated with IL-2–PE40 in fact showed no clinical or histologic evidence of arthritis at the end of the study. Control fusion proteins that lacked either a membrane-binding domain or an enzymatically inactive toxin domain failed to suppress adjuvant arthritis. Another group earlier showed than an anti-IL-2R antibody could block the adoptive transfer of adjuvant arthritis with spleen cells (71). However, in marked contrast to the high efficacy of IL-2–PE40, the particular anti-IL-2R antibody failed to suppress adjuvant arthritis (71). This may have been due to early development of antixenogeneic antibodies or to ex-cess IL-2 production in this disease out-competing the anti-IL-2R antibody for binding to the IL-2R. The administration of IL-2–PE40 immunotoxin in rats IP, however, led to the development of ascites in the injected animals (70). This could have been due to the "capillary leak" syndrome noticed earlier in IL-2 im-munotherapy in humans (70,72). This side effect has to be kept in mind in plann-ing future immunotherapy with IL-2 toxins.

Perhaps the best compromise in the future treatment of human autoimmune diseases could be the use of the recently described recombinant immunotoxin anti-Tac (Fv)-PE40 (73). This fusion protein combines the smallest binding unit (Fv fragment) of an anti-human IL-2R antibody and PE40. The variable regions of the heavy and light chains of a monoclonal antibody to the p55 subunit of the human IL-2R [anti-Tac (45)] have been joined in peptide linkage to PE40 (lack-ing the membrane binding region) by recombinant techniques. This fusion cosntruct has been shown to be cytotoxic to two IL-2R-positive human cell lines but had no effect on IL-2R-negative cells in vitro. In fact, this latest anti-Tac (Fv)-PE40 construct has been shown to be more cytotoxic in vitro to an IL-2R$^+$ human cell line than IL-2–PE40 (73).

IV. CONCLUSIONS

The unique expression of a high-affinity form of IL-2R only on activated T cells but not on resting or memory cells has allowed a more selective and specific form of immunotherapy. IL-2R-targeted therapy has proven to be useful in the treat-ment of autoimmune diseases in experimental animals. As in allograft rejection, a hyperreactive IL-2–IL-2R system is probably involved in the im-munopathogenesis of a number of autoimmune diseases in both animals and humans (74). Early results of the use of anti-IL-2R antibodies in clinical situations have been very encouraging. IL-2R-targeted immunotherapy holds a promising approach to the selective immunosuppression of human autoimmune diseases.

REFERENCES

1. Trentham, D.E., Townes, A.S., and Kang, A.H. (1977). Autoimmunity to type II collagen: an experimental model of arthritis. J. Exp. Med. 146:857.
2. Courtenay, J.S., Dallman, M.J., Dayan, A.D., Martin, A., and Mosedale, B. (1980). Immunization against heterologous type II collagen induces arthritis in mice. Nature 283:666.
3. Wooley, P.H., and Chapdelaine, J.M. (1987). Immunogenetics of collagen-induced arthritis. CRC Crit. Rev. Immunol. 8:23.
4. Wooley, P.H., Luthra, H.S., Stuart, J.M., and David, C.S. (1981). Type II collagen-induced arthritis in mice. I. Major histocompatibility complex (I region) linkage and antibody correlates. J. Exp. Med. 154:688.
5. Griffiths, M.M., Eichwald, E.J., Martin, J.H., Smith, C.B., and DeWitt, C.W. (1981). Immunogenetic control of experimental type II collagen-induced arthritis. I. Susceptibility and resistance among inbred strains of rats. Arthritis Rheum. 24:781.
6. Stastny, P. (1978). Association of B-cell alloantigen DRw4 with rheumatoid arthritis. N. Engl. J. Med. 298:869.
7. Mathis, D.J., Benoist, C., Williams, V.E., Kanter, M., and McDevitt, H.O. (1983). Several mechanisms can account for defective E_α gene expression in different mouse haplotypes. Proc. Natl. Acad. Sci. USA 80:273.
8. Holmdahl, R., Klareskog, L., Andersson, M., and Hansen, C. (1986). High antibody response to autologous type II collagen is restricted to H-2^q. Immunogenetics 24:84.
9. Wooley, P.H., Luthra, H.S., Griffiths, M.M., Stuart, J.M., Huse, A., and David, C.S. (1985). Type II collagen-induced arthritis in mice. IV. Variations in immunogenetic regulation provide evidence for multiple arthritogenic epitopes on the collagen molecule. J. Immunol. 135:2443.
10. Holmdahl, R., Jansson, L., Larsson, E., Rubin, K., and Klareskog, L. (1986). Homologous type II collagen induces chronic and progressive arthritis in mice. Arthritis Rheum. 29:106.
11. Holmdahl, R., Jansson, L., Gullberg, D., Rubin, K., Forsberg, P.O., and Klareskog, L. (1985). Incidence of arthritis and autoreactivity of anti-collagen antibodies after immunization of DBA/1 mice with heterologous and autolous collagen II. Clin. Exp. Immunol. 62:639.
12. Banerjee, S., Haqqi, T.M., Luthra, H.S., Stuart, J.M., and David, C.S. (1988). Possible role of V_β T cell receptor genes in susceptibility to collagen-induced arthritis in mice. J. Exp. Med. 167:832.
13. Stuart, J.M., and Dixon, F.J. (1983). Serum transfer of collagen-induced arthritis in mice. J. Exp. Med. 158:378.
14. Wooley, P.H., Luthra, H.S., Krco, C.J., Stuart, J.M., and David, C.S. (1984). Type II collagen-induced arthritis in mice. II. Passive transfer and suppression by intravenous injection of anti-type II collagen antibody or free native type II collagen. Arthritis Rheum. 27:1010.

15. Wooley, P.H., Luthra, H.S., Singh, S.K., Huse, A., Stuart, J.M., and David, C.S. (1984). Passive transfer of arthritis in mice by human anti-type II collagen antibody. Mayo Clin. Proc. 59:737.

16. Klareskog, I., Holmdahl, R., Larsson, E., and Wigzell, H. (1983). Role of T-lymphocytes in collagen II induced arthritis in rats. Clin. Exp. Immunol. 51:117.

17. Takagishi, K., Kaibara, N., Hotokebuchi, T., Arita, C., Morinaga, M., and Arai, K. (1985). Serum transfer in congenitally athymic nude rats. J. Immunol. 134: 3864.

18. Steinman, L., Rosenbaum, J.T., Sriram, S., and McDevitt, H.O. (1981). In vivo effects of antibodies to immune response gene products: Prevention of experimental allergic encephalitis. Proc. Natl. Acad. Sci. USA 78:7111.

19. Adelman, H.E., Watling, D.L., and McDevitt, H.O. (1983). Treatment of (NZB × NZW)F$_1$ disease with anti-Ia monoclonal antibodies. J. Exp. Med. 158:1350.

20. Vladutiu, A., and Steinman, L. (1984). Inhibition of experimental allergic thyroiditis in mice by monoclonal anti-I-A Fed. Proc. 43:1991.

21. Wooley, P.H., Luthra, H.S., Lafuse, W.P., Huse, A. Stuart, J.M., and David, C.S. (1985). Type II collagen-induced arthritis in mice. III. Suppression of arthritis using monoclonal and polyclonal anti-Ia antisera. J. Immunol. 134:2366.

22. Waldor, M., Hardy, R. Hayakawa, K., Steinman, L., and Herzenberg, L. (1984). Disappearance and reappearance of B cells following in vivo treatment with monoclonal anti-I-A antibody. Proc. Natl. Acad. Sci. USA 81:2855.

23. Frelinger, J.H., Niederhuber, J.E., David, C.S., and Shreffler, D.C. (1974). Evidence for the expression of Ia (H-2-associated) antigen on thymus derived lymphocytes. J. Exp. Med. 140:1273.

24. Rosenbaum, J.T., Adelman, N.E., and McDevitt, H.O. (1981). In vivo effects of antibodies to immune response gene products. I. Haplotype specific suppression of humoral immune responses with a monoclonal anti-I-A antibody. J. Exp.Med. 154:1694.

25. Sriram, S., and Steinman, L. (1983). Anti-Ia antibody suppresses active encephalomyelitis: treatment model for diseases linked to Ir genes. J. Exp. Med. 158:1362.

26. Perry, L.L., and Greene, M.I. (1982). Conversion of immunity to suppression by in vivo administration of I-A subregion specific antibodies. J. Exp. Med. 156: 480.

27. Steinman, L., Schwartz, G., Waldor, M., O'Hearn, M., Lim, M., and Sriram, S. (1984). Genetic specific and antigen specific strategies for the induction of suppressor T cells to myelin basic protein. In: EAE: A Good Model for MS. Kies, M., ed. Alan R. Liss, New York.

28. Sprent, J. (1980). Effect of blocking helper T cell induction in vivo with anti-Ia antibodies: Possible role of I-A/E hybrid molecules as restriction elements. J. Exp. Med. 152:996.

29. Clot, J., and Sany, J. (1984). Anti-Ia-like antibodies: Preliminary use in rheumatoid arthritis. Immunol. Today 5:126.

30. Combe, B., Cosso, B., Clot, J., Bonneau, M., and Sany, J. (1985). Human placenta-eluted gammaglobulin in immunomodulating treatment of rheumatoid arthritis. Am. J. Med. 78:920.

31. Holmdahl, R., Klareskog, L., Rubin, K., Bjork, J., Smedegard, G., Jonsson, R., and Andersson, M. (1986). Role of T lymphocytes in murine collagen arthritis. Agents Actions 19:295.

32. Stuart, J.M., Townes, A.S., and Kang, A.H. (1984). Collagen autoimmune arthritis. Annu. Rev. Immunol. 2:199.

33. Morgan, K., Clague, R.B., Shaw, M.J., Firth, S.A., Twose, T.M., and Holt, P.J.L. (1981). Native type II collagen-induced arthritis in the rat: The effect of complement depletion by cobra venom factor. Arthritis Rheum. 24:1356.

34. Holmdahl, R., Rubin, K., Klareskog, L., Dencker, L., Gustafsson, G., and Larson, E. (1985). Appearance of different lymphoid cells in synovial tissue and in peripheral blood during the course of collagen-II-induced arthritis in rats. Scand. J. Immunol. 21:197.

35. Helfgott, S.M., Dynesius-Trentham, R., Brahn, E., and Trentham, D.E. (1985). An arthritogenic lymphokine in the rat. J. Exp. Med. 162:1531.

36. Holmdahl, R., Klareskog, L., Rubin, K., Larson, E., and Wigzell, H. (1985). T lymphocytes in collagen II-induced arthritis in mice. Characterization of arthritogenic collagen II-specific T cell lines and clones. Scand. J. Immunol. 22:295.

37. Brahn, E., and Trentham, D.E. (1989). Experimental synovitis induced by collagen-specific T cell lines. Cell. Immunol. 118:491.

38. Ranges, G.E., Sriram, S., and Cooper, S.M. (1985). Prevention of type II collagen-induced arthritis by in vivo treatment with anti-L3T4. J. Exp. Med. 162:1105.

39. Robb, R.J., Munch, A., and Smith, K.A. (1981). T cell growth factors: Quantification, specificity, and biological relevance. J. Exp. Med. 154:1455.

40. Herrman, F., Canistra, S.A., Levine, H., and Griffin, J.D. (1985). Expression of interleukin 2 receptors and binding of interleukin 2 by gamma interferon-induced human leukemic and normal monocytic cells. J. Exp. Med. 162:1111.

41. Smith, K.A. (1988). Interleukin-2: Inception, impact, and implications. Science 240:1169.

42. Teshigawara, K., Wang, H.M., Kato, K., and Smith, K.A. (1987). Interleukin 2 high-affinity receptor expression requires two distinct binding proteins. J. Exp. Med. 165:223.

43. Tsudo, M., Kitamura, F., and Miyasaka, M. (1989). Characterization of the interleukin 2 receptor β chain using three distinct monoclonal antibodies. Proc. Natl. Acad. Sci. USA 86:1982.

44. Diamantstein, T. and Osawa, H. (1986). The interleukin-2 receptor, its physiology and a new approach to a selective immunosuppressive therapy by anti-interleukin-2 receptor monoclonal antibodies. Immunol. Rev. 92:5.

45. Uchiyama, T., Broder, S., and Waldmann, T.A. (1981). A monoclonal antibody (anti-Tac) reactive with activated and functionally mature human T cells. J. Immunol. 126:1293.

46. Osawa, H., and Diamantstein, T. (1983). The characteristics of a monoclonal antibody that binds specifically to rat T-lymphoblasts and inhibits IL-2 receptor functions. J. Immunol. 130:51.

47. Gaulton, G.N., Bangs, J., Maddock, S., Springer, T., Eardley, D.D., and Strom, T.B. (1985). Characterization of a monoclonal rat anti-mouse IL-2 receptor antibody

and its use in the biochemical characterization of the murine IL-2 receptor. Clin. Immunol. Immunopathol. 36:18.

48. Malek, T.R., Robb, R.J., and Shevach, E.M. (1983). Identification and initial characterization of a rat monoclonal antibody reactive with the murine interleukin-2 receptor-ligand complex. Proc. Natl. Acad. Sci. USA 80:5694.

49. Mouzaki, A., Volk, H., Osawa, H., and Diamantstein, T. (1989). Blocking of interleukin-2 (IL-2) binding to the IL-2 receptor is not required for the in vivo action of anti-IL-2 receptor monoclonal antibody (mAb). I. The production, characterization and in vivo properties of a new mouse anti-rat IL-2 receptor mAb that reacts with an epitope different to the one that binds to IL-2 and the mAb ART-18. Eur. J. Immunol. 17:335.

50. Malek, T.R., Ortega, G.R., Jakway, J.P., Chan, C., and Shevach, E.M. (1984). The murine IL-2 receptor. II. Monoclonal anti-IL-2 receptor antibodies as specific inhibitors of T cell function in vitro. J. Immunol. 133:1976.

51. Kirkman, R.L., Barrett, L.V., Gaulton, G.N., Kelley, V.E., Ythier, A., and Strom, T.B. (1985). Administration of an anti-interleukin-2 receptor monoclonal antibody prolongs cardiac allograft survival in mice. J. Exp. Med. 162:358.

52. Granstein, R.D., Goulston, C., and Gaulton, G.N. (1986). Prolongation of murine skin allograft survival by immunologic manipulation with anti-interleukin 2 receptor antibody. J. Immunol. 136:898.

53. Soulillou, J.P. Peyronnet, P., LeMauff, B., Hourmant, M., Olive, D., Mawas, C., DeLaage, M., Hirn, M., and Jacques, Y. (1987). Prevention of rejection of kidney transplants by monoclonal antibody directed against interleukin-2 receptor. Lancet 1:1339.

54. Ortega, G.R., Robb, R.J., Shevach, E.M., and Malek, T.R. (1984). The murine IL-2 receptor. I. Monoclonal antibodies that define distinct functional epitopes on activated T cells and react with activated B cells. J. Immunol. 133:1970.

55. Banerjee, S., Luthra, H.S., Stuart, J.M., and David, C.S. (1987). Immunotherapy of type II collagen induced arthritis in mice with an anti-IL-2 receptor antibody. Arthritis Rheum. 30:s19.

56. Banerjee, S., Wei, B.-Y., Hillman, K., Luthra, H.S., and David, C.S. (1988). Immunosuppression of collagen-induced arthritis in mice with an anti-IL-2 receptor antibody. J. Immunol. 141:1150.

57. Watson, W.C., and Townes, A.S. (1985). Genetic susceptibility to murine collagen II autoimmune arthritis. Proposed relationship to the IgG_2 autoantibody subclass response, complement C5, major histocompatibility complex (MHC) and non-MHC loci. J. Exp. Med. 162:1878.

58. Kelley, V.L., Gaulton, G.N., Hattoti, M., Ikegami, H., Eisenbarth, G., and Strom, T.B. (1988). Anti-interleukin-2 receptor antibody suppresses murine diabetic insulitis and lupus nephritis. J. Immunol. 140:59.

59. Kyle, V., Coughlan, R.J., Tighe, H., Waldmann, H., and Hazleman, B.L. (1989). Beneficial effect of monoclonal antibody to interleukin-2 receptor on activated T cells in rheumatoid arthritis. Ann Rheum. Dis. 48:429.

60. Kelley, V.E., Gaulton, G.N., and Strom, T.B. (1987). Inhibitory effects of anti-interleukin 2 receptor and anti-L3T4 antibodies on delayed-type hypersensitivity: The role of complement and epitope. J. Immunol. 138:2771.

61. Volk, H.D., Josimovic-Alasevic, O., Gross, M., and Diamantstein, T. (1989). The therapeutic efficacy of an anti-IL-2 receptor monoclonal antibody correlates with an increase in serum soluble IL-2 receptor levels. Clin. Exp. Immunol. 76:121.

62. Schneider, T.M., Kupiec-Weglinski, J.W., Towpik, E., Padberg, W., Araneda, D., Diamantstein, T., Strom, T.B., and Tilney, N.C. (1986). Development of suppressor lymphocytes during acute rejection of rat cardiac allografts and preservation of suppression by anti-IL-2 receptor monoclonal antibody. Transplantation 42:191.

63. Kupiec-Weglinski, J.W., Diamantstein, T., Tilney, H.L., and Strom, T. B. (1986). Therapy with monoclonal antibody to interleukin-2 receptor spares suppressor T cells and prevents or reverses acute allograft rejection in rats. Proc. Natl. Acad. Sci. USA 83:2624.

64. Tanaka, K., Turka, L.A., Veda, H., Diamantstein, T., Milford, E.L., Carpenter, C.B., Tilney, N.L., and Kupiec-Weglinski, J.W. (1989). Selective sparing of T suppressor cells by anti-interleukin-2 receptor monoclonal antibodies (IL-2R mAbs) in vitro correlates with their therapeutic effects in vivo. Transplant. Proc. 21:475.

65. Stefano, R.D., Mouzaki, A., Araneda, D., Diamantstein, T., Tilney, N.L., and Kupiec-Weglinski, J.W. (1988). Anti-interleukin-2 receptor monoclonal antibodies spare phenotypically distinct T suppressor cells in vivo and exert synergistic biological effect. J. Exp. Med. 167:1981.

66. Kresina, T.F., and Finegan, C.G. (1986). Restricted expression of anti-type II collagen antibody isotypes in mice suppressed for collagen-induced arthritis. Ann. Rheum. Dis. 45:60.

67. Lorberboum-Galski, H., Fitzgerald, D., Chaudhary, V., Adhya, A., and Pastan, I. (1988). Cytotoxic activity of an interleukin-2 pseudomonas exotoxin chimeric protein produced in Escherichia coli. Proc. Natl. Acad. Sci. USA 85:1922.

68. Williams, D.P., Parker, K., Bacha, P., Bishai, W., Borowski, M., Genbauffe, F., Strom, T.B., and Murphy, J.R. (1987). Diphtheriotoxin receptor binding domain substitution with interleukin-2: Genetic construction and properties of a diphtheria toxin-related interleukin 2 fusion protein. Protein Eng. 1:493.

69. Bacha, P., Williams, D.P., Waters, C., Williams, J.M., Murphy, J.R., and Strom, T.B. (1988). Interleukin 2 receptor-targeted cytotoxicity. Interleukin-2 receptor-mediated action of a diphtheria toxin-related interleukin 2 fusion protein. J. Exp. Med. 167:612.

70. Case, J.P., Lorberboum-Galski, H., Lafyatis, R., Fitzgerald, D., Wilder, R.L., and Pastan, I. (1989). Chimeric cytotoxin IL2-PE40 delays and mitigates adjuvant-induced arthritis in rats. Proc. Natl. Acad. Sci. USA 86:287.

71. Stunkel, K.G., Theisen, P., Mouzaki, A., Diamantstein, T., and Schlumberger, H.D. (1988). Monitoring of interleukin 2 receptor (IL-2R) expression in vivo and studies on an IL-2R-directed immunosuppressive therapy of active and adoptive adjuvant-induced arthritis in rats. Immunology 64:683.

72. Rosenstein, M., Ettinghausen, S.E., and Rosenberg, S.A. (1986). Extravasation of intravascular fluid mediated by the systemic administration of recombinant interleukin 2. J. Immunol. 137:1735.

73. Chaudhary, V.K., Queen, C., Junghans, R.P., Waldmann, T.A., Fitzgerald, D.J., and Pastan, I. (1989). A recombinant immunotoxin consisting of two antibody variable domains fused to pseudomonas exotoxin. Nature 339:394.
74. Kroemer, G., and Wick, G. (1989). The role of interleukin 2 in autoimmunity. Immunol. Today 10:246.

14

Anti-L3T4 Antibody Therapy in Systemic Lupus Erythematosus

Nancy L. Carteron and David Wofsy
Veterans Administration Medical Center and the University of California, San Francisco, California

I. INTRODUCTION

Monoclonal antibodies (MAb) directed against distinct lymphocyte subsets have been used in vivo to deplete selected cells and thereby examine the function of these cells in immune responses (1–8). During the past several years, we have been using MAb directed against a specific T cell subset, the T helper (T_H) cell, to determine the role of this subset in autoimmunity (4,7,9,10). Our studies have utilized NZB × NZW F_1 (B/W) mice, which spontaneously develop an autoimmune disease similar to systemic lupus erythematosus (SLE) in humans (11–13). Through these studies, we hope to achieve two goals. First, by depleting or interfering with the function of T_H cells, we hope to determine the contribution of these cells to the pathogenesis of such autoimmune diseases as SLE. Second, by identifying the cells that promote autoimmunity, we hope to develop new approaches to therapy that utilize MAb as therapeutic agents.

II. MURINE MODELS FOR SYSTEMIC LUPUS ERYTHEMATOSUS

Several strains of mice have been developed that serve as models for SLE. These include B/W, MRL/lpr, and BXSB mice (12,13). All these strains develop anti-DNA antibodies and immune complex glomerulonephritis, but the B/W model

most closely resembles SLE in humans with respect to disease manifestations and
the predilection for more severe illness in females (11–13). Moreover, the immunologic abnormalities present in B/W mice closely parallel the immunologic
abnormalities in humans with SLE. These include the development of T lymphopenia (4,14,15), impaired suppressor T cell function (14,16–18), reduced
cytokine production (19–21), polyclonal B cell activation (22,23), and defective
immune clearance (24,25). These similarities suggest that SLE in humans and
SLE in B/W mice share common pathogenetic mechanisms. Thus, studies in B/W
mice may provide insight into the pathogenesis of SLE and guide the development of new treatment strategies.

III. T CELL REGULATION OF IMMUNITY

Our studies have utilized the fact that mature (extrathymic) T cells can be divided into two mutually exclusive subsets based on their surface antigens (26–28).
In mice, these subsets can be distinguished by the expression of either L3T4 or
Lyt-2 (28–32). L3T4$^+$ cells and Lyt-2$^+$ cells are often referred to as "helper-
inducer" and "suppressor/cytotoxic" cells, respectively (26–29,32), but both
subsets may be functionally heterogeneous (33). These subsets can be distinguished
more precisely based on their mechanism of interaction with antigen presenting
cells (APC). L3T4$^+$ and Lyt-2$^+$ cells recognize antigen (Ag) exclusively in
association with class II major histocompatibility antigens (MHC II) (30–35) or
class I major histocompatibility antigens (MHC I) (30,34–36) on APC,
respectively.

Both L3T4$^+$ and Lyt-2$^+$ cells play important roles in immune regulation.
L3T4$^+$ cells promote B cell activation and contribute to the induction of suppressor and cytotoxic T cells (35); Lyt-2$^+$ cells suppress immunity or mediate
cytotoxicity (28). MAb directed against L3T4 or Lyt-2 can modulate the function of cells that bear these Ag. MAb to L3T4 block antigen-induced clonal proliferation and the release of interleukin-2 by MHC II-restricted T cell clones (32).
Anti-L3T4 also inhibits the binding of cloned T cells to MHC II$^+$ cells implying that L3T4 may bind to MHC II (32). However, prevention of binding to MHC
II is not the sole mechanism through which anti-L3T4 inhibits T cell function,
because anti-L3T4 can also inhibit T cell function in the absence of MHC II$^+$
cells (37–40). This suggests that L3T4 may transmit an inhibitory signal or block
a stimulatory signal to T cells. These observations form the basis for our attempts
to suppress murine lupus with MAb to L3T4 (4,7,9,10,41).

Mechanisms of T cell regulation in mice are highly conserved in humans (26,27),
in whom the CD4 surface Ag is homologous to L3T4 in mice (29,30,34,42).
Like antibodies to L3T4, antibodies to CD4 block MHC II-dependent T cell
responses (43). These observations suggest that the effects of anti-CD4 in humans
may parallel the effects of anti-L3T4 in mice.

IV. EFFECTS ON ANTI-L3T4 ON MURINE LUPUS

A. Chronic Administration of Anti-L3T4 Prevents Murine Lupus

We proposed that since L3T4$^+$ cells play a central role in promoting immune responses, MAb directed against L3T4$^+$ cells might inhibit T cell responses that result in autoimmunity. To test this hypothetisis, we initially treated 10 female B/W mice with weekly intraperitoneal injections (2 mg per mouse per week) of a rat IgG$_{2b}$ MAb to L3T4 produced by hybridoma GK1.5 (4). B/W mice spontaneously develop clinical signs of autoimmune disease between 5 and 6 months of age (12). Therefore, treatment was begun at age 4 months, before the onset of overt autoimmune disease, to determine whether the development of autoimmunity could be prevented. Weekly therapy was continued until age 12 months. There were two control groups: one group received weekly injections (2 mg) of purified, nonimmune rat IgG; the other group received weekly injections of saline.

Circulating Lymphocytes

Treatment of B/W mice with weekly anti-L3T4 MAb produced a profound and sustained depletion in circulating L3T4+ lymphocytes (Fig. 1A). Circulating L3T4$^+$ cells were reduced by 90% after 1 week of treatment. Staining with fluorescein-conjugated anti-Thy-1.2 MAb and anti-Lyt-2 showed that, after 1 week of treatment, >90% of peripheral T cells in treated mice expressed Lyt-2, indicating that the reduction in L3T4$^+$ cells reflected target cell depletion rather than antigenic modulation. The effect of treatment was limited to the L3T4$^+$ cell population. The number of circulating B cells and Lyt-2$^+$ T cells remained stable in mice treated with anti-L3T4 (Fig. 1B and C).

Control B/W mice developed a spontaneous age-dependent decline in circulating T lymphocytes (Fig. 1A and B), whereas circulating B lymphocytes remained relatively constant (Fig. 1C). Although T cell counts in the control groups fell by approximately 50% between age 4 and 8 months, L3T4$^+$ cells and Lyt-2$^+$ cells were equally affected, and therefore, the L3T4/Lyt-2 (helper-suppressor) ratio remained constant (Fig. 1D). In contrast, mice treated with anti-L3T4 had selective depletion of L3T4$^+$ cells, resulting in a dramatic reversal of the L3T4–Lyt-2 ratio (Fig. 1D).

Autoimmunity

Continual treatment of B/W mice with anti-L3T4 MAb markedly inhibited the production of antibodies to double-stranded DNA (dsDNA, Fig. 2). Although treated mice developed low levels of anti-dsDNA antibodies during the first 2 months of therapy, the titers remained low during the course of therapy. At age 8 months, the peak titers were reduced from a mean of 1:2200 in control mice treated with saline to 1:270 in mice treated with anti-L3T4 (>80% inhibition).

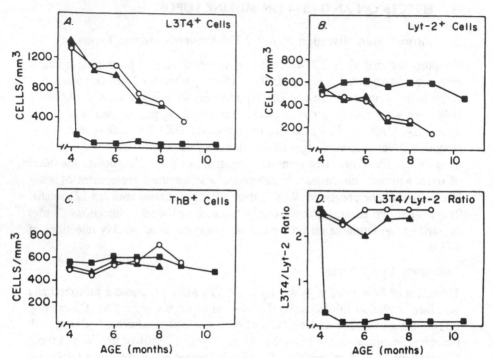

Figure 1 Circulating lymphocytes from groups of 10 B/W females treated beginning at age 4 months with weekly injections of MAb to L3T4 (■), nonimmune rat IgG (▲), or saline (○). Treatment with anti-L3T4 selectively depleted L3T4$^+$ cells. In contrast, control mice spontaneously developed progressive T lymphocytopenia involving L3T4$^+$ and Lyt-2$^+$ cells. Helper T cells, suppressor-cytotoxic T cells, and B cells were identified using fluorescein-conjugated anti-L3T4 MAb (A), anti-Lyt-2 (B), and anti-ThB (C), respectively. The relative proportion of L3T4$^+$ and Lyt-2$^+$ T cells is shown in D. (Reproduced from the Journal of Experimental Medicine 161:378–391,1985, by copyright permission of the Rockefeller University Press.)

The inhibition of anti-dsDNA antibodies was not a nonspecific effect of administering IgG antibodies, since control mice that received nonimmune rat IgG developed a peak mean titer of 1:1500, which was comparable to that in the saline control group. The reduction in anti-dsDNA antibodies did not reflect a generalized reduction in total Ig levels in treated mice (4).

The reduction in anti-dsDNA antibodies in mice treated with anti-L3T4 was associated with a significant reduction in renal disease, as assessed by both blood urea nitrogen (BUN) and proteinuria measurements. At 9 months of age, the mean BUN in mice treated with saline rose to 38.0 ± 11.6 mg/dl, compared to

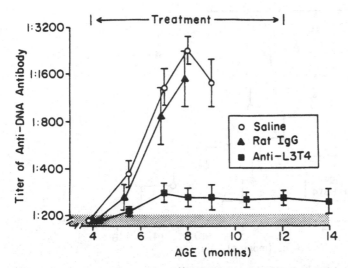

Figure 2 Geometric mean titer ($\frac{\times}{+}$ SEM) of antibodies to double-stranded DNA in B/W females treated beginning at age 4 months with weekly injections of MAb to L3T4 (■), nonimmune rat IgG (▲), or saline (O). The shaded area indicates the titer of anti-DNA antibodies in normal (C57BL/6) mice. (Adapted from the Journal of Experimental Medicine 161:378-391,1985, by copyright permission of the Rockefeller University Press.)

14.3 ± 0.9 mg/dl in mice treated with anti-L3T4 ($p < 0.01$). Significant proteinuria (≥ 100 mg/dl) developed in 90% of control mice but only in 20% of the mice treated with anti-L3T4 (4). Renal failure occurred earliest in the mice treated with nonimmune rat IgG, perhaps due to the host immune response to rat Ig. Examination of renal histopathology in subsequent studies confirmed the dramatic beneficial effects of anti-L3T4 (9).

The reduction in autoantibody production and the prevention of renal failure in mice treated with anti-L3T4 resulted in prolonged survival (Fig. 3). When treatment was stopped at age 12 months, 90% of the treated mice were alive, compared to 18% in the group that received saline and 0% in the group that received nonimmune rat IgG. At age 18 months, 6 months after stopping therapy, 80% of the treated mice were still alive.

Host Immune Response to Treatment

One of the obstacles to the use of MAbs as therapeutic agents in humans has been the development of a host immune response to the foreign MAb (44–48). This host immune response has been a major problem in targeting neoplastic cells (44,45) and has limited the use of anti-CD3 MAb (OKT3) to a single course in the treatment of renal allograft rejection (46,47). In contrast to previously used

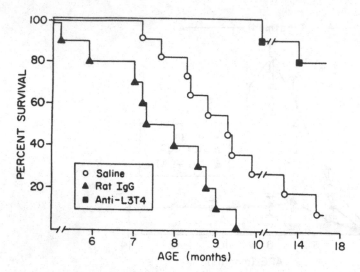

Figure 3 Survival of female B/W mice treated beginning at age 4 months with weekly injections of MAb to L3T4 (■), nonimmune rat IgG (▲), or saline (O). (Adapted from the Journal of Experimental Medicine 161:378–391, 1985, by copyright permission of the Rockefeller University Press.)

xenogeneic MAb, the high-dose regimen of rat anti-L3T4 used in our studies did not elict a substantial host immune response (Fig. 4). Of 10 treated mice, 7 never developed antibodies to rat Ig, even after 8 months of weekly challenges, and the remaining 3 mice developed only low titers of antirat antibody several months into therapy. In marked contrast, nonimmune rat IgG elicited a strong immune response in control mice (Fig. 4). In fact, the host immune response to rat IgG may have accelerated mortality in this control group (Fig. 3). The ability to administer anti-L3T4 without inducing a host immune response prevents the rapid clearance of the MAb by host antibodies, thereby prolonging the therapeutic benefits. The lack of a host immune response also minimizes the adverse side effects, such as serum sickness and chronic immune complex deposition, that can occur during chronic administration of a foreign antibody.

B. Treatment with Anti-L3T4 Reverses Murine Lupus

Our initial studies in B/W mice showed that L3T4$^+$ T helper cells play a central role in autoimmune disease. However, these studies did not have direct therapeutic implications because administration of anti-L3T4 was started before the development of overt clinical disease (4). Therefore, to determine if treatment with anti-L3T4 could improve murine lupus in B/W mice after disease had

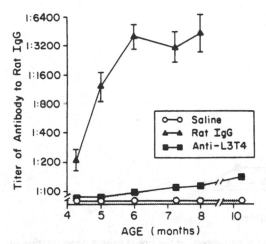

Figure 4 Geometric mean titer ($\overset{\times}{\div}$ SEM) of antibodies to rat Ig in B/W mice treated beginning at age 4 months with weekly injections of rat MAb to L3T4 (■), nonimmune rat IgG (▲), or saline (○). The shaded area indicates assay results using normal sera as negative controls. (Reproduced from the Journal of Experimental Medicine 161: 378–391,1985, by copyright permission of the Rockefeller University Press.)

developed, we monitored a cohort of B/W female mice until age 7 months, by which time all the mice had high titers of anti-dsDNA antibodies, the majority had clinical evidence of renal disease, and 20% had already died (7). The surviving mice were then divided into matched groups based on autoantibody levels and degree of proteinuria, and weekly treatment with either anti-L3T4 (2 mg per mouse per week) or saline was begun.

Circulating Lymphocytes

Weekly injections of anti-L3T4 reduced circulating L3T4$^+$ cells by 10% after 1 week, by 55% after 4 weeks, by 75% after 8 weeks, and eventually by >90% after 12 weeks (Fig. 5). This gradual depletion of target cells contrasts with the rapid depletion observed in our previous studies (Fig. 5). The decreased clearance of L3T4$^+$ cells was not due to inadequate therapy (7) but apparently to a defect in immune clearance of antibody-coated cells. Similar defects in the clearance of antibody-coated cells have been reported in lupus-prone MRL/lpr mice (49) and in humans with SLE (24,25).

Autoimmunity

Despite the delay in target cell clearance, treatment with anti-L3T4 had an immediate effect on autoimmunity. Before starting therapy, the concentration of

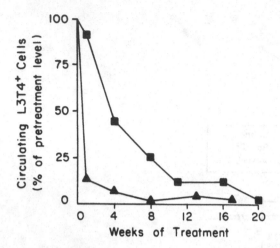

Figure 5 Circulating L3T4+ cells as a percentage of the pretreatment concentration in female B/W mice treated with weekly injections of anti-L3T4 beginning at age 7 months (■). Shown for comparison is the rate of target cell depletion in B/W mice treated with weekly injections of anti-L3T4 beginning at age 4 months (▲). (Reproduced from D. Wofsy and W.E. Seaman, Reversal of advanced murine lupus in NZB/NZW F_1 mice by treatment with monoclonal antibody to L3T4. J. Immunol. 138:3247–3253, 1987, by copyright permission of the American Association of Immunologists.)

anti-dsDNA antibodies had been increasing in both experimental groups (Fig. 6). During the treatment course, the mean titer continued to rise in the saline control group, but in the group that received anti-L3T4, the concentration of anti-dsDNA antibodies immediately plateaued and then dramatically fell. After 2 months of therapy, the mean anti-dsDNA titer in the control group was 1:1300, compared to 1:250 in the anti-L3T4-treated group ($p < 0.02$).

The decrease in anti-dsDNA antibody levels was not secondary to a reduction in total Ig levels in anti-L3T4-treated mice (7). The mean IgG concentration was not significantly different in mice treated with anti-L3T4, and the mean IgM concentration gradually increased compared to pretreatment levels (7). A similar increase in IgM levels was observed previously when 4-month-old B/W mice were treated with anti-L3T4 (4).

Treatment of advanced autoimmunity with anti-L3T4 also had a beneficial effect on renal disease (7) as measured by BUN and proteinuria (Fig. 7). Before initiation of treatment, 7 of 12 mice in each group (58%) had significant proteinuria (≥ 100 mg/dl). By age 11 months, after 4 months of therapy, all the control mice had developed significant proteinuria. In marked contrast, only 4 of 12 treated

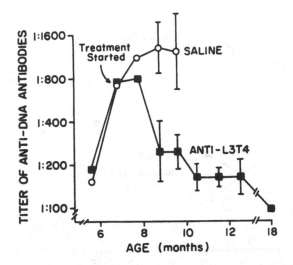

Figure 6 Geometric mean titer ($\stackrel{\times}{\div}$ SEM) of antibodies to double-stranded DNA in female B/W mice treated with weekly injections of anti-L3T4 (■) or saline (○) beginning at age 7 months. (Adapted from D. Wofsy and W.E. Seaman, Reversal of advanced murine lupus in NZB/NZW F_1 mice by treatment with monoclonal antibody in L3T4. J. Immunol. 138:3247–3253, 1987, by copyright permission of the American Association of Immunologists.)

mice had proteinuria (33%, $p < 0.005$ compared with control mice). Similarly, progressive azotemia developed in 80% of the control mice compared to 17% of the anti-L3T4-treated mice ($p < 0.02$) (7).

These data show that anti-L3T4 therapy inhibits the progression of lupus nephritis in B/W mice. However, they do not establish whether therapy can actually reverse the clinical signs of autoimmune renal disease. To address this issue, we reviewed the course of renal disease in nine long-term survivors of anti-L3T4 therapy. Before treatment was started, five of the nine mice (56%) had developed proteinuria. However, after 5 months of therapy, only one of the treated mice (11%) had proteinuria (Fig. 8). Thus, treatment with anti-L3T4 can improve renal disease even after damage has occurred. This conclusion has since been confirmed directly by comparison of renal histopathology before and after treatment with anti-L3T4 (unpublished data).

The improvement in renal function observed in the mice treated with anti-L3T4 was reflected by a marked improvement in their survival compared to control B/W mice. Of the original cohort of B/W mice, 20% died before treatment was begun at age 7 months (Fig. 9). Mice in the control group continued to die at a rapid rate, leading to a mortality of 83% by 12 months of age. In marked

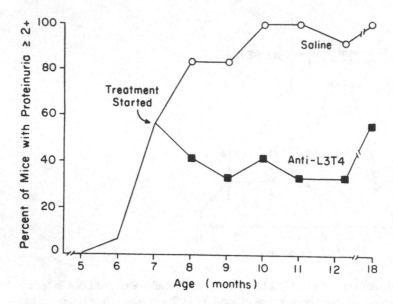

Figure 7   Frequency of proteinuria $\geq 2^+$ (100 mg/dl) in female B/W mice treated with weekly injections of anti-L3T4 (■) or saline (○) beginning at age 7 months. To reflect accurately the development of renal disease in all mice, each point represents the current level of proteinuira in surviving mice as well as the last measurement of proteinuria in deceased mice. (Adapted from D. Wofsy and W.E. Seaman, Reversal of advanced murine lupus in NZB/NZW F_1 mice by treatment with monoclonal antibody to L3T4. J. Immunol. 138:3247–3253, 1987, by copyright permission of the American Association of Immunologists.)

contrast, the anti-L3T4-treated mice had a mortality of 25% at age 12 months ($p < 0.02$). These observations establish conclusively that treatment with anti-L3T4 can retard murine lupus even after the disease is fully active.

C. Effects of Anti-L3T4 on the Histopathology of Target Organs

To determine the effect of treatment with anti-L3T4 on the histopathology of autoimmune disease, groups of 10 B/W female mice were treated with weekly injections of either anti-L3T4 (2 mg per mouse) or saline from age 5 months until age 8 months (9,10). Surviving mice were then sacrificed to examine the composition of the lymphoid organs and the histologic manifestations of murine lupus in the kidneys, salivary glands, liver, and lungs (9). Selected mice from each group were also used for immunohistochemical analysis of spleen, lymph nodes, and thymus (10).

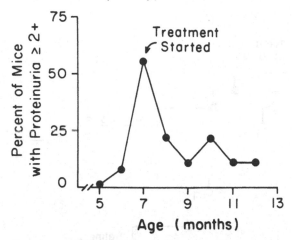

Figure 8 Evolution of renal disease in long-term survivors of treatment with anti-L3T4. The percentage of mice with proteinuira ≥ 2$^+$ (100 mg/dl) is shown. (Adapted from D. Wofsy and W.E. Seaman, Reversal of advanced murine lupus in NZB × NZW F$_1$ mice by treatment with monoclonal antibody to L3T4. J. Immunol. 138:3247–3253, 1987, by copyright permission of the American Association of Immunologists.)

Lymphoid Organs

Progressive splenomegaly and lymphadenopathy were prominent features in control B/W mice (12). The majority of the T cells in both the spleen and lymph nodes were L3T4$^+$ cells, although B cells and Lyt-2$^+$ T cells were also present (10). These lymphocytes were organized into secondary follicles with germinal centers that contained an unusual population of L3T4$^+$/Thy-1.2$^-$ cells (10). These L3T4$^+$/Thy-1.2$^-$ cells constituted up to 25% of the L3T4$^+$ cells in aged B/W mice (10). Treatment with anti-L3T4 resulted in the depletion of >95% of L3T4$^+$ cells from the spleen and lymph nodes of B/W mice (Table 1), as had been observed in the peripheral blood (see Fig. 1). Chronic administration of anti-L3T4 prevented both the development of lymphoproliferation and the generation of secondary lymphoid follicles (10).

The thymuses of the control B/W mice were also markedly abnormal. Thymic abnormalities included (1) enlarged medulla, with increased number of B cells compared to nonautoimmune mice; (2) atrophied cortex; and (3) the presence of thymomas (10). Treatment with anti-L3T4 prevented all these abnormalities (10). In mice treated with anti-L3T4, the L3T4 antigen in the outer cortex was covered by the administered MAb, and modulation of antigen density was also evident (10). The administered antibody did not penetrate the inner cortex (10). In contrast to the depletion of L3T4$^+$ cells from the spleen and lymph nodes of

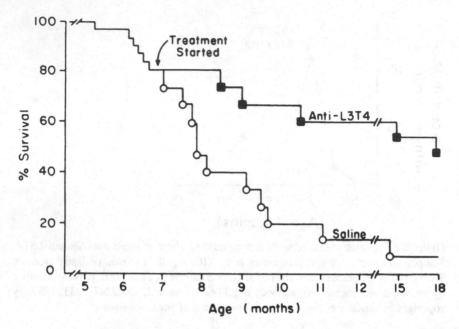

Figure 9 Survival of female B/W mice treated with weekly injection of anti-L3T4 (■) or saline (○) beginning at age 7 months. As shown, 20% of the original cohort of 30 mice died before initiation of therapy. (Adapted from D. Wofsy and W.E. Seaman, Reversal of advanced murine lupus in NZB/NZW F_1 mice by treatment with monoclonal antibody to L3T4. J. Immunol. 138:3247–3253, 1987, by copyright permission of the American Association of Immunologists.)

mice treated with anti-L3T4, $L3T4^+$ cells were not depleted from the thymus (10). Persistence of $L3T4^+$ thymocytes most likely accounts for the repopulation of the peripheral circulation with $L3T4^+$ cells that occurs after cessation of treatment.

Kidney and Other Sites of Immunopathology

As discussed earlier, B/W mice develop progressive renal failure that can be prevented and/or reversed by anti-L3T4 treatment (4,7). Apparently this renal failure is secondary to immune complex glomerulonephritis; however, cellular immune mechanisms may also play a role in this process (50). Control B/W mice had large lymphocytic infiltrates that occurred primarily under the renal calyx epithelium. Lymphocytes were also scattered throughout the interstitium and were present surrounding arterioles and venules (9). Glomeruli were hypertrophied and contained large amounts of IgG and C3. Treatment with anti-L3T4

Table 1 Composition of the Lymphoid Organs in B/W Mice Treated with Anti-L3T4

Treatment	Cell count[a] (cells × 10^{-7})	Lymphocyte subsets (% of cells)[b]			
		B cells	T cells	L3T4[+]	Lyt-2[+]
Spleen					
Saline	23.5 ± 4.9	35 ± 10	35 ± 1	30 ± 2	9 ± 1
Anti-L3T4	6.4 ± 0.5[c]	45 ± 3	30 ± 4	<5[e]	28 ± 2[c]
Inguinal node					
Saline	2.6 ± 0.9	22 ± 7	68 ± 7	49 ± 6	22 ± 1
Anti-L3T4	0.9 ± 0.8[d]	21 ± 4	79 ± 3	<5[e]	67 ± 6[c]
Thymus					
Saline	2.7 ± 1.5	11 ± 2	72 ± 8	64 ± 8	51 ± 8
Anti-L3T4	9.6 ± 3.4[d]	2 ± 1[c]	91 ± 4[d]	>90[f]	84 ± 1[c]

[a]Female B/W mice received weekly IP injections of MAb to L3T4 (2 mg) or saline (200 μl) from age 5 months until sacrifice at age 8 months. Spleen cell counts indicate the mean ± SEM of spleens from nine mice treated with anti-L3T4 and five mice treated with saline. All other data were obtained from four mice per group.
[b]Lymphocyte subsets as a percentage of total mononuclear cells were identified by flow cytometry using anti-B220 to identify B cells, anti-Thy-1.2 to identify T cells, and anti-L3T4 and anti-Lyt-2 to identify T cell subsets. Cells were also stained with antirat x chain (MAR 18.5) to identify L3T4[+] cells that were coated with the rat MAb used for treatment.
[c]$p < 0.01$ compared to control group.
[d]$p < 0.05$ compared to control group.
[e]L3T4[+] cells could not be detected in the spleen or inguinal lymph node either by staining with anti-L3T4 or by staining with MAR 18.5. Dual-color fluorescence analysis with anti-Thy-1.2 and anti-Lyt-2 confirmed the absence of Thy-1.2[+]/Lyt-2[-] (L3T4[+]) cells.
[f]Weak expression of L3T4 by most thymocytes was detected by staining with MAR 18.5.
Source: Adapted from The Journal of Autoimmunity 1:415–431, 1988, by copyright permission of the Academic Press.

substantially reduced immune complex deposition, and markedly inhibited the lymphocytic infiltration and vasculitis (Fig. 10).

Like SLE in humans, murine lupus in B/W mice affects multiple organs (11,12). The pathology includes lymphocytic infiltration of salivary glands similar to Sjögren's syndrome (11,51–53), and interstitial lung disease (11,12). Control B/W mice had large lymphocytic infiltrates in their salivary glands and lungs; only small focal infiltrates were present in the liver (9). Treatment with anti-L3T4 markedly decreased the lymphocytic infiltration of the salivary glands and completely prevented lymphocytic infiltration of the liver. Lymphocytes were still present in the lungs of treated mice, although they were somewhat decreased (9). These observations suggest that treatment with anti-L3T4 has beneficial effects on both autoantibody production and resultant immune complex deposition and on tissue damage due to cellular infiltration.

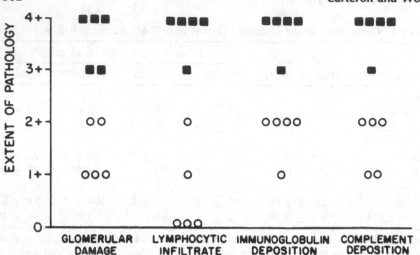

Figure 10 Extent of renal pathology in female B/W mice treated from age 5 months to age 8 months with either anti-L3T4 (O) or saline (■). Tissue sections were coded and evaluated by observers who did not know the treatment status of the mice. (Reproduced from the Journal of Autoimmunity 1:415–431,1988, by copyright permission of the Academic Press.)

V. EFFECTS OF F(ab')₂ FRAGMENTS OF ANTI-L3T4 ON MURINE LUPUS

The studies already reviewed utilized intact anti-L3T4 and were therefore associated with profound depletion of L3T4$^+$ cells (4,7,9,10). However, depletion of the T_H cells may not have been the sole mechanism by which anti-L3T4 exerted its beneficial effects on autoimmunity. If depletion of L3T4$^+$ T_H cells were necessary for the beneficial effects, then the potential use of anti-L3T4 (or anti-CD4) as a therapeutic agent would necessarily be complicated by a prolonged inhibition of normal immune function due to prolonged depletion of T_H cells. This prolonged immune suppression might result in an unacceptably high incidence of side effects, such as infection. We previously showed that depletion of L3T4$^+$ cells was not the sole mechanism by which anti-L3T4 inhibits humoral immunity in normal mice (54). These studies utilized F(ab')₂ fragments of anti-L3T4, which lack the Fc portion of the antibody molecule required for recognition and removal of antibody-coated cells by the mononuclear phagocyte system (55,56). The observation that F(ab')₂ fragments of anti-L3T4 could inhibit normal immunity without depleting L3T4$^+$ cells suggested that F(ab')₂ anti-L3T4 might inhibit autoimmunity as well.

The first attempts to treat B/W mice with F(ab')₂ anti-L3T4 were complicated by the development of a host immune response to the rat MAb fragments (Fig. 11).

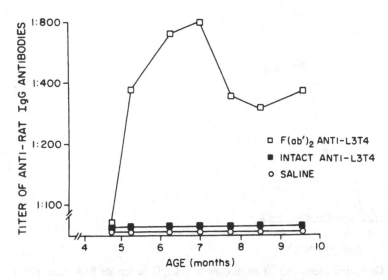

Figure 11 Geometric mean titer of antibodies of rat IgG in female B/W mice treated with F(ab')₂ anti-L3T4 (□), intact anti-L3T4 (■), or saline (○) from age 5 to 9 months. (Reproduced from N.L. Carteron, C. L. Schimenti, D. Wofsy, Treatment of murine lupus with F(ab')₂ fragments of monoclonal antibody to L3T4. J. Immunol. 142:1470–1475, 1989, by copyright permission of the American Association of Immunologists.)

In these studies, mice treated with the fragments developed serum sickness and had no improvement in their survival compared to control mice (41). Thus, the development of a host immune response prevented the beneficial effects of the therapeutic MAb. A similar host immune response has complicated attempts to treat nonhuman primates (57) and humans (58) with mouse MAb to CD4. Recent observations in our laboratory suggest a way to prevent this host immune response. We and others found that high doses of intact rat MAb to L3T4 could induce tolerance to itself and to certain other Ag in normal mice (8,59,60). Therefore, we administered a single tolerizing dose of intact anti-L3T4 (1 mg) at age 2 months, allowed the L3T4⁺ cells to recover, and then began treatment at age 4 months with F(ab')₂ anti-L3T4 (0.5 mg three times per week). The initial tolerizing dose of intact anti-L3T4 prevented the development of a host immune response during the entire 10 month treatment course (Fig. 12).

Chronic administration of F(ab')₂ anti-L3T4 did not deplete L3T4+ cells from the circulation (Fig. 13A). Mice treated with F(ab')₂ anti-L3T4 had low concentrations of anti-dsDNA antibody, did not develop renal disease (Fig. 13B), and had improved survival (Fig. 13C) relative to control mice (41). The beneficial

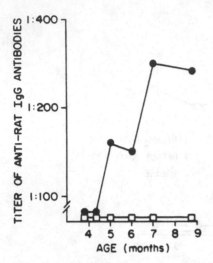

Figure 12 Geometric mean titer of antibodies of rat IgG in female B/W mice either tolerized with a single dose of intact rat anti-L3T4 (□) or given saline (●) at age 2 months followed by treatment with F(ab')$_2$ anti-L3T4 three times per week beginning at age 4 months. (Reproduced from N.L. Carteron, C.L. Schimenti, and D. Wofsy, Treatment of murine lupus with F(ab')$_2$ fragments of monoclonal antibody to L3T4. J. Immunol. 142:1470–1475, 1989, by copyright permission of the American Association of Immunologists.)

effects of F(ab')$_2$ anti-L3T4 were equivalent to those achieved with intact anti-L3T4 (Fig. 13). The tolerizing dose, by itself, was not sufficient to produce the beneficial effects on autoimmunity (41). These findings demonstrate that the beneficial effects of anti-L3T4 on autoimmunity do not depend solely on the depletion of L3T4$^+$ cells. Moreover, the MAb fragments are cleared and normal immunity restored within 72 after cessation of therapy (Ref. 61 and unpublished data). Therefore, the use of F(ab')$_2$ anti-L3T4 offers an immediately reversible approach to therapy. These studies suggest that altering the function of T$_H$ cells may offer a more specific and less toxic therapy than current cortiocosteroid and/or cytotoxic drugs for the treatment of autoimmune diseases.

VI. CLINICAL IMPLICATIONS

Since L3T4 in mice is homologous to CD4 in humans, our studies suggest that anti-CD4 MAb or its fragments may be beneficial in the treatment of autoimmune diseases in humans. This possibility is further supported by studies showing

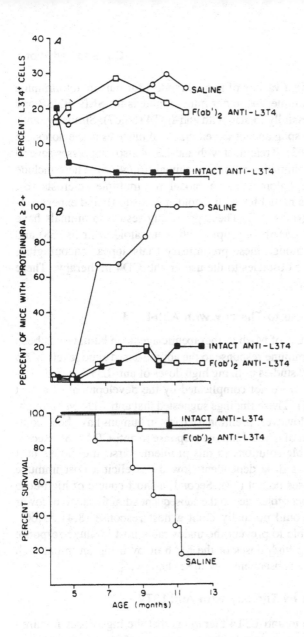

Figure 13 Groups of 6–10 female B/W mice were tolerized with a single dose of intact rat anti-L3T4 at age 2 months to facilitate subsequent treatment with F(ab')$_2$ anti-L3T4 (□), intact anti-L3T4 (■), or saline (○) beginning at age 4 months. (A) Concentration of circulating L3T4$^+$ cells. (B) Frequency of proteinuria $\geq 2^+$ (100 mg/dl). (C) Percentage survival. (Reproduced from N.L. Carteron, C.L. Schimenti, and D. Wofsy, Treatment of murine lupus with F(ab')$_2$ fragments of monoclonal antibody to L3T4. J. Immunol. 142:1470–1475, 1989, by copyright permission of the American Association of Immunologists.)

that anti-L3T4 is effective in a variety of animal models for human autoimmune diseases (6,62–65). For example, two other murine models for SLE, BXSB and MRL/lpr mice can be successfully treated with anti-L3T4 (66,67). Similarly, anti-L3T4 treatment inhibits the spontaneous development of diabetes in the nonobese diabetic (NOD) mouse (62,63). Treatment with anti-L3T4 also suppresses several experimentally induced autoimmune diseases in animals (6,64,65). These include experimental allergic encephalomyelitis, a model for multiple sclerosis (6); collagen-induced arthritis, a model for rheumatoid arthritis (64); and experimentally induced myasthenia gravis (65). These promising results in animals have prompted trials of anti-CD4 MAb in people with rheumatoid arthritis (68) and multiple sclerosis (58). Although these preliminary trials appear encouraging, two problems present major obstacles to the use of anti-CD4 in therapy. These problems are discussed here.

A. Host Immune Response to Therapy with Anti-L3T4

One of the obstacles to the use of MAb as therapeutic agents in humans has been the development of a host immune response to the administered xenogeneic MAb (44–48). Surprisingly, early studies utilizing high doses of anti-L3T4 in both normal and autoimmune mice were not complicated by the development of a host immune response (3,4,7,67). These findings suggested that anti-CD4 MAb might not elicit a host response. However, preliminary trials in humans have been complicated by the development of a host immune response to anti-CD4 (58). Recent findings suggest two possible solutions to this problem. First, the mouse host response to rat anti-L3T4 is dose dependent: low doses elicit a host immune response, whereas high doses do not (54). Second, a short course of high-dose therapy with anti-L3T4 induces tolerance to the subsequent administration of lower doses of anti-L3T4 that would normally elicit a host response (8,41,59,60). Therefore, it may be possible to prevent the undesirable host immune response to anti-CD4 either by using high doses of the MAb or by using an initial high dose to induce tolerance to subsequent low-dose therapy.

B. Immune Suppression by Therapy with Anti-L3T4

The second major obstacle to anti-L3T4 therapy is that the high doses required to prevent the host immune response to the MAb are profoundly immunosuppressive. High doses of anti-L3T4 markedly deplete L3T4$^+$ cells (Fig. 1A and Table 1), block primary and secondary humoral immune responses (3,54,69,70), and diminish cellular immune responses (71). Substantial depletion of L3T4$^+$ cells and, thus, inhibition of normal immune function persist for a prolonged period after stopping therapy (69,72). This prolonged suppression of normal immunity may preclude anti-CD4 therapy in humans.

Recent studies in our laboratory have shown that sustained suppression of normal immunity by anti-L3T4 may be avoidable (41,54,61). As discussed earlier, we find that F(ab')$_2$ fragments of anti-L3T4 can inhibit immune function (41,54,61) without depleting L3T4$^+$ cells. Thus, the effects of F(ab')$_2$ anti-L3T4 on normal immunity are immediately reversible upon stopping therapy (61). These findings suggest that F(ab')$_2$ fragments, or other MAb preparations that do not deplete target cells, may provide a readily reversible approach to anti-CD4 therapy in autoimmunity.

VII. CONCLUSION

Currently, there is no safe and reliable treatment for SLE or for other serious autoimmune diseases. Severe cases usually require treatment with corticosteroids and/or cytotoxic drugs, which frequently are inadequate and can cause serious immediate and long-term complications. These therapies are not restricted in their effects to cells of the immune system but are toxic to a broad range of cells throughout the body. The studies discussed in this chapter suggest an alternative approach to the treatment of autoimmune disease that is restricted in its effect to a specific subset of lymphocytes that express L3T4. MAb directed against the L3T4 Ag on T_H cells inhibit autoimmune disease in animal models for diabetes mellitus, multiple sclerosis, rheumatoid arthritis, and myasthenia gravis, as well as SLE. Because L3T4 in mice is homologous to CD4 in humans, this approach to therapy may be useful in humans with severe autoimmune disease.

REFERENCES

1. Cosimi, A.B., Colvin, R.B., Burton, R.C., Rubin, R.H., Goldstein, G., Kung, P.C., Hansen, W.P., Delmonico, F.L., and Russell, P.S. (1981). Use of monoclonal antibodies to T-cell subsets for immunologic monitoring and treatment in recipients of renal allografts. N. Engl. J. Med. 305:308.
2. Ledbetter, J.A., and Seaman, W.E. (1982). The Lyt-2, Lyt-3 macromolecules: Structural and functional studies. Immunol. Rev. 68:197.
3. Cobbold, S.P., Jayasuriya, A., Nash, A., Prospero, T.D., and Waldmann, H. (1984). Therapy with monoclonal antibodies by elimination of T-cell subsets in vivo. Nature 312:548.
4. Wofsy, D., and Seaman, W.E. (1985). Successful treatment of autoimmunity in NZB/NZW F$_1$ mice with monoclonal antibody to L3T4 J. Exp. Med. 161:378.
5. Wofsy, D., Ledbetter, J.A., Hendler, P.L., and Seaman, W.E. (1985). Treatment of murine lupus with monoclonal anti-T cell antibody. J. Immunol. 134:852.
6. Waldor, M.K., Sriram, S., Hardy, R., Herzenberg, L.A., Herzenberg, L.A., Lanier, L., Lim, M., and Steinman, L. (1985). Reversal of experimental allergic encephalomyelitis with monoclonal antibody to a T-cell subset marker. Science 227:415.

7. Wofsy, D., and Seaman, W.E. (1987). Reversal of advanced murine lupus in NZB/NZW mice by treatment with monoclonal antibody to L3T4. ˙. Immunol. 138:3247.

8. Gutstein, N.L., Seaman, W.E., Scott, J.H., and Wofsy, D. (1986). Induction of immune tolerance by administration of monoclonal antibody to L3T4. J. Immunol. 137:1127.

9. Wofsy, D., Chiang, N.Y., Greenspan, J.S., and Ermak, T.H. (1988). Treatment of murine lupus with monoclonal antibody to L3T4. I. Effects on the distribution and function of lymphocyte subsets and on the histopathology of autoimmune disease. J. Autoimmun. 1:415.

10. Ermak, T.H., Steger, H.J., and Wofsy, D. (1989). Treatment of murine lupus with monoclonal antibody of L3T4. II. Effects on immunohistopathology of thymus, spleen, and lymph node. Lab. Invest. 61:447.

11. Howie, J.B., and Simpson, L.O. (1976). The immunopathology of the NZB mice and their hybrids. In: Textbook of Immunopathology. Meissner, P.S., and Mueller-Eberhard, H., eds. Grune and Stratton, New York, p. 247.

12. Andrews, B.S., Eisenberg, R.A., Theofilopoulos, A.N., Izui, S., Wilson, C.B., McConahey, P.J., Murphy, E.D., Roths, J.B., and Dixon, F.J. (1978). Spontaneous murine lupus-like syndromes. I. Clinical and immunological manifestations in several strains. J. Exp. Med. 148:1198.

13. Steinberg, A.D., Raveche, E.S., Laskin, C.A., Smith, H.R., Santoro, T., Miller, M.L., and Plotz, P.H. (1984). Systemic lupus erythematosus: Insights from animal modes. Ann. Intern. Med. 100:714.

14. Fauci, A.S., Steinberg, A.D., Haynes, B.F., and Whalen, G. (1978). Immunoregulatory aberrations in systemic lupus erythematosus. J. Immunol. 121:1473.

15. Morimoto, C., Reinherz, E.L., Schlossman, S.F., Schur, P.H., Mills, J.A., and Steinberg, A.D. (1980). Alterations in immunotherapy T cell subsets in active systemic lupus erythematosus. J. Clin. Invest. 66:1171.

16. Krakauer, R.S., Waldmann, T.A., and Strober, W. (1976). Loss of suppressor T cells in adults NZB/NZW mice. J. Exp. Med. 144:662.

17. Miller, K.B., and Schwartz, R.S. (1979). Familial abnormalities of suppressor-cell function in systemic lupus erythematosus. N. Engl. J. Med. 301:803.

18. Steinberg, A. D.(1974). Pathogenesis of autoimmunity in New Zealand mice. Loss of thymic suppressor function. Arthritis Rheum. 17:11.

19. Altman, A., Theofilopoulos, A.N., Weiner, R., Katz, D.H., and Dixon, F.J. (1981). Analysis of T cell function in autoimmune murine strains. J. Exp. Med. 154:791.

20. Dauphinee, M., Kipper, S., Wofsy, D., and Talal, N. (1981). Interleukin 2 deficiency is a common feature of autoimmune mice. J. Immunol. 127:2483.

21. Linker-Israeli, M., Bakke, R.C., Kitridou, S., Gendler, S., Gillis, S., and Horowitz, D.A. (1983). Defective production of interleukin 1 and interleukin 2 in patients with systemic lupus erythematosus. J. Immunol. 130:2651.

22. Blaese, R.M., Grayson, J., and Steinberg, A.D. (1980). Elevated immunoglobulin-secreting cells in the blood of patients with active systemic lupus erythematosus: Correlation of laboratory and clinical assessment of disease activity. Am. J. Med. 69:345.

23. Klinman, D.M., and Steinberg, A.D. (1987). Systemic autoimmune disease arises from polyclonal B cell activation. J. Exp. Med. 165:1755.

24. Frank, M.M., Hamburger, M.I., Lawley, T.J., Kimberly, R.P., and Plotz, P.H. (1979). Defective reticuloendothelial system Fc-receptor function in systemic lupus erythematosus. N. Engl. J. Med. 300:518.
25. Shear, H.L., Roubinian, J.R., Gil, P., and Talal, N. (1981). Clearance of sensitized erythrocytes in NZB/NZW mice. Effects of castration and sex hormone treatment. Eur. J. Immunol. 11:776.
26. Reinherz, E.L., and Schlossman, S.F. (1980). The differentiation and functions of human T lymphocytes. Cell 19:821.
27. Ledbetter, J.A., Evans, R.L., Lipinski, M., Cunningham, C., Good, R.A., and Herzenberg, L.A. (1981). Evolutionary conservation of surface molecules that distinguish T lymphocyte helper/inducer and cytotoxic/suppressor subpopulations in mouse and man. J. Exp. Med. 153:310.
28. Ledbetter, J.A., Rouse, R.V., Micklem, H.S., and Herzenberg, L.A. (1980). T cell subsets defined by expression of Lyt-1,2,3 and Thy-1 antigens. Two parameter immunofluorescence and cytotoxicity analysis with monoclonal antibodies modified current views. J. Exp. Med. 152:280.
29. Dialynas, D.P., Quan, Z.S., Wall, K.A., Pierres, A., Quintans, J., Loken, M.R., Pierres, M., and Fitch, F.W. (1983). Characterization of the murine T cell surface molecule, designated L3T4, identified by monoclonal antibody GK1.5: Similarity of L3T4 to the human Leu-3/T4 molecule. J. Immunol. 131:2445.
30. Swain, S.L. (1983). T cell subsets and the recognition of MHC class. Immunol. Rev. 74:129.
31. Dialynas, D.P. Wilde, D.B., Marrack, P., Pierres, A., Wall, K.A., Harran, W., Otten, G., Loken, M.R., Pierres, M., Kappler, J., and Fitch, F.W. (1983). Characterization of the murine antigenic determinant, designated L3T4a, recognized by monoclonal antibody GK1.5: Expression of L3T4a by functional T cell clones appears to correlate primarily with class II MHC antigen reactivity. Immunol. Rev. 74:29.
32. Wilde, D.B., Marrack, P., Kappler, J., Dialynas, D., and Fitch, F.W. (1983). Evidence implicated L3T4 in class II MHC antigen reactivity: Monoclonal antibody GK1.5 (anti-L3T4a) blocks class II MHC antigen-specific proliferation, release of lymphokines, and binding by cloned murine helper T lymphocyte lines. J. Immunol. 131:2178.
33. Rosenberg, A.S., Mizuochi, T., Sharrow, S.O., and Singer, A. (1987). Phenotype specificity, and function of T cell subsets and T cell interactions involved in skin allograft rejection. J. Exp. Med. 165:1296.
34. Swain, S.L., Dialynas, D.P., Fitch, F.W., and English, M. (1984). Monoclonal antibody to L3T4 blocks the function of T cell specific for class 2 major histocompatibility complex antigens. J. Immunol. 132:1118.
35. Greenstein, J.L., Kappler, J., Marrack, P., and Burakoff, S.J. (1984). The role of L3T4 in recognition of Ia by a cytotoxic, H-2D^d-specific T cell hybridoma. J. Exp. Med. 159:1213.
36. Swain, S.L. (1981). Significance of Lyt phenotypes: Lyt-2 antibodies block activities of T cells that recognize class I major histocompatibility complex antigens regardless of their function. Proc. Natl. Acad. Sci USA 78:7101.

37. Wassmer, P.J., Chan, C., Logdberg, L., and Shevach, E.M. (1985). Role of the L3T4-antigen in T cell activation. II. Inhibition of T cell activation by monoclonal anti-L3T4 antibodies in the absence of accessory cells. J. Immunol. 1335:2237.

38. Tite, J., Sloan, A., and Janeway, C.A., Jr. (1986). The role of L3T4 in T cell activation: L3T4 may be both an Ia-binding protein and a receptor that transduces a negative signal. J. Mol. Cell. Immunol. 2:179.

39. Owens, T., and Fazekas de St. Groth, B. (1987). Participation of L3T4 in T cell activation in the absence of class II major histocompatibility antigens. Inhibition by anti-L3T4 antibodies is a function of epitope density and mode of presentation of anti-receptor antibody. J. Immunol. 138:2402.

40. Pont, S., Regnier-Vigouroux, A., Marchetto, S., and Pierres, M. (1987). Acccessory molecules and T cell activation. II. Antibody binding of L3T4a inhibitis Ia-independent mouse T cell proliferation. Eur. J. Immunol. 17:429.

41. Carteron, N.L., Schimenti, C.L., and Wofsy, D. (1989). Treatment of murine lupus with F(ab')₂ fragments of monoclonal antibody to L3T4: Suppression of autoimmunity does not depend on T helper cell depletion. J. Immunol. 142:1470.

42. Meuer, S.C., Schlossman, S.F., and Reinherz, E.L. (1982). Clonal analysis of human T lymphocye subsets: T4⁺ and T8⁺ effector T cells recognize products of different major histocompatibility complex regions. Proc. Natl. Acad. Sci. USA 79:4395.

43. Spits, H., Borst, J., Terhorst, C., and deVries, J.W. (1982). The role of T cell differentiation markers in antigen-specific and lectin-dependent cellular cytotoxicity mediated by T8⁺ and T4⁺ human cytotoxic T cell clones directed at class I and class II MHC antigens. J. Immunol. 129:1563.

44. Lowder, J.N., and Levy, R. (1985). Monoclonal antibodies—therapeutic and diagnostic uses in malignancy. West J. Med. 143:810.

45. Meeker, T.C., Lowder, J., Maloney, D.G., Miller, R.A. Thielemans, K., Warnke, R., and Levy, R. (1985). A clinical trial of anti-idiotypic therapy of B cell malignancy. Blood 65:1349.

46. Burton, R.C., Cosimi, A.B., Colvin, R.B., Rubin, R.H., Delmonico, F.L., Goldstein, G., and Russel, P.S. (1982). Monoclonal antibodies to human T cell subsets: Use of immunological monitoring and immunosuppression in renal transplantation. J. Clin. Immunol. 2:1425.

47. Ortho Multicenter Transplant Group (1985). A randomized clinical trial of OKT3 monoclonal antibody for acute rejection of cadaveric renal transplants. N. Engl. J. Med. 313:337.

48. Chatenoud, L. (1986). The immune response against therapeutic monoclonal antibodies. Immunol. Today 7:367.

49. Seaman, W.E., Wofsy, D., Greenspan, J.S., and Ledbetter, J.A. (1983). Treatment of autoimmune MRL/1pr mice with monoclonal antibody to Thy-1.2: A single injection has sustained effects on lymphoproliferation and renal disease. J. Immunol. 130:1713.

50. Atkins, R.C., Holdsworth, S.R., Hancock, W.W., Thomson, N.M., and Glasgow, E.F. (1982). Cellular immune mechanisms in human glomerulonephritis: The role of mononuclear leukocytes. Springer Semin. Immunopathol. 5:269.

51. Kessler, H.S. (1968). A laboratory models for Sjögren's syndrome. Am. J. Pathol. 52:671.

52. Jonsson, R., Tarkowski, A., Bäckman, K., and Klareskog, L. (1987). Immunohistochemical characterization of sialadenitis in NZB × NZW F_1 mice. Clin. Immunol. Immunopathol. 42:93.

53. Chou, S.T., and Herdson, P.D. (1969). Histological and fine structural abnormalities of the livers of NZB × NZW F_1 mice. Br. J. Pathol. 50:250.

54. Gutstein, N.L., and Wofsy, D. (1986). Administration of F(ab')$_2$ fragments of monoclonal antibody to L3T4 inhibits humoral immunity in mice without depleting L3T4 cells. J. Immunol. 137:3414.

55. Frank, M.H., Lawley, T.J., Hamburger, M.I., and Brown, E.J. (1983). Immunoglobulin G Fc receptor-mediated clearance in autoimmune diseases. Ann. Intern. Med. 98:206.

56. Englefreit, C.P., von dem Borne, A.E.G., Fleer, A., van der Meulen, F.W., and Roos, D. (1980). In vivo destruction of erythrocytes by complement-binding and non complement-binding antibodies. Prog. Clin. Biol. Res. 43:213.

57. Jonker, M., Neuhaus, P., Zurcher, C., Fucello, A., and Goldstein, G. (1985). OKT4 and OKT4A antibody treatment as immunosuppression for kidney transplantation in rhesus monkeys. Transplantation 39:247.

58. Hafler, D.A., Ritz, J., Schlossman, S.F., and Weiner, H.L. (1988). Anti-CD4 and anti-CD2 monoclonal antibody infusions in subjects with multiple sclerosis: Immunosuppressive effects and human anti-mouse responses. J. Immunol. 141:131.

59. Benjamin, R.J., and Waldmann, H. (1986). Induction of tolerance by monoclonal antibody therapy. Nature 320:449.

60. Benjamin, R.J., Cobbold, S.P., Clark, M.R., and Waldmann, H. (1986). Tolerance to rat monoclonal antibodies—implications for seratherapy. J. Exp. Med. 163:1539.

61. Carteron, N.L., Wofsy, D., and Seaman, W.E. (1988). Induction of immune tolerance during administration of monoclonal antibody to L3T4 does not depend on depletion of L3T4$^+$ cells. J. Immunol. 140:713.

62. Koike, T., Itoh, Y., Ishi, T., Ito, I., Takabayashi, K., Marumaya, N., Tomioka, H., and Yoshida, S. (1987). Preventive effect of monoclonal anti-L3T4 antibody on development of diabetes in NOD mice. Diabetes 36:539.

63. Shizuru, J.A., Taylor-Edwards, C., Banks, B.A., Gregory, A.K., and Fathman, C.G. (1988). Immunotherapy of the nonobese diabetic mouse: treatment with an antibody of T-helper lymphocytes. Science 240:659.

64. Ranges, G.E., Sriram, S., and Cooper, S.M. (1985). Prevention of type II collagen-induced arthritis by in vivo treatment with anti-L3T4. J. Exp. Med. 162:1105.

65. Christadoss, P., and Dauphinee, M.J. (1986). Immunotherapy for myasthenia gravis: A murine model. J. Immunol. 136:2437.

66. Santoro, T.J., Portanova, J.P., and Kotzin, B.L. (1988). The contribution of L3T4$^+$ T cells to lymphoproliferation and autoantibody production of MRL-1pr/lpr mice. J. Exp. Med. 167:1713.

67. Wofsy, D. (1986). Administration of monoclonal anti-T cell antibodies retards murine lupus in BXSB mice. J. Immunol. 136:4554.

68. Herzog, C., Walker, C., Pichler, W., Aeschlimann, A., Wassmer, P., Stockinger, H., Knapp, W., Riber, P., and Muller, W. (1987). Monoclonal anti-CD4 in arthritis. Lancet 2:1461.

69. Wofsy, D., Mayes, D.C., Woodcock, J., and Seaman, W.E. (1985). Inhibition of humoral immunity in vivo by monoclonal antibody to L3T4: Studies with soluble antigens in intact mice. J. Immunol. 135:1698.
70. Goronzy, J., Weyand, C.M., and Fathman, C.G. (1986). Long-term humoral unresponsiveness in vivo, induced by treatment with monoclonal antibody against L3T4. J. Exp. Med. 164:911.
71. Woodcock, J.W., Wofsy, D., Eriksson, E., Scott, J.H., and Seaman, W.E. (1986). Rejection of skin grafts and generation of cytotoxic T cells by mice depleted of L3T4+ cells. Transplantation 42:636.
72. Wofsy, D., and Seaman, W.E. (1986). Analysis of the function of L3T4+ T cells by in vivo treatment with monoclonal antibody to L3T4. Surv. Immunol. Res. 5:97.

15

Autoreactive B Cells in Collagen-Induced Arthritis

Rikard Holmdahl
Uppsala University, Uppsala, Sweden

I. INTRODUCTION

One approach to study the development of autoimmune arthritis has been to induce disease by immunization with joint-specific molecules in experimental animals. Hitherto, both type II collagen (CII) (1) and cartilage proteoglycan (2,3) have shown to be arthritogenic using this approach. Severe polyarthritis can be induced in a number of various species, such as mice (4), rats (1), and monkeys (5), after intradermal immunization with CII. The successful induction of autoimmune diseases with CII is, at a first glance, somewhat surprising, since CII is abundant in the body and probably accessible for recognition by the immune system as a self protein. It is one of the major structural components of joint hyaline cartilage, fibrous cartilage in the spine, and elastic cartilage in external ear and is present in the vitreous body of the eye (6,7). Although cartilaginous tissue are not vascularized and therefore not penetrated by lymphoid cells, CII is accessible to many different types of scavenger cells: such cells are in the joints present in the synovial lining layer. It is likely, although not directly demonstrated, that synovial cells of bone marrow origin (8), such as macrophages and dendritic cells, pick up cartilage antigens that will be processed to peptides, bound to class II molecules, and migrate to draining lymph nodes as has been shown for dendritic cells in the epidermis (9). Hence, autoantigenic peptide from CII may also be in the lymph nodes, where they can be presented to lymphocytes. In addition, antibodies have access to cartilage since anti-CII autoantibodies bind to cartilage in vivo as has been demonstrated by injection of polyclonal antiserum (10) and syngeneic monoclonal antibodies (11). Thus, it is likely that CII is accessible to the immune system during ontogeny and in adult life. In conclusion, it can be anticipated that CII is a self protein that may be recognized by the immune system as a self protein, both by the peripheral immune system and possibly also during thymic maturation. Therefore, CII must be regarded as a true self protein, not with "nonself" properties as can be postulated for a self protein localized in immunopriviliged sites. Nevertheless, both arthritis and an autoimmune response develop after immunization with heterologous as well as autologous CII. Furthermore, auto-CII-reactive lymphocytes and circulating anti-CII antibodies may already be present in the functional repertoire of naive as well as CII-immunized animals (12–14). To understand the pathogenesis of CIA we start by raising questions about the physiologic role of these "natural" autoreactive lymphocytes and how these are activated and subsequently how they may induce and/or perpetuate the disease. We discuss here the origin and the role of B cells reactive with CII in CIA.

II. INDUCTION OF CIA AND ANTIBODY RESPONSES TO CII

The anti-CII antibody response and development of arthritis have been extensively characterized in collagen-induced arthritis (CIA)-susceptible mouse and rat strains. CII derived from several different animal species can effectively induce CIA in mice and rats after immunization (15–20). From these experiments it can be concluded that two different forms of CIA are discernible. The first form can be induced with heterologous CII derived from various sources— heterologus CIA (HCIA)—and is clinically characterized by an acute onset and severe arthritis but lacks a progression to active arthritis. The other form can be induced after immunization with autologous CII—autologous CIA (ACIA)— and is clinically characterized by a chronic development of active arthritis.

A. CIA Induced with Heterologous CII

Immunization with several different heterologous CII (rat, chick, porcine, bovine, and human) induces polyarthritis in the DBA/1 mouse (Table 1) (4,16–19). There is a sudden onset of acute arthritis in one or more paws, with severe swelling and erythema, 3–4 weeks after immunization. Activated T cells appear in the earliest detectable arthritic lesions, as elucidated with immunohistochemical techniques, before the swelling of the joints and may play an important permissive role for the development of arthritis (21).

The subsequent acute swelling of the paws is most likely dependent on soft tissue edema and infiltration of inflammatory cells, mainly composed of

Table 1 Development of Arthritis and Serum Levels of Anti-CII Antibodies in DBA/1 Male Mice 14 Weeks After Immunization with CII Derived from Various Species[a]

| Immunogen | n | Incidence of arthritis (%) | Levels of Antibodies (μg/ml) reactive with | |
			Immunogenic CII	Mouse CII
Mouse CII	31	33	5	5
Rat CII	40	90	52	32
Chick CII	51	76	64	10
Bovine CII	38	68	25	8
Human CII	82	71	62	20

[a]A monoclonal anti-CII antibody (CIIB1) is used as standard for estimation of anti-CII antibody levels. This standard gives approximately five times lower antibody levels compared with the subsequently used polyclonal anti-CII antibody standard.
Source: From Ref. 19.

granulocytes. Gradually this inflammatory synovium is transformed to a pannuslike tissue, with a larger content of macrophages and fibroblasts, eroding the cartilage and bone tissue. Inflammatory activity lasts for a couple of weeks, and the end result is usually fibrous or cartilaginous ankylosis or other deformities of the affected joints but no signs of inflammatory activity or recrudescence of arthritis. In rats, for example the Lewis strain, which is susceptible to arthritis after immunization with heterologous CIIs from a number of different species (chick, bovine, deer, human, and porcine CII) (1,15,22–25), the onset of arthritis occurs 2 weeks after immunization, thus somewhat earlier compared with HCIA in mice. Also in the rat the onset of the disease is acute, with severe swelling, and the disease ends after a few weeks with a silent fibrosis in the joints. From these observations in mice and rats there is no evidence for a chronic development of arthritis and therefore no need to postulate the occurrence of autoimmune self-perpetuative mechanisms in the HCIA model. The inducing arthritogenic cells may have been actively downregulated; alternatively, these cells become anergic as a result of lack of stimulation after the disappearance of the injected heterologous CII.

Most mouse and rat strains susceptible to CIA after immunization with heterologous CII also develop a strong antibody response to CII. This anti-CII response is largely specific for type II and possesses only minor cross-reactivity with type I or other types of collagens (17,26,27). In contrast to the antibody response after immunization with type I collagen (28), the anti-CII antibody response is widely cross-reactive between CII obtained from different species, including autologous CII. Thus a strong autoantibody response to CII is evoked after immunization with heterologous CII in rats and mice (exemplified in Table

1). An obvious, but important, conclusion from these findings is that B cells reactive with autologous CII are not deleted from the funtional repertoire.

As to the question of whether the anti-CII autoantibody response is correlated with the development of arthritis in individual animals, there is no evidence for such a linkage. No correlation can be found between the total levels of anti-CII antibody responses and the incidence of severity of arthritis in mice (29) or rats (30).

The next question to arise is whether a correlation exists between a certain isotype of anti-CII antibodies and the development of arthritis. Although some evidence for a critical involvement of IgG_{2a} anti-CII antibodies for the development of HCIA in both mice and rats has been reported (31,32), these findings may be complex to interpret since the corresponding isotype to mouse IgG_{2a} is rat IgG_{2b} rather than rat IgG_{2a} (33,34). Furthermore, in recent experiments, we have not been able to reproduce the earlier observed correlation between serum levels of IgG_{2a} antibodies reactive with heterologous CII and incidence or severity to arthritis by assaying the levels of serum antibodies reactive with autologous CII (Jansson et al., J. Autoimmunity (1990) 3:257).

One of the most interesting questions is whether there are any specific arthritogenic epitopes on the autologous CII molecule recognized by anti-CII antibodies The presence of antibody-defined epitopes on the CII molecule can be demonstrated by employing monoclonal antibodies in inhibition solid-phase assays. Using such assays some of the epitopes are more frequently recognized by antibodies in serum from mice with arthritis compared to serum antibodies from nonarthritic mice, although this correlation was found using pooled serum (27). In fact, analysis of the fine specificity of the anti-CII antibody response in individual mice after immunization with rat CII shows that the antibody response is often restricted to one of the major epitopes, and individual arthritic mice can be found that produce such an immunodominant response to each of the defined major epitopes (Table 2). These epitopes are located on different peptides produced after cyanogen-bromide digestion of CII (CII CB-peptides, in preparation). More definite evidence for the involvement of certain arthritogenic epitopes in the development of HCIA have been reported by Terato et al. (35). These authors immunized DBA/1 mice with CB peptides derived from chick CII and found only CB11 to be arthritogenic and, in addition, that the antibody response to CB11 cross-reacted well with mouse CII. Thus, epitopes on chick CII CB11 peptides seem to be of importance for the development of HCIA, although it is not clear whether these epitopes are recoginzed by T cells or only by antibodies. Another problem is that CB11 is a large peptide comprising one-third of the CII α1 chain, and in addition, it is possible that the immune response to CII obtained from species other than chick are predominantly directed to peptides other than CB11. Thus, as yet no specific antibody-defined epitopes on the CII molecule that play a role in the development of CIA induced with heterologous CII have been possible to define.

Table 2 CII Epitope Specificity of Antibodies in Serum Obtained from Arthritic DBA/1 Mice Immunized with Rat CII[a]

Mouse	Arthritc scores	CII epitopes				
		C1	C2	E8	B1	F4
M2	6	**248**	0	0	40	130
M3	2	0	3	**58**	60	0
M4	8	20	35	0	70	**200**
F8	6	0	8	**200**	40	110
F9	2	17	14	0	40	**340**
F11	8	14	**260**	0	0	90
F20	6	28	73	0	**120**	59
F21	8	0	11	0	40	**160**
F24	5	0	0	0	0	**200**
F25	5	5	0	0	**250**	100
F26	2	19	6	0	40	**1000**
F27	4	3	0	**236**	40	120
F28	1	**212**	0	15	0	150
F31	1	0	8	42	50	**250**
F36	2	0	46	0	40	70

[a]All mice were bled within 1 week after onset of arthritis. Binding to the different epitopes, designated C1, C2, E8, B1, and F2, was measured with an inhibition ELISA described earlier and expressed in μg/ml (13,27). The immunodominant response is indicated in bold type.

B. CIA Induced with Autologous CII

Immunization with autologous CII can effectively induce arthritis in certain strains of rats and mice. In the DBA/1 mouse the onset is relatively late and the first signs of acute joint swelling usually appear 4–12 weeks after immunization (36–38). In the DA rat, arthritis develops earlier and the first signs regularly appear around 2 weeks after immunization (20). In contrast to the arthritis induced with heterologous CII, the ACIA disease in both DBA/1 mice and DA rats follows a chronic course, which adds many interesting clinical characteristics. Thus, several relapses of arthritis can be observed and the activity of the disease in some animals never subsides (observation period is about 1 year after immunization, unpublished observation). Furthermore, in the rat, symmetrical involvement of relapsing arthritis in peripheral metacarpo/tarsophalangeal (MP) and proximal interphalangeal (PIP) joints has been observed (20). The chronic character of active arthitis can also be observed by histopathologic analysis of joints in which inflammatory cellular infiltrates and pannus tissue, as well as fibrous and cartilaginous ankylosis, occur simultaneously (20,36).

The antibody response after immunization with autologous CII is relatively weak and does not correlate with the development of arthritis (20,36–38). In the

DBA/1 mouse the strongest anti-CII autoantibody response develops in females despite that females are relatively resistant to the induction ACIA (36). Furthermore, certain individual mice develop arthritis but no detectable anti-CII autoantibodies in serum (39). In the DA rat, a somewhat stronger autoantibody response to CII develops, and also in this case no correlation with arthritis is found (20). In contrast to mice, there is a female preponderance for development of arthritis in the rat (40). The influence of gender in the ACIA is schematically presented in Table 3. From the findings already discussed it can be anticipated that antibody-mediated mechanisms do not play an important effector role in the pathogenesis of ACIA disease as is likely for the pathoagenesis of HCIA.

III. IMMUNOGENETICS

In rat and mouse species, only certain inbred strains are susceptible to the induction of CIA, suggesting a genetic linkage of CII responsiveness. Susceptibility for CIA is inherited polygenically, and there is evidence for at least four gene loci of importance: genes within MHC (16,18,39,41), V genes coding for T cell receptors (42–44), complement genes (31,45), and possibly genes on sex chromosomes (29).

A. Major Histocompatibility Complex

Development of CIA and anti-CII antibody responses after immunization with CII in both rats (15) and mice (16,18,39,41) is linked to MHC genes. The larger polymorphism in the mouse, compared with rats, has allowed a more detailed analysis of the involvement of particular MHC molecules for CII responsiveness. Development of arthritis after immunization with heterologous (16,18,41) or autologous CII (39) is restricted to mouse strains of H-2^q, H-2^q related, or H-2^r haplotypes (summarized in Table 3). By using mouse strains recombinant at the MHC region it has been shown that CIA susceptibility is associated with genes in the class II region (16,18). The H-2^q linkage of susceptibility to CIA is of particular interest since the H-2^q and H-2^p haplotypes are very closely related and

Table 3 Summary of Anti-CII Antibody Responses and Arthritis Susceptibility in Both Sexes of Rats and Mice Immunized with Autologous CII

	Mice (DBA/1		Rats (DA)	
Arthritis[a]	+	+ + +	+ + + + +	+ + +
Anti-CII antibody response[b]	+	+	+ + + + +	+ + + +

[a]Each + represents approximately 20% arthritis.
[b]Each + represents approximately 20 μg/ml anti-CII anibodies in serum.
Source: From Refs. 19, 20, and 36–38.

possess only minor differences on the expressed A_β chains since the A^α chain has been shown to be identical by tryptic fingerprint analysis (46). Furthermore, only I-A but not I-E molecules are expressed in the H-2^q haplotype (47). In contrast, H-2^r haplotypes express I-E molecules and also express I-A molecules not related to 1-A^q (18,48), indicating that the CIA disease in H-2^r haplotype mice is dependent on different molecular interactions at the T cell MHC level compared with CIA disease in H-2^q mice. Accordingly, B10RIII (H- 2^r) have been shown to develop a strong anti-CII antibody response and CIA only after immunization with bovine and porcine CII but not with chick, rat, or human CII (18). In contrast, a B10 congenic strain of the H-2^q haplotype, B10Q, develops a strong anti-CII antibody response as well as CIA after immunization with heterologous CII tested thus far: chick, bovine, porcine, human, and rat CII (16,18).

We have analyzed the anti-CII autoantibody response and the development of arthritis in a number of inbred mouse strains of different H-2 haplotypes. In these experiments we immunized the animals with various heterologous as well as autologous CIIs. Based on the responsiveness to autologous and heterologous CII the mice could be divided into three groups (results are summarized in Tables 4 and 5).

1. H-2^q and H2^r haplotypes (DBA/1, NFR/N, B10G, and B10RIII). Immunization with autologous CII led to the development of both an anti-CII autoantibody response and CIA. In addition, immunization with heterologous CII

Table 4 MHC Linkage of Anti-CII Antibody Responses[a]

Strain	H-2	Anti-CII autoantibody serum levels (μg/ml) after immunization with			
		Chick-CII	Bovine CII	Rat CII	Mouse CII
DBA/1	q	62	234	120	11
NFR/N	q	83	315	98	0
B10G	q	25	628	47	6
B10P	p	8	0	2	0
B10KEA5	w5	12	24	9	0
B10SAA48	w3	6	7	12	13
B10CAS2	w17	11	2	2	4
B10RIII	r	nd	261	2	7
B10	b	5	177	13	0
B10D2	d	2	0	9	0

[a]Levels of anti-CII autoantibodies 15 weeks after immunization with CII derived from different species (39,41). Purified polyclonal DBA/1 anti-CII antibodies are used as standard for estimation of anti-CII antibody levels.

Table 5 MHC Linkage of Susceptibility to CIA[a]

Strain	H-2	Incidence of arthritis after immunization with			
		Chick-CII	Bovine CII	Rat CII	Mouse CII
DBA/1	q	9/10	10/10	10/10	8/9
NFR/N	q	6/8	3/5	5/10	4/4
B10G	q	4/12	4/9	3/10	0/10
B10P	p	0/10	0/12	0/10	0/12
B10KEA5	w5	0/9	0/4	0/10	0/3
B10SAA48	w3	1/11	0/5	0/10	2/7
B10CAS2	w17	1/11	2/6	2/10	0/7
B10RIII	r	ND	4/6	0/10	3/6
B10	b	0/11	0/3	0/10	0/4
B10D2	d	0/6	0/5	0/10	0/6

[a]Incidence of arthritis 15 weeks after immunization with CII derived from various species (39,41). Occurrence of arthritis induced with heterologous CII has been recorded after macroscopic examination and arthritis induced with mouse CII with both macroscopic and microscopic examination.

induced a stronger autoantibody response and a more severe arthritis than after immunization with mouse CII. These findings indicate that one or more determinants present only on heterologous CII (for H-2^r on bovine, but not chick, human, or rat CII) are detected by T cells capable of helping B cells producing antibodies cross-reactive with mouse CII. Thus, both T cells reactive with autologous CII and T cells reactive with heterologous CII may be activated in these strains.

2. H-2^{w3}, H-2^{w17} (B10SAA48 and B10CAS2). Immunization of these mice with autologous CII produced low levels of anti-CII autoantibodies and low frequencies of arthritis. The response to heterologous CII was of equal magnitude, implying that the determinants seen are identical. Thus, only autoreactive T cells detecting an epitope common to autologous and certain heterologous CII may be activated in these strains.

3. H-2^p, H-2^{w5}, H-2^b, H-2^d (B10P, B10KEA5, B10, B10D2). Immunization of mice from these strains with autologous CII induced neither an anti-CII antibody production nor arthritis. Immunization with various heterologous CII induced an anti-CII autoantibody response in all strains, although the magnitude of this response was variable. In some cases, for example B10 immunized with bovine CII, a strong autoantibody response to CII was seen, but none of these mice developed arthritis. Thus, only T cells exclusively reactive with various heterologous CII, but not with autologous CII, can be activated in these strains.

In addition, it is clear from the sets of experiments described here that other, non-MHC genes influence the susceptibility to CIA as well as the antibody response to CII. This was most clearly demonstrated by the observed differences between the three H-2^q strains, DBA/1, NFR/N, and B10G (see also Refs. 29, 39, and 41), and by analysis of the genetic susceptibility to CIA in the rat (15).

Taken together, immunogenetic analysis suggests that a critical requirement for the development of CIA is the activation of T helper cells reactive with autologous CII. Immunization with heterologous CII may in addition activate T cells specific for heterologous CII. These nonself reactive T cells may enhance a strong autoantibody response to CII, presumably via activation of B cells producing antibodies detecting species cross-reactive epitopes on CII.

B. T Cell Receptor V Genes

Further evidence for the involvement of CII-reactive T cells has recently been reported by David and coworkers. With F$_1$ hybridization and backcross experiments they found that the H-2^q haplotype SWR and AU mice are not susceptible to CIA because of a large genomic deletion in the T cell receptor V$_\beta$ region (42,43). However, the resistance of the SWR mice seems also to partly depend on complement factors since this mouse is C5 deficient (45). Accordingly, backcrosses of SWR to C5-deficient but TCR-V$_\beta$-nondeleted strains were susceptible to arthritis but had a significantly delayed onset of disease (44). The resistance to CIA in SWR mice may, however, also be dependent on the influence of other genes not related to TCR or C5. This was found in a recent analyses of (SWR×DBA/1)F2 mice (106). Moreover, in vivo depletion of T cells expressing some of the proposed TCR Vβ-elements (β8.1,2 and β6) do not affect the course of CIA in DBA/1 mice (107). Thus, the influence by TCR V genes is challenging but not yet precisely determined.

C. Complement Genes

The availability of specific deletion of C5 genes in a large number of inbred mouse strains has given valuable information on the important role of complement in the development of CIA induced with heterologous CII. Thus, the lack of C5 induces a delay or inhibition of the CIA disease (31,44,45), and this effect seems to affect the effector pathways of antibody-mediated induction of disease since serum-transferred arthritis is only effective in C5-competent but not C5-deficient strains (49).

IV. THE ROLE OF T CELLS IN THE PATHOGENESIS OF CIA

T cell-deficient rats (50) or mice (Table 6) do not develop a CII immune response or CIA after immunization with CII, clearly demonstrating the critical role of

Table 6 Anti-CII Antibody Response and Development of CIA Dependent on T Cells[a]

Mouse strain	n	Anti-CII autoantibody serum levels (mean μg/ml ± SD)	Number with arthritis
+/+	5	393 ± 322	3
+/nu	5	246 ± 164	5
nu/nu	4	0	0

[a]Comparison of the antibody response and CIA development in nude, nude/+, and +/+ NFR/N mice 6 weeks after immunization with rat CII. Purified polyclonal DBA/1 anti-CII antibodies are used as a standard for estimation of anti-CII antibody levels.

T cells both for the development of the disease and for the production of anti-CII autoantibodies. Immunization with heterologous CII not only induces a strong autoantibody response to CII in susceptible animals but also a delayed-type hypersensitivity reaction after challenge with CII in the ears (17,23,51–53). Furthermore, a CII-specific proliferative response can be measured in lymph node cells cultured in vitro (17,23–26). It is likely that the activation of CII-reactive T cells occurs in the lymph nodes that drain the immunization site. Such T cells become competent to various effector functions, such as helping B cells to produce anti-CII autoantibodies and migration to tissues where the corresponding antigen is present. In the DTH reaction in the ear antigen-specific T cells migrate after antigen challenge, and it is possible that similar phenomena occur in the joints, provided that autoreactive T cells have been activated and migrated to the joints. In the joints these autoreactive T cells may permit the activation of various mesenchymal cells by secretion of interleukins, such as interferon-γ.

We have investigated the earliest developing cellular events in the joints after immunization with rat CII. Paws from DBA/1 mice were analyzed immediately before the onset of clinically apparent but after the development of microscopic visible pathologic changes in the synovium. This demonstrated that few, but significant, numbers of IL-2 receptor expressing CD4+ T cells, together with increased expression of class II antigens on synovial cells, appeared in distinct foci in the synovium (21). Very few granulocytes or B cells were present in these foci. It is tempting to speculate that these few T cells have been activated by CII and subsequently secrete macrophage and fibroblast activating interleukins, such as interferon-γ, and thereby initiate the development of arthritis. In accordance with this hypothesis we have recently found that local treatment with recombinant interferon-γ of DBA/1 mice, shortly after CII immunization, triggers the earlier onset of arthritis with greater severity (54). The joints from interferon-γ-treated arthritic mice contain substantial number of infiltrated CD4+ T cells and synovial cells intensively expressing class II molecules.

Although CIA is clearly a T cell-dependent disease, the pathologically active T cell clones have not as yet been isolated and characterized. The epitope specificity, interleukin production, or regulatory properties of these cells are not known. However, it is known that (1) depletion of $CD4^+$ T cells before immunization abrogates CIA (55,56) (2) transfer of $CD4^+$ CII-reactive T cells induces arthritis (57–60), and (3) various T cell-produced interleukins promote the development of arthritic disease (54,61,62). It is likely that activated T cells regulate two different processes of importance to the pathogenesis of CIA. First, activated T cells located in the joints can, via secretion of interleukins, permit and promote joint inflammation and erosion of cartilage and bone. Second, they can help B cells to produce autoantibodies that can immunoprecipitate in the joints and promote migration of neutrophils and development of acute edema in the joints. Although there is some evidence for both processes and for synergism between these two processes (63,64), we do not have exact knowledge of their relative importance in CIA.

V. ROLE OF B CELLS IN THE PATHOGENESIS OF CIA

One bit of evidence for the involvement of B cell-mediated effector functions in the pathogenesis of CIA is the dependence of functional complement for the development of CIA induced with heterologous CII. It was demonstrated early that depletion of C3 with cobra venom factor in rats delayed the onset of arthritis as long as the C3 levels were suppressed (65). Furthermore, genetically determined C5 deficiency in mice delays or abrogates the development of CIA (31). Histopathologic analysis of joints shortly after the onset of arthritis is also compatible with an antibody- or immune complex-mediated type of disease, with deposition of complement and antibodies on joint surfaces, development of edema, and infiltration of large numbers of polymorphic neutrophilic cells (21,22,32).

A pathogenic role of humoral components has been directly demonstrated by several groups using passive transfer experiments (32,66–68). Syngeneic serum concentrates corresponding to 4 ml immune anti-CII serum in the rat and 3 ml in the mouse induced acute arthritis 24–48 after injection in naive recipients (66–69). In contrast to the actively induced CIA, the anti-CII serum-induced arthritis is transient, with no persistent destructive changes in the joints. It is likely that anti-CII antibodies play a crucial role in the passively transferred disease since serum antibodies purified on CII-Sepharose are effective in inducing arthritis after injection of 12 mg immunoglobulin in naive rats (32). Furthermore, deposits of C3 and immunoglobulin could be demonstrated on cartilage surfaces. Treatment of rats with cobra venom factor decomplemented cartilage surfaces and abrogated the development of arthritis after transfer of the anti-CII antibody fraction (32). It is likely that the effector part of the passively induced arthritis is not dependent on functional T cells. First, athymic nude rats are susceptible to passively (70) but not actively induced arthritis (50). Second, the anti-CII serum-induced arthritis is not restricted to MHC since passive arthritis can be induced in mouse strains with MHC haplotypes not susceptible to conventionally induced CIA (67). These findings suggest that the effector part of the arthritis induced with anti-CII antibody containing serum is a T cell-independent, complement-dependent type of arthritis mediated by precipitation of immune complexes containing anti-CII antibodies in the joints. In accordance with this view is the immunohistopathologic finding of infiltration of large numbers of infiltrated granulocytes, very few T cells, and a relatively sparse class II expression on cells within the inflammatory lesions (12).

Although antibody-mediated mechanisms are of great importance in the development of CIA, we have very limited knowledge about the specificity of pathogenic antibodies. Attempts to induce arthritis by injecting monoclonal anti-CII antibodies have been largely unsuccessful in both mice (27) and rats (71). We have studied the pathogenicity of a series of syngeneic monoclonal anti-CII autoantibodies in DBA/1 mice (Refs. 11 and 27 and unpublished results). Injection of large amounts (0.5–5 mg per mouse) of antibodies of various IgG subclasses and with high affinity to mouse CII and to cartilage induces only limited hyperplasia of synovium and failed to induce granulocyte infiltration and edema formation as is reproducively found after transfer with anti-CII serum. These monoclonal antibodies react with five to seven of the most invariably detected epitopes on the CII molecule. A mixture of these monoclonal antibodies, detecting different epitopes, was also ineffective in producing arthritis. Although it is still possible that we have not yet found an antibody detecting a specific arthritogenic epitope, we favor the idea that the presence of anti-CII antibodies is not solely enough for the induction of passively induced arthritis. We suggest that the formation of immune complexes, precipitating in the joints, is a necessary requirement. Therefore, polyclonal anti-CII antibody preparations, effective to induce arthritis, may also contain other antibody specificities of importance to the formation of immune complexes.

VI. ORIGIN OF AUTOREACTIVE ANTI-CII B CELLS

The anti-CII antibody response is mainly a T cell-dependent process; specificities and isotype usage of the antibody response therefore also reflects activation of T cells reactive with the immunogen and/or reactive with autologous CII present in joint cartilage in vivo.

A. The Primary Immune Response

A characteristic of the CIA model induced with heterologous CII is the strong activation of autoantibody-producing B cells. Immunization with rat CII in high responder DBA/1 mice induces activation of large numbers of autoantibody-producing B cells as early as 9–11 days after immunization (13,14,72,73). In fact, approximately 20% of all antibody-producing B cells in a DBA/1 popliteal lymph node produce anti-CII reactive antibodies 9 days after immunization with rat CII. The overwhelming majority of these B cells produce IgG specific for mouse CII. The anti-CII-reactive B cells produce antibodies encoded from several different V_H and V_L genes (14), and they have no Ly-1$^+$ (CD5) mRNA message as determined with Northern blotting (Mayer et al., in preparation). The latter finding is in contrast to most autoantibody-producing B cells in certain lupus autoimmune mouse strains (74).

In contrast, a very weak antibody response in serum and no B cells in the draining lymph nodes can be detected after immunization with autologous CII in DBA/1 mice (Mo et al. in preparation). A reasonable explanation may be that T cells exclusively reactive with heterologous CII are activated after immunization with rat CII but not after immunization with mouse CII. However, the very strong B cell response after a primary immunization with rat CII also indicates that B cells have already been primed to CII reactivity in vivo before immunization. Such a possibility is of utmost importance since it indicates an ongoing autoimmune process in the naive DBA/1 mouse. Such a process may be part of a physiologic network of autoreactive lymphocytes controlling each other in idiotypic interrelationships and maintaining natural activation of the immune system. It may also refect regulatory cells of importance of control autoreactive T cells activated with CII accessible to the immunes system, which obviously not have been deleted in the thymus. The specificity and functional properties of B cells activated in a primary immunization with heterologous CII is therefore of importance.

B. Connectivity of the Anti-CII Antibody Response

We are studying specificities and phenotypes of large number of B cells in primed lymph nodes utilizing both ELISPOT (enzyme-linked immunospot) assays, presumably detecting high antibody-secreting plasma cells, and hybridoma collections, representing a selected population of B cells in the lymphoblastoid stage. With both ELISPOT techniques and hybridoma collections obtained from DBA/1 lymph nodes after primary immunizations with heterologous CII, very high frequencies of IgG anti-CII-producing B cells have been recorded. With the hybridoma collection method it is also possible to study cross-reactivities, CII fine specificity, Ig isotypes, and also V genes used by the autoreactive anti-CII hybridomas (see earlier). One of the most challenging findings is the pattern of cross-reactive binding to other self antigens by the CII-reactive hybridomas.

Approximately 10% of the isolated hybridomas produce multispecific IgM antibodies binding to a large number of self and nonself antigens, a frequency constantly found in hybridoma collections from various antigens, native rat CII, ovalbumin, or denatured rat CII. In hybridomas obtained from CII immunization we have also found those that produce antibodies cross-reactive between CII and

IgG-Fc and others between CII and IgG-Fab, indicating a specific relationship between CII reactivity and rheumatoid factor specificity. Similar observations have also recently been made by others (75). We have also produced hybridomas from spleens of arthritis DBA/1 mice after immunization with CII–anti-CII immune complexes. These hybridomas represent a very interesting collection of different cross-reactive specificities, as illustrated in Fig. 1. Two monoclonal rheumatoid factors were isolated, one with a double specificity for IgG-Fc and CII and the other a double specificity for IgG-Fc and a cross-reactive idiotope present on many anti-CII antibodies (76,77). In addition, a third type of anti-CII antibody cross-reacts with the collagenous part of C1q (78). Interestingly, rheumatoid factors can also be measured in serum from DBA/1 mice immunized with autologous or heterologous CII (Fig. 2) using the DIGELISA (diffusion in gel ELISA) technique (77). Also, in guinea pigs rheumatoid factors and anti-F(ab′)$_2$ antibodies can be demonstrated in serum after immunization with CII (79). These unique properties of the anti-CII immune response may have important bearing for the understanding of the pathogenesis of CIA and possibly also RA. First, it is possible that immune complexes between various autoantibodies, CII, and complement factors precipitate in the joints and promote arthritis, thus giving a satisfactory hypothetical explanation for the passively transferred arthritis. Second, B cells with these specificities may have important regulatory roles for the CII

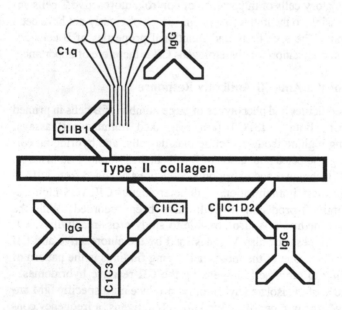

Figure 1 Cross-reactivities by monoclonal antibodies derived from a fusion of B cells from CII-immunized arthritic DBA/1 mice. (From Ref. 76.)

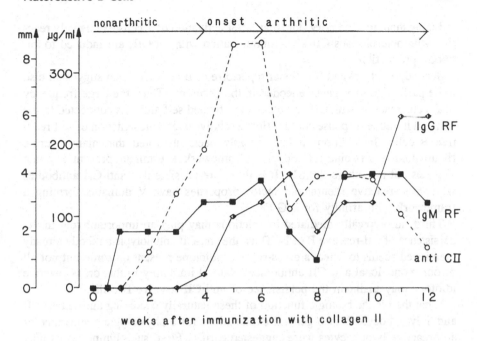

Figure 2 Production of IgG and IgM rheumatoid factors reactive with rabbit IgG (estimated with DIGELISA) and anti-CII antibodies (estimated with ELISA) in serum of DBA/1 mice after immunization with rat CII.

autoimmunity and development of CIA. Such B cells may be triggered by the formation of immune complexes and degradation of CII in situ and play a role as antigen presenting cells for autoreactive T cells.

C. Origin of Autoreactive B Cells Connected to CII Reactivity

From these findings it can be concluded that B cells with anti-CII reactivity are present in the functional immune repertoire of CIA-susceptible mouse strains. In addition, the anti-CII antibody response is connected with cross-reactive responses to other self antigens, such as IgG-Fc (rheumatoid factors), C1q, and anti-CII idiotypes. Concerning the mechanisms leading to the generation of autoreactive lymphocytes, we prefer to speculate along three alternative and un-contradictory lines of reasoning.

First, autoreactive T cells stimulated and tolerized with autologous CII may be a natural part of the immune system in mice with certain H-2 haplotypes, such as H-2q. These autoreactive T cells may also interact with CII-reactive B cells, inducing them to a memory state that, after activation of T cells exclusively reactive with heterologous CII after immunization with rat CII, are induced to antibody production.

Second, a natural and functional repertoire of B cells has been suggested also to be partly due to V genes encoded in the germline. Thus, the large frequency of B cells reactive with CII and other investigated self antigens connected to the anti-CII immune response could reflect a relative overrepresentation of self reactive B cells. In addition, it has recently been suggested that many murine rheumatoid factors bind IgG-Fc with a framework determinant present on some V genes but not others (80,81). It is therefore possible that anti-CII antibodies with cross-reactive rheumatoid factor properties have V domains forming a framework with affinity for IgG-Fc.

Third, idiotypically mediated interactions may play an important role in the persistence of CII-reactive B cells. Thus, the anti-CII antidiotypic antibody already mentioned seems to detect a cross-reactive idiotope present on some but not all of our monoclonal anti-CII antibodies. Natural immunity to this cross-reactive idiotope may maintain the persistence of anti-CII-reactive B cells.

What then is the biologic function of these naturally occurring autoreactive B and T lymphocytes? Two general explanations for a physiologic occurrence of autoreactive lymphocytes were suggested earlier. First, such lymphocytes may be of importance in the continuous stimulation and survival of the immune system (83,83); second, certain autoreactive lymphocytes may have important roles in cleaning the body of tissue garbage (84). From the accessibility of CII and the continuous degradation of cartilage it is easy to imagine such a role for the autoreactive lymphocytes described here. The price to be paid is the risk of development of autoimmune arthritis in certain genetically predisposed individuals.

VII. REGULATORY ROLE OF B CELLS AND VACCINATION WITH ANTIBODIES

One early and very important observation made by Staines and coworkers (85) was that anti-CII serum given immediately before immunization with heterologous CII abrograted the development of CIA in rats. Interestingly, administration of immune complexes between CII and anti-CII serum was even more effective and could vaccinate the rats from HCIA when given more than 1 week before immunization. Furthermore, rats that have recovered from arthritis induced with anti-CII immune serum are resistant to a second attempt to induce passive arthritis or against actively induced CIA by immunization with heterologous CII (71,86,87). In addition, the passively induced arthritis persists for less than a week despite the presence of antibodies and complement on cartilage surfaces up to 16 days. Thus, the transient arthritis after injection of anti-CII antibodies is more likely terminated by regulatory forces than elimination of the anti-CII antibodies. Furthermore, it is tempting to suggest that the downregulation of active arthritis in CIA induced with heterologous CII, in contrast to CIA induced with autologous CII in which a chronic form of arthritis develops, is influenced by anti-CII antibody-mediated downregulation of arthritis.

Several lines of evidence indicate that the vaccinating effect of anti-CII antibodies is controlled by T cells. For instance, thymus-deficient nude rats or T cell-depressed cyclosporin-treated rats cannot be vaccinated with anti-CII antibodies (87,88). Also, the mouse is susceptible to anti-CII antibody-mediated vaccination (66). We have recently observed that only polyclonal anti-CII antibodies are able to vaccinate, but not a number of different monoclonal anti-CII antibodies (unpublished results), indicating that the vaccinating effect is triggered either by very rare antibodies in the polyclonal antibody preparation or by other antibodies or immune complexes in these preparations, as was earlier discussed for the arthritogenicity of anti-CII antibodies. Such immune complexes may be efficiently bound to antigen presenting cells and presented to anti-idiotypic regulatory T cells. It is interesting to tnate that a cross-reactive idiotope is present on our monoclonal anti-CII antibodies (77), and we are at present investigating the regulatory effects of an antibody detecting this cross-reactive idotope. Other groups have also described cross-reactive idiotopes present on anti-CII antibodies (89), and it has also been possible to downregulate murine HCIA with rabbit anti-idiotypic antibodies to anti-CII antibodies (90).

VIII. IMPLICATIONS FOR STUDIES OF RHEUMATOID ARTHRITIS

The onset of rheumatoid arthritis is usually acute and develops with a chronic and progressive course (91). Chronic inflammation develops in the joints, with destruction of cartilage and bone tissue. We discuss rheumatoid disease from the standpoint that tolerance to an unknown autoantigen has been broken and that the chronic process is maintained by self perpetuative mechanisms.

A. Immunogenetics

Susceptibility to RA is to a large extent genetically determined. First, females are more often affected than males, a sex linkage that cannot easily be explained by the actions of sex hormones since estrogens have been found to protect against disease (92). It is possible that sex chromosomes may be of importance to the observed sex linkage. Second, the susceptibility to RA is linked to MHC class II genes coding for HLA-DR4 and HLA-DR1, and this linkage is even closer when specific determinants on the class II molecules are defined. Thus, a strong correlation has been found with HLA-Dw4 and Dw14 subtypes of DR4 that have sequence similarities at position 70–71 on the DRB chain (93). The observed MHC class II linkage is a strong indication that RA is a T cell-mediated immunospecific disease.

B. T Cell-Mediated Autoimmunity

Several lines of data indicate that a local T cell activation against as-yet-unknown antigens occurs in the synovial tissue in RA. Thus immunohistochemical studies have demonstrated a multitude of class II antigen-expressing and potential antigen presenting cells in the rheumatoid synovial tissue (94,95). T cells, particulary $CD4^+$ T "helper" cells, are present in close proximity to class II antigen-expressing cells. Thus, a cellular basis for local class II-restricted T cell activated exists. Evidence that T cells in the synovial tissue are activated to a larger extent than T cells in the synovial fluid or in peripheral blood has been provided from the observations of increased expression of class II molecules and IL-2 receptors on synovial T cells from patients with active RA (94,96,97). Synovial lining cells of macrophages and fibroblasts as well as endothelial cells, express class II molecules, probably as a result of actions of interferon-γ produced by the activated T cells (98). As to the specificity of the activated T cells in synovium, very limited information has emerged. However, cellular reactivities against various mycobacterial fractions (99) as well as to collagen (100) have been reported. Recently, isolation of CII-reactive T cell clones from a rheumatoid synovium was demonstrated (101).

C. B Cell-Mediated Autoimmunity

RA is also characterized by activation of autoreactive B cells, and immune complexes precipitating in the joints is belived to be an important contributing factor in the pathogenesis (102). A hallmark of RA is the production of rheumatoid factors. This is an autoimmune reaction toward autologous IgG that has been shown to be dependent on activated T helper cells (103). Also, the occurrence of autoantibodies with other specificities, for example against such cartilage structures as CII, has been demonstrated (104,105). These autoantibodies have been shown to form immune complexes locally in the joints (104,105). It is likely that interferon-γ and other T cell-derived interleukins, as well as immune complexes formed by the locally produced immunoglobulins and autoantigens, contribute to the activation of synovial macrophages and fibroblasts in the synovial tissue and granulocytes in the synovial fluid.

D. The Future

The most challenging question for the study of rheumatoid arthritis concerns the specificity of the immune reactions that initiate and perpetuate the autoimmune pathology. These reactions are most likely dependent on both activated autoreactive T cells and certain autoreactive B cells. Thus, immune-specific lymphocytes are of importance for both delayed hypersensitivity and immune complex-mediated pathogenetic mechanisms. One of the most pertinent questions now is to determine the specificity of these activated lymphocytes infiltrating in the synovial tissue during rheumatoid disease. It is also possible that the critical interactions and occurrence of autoreactive T cells and B cells are localized to the lymph nodes draining the actively affected joints, although only very limited studies have been performed on such lymph nodes in RA. The isolation of lymphocytes with critical specificities may prove to be a complicated task, however. First, the activated lymphocytes are not monoclonal but rather polyclonal or possibly oligoclonal in origin, and few of them can be postulated to have direct importance in the initiation and perpetuation of the disease. Second, we will have difficulty in proving the pathogenicity of a given isolated lymphocyte. Third, we have limited basic knowledge on how autoreactive T cells and B cells are regulated in vivo; for instance, it may not be the presence per se of autoreactive lymphocytes but rather a failure to regulate such normally occurring cells that is the pathologic event. We think that experimental models for RA are useful for studies of basic mechanisms and the importance of specific autoimmune reactions for the development of arthritis, although they cannot be directly applied to human diseases.

IX. CONCLUDING REMARKS AND POSSIBLE THERAPEUTIC STRATEGIES

The CIA model is well suited to studies of immunogenetic and pathogenetic requirements for the development of autoimmune arthritis. Activation of autoreactive T helper and/or T inflammatory cells in high-responder animals may trigger two different pathways that may synergize in the induction of arthritis. One is a T cell-mediated activation of macrophages and fibroblasts in the joints, leading to a destructive delayed-type hypersensitivity reaction. The other is the formation of immune complexes in the joints, consisting of anti-CII autoantibodies and rheumatoid factors. These immune complexes precipitate in the joints and activate the complement cascades and granulocyte infiltration, as well as destructive macrophages. It is easy to imagine that both these pathogenetic events may also occur in RA, and therefore CIA may be a useful model for studies of pathogenetic mechanisms leading to arthritis. In such studies the CIA model provides opportunities for characterization of the immunospecific reactions leading to arthritis. B cells activated in the CIA disase have importance in both effector functions and regulatory effects on the development of disease. This may enable us to define the idiotopes of importance to immunoregulation and the requirements for treatment of animals with idiopeptides or antibodies against cross-reactive idiotopes. In parallel, a similar detailed characterization of the autoantibody response in RA should be carried out and compared with the immune response in CIA. We do not believe that identical specificities are involved in RA and CIA disease, but it may be valuable to use the CIA model to develop new therapeutic strategies and to develop a deeper understanding of autoimmunity leading to arthritis.

ACKNOWLEDGMENTS

This work was supported by the Swedish Medical Research Council, Craaford Foundation, King Gustav V's 80-year Foundation, the Nanna Swartz Foundation, and Riksförbundet mot Reumatism. I also thank Kristofer Rubin, Mikael Andersson, Lotta Jansson, John Mo, Tom Goldschmidt, Vivianne Malmström, and Mikael Karlsson for contributing unpublished material and for critical reading of the manuscript.

REFERENCES

1. Trentham, D.E., Townes, A.S., and Kang, A.H. (1977). Autoimmunity to type II collagen: An experimental model of arthritis. J. Exp. Med. 146:857.
2. Glant, T.T., Mikecz, K., Aroumanian, A., Poole A.R. (1987). Proteoglycan-induced arthritis in Balb/c mice. Arthritis Rheum. 30:201–212.
3. Mikecz, K., Glant, T.T., and Poole, A.R. (1987). Immunity to cartilage proteoglycans in Balb/c ice with progressive polyarthritis and ankylosing spondylitis induced by injection of human cartilage proteoglycan. Arthritis Rheum. 30:306.
4. Courtenay, J.S., Dallman, M.J., Dayan, A.D., Martin, A., and Mosedal, B. (1980). Immunization against heterologous type II collagen induces arthritis in mice. Nature 283:666.
5. Yoo, T.J., Kim, S.Y., Stuart, J.M., Floyd, R.A., Olson, G.A., Cremer, M.A., and Kang, A.H. (1988). Induction of arthritis in monkeys by immunization with type II collagen. J. Exp. Med. 168:777.
6. Heinegård, D., and Paulsson, M. (1987). Cartilage. Methods Enzymol. 145:336.
7. Stuart, J.M., Cremer, M.A., Dixit, S.N., Kang, A.H., and Townes, A.S. (1979). Collagen induced arthritis in rats. Comparison of vitreous and cartilage-derived collagens. Arthritis Rheum. 22:347.
8. Klareskog, L., Forsum, U., and Wigzell, H. (1982). Murine synovial intima contains I-A, I-E/C positive bonemarrow-derived cells. Scand. J. Immunol. 15:509.
9. Silberberg-Sinakin, I., Gigli, I., Baer, R.L., and Thorbecke, G.J. (1980). Langerhans cells: Role in contact hypersensitivity and relationship to lymphoid dendritic cells and to macrophages. Immunol. Rev. 53:203.
10. Stuart, J.M., Cremer, M.A., Townes, A.S., and Kang, A.H. (1982). Type II collagen-induced arthritis in rats. Passive transfer with serum and evidence that IgG anti-collagen antibodies can cause arthritis. J. Exp. Med. 155:1.
11. Jonsson, R., Karlsson, A.L., and Holmdahl, R. (1989). Demonstration of immune-reactive sites on cartilage after in vivo administration of biotinylated anti-type II collagen antibodies. J. Histochem. Cytochem. 37:265.
12. Holmdahl, R., Andersson, M., Enander, I., Goldschmidt, T., Jansson, L., Larsson, P., Nordling, C., and Klareskog, L. (1988). Nature of the type II collagen autoimmunity in mice. Int. J. Immunol. 4:49.
13. Holmdahl, R., Andersson, M., and Tarkowski, A. (1987). Origin of the autoreactive anti-type II collagen response. I. Frequency of specific and multispecific B cells in primed murine lymph nodes. Immunology 61:369.

14. Holmdahl, R., Bailey, C., Enander, I., Mayer, R., Klareskog, L., Moran, T., and Bona, C. (1989). Origin of the autoreactive anti type II collagen response. II. specificities, isotypes and usage of V gene families of anti-type II collagen autoantibodies. J. Immunol. 142:1881.

15. Griffiths, M.M., and Dewitt, C.W. (1981). Immunogenetic control of experimental collagen-induced arthritis in rats. II. ECIA susceptibility and immune response to type II collagen (calf) are linked to RT1. J. Immunogenet. 8:463.

16. Wooley, P.H., Luthra, H.S., Stuart, J.M., and David, C.S. (1981). Type II collagen induced arthritis in mice. I. Major histocompatibility complex (I-region) linkage and antibody correlates. J. Exp. Med. 154:688.

17. Stuart, J.M., Townes, A.S., and Kang, A.H. (1982). Nature and specificity of the immune response to collagen in type II collagen induced arthritis in mice. J. Clin. Invest. 69:673.

18. Wooley, P.H., Luthra, H.S., Lafuse, W.P., Huse, A., Stuart, J.M., and David, C.S. (1985). Type II collagen induced arthritis in mice. IV. Variations in immunogenetic regulation provide evidence for multiple arthritogenic epitopes on the collagen molecule. J. Immunol. 135:2443.

19. Holmdahl, R., Jansson, L., Gullberg, D., Rubin, K., Forsberg, P.O., and Klareskog, L. (1985). Incidence of arthritis and autoreactivity of anti-collagen antibodies after immunization of DBA/1 mice with heterologous and autologous collagen II. Clin. Exp. Immunol. 62:639.

20. Larsson, P., Kleinau, S., Holmdahl, R., and Klareskog, L. (1990). Autologous collagen-II induced arthritis in rats. Demonstration of clinically distinct forms of arthritis in two strains of rats. Arthritis Rheum. 33:693.

21. Holmdahl, R., Jonsson, R., Larsson, P., and Klareskog, L. (1988). Early appearance of activated CD4 positive T lymphocytes and Ia-expressing cells in joints of DBA/1 mice immunized with type II collagen. Lab. Invest. 58:53.

22. Caulfield, J.P., Hein, A., Dynesius-Trentham, R., and Trentham, D.E. (1982). Morphologic demonstration of two stages in the development of type II collagen-induced arthritis. Lab. Invest. 46:321.

23. Stuart, J.M., Cremer, M.A., Kang, A.H., and Townes, A.S. (1979). Collagen induced arthritis. Evaluation of early immunological events. Arthritis Rheum. 22:1344.

24. Holmdahl, R., Rubin, K., Klareskog, L., Dencker, L., Gustafsson, G., and Larsson, E. (1985). Appearance of different lymphoid cells in synovial tissue and in peripheral blood during the course of collagen II-induced arthritis in rats. Scand. J. Immunol. 21:197.

25. Kakimoto, K., Hirofuji, T., and Koga, T. (1984). Specificity of anti-type II collagen antibody response in rats. Clin. Exp. Immunol. 57:57.

26. Trentham, D.E., Townes, A.S., Kang, A.H., and David, J.R. (1978). Humoral and cellular sensitivity to collagen in type II collagen induced arthritis in rats. J. Clin. Invest. 61:89.

27. Holmdahl, R., Rubin, K., Klareskog, L., Larsson, E., and Wigzell, H. (1986). Characterization of the antibody response in mice with type II collagen-induced arthritis, using monoclonal anti-type II collagen antibodies. Arthritis Rheum. 29:400.

28. Nowack, H., Hahn, E., and Timpl, R. (1975). Specificity of the antibody response in inbred mice to bovine type I and type II collagen. Immunology 29:621.

29. Holmdahl, R., Jansson, L., and Andersson, M. (1986). Female sex hormones suppress development of collagen-induced arthritis in mice. Arthritis Rheum 29:1501.

30. Carlson, R.P., Blazek, E.M., Datko, L.J., and Lewis, A.J. (1984). Humoral and cellular immunological responses in collagen-induced arthritis in rats: Their correlation with severity of arthritis. J. Immunopharmacol. 6:379.

31. Watson, W.C., and Townes, A.S. (1985). Genetic susceptibility to murine collagen II autoimmune arthritis. Proposed relationship to the IgG_2 autoantibody subclass response, complement C5, major histocompatibility complex (MHC) and non-MHC loci. J. Exp. Med. 162:1878.

32. Kerwar, S.S., Englert, M.E., McReynolds, R.A., Landes, M.J., Lloyd, J.M., Oronsky, A.L., and Wilson, F.J. (1983). Type II collagen-induced arthritis. Studies with purified anticollagen immunoglobulin. Arthritis Rheum. 26:1120.

33. Denham, S., Barfoot, R., and Jackson, E. (1987). A receptor for monomeric IgG2b on rat macrophages. Immunology 62:69.

34. Füst, G., Medgyesi, G.A., Bazin, H., and Gergley, J. (1980). Differences in the ability of the rat IgG subclasses to consume complement in homologous and heterologous serum. Immunol. Lett. 1:249.

35. Terato, K., Hasty, K.A., Cremer, M.A., Stuart, J.M., Townes, A.S., and Kang, A.H. (1985). Collagen-induced arthritis in mice. Localization of an arthritogenic determinant to a fragment of the type II collagen molecule. J. Exp. Med. 162:637.

36. Holmdahl, R., Jansson, L., Larsson, E., Rubin, K., and Klareskog, L. (1986). Homologous type II collagen induces chronic and progressive arthritis in mice. Arthritis Rheum. 29:106.

37. Boissier, M.C., Feng, X.Z., Carlioz, A., Roudier, R., and Fournier, C. (1987). Experimental autoimmune arthritis in mice. I. Homologous type II collagen is responsible for self-perpetuating chronic polyarthritis. Ann. Rheum. Dis. 46:691.

38. Boissier, M.C., Carlioz, A., and Fournier, C. (1988). Experimental autoimmune arthritis in mice. II. Early events in the elicitation of the autoimmune phenomenon induced by homologous type II collagen. Clin. Immunol. Immunopathol. 48:225.

39. Holmdahl, R., Klareskog, L., Andersson, M., and Hansen, C. (1986). High antibody response to autologous type II collagen is restricted to H-2q. Immunogenetics 24:84.

40. Larsson, P., Klareskog, L., and Holmdahl, R. (1989). Demonstration of female preponderance as well as estrogen-induced disease suppression in autologous collagen II arthritis in rats. Submitted for publication.

41. Holmdahl, R., Jansson, L., Andersson, M., and Larsson, E. (1988). Immunogenetics of type II collagen autoimmunity and susceptibility to collagen arthritis. Immunology 65:305.

42. Banerjee, S., Haqqi, T.M., Luthra, H.S., Stuart, J.M., and David, C.S. (1988). Possible role of V_β T cell receptor genes in susceptibility to collagen-induced arthritis in mice. J. Exp. Med. 167:832.

43. Haqqi, T.M., Banerjee, S., Jones, W.L., Anderson, G., Behlke, M.A., Loh, D.Y., Luthra H.S., and David, C.S. (1989). Identification of T-cell receptor V_β deletion mutant mouse strain AU/ssJ (H-2q) which is resistant to collagen-induced arthritis. Immunogenetics 29:180.

44. Banerjee, S., Anderson, G.D., Luthra, H.S., and David, C.S. (1989). Influence of complement C5 and V_β T cell receptor mutations on susceptibility to collagen-induced arthritis in mice. J. Immunol. 142:2237.

45. Fujita, M., Mishima, M., Iwabuchi, K., Katsume, C., Gotohda, T., Ogasawara, K., Mizuno, Y., Good R.A., and Onoe, K. (1989). A study on type II collagen-induced arthritis in allogeneic bone marrow chimaeras. Immunology 66:422.

46. Peck, A.B., Darby, B., and Wakeland, E.K. (1983). Variant class II molecules from H-2 haplotypes in wild mouse populations: Functional characteristics of closely related class II gene products. J. Immunol. 131:2432.

47. Tacchini-Cottier, F.M., and Jones, P.P. (1988). Defective E-beta expression in three mouse H-2 haplotypes results from aberrant RNA splicing. J. Immunol. 141:3647.

48. Klein, D., Zaleska-Rutczynska, Z., Davis, W.C., Figueroa F., and Klein, J. (1987). Monoclonal antibodies specific for mouse class I and class II MHC determinants. Immunoenetics 25:351.

49. Watson, W.C., Brown, P.S., Pitcock, J.A., and Townes, A.S. (1987). Passive transfer studies with type II collagen antibody in B10.D2/old and new line and C57B1/6 normal and beige (Chediak-Higashi) strains: Evidence of important roles for C5 and multiple inflammatory cell types in the development of erosive arthritis. Arthritis Rheum 30:460.

50. Klareskog, L., Holmdahl, R., Larsson, E., and Wigzell, H. (1983). Role of T lymphocytes in collagen II induced arthritis in rats. Clin. Exp. Immunol. 51:117.

51. Butler, L., Simmons, B., Zimmerman, J., DeRiso, P., and Phadke, K. (1986). Characteristics of cellular immune response to collagen type I or collagen type II. Cell. Immunol. 100:314.

52. Holmdahl, R., and Jansson, L. (1988). Estrogen induced suppression of collagen arthritis. III. Adult thymectomy does not affect the course of arthritis or the estrogen mediated suppression of T cell immunity. Brain Behav. Immun. 2:123.

53. Farmer, L.M., Watt, G., Glatt, M., Blaettler, A., Loutis, N., and Feige, U. (1986). Delayed type hypersensitivity (DTH) to type II collagen (CII) in DBA-1 mice. Clin. Exp. Immunol 65:329.

54. Mauritz, N.J., Holmdahl. R., Jonsson, R., der Meide, P., Scheynius, A., and Klareskog, L. (1988). Treatment with interferon gamma triggers onset of collagen arthritis in mice. Arthritis Rheum. 31:1297.

55. Ranges, G.E., Sriram, S., and Cooper, S.M. (1985). Prevention of type II collagen-induced arthritis by in vivo treatment with anti-L3T4 J. Exp. Med. 162:1105.

56. Hom, J.T., Butler, L.D., Riedl, P.E., and Bendele, A.M. (1988). The progression of the inflammation in established collagen-induced arthritis can be altered by treatment swith immunological or pharmacological agents which inhibit T cell activities. Eur. J. Immunol. 18:881.

57. Ranges, G.E., Fortin, S., Barger, M.T., Sriram, S., and Cooper, S. (1988). In vivo modulation of murine collagen induced arthritis. Int. Rev. Immunol. 4:83.

58. Holmdahl, R., Klareskog, L., Rubin, K., Larsson, E., and Wigzell, H. (1985). T lymphocytes in collagen II-induced arthritis in mice. Characterization of arthritogenic collagen II-specific T cell lines and clones. Scand. J. Immunol.22:295.

59. Holmdahl, R., Klareskog, L., Rubin, K., Björk, J., Smedegård, G., Johnsson, R., and Andersson, M. (1986). Role of T lymphocytes in murine collagen induced arthritis. Agents Actions 19:1.

60. Kakimoto, K., Katsuki, M., Hirofuji, T., Iwata, H., and Koga, T. (1988). Isolation of T cell line capable of protecting mice against collagen-induced arthritis. J. Immunol. 140:78.

61. Helfgot, S.M., Dynesius-Trentham, R.E., Brahn, E., and Trentham, D.E. (1985). An arthritogenic lymphokine in the rat. J. Exp. Med. 162:1531.

62. Helfgott, S.M., Kieval, R.I., Breedveld, F.C., Brahn, E., Young, C.T., Dynesius-Trentham, R., and Trentham, D. (1988). Detection of arthritogenic factor in adjuvant arthritis. J. Immunol. 140:1838.

63. Seki, N., Sudo, Y., Yoshioka, T., Sugihara, S., Fujitsu, T., Sakuma, S., Ogawa, T., Hamaoka, T., Senoh, H., and Fujiwara, H. (1988). Type II collagen induced murine arthritis. I. Induction and perpetuation of arthritis require synergy between humoral and cell-mediated immunity. J. Immunol. 140:1477.

64. Taurog, J.D., Kerwar, S.S., McReynolds, R.A., Sandberg, G.P., Leary, S.L., and Mahowald, M.L. (1985). Synergy between adjuvant arthritis and collagen-induced arthritis in rats. J. Exp. Med. 162:962.

65. Morgan, K., Clague, R.B., Shaw, J.J., Firth, S.A., Twose, T.M., and Holt, P.J.L. (1981). Native type II collagen-induced arthritis in the rat. The effect of complement depletion by cobra venom factor. Arthritis Rheum. 24:1356.

66. Wooley, P.H., Luthra, H.S., Krco, C.J., Stuart, J.M., and David, C.S. (1984). Type II collagen induced arthritis in mice. II Passive transfer and suppression by intravenous injection of anti-type II collagen antibody or free native type II collagen. Arthritis Rheum. 27:1010.

67. Stuart, J.M., and Dixon, F.J. (1983). Serum transfer of collagen induced arthritis in mice. J. Exp. Med. 158:378.

68. Stuart, J.M., Cremer, M.A., Townes, A.S., and Kang, A.H.(1982). Type II collagen-induced arthritis in rats. Passive transfer with serum and evidence that IgG anti-collagen antibodies can cause arthritis. J. Exp. Med. 155:1.

69. Stuart, J.M., Tomoda, K., Yoo, T.J., Townes, A.S., and Kang, A.H. (1983). Serum transfer of collagen-induced arthritis. II. Identification and localization of autoantibody to type II collagen in donor and recipient rats. Arthritis Rheum. 26:1237.

70. Takagishi, K., Kaibara, N., Hotokebuchi, T., Arita, C., Morinaga, M., and Arai, E. (1985). Serum transfer of collagen arthritis in congentically athymic nude rats. J. Immunol. 134:3864.

71. Kerwar, S.S., and Oronsky, A.L. (1988). Passive collagen induced arthritis induced by anticollagen IgG. Int. Rev. Immunol. 4:17.

72. Holmdahl, R., Moran, T., and Andersson, M. (1985). A rapid and efficient immunization protocol for production of monoclonal antibodies reactive with autoantigens. J. Immunol. Methods 83:379.

73. Holmdahl, R., Andersson, M., and Jansson, L. (1987). A method for the analysis of a large number of specific and multispecific B cell hybridomas derived from primary immunized lymph nodes. Hybridoma 6:197.

74. Hayakawa, K., Hardy, R.R., Parks, D.R., and Herzenberg, L.A. (1983). The Ly-1 B cell subpopulation in normal, immunodefective and autoimmune mice. J. Exp. Med. 157:202.

75. Punjabi, C.J., Wood, D.D., and Wooley, P.H. (1988). A monoclonal anti-type II collagen antibody with cross-reactive anti-Ig activity specific for the $F(ab)_2$ fragment. J. Immunol. 141:3819.

76. Holmdahl, R., Nordling, C., Rubin, K., Tarkowski, A., and Klareskog, L. (1986). Generation of monoclonal rheumatoid factors after immunization with collagen II-anticollagen II immune complexes. Scand. J. Immunol. 24:197.

77. Holmdahl, R., Tarkowski, A., Nordling, C., Rubin, K., and Klareskog, L. (1987). Connection between autoimmunity to cartilage type II collagen and rheumatoid factor production. Monogr. Allergy 22:71.

78. Heinz, H.P., Rubin, K., Loos, M., and Laurell, A.B. (1989). Common epitopes in C1q and collagen type II. Mol. Immunol. 26:163.

79. Wolf, B., Bashey, R.I., Newton, C.D., and Jimenez, S.A.(1986). Development of rheumatoid factors and anti-$F(ab)_2$ antibodies in guinea pigs immunized with type II collagen. Int. Arch. Allergy Appl. Immunol. 80:214.

80. Shlomchik, M., Nemazee, D., VanSnick, J., and Weigert, M. (1987). Variable region sequences of murine IgM anti-IgG monoclonal antibodies (rheumatoid factors). II. Comparison of hybridomas derived by lipopolysaccharide stimulation and secondary protein immunization. J. Exp. Med. 165:970.

81. Shlomchik, M.J., Nemazee, D.A., Sato, V.L., VanSnick, J., Carson, D.A., and Weigert, M.G. (1986). Variable region sequences of murine IgM anti-Ig monoclonal autoantibodies (rheumatoid factors). A structural explanation for the high frequency of IgM anti-IgG B cells. J. Exp. Med. 164:407.

82. Huez, F., Sciard-Larsson, E.L., Pereira P., Portnoi, D., and Coutinho, A. (1988). T cell dependence of the "natural" autoreactive B cell activation in the spleen of normal mice. Eur. J. Immunol. 18:1615.

83. Pereira, P., Larsson, E., Forni, L., Bandeira, A., and Coutinho, A. (1985). Natural effector T lymphocytes in normal mice. Proc. Natl. Acad. Sci. USA 82:7691.

84. Grabar, P. (1975). Autoantibodies and immunological theories: An analytical review. Clin. Immunol. Immunopathol. 4:453.

85. Staines, N.A., Hardingham, T., Smith, M., and Henderson, B. (1981). Collagen-induced arthritis in the rat: Modification of immune and arthritic responses by free collagen and immune anti-collagen antiserum. Immunology 44:737.

86. Englert, M., McReynolds, R.A., Landes, M.J., Oronsky, A.L., and Kerwar, S.S. (1985). Pretreatment of rats with anticollagen IgG renders them resistent to active type II collagen arthritis. Cell. Immunol. 90:258.

87. Takagishi, K., Hotokebuchi, T., Arai, K., Arita, C., and Kaibara, N. (1988). Collagen arthritis in rats—the importance of humoral immunity in the initiation of the disease and perpetuation of the disease by suppressor T cells. Int. Rev. Immunol.4:35.

88. Kaibara, N., Arai, K., Arita, C., Hotokebuchi, T., and Takagishi, K. (1986). Treatment with cyclophosphamide reverses acquired resistance to collagen arthritis subsequent to recovery from passive arthritis. Cell. Immunol. 101:643.

89. Nagler-Andersson, C., VanVollenhoven, R., Gurish, M.F., Bober, L.A.A., Siskind, G.W., and Thorbecke, G.J. (1988). A crossreactive idiotype on anti-collagen antibodies in collagen-induced arthritis: Identification and relevance to disease. Cell. Immunol. 113:447.

90. Arita, C., Kaibara, N., Jingushi, S., Takagishi, K., Hotokebuchi, T., and Arai, K. (1987). Suppression of collagen arthritis in rats by heterologous anti-idiotypic antisera against anticollagen antibodies. Clin. Immunol. Immunopathol. 43:374.

91. Lotz, M., and Vaughan, J.H. (1988). Rheumatoid Arthritis. Vol. II. Little, Brown, Boston, p. 1365.

92. Vandenbroucke, J.P., Valkenburg, H.A., Boersma, J.W., Cats, A., Festen, J.J.M., Huber-Bruning, O., and Rasker, J.J. (1982). Oral contraceptives and rheumatoid arthritis: Further evidence for a preventive effect. Lancet 2:839.

93. Nepom, G.T., Byers, P., Seyfried, C., Healey, L.A., Wilske, K.R., Stage, D., and Nepom, B.S. (1989). HLA genes associated with rheumatoid arthritis. Identification of susceptibility alleles using specific oligonucleotide probes. Arthritis Rheum. 32:15.

94. Klareskog, L., Forsum, U., Scheynius, A., Kabelitz, D., and Wigzell, H. (1982). Evidence in support of a self-perpetuating HLA-DR dependent delayed-type hypersensitivity reaction in rheumatoid arthritis. Proc. Natl. Acad. Sci. USA 79:3632.

95. Janossy, G., Panai, G., Duke, O., Bofill, M., Poulter, L. W., and Goldstein, G. (1981). Rheumatoid arthritis: A disease of T lymphocyte/macrophage immunoregulation. Lancet 2:839.

96. Burmester, G.R., Jahn, B., Gramatzki, M., Zacher, J., and Kalden, J.R. (1984). Activated T cells in vitro and in vivo: Divergence in expression of Tac and Ia antigens in the noblastoid small T cells of inflammation and normal T cells activated in vitro. J. Immunol. 133:1230.

97. Buchan, G., Barrett, K., Fujita, T., Taniguchi, T., Maini, R., and Feldmann, M. (1988). Detection of activated T cell products in the rheumatoid joint using cDNA probes to interleukin-2 (IL-2), IL-2 receptor and IFN-gamma. Clin. Exp. Immunol. 71:295.

98. Scher, M.G., Beller, D.I., and Unanue, E.R. (1980). Demonstration of a soluble mediator that induces exudates rich in Ia-positive macrophages. J. Exp. Med. 152:1684.

99. Palacios-Boix, A.A., Estrada, G.I., Colston, M.J., and Panayi, G.S. (1988). HLA-DR4 restricted lymphocyte proliferation to a mycobacterium tuberculosis extract in rheumatoid arthritis and healthy subjects. J. Immunol. 140:1844.

100. Trentham, D.E., Dynesius, R.A., Rocklin, R.E., and David, J.R. (1978). Cellular sensitivity to collagen in rheumatoid arthritis. N. Engl. J. Med. 299:327.

101. Londei, M., Savill, C.M., Verhoef, A., Brennan, F., Leech, Z.A., Duance, V., Maini, R.N., and Feldmann, M. (1989). Persistence of collagen type II-specific T-cell clones in the synovial membrane of a patient with rheumatoid arthritis. Proc. Natl. Acad. Sci. USA 86:636.

102. Zvaifler, N.J. (1973). The immunopathology of joint inflammation in rheumatoid arthritis. Adv. Immunol. 16:265.

103. Carson, D.A., Chen, P.P.,Fox, R.I., Kipps, T.J., Jirik, F., Goldfien, R.D., Silverman, G., Radou, V., and Fong, S. (1987). Rheumatoid factor and immune networks. Annu. Rev. Immunol. 5:109.

104. Clague, R.B., and Moore, L.J. (1984). IgG and IgM antibody to native type II collagen in rheumatoid arthritis serum and synovial fluid. Evidence for the presence of collagen-anticollagen immune complexes in synovial fluid. Arthritis Rheum. 27:1370.

105. Jasin, H.E. (1985). Autoantibody specificities of immune complexes sequestered in articular cartilage of patients with rheumatoid arthritis and osteoarthritis. Arthritis Rheum. 28:241.

106. Andersson, M., Goldschmidt, T.J., Michaelsson, E., Larsson, A., and Holmdahl, R. (1990). T cell receptor Vβ haplotype and complement C5 play no significant role for the resistance to collagen-induced arthritis in the SWR mouse. Submitted for publication.

107. Goldschmidt, T.J., Jansson, L., and Holmdahl, R. (1990). In vivo elimination of T cells expressing specific T cell receptor Vβ chains in mice susceptible to collagen-induced arthritis. Immunology 69:508.

16

Antiproteoglycan Antibodies in Experimental Spondylarthritis

Tibor T. Glant and Katalin Mikecz
Rush-Presbyterian–St. Luke's Medical Center, Chicago, Illinois and the University of Medicine, Debrecen, Hungary

Edit Buzás
University of Medicine, Debrecen, Hungary

Eric Dayer
Institut Central des Hôpitaux Valaisans, Sion, Switzerland

A. Robin Poole
Shriners Hospital for Crippled Children and McGill University, Montreal, Quebec, Canada

I. IMMUNOPATHOLOGY OF CARTILAGE PROTEOGLYCANS IN HUMANS AND ANIMALS

Proteoglycans and collagens are the major components of the extracellular matrix of articular cartilage, which is synthesized and maintained by a relatively sparse population of chondrocytes. Most of these proteoglycans are large molecules of high density that bind to hyaluronic acid to form macromolecular aggregates (1–4). The proteoglycan core protein to which glycosaminoglycan chains of chondroitin sulfate and keratan sulfate are attached together with O-linked and N-linked oligosaccharides is highly antigenic (5–8), but epitopes on core protein are frequently masked by the negatively charged glycosaminoglycan side chains.

Although immunity to cartilage proteoglycans has been less extensively studied than immunity to collagen, cartilage proteoglycans are currently considered a causal factor in experimental inflammatory joint diseases and a potential causal factor in human rheumatoid diseases. Both humoral and cellular immunity to allogeneic cartilage proteoglycans have occasionally been detected in patients with rheumatoid arthritis, juvenile rheumatoid arthritis, and relapsing chondritis (9–15). It is of special interest that cellular immunity to adult cartilage proteoglycans has been detected quite frequently in patients with ankylosing spondylitis (11–13,16). Moreover, we have succeeded in isolating proteoglycan-specific T cell lines and clones from these patients (17,18). The specificity of these autoreactive T helper lymphocytes is probably related to core protein epitope(s) localized in the chondroitin sulfate attachment region of the human proteoglycan molecule (17,18).

Experimental animal models of inflammatory arthritis have provided important advances in understanding the possible mechanisms for human diseases and in developing therapeutic agents for treatment in human diseases. The most frequently studied experimental models are those induced by type II collagen or mycobacterial adjuvant (19,20). Although their pathologic mechanisms are different (21) and are not fully understood, both of them may be sustained by genetically controlled autoimmune responses to cartilage matrix components (22–26). Type II collagen-induced arthritis can be elicited in susceptible strains of rats (27,28), mice (29), and monkeys (30) by immunization with *native* type II collagen in complete or incomplete adjuvant. Adjuvant (or reactant) arthritis can be established in rats by a single intradermal injection of mycobacterial cell wall peptidoglycans in oil (i.e., with complete Freund's adjuvant). Recent studies indicate that cartilage proteoglycans may participate in the development of adjuvant arthritis, suggesting some molecular mimicry exhibited by cartilage proteoglycans to bacterial components (31–35).

Experimental arthritis can also be produced by intra-articular injection of antigen into previously sensitized animals (36). The chronic synovitis that develops appears to be caused by a local delayed hypersensitivity. The type of antigen or the animal species used is less important than the titer of circulating antibody (20,37–41), suggesting that a vigorous immune response to the injected antigen is required. The resulting cartilage degradation, however, can be counterbalanced by extensive synthesis of new matrix during postinjection recovery (41–43). A single intra-articular injection of either homologous or heterologous proteoglycans into antigen-sensitized animals or of antibodies to cartilage matrix components produces a local inflammatory arthritis that leads to severe deterioration of articular cartilage (41,42,44–50). On the other hand, a chronic inflammation process in joints produces cartilage degradation that is often not repaired and is usually accompanied by autoantibody production to host cartilage proteoglycans or type II collagen (41,42,46,47,49,51).

II. PROTEOGLYCAN-INDUCED POLYARTHRITIS AND SPONDYLITIS IN Balb/c MICE

A. Etiopathogenesis of Proteoglycan-Induced Arthritis

Recently we found that immunization of Balb/c mice with fetal human proteoglycan depleted of chondroitin sulfate can produce progressive polyarthritis and ankylosing spondylitis (52). This disease developed *in all female Balb/c mice* when human fetal or newborn proteoglycans were injected intraperitoneally in either complete or incomplete Freund's adjuvant (52–55). The initial external symptoms of joint inflammation (swelling and redness) appear after the third, fourth, or fifth intraperitoneal injection of antigen, depending on the Balb/c colony and the proteoglycan preparation used. This mouse model shows many similarities to human rheumatoid arthritis and ankylosing spondylitis as indicated by such clinical assessments as radiographic analysis, scintigraphic bone scans, and histopathologic studies of diarthrodial joints and spine (52). During the early phases, perivascular concentration of mononuclear cells and polymorphonuclear leukocytes occurred, which was followed by "tumorlike" proliferation of synovial cells (Fig. 1). The arthritis often starts as a bilateral, polyarticular synovitis in small peripheral joints and becomes progressive, with extensive erosion of cartilage and bone within the joint. The axial skeleton is also involved. Lumbar spine and proximal intervertebral disks of the tail are most frequently exposed to inflammatory and degenerative changes (52). It is of special interest that the inflammatory process starts adjacent to the disk and may involve periostitis, tendonitis, and myositis. This is followed by invasion of the disk. About 50% of sacroiliac joints are also involved in degenerative processes (Fig. 2). Other cartilages, such as those in the ribs, ears, or respiratory tract, are never exposed to the inflammatory process, with the exception of the growth plate, which is often eroded (52). However, slight tendonitis and nodular lesions on periarticular areas, skin rashes, and transient diarrhea are common.

The development of the disease in Balb/c mice is dependent upon the expression of both cell-mediated and humoral immunity to host mouse cartilage proteoglycan (54). Autoantibodies react with the immunizing fetal human proteoglycan and cross-react with both native and degraded proteoglycans of mouse cartilage (54–56).

This proteoglycan-induced arthritis can be passively transferred to irradiated normal (nonimmunized) syngeneic mice using lymphocytes from arthritic mice stimulated either in vivo or in vitro with chondroitinase ABC-treated fetal human proteoglycan (57). The appearance of autoantibodies in the sera of animals with either primary or passively transferred arthritis precedes the development of the

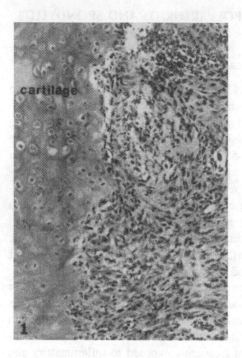

Figure 1 Erosion of cartilage by proliferating synovial cells 3 weeks after the onset of arthritis. Hematoxylin and eosin, × 240.

first clinical symptoms by a few days. Transfer of arthritis, however, never occurred after injection of sera alone from arthritic animals, when sera from arthritic animals were used with lymphocytes from nonarthritic animals, or when lymphocytes from arthritic animals were adminstered with "nonarthritogenic" antigens, such as fetal calf proteoglycan (57), but the rate of the development of arthritis was enhanced by sera from arthritic mice. Also, antibodies to mouse proteoglycan always accompany the development of the transferred arthritis and are not usually seen in those animals that do not develop arthritis. These results and those observed with subpopulations of lymphocytes from arthritic animals and the negative results obtained by the immunization of nude mice of Balb/c origin strongly suggest that the pathomechanism of this proteoglycan-induced arthritis requires the participation of both T cells and B cells and that an antibody-dependent T cell-mediated reaction creates the pathologic basis of this organ-specific inflammatory process.

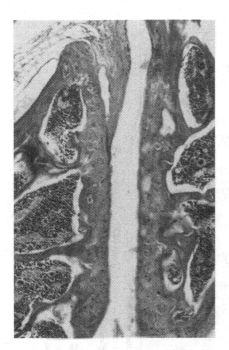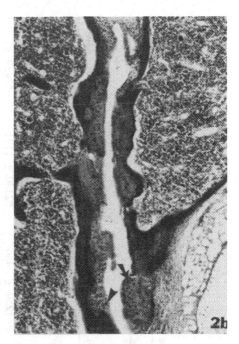

Figure 2 Vertical section of sacroiliac joints of control (a) and arthritic (b) animals on week 38 of experiment. Arthritic animal developed arthritis on week 12. Narrowed joint space and rough articular surfaces are produced by osteophyte (arrow) and proliferative synovial tissue (arrowheads) that erodes articular cartilage. Hematoxylin and eosin, ×120.

B. Genetic Background of Proteoglycan-Induced Arthritis

Murine strains (listed in Table 1) with H-2^d or different haplotypes treated in the same way showed that arthritis could only be produced in Balb/c mice, although Balb/c, C3H, and NZB/j strains proved to be equally high responders to fetal human cartilage proteoglycan in terms of both cellular reactivity (54) and antibody production (Table 1). Acquired cellular immune responses to fetal human-proteoglycan in murine strains, however, were very divergent: significantly increased (p < 0.001) in Balb/c, DBA/2, C57B1/6, and C3H mice but hardly detected in BDP/j and SWR/j animals (54). Cellular reaction to chondroitinase ABC-digested fetal human proteoglycan was significantly higher than to native proteoglycan (p < 0.01) in all high-responder strains. The cellular immune response to chondroitinase ABC-digested fetal human proteoglycan in DBA/2 mice

Table 1 Serum Antibody Levels to Cartilage Proteoglycans in Inbred Mouse Strains, CDF$_1$ Hybrid (Balb/c and DBA/2 Parents), and Nude Mice (Balb/c Origin) Immunized with Chondroitinase ABC-Digested Fetal Human Cartilage Proteoglycan[a]

Mouse strain	Haplotype H-2	Incidence of arthritis	Antibody titer (cpm) to			
			Intact mouse proteoglycan (1:500)	Chase ABC	Intact fetal human proteoglycan (1:2500 or *1:10,000)	Chase ABC
BALB/c	d	18/18	1410 ± 366	2316 ± 933	*2866 ± 846	*3246 ± 1220
Nude	d	0/14	ND	ND	ND	ND
CDF1	d	0/24	1110 ± 584	2120 ± 1004	*636 ± 188	*1313 ± 160
DBA/2	d	0/8	ND	ND	752 ± 555	889 ± 451
NZB/j	d	2/8	432 ± 120	1250 ± 446	*2130 ± 1121	*2429 ± 861
C56BL/6	b	0/8	ND	312 ± 196	456 ± 252	745 ± 318
C3H	k	0/8	146 ± 98	1512 ± 1024	*3110 ± 1845	*3659 ± 1588
AKR/j	k	0/8	ND	ND	203 ± 212	604 ± 754
SWR/j	r	0/8	ND	ND	886 ± 635	1515 ± 1279
BDP/j	p	0/8	ND	ND	92 ± 158	394 ± 337
MRL/1	k	0/8	ND	ND	ND	156 ± 137

[a]Values are the mean cpm ± SD. Chase = chondroitinase ABC-digested cartilage proteoglycan.
Animals were immunized with chondroitinase ABC-digested fetal human cartilage proteoglycan (400 μg total antigen protein) as described (52,54). Serum samples were collected by retro-orbital puncture weekly or before each booster injection, and they were bled on weeks 14–16. MRL/1 mice were killed during weeks 13–14.
Titers of antibodies were determined in solution radioimmunoassay using 125I-labeled cartilage proteoglycans (specific activity 89–94 μCi/mg proteoglycan protein) and 10,000 cpm in 50 μl per assay was used in each experiment; 100 μl of 1:500 (for mouse proteoglycan) and 1:2500 or *1:10,000 dilutions of sera (for human proteoglycan) were used. ND, not detected down to 1:100 serum dilution.

was more pronounced (stimulation index SI = 24.4 ± 2.9 SD; n = 14) than in Balb/c mice (SI = 17.8 ± 3.6 SD; N = 38), but DBA/2 animals did not develop arthritis. CDF1 mice (F_1 hybrids of Balb/c and DBA/2 parents, both expressing the H-2^d haplotype) showed high antibody titer (Table 1) and cellular reaction (SI = 16.8 ± 6.8 SD; n = 45) to chondroitinase ABC-digested fetal human proteoglycan and, in some experiments (see Ref. 54 and Table 1), autoantibodies to mouse proteoglycan without clinical or histopathologic evidence of arthritis. Susceptibility, however, "returned" in 18% of their F_2 hybrids. Only MRL/1 mice showed modest lymphoid cell proliferation in the synovial layer as early as weeks 13–14, which might be the consequence of the spontaneous development of arthritis characteristic of this murine strain (58–60). It is important to note that only Balb/c mice expressed natural ("preimmune") cellular reactivity to mouse proteoglycan depleted of chondroitin sulfate (54). This was not observed in CDF$_1$ hybrid animals (SI = 1.9 ± 0.8 SD; n = 45) but was detected in 29% of CDF$_2$ mice (SI = 6.8 ± 0.9 SD; n = 13 of 45).

Finally, an important observation was that the susceptibility of different Balb/c colonies were also variable. For example, 250–350 µg protein of chondroitinase ABC-digested fetal human cartilage proteoglycan consistently produced arthritis (149 of 152 immunized animals) in Balb/c mice of the Charles River colony (Montreal), but Balb/c mice from Jackson Laboratories (Maine) or MRC (London) developed arthritis only after the inoculation of 450–500 µg antigen-protein. Moreover, Charles River animals from Frankfurt lost their susceptibility to arthritis, although there was no significant difference observed between Balb/c colonies in either antibody production or cellular reactivity. Thus, we suppose that the H-2^d haplotype alone does not define this susceptibility, or yet unknown differences within the MHC complex (61) basically determine the susceptibility of murine strains.

C. Proteoglycans with Arthritogenic Potential and Antiproteoglycan Antibodies in Balb/c Mice

Although fetal human and calf proteoglycans have many biochemical and immunologic similarities (8,62–70), calf proteoglycan treated and administered in the same way did not produce arthritis in Balb/c mice (18,52,53,55). Thus, we suppose that the arthritogenic structures are related to portions of the core protein in fetal human proteoglycans that become accessible after the chondroitin sulfate side chains are removed. Intact (nondigested) and chondroitinase ABC-digested large aggregating cartilage proteoglycans from nine different species were used to immunize Balb/c mice (55,71). Chondroitinase-digested proteoglycans of human fetal and newborn articular cartilages and chondroitinase-digested proteoglycans of human osteophyte, fetal pig articular cartilage, and human chondrosarcoma were the only ones able to induce arthritis consistently (Table 2).

Table 2 Incidence of Arthritis and Immune Responses in Balb/c Mice Immunized with Cartilage Proteoglycans[a]

Experimental groups	Incidence of arthritis (number of positive/total number) tested	Antibody titer (cpm) to				Stimulation index (SI), mouse proteoglycan (intact)
		Antigen used for immunization (1:2000)	Fetal human proteoglycan Chase ABC (1:2000)	Mouse proteoglycan Intact (1:500)	Chase ABC (1:500)	
1. Control group (PBS + FCA)	0/24	ND	ND	ND	ND	1.22 ± 0.31
Animals immunized with chondroitinase ABC-digested proteoglycans						
2. Fetal human articular (24–27 weeks)	12/12	3642 ± 1041	3462 ± 1142	1116 ± 137	1357 ± 142	5.24 ± 0.72
3. Newborn human articular	8/9	2120 ± 1024	1840 ± 900	1157 ± 987	1123 ± 112	5.02 ± 0.34
4. Chondrophyte (human osteophyte)	5/5	3439 ± 339	3309 ± 197	1152 ± 430	1938 ± 540	5.28 ± 0.92
6. Human chondrosarcoma	2/2	2916 ± 1320	3012 ± 1457	863 ± 242	1243 ± 657	4.86 ± 1.44
7. Fetal pig articular	5/7	2429 ± 540	1626 ± 330	251 ± 231	654 ± 272	8.62 ± 2.26
8. Newborn canine	3/8	3372 ± 575	2158 ± 607	515 ± 334 (4)	919 ± 475	4.81 ± 0.66
9. Chicken sternal	*1/12	2155 ± 1560	1757 ± 985	1322 ± 1041	916 ± 638	3.26 ± 0.92
10. Newborn lamb articular	0/6	2625 ± 1310	1842 ± 781	80 (2)	300 ± 254	1.96 ± 0.42
11. Fetal calf (21 weeks)	0/16	2232 ± 1180	1493 ± 8493	ND	ND	1.26 ± 0.27

[a]Animals were immunized intraperitoneally with chondroitinase ABC-digested proteoglycans as described (52,54) (Total: 400 μg antigen protein.) Serum samples collected weekly from the retro-orbital venous plexus were tested for antibodies by direct radioimmunoassay using ^{125}I-labeled proteoglycans on week 30. Dilution of sera is indicated in parentheses. Animals were bled on weeks 32–38 of experiment. Forepaws, one knee joint, and the proximal part of the tail of each animal were histologically examined. (*Synovitis was detected only histologically.) Numbers in parentheses (groups 8 and 10) indicate the number of animals that produced autoantibodies to mouse cartilage proteoglycan. Spleen cells were tested for in vitro lymphocyte stimulation with immunizing antigen, fetal human proteoglycans (both intact and chondroitinase ABC-digested, chase ABC, data not shown), and newborn native mouse proteoglycans (stimulation indices SI are indicated). ND = antibody was not detected. SI expressed as a ratio of cpm of incorporated [^{3}H]thymidine in cultures in the presence and absence of antigen. Data of animals immunized with native (nondigested) proteoglycans or proteoglycans isolated from mature and newborn rabbit and guinea pig cartilages are not shown. None of these animals developed arthritis or antibodies to mouse proteoglycan.

Animals immunized with intact cartilage proteoglycans (i.e., not digested with chondroitinase ABC) never developed arthritis and only occasionally autoantibodies (data not shown).

The in vitro lymphocyte stimulation by intact mouse cartilage proteoglycan, the serum autoantibody titer to mouse cartilage proteoglycan, and the incidence of arthritis showed correlations. Despite this positive correlation, neither antibody titer nor cellular reactions either to fetal human or mouse cartilage proteoglycan (alone or together) cannot be designated as single risk factor(s) for arthritis. For example, immunization with proteoglycans of either chicken sternal or newborn canine articular cartilage produced higher antibody levels to mouse proteoglycan than the fetal pig articular cartilage, but the incidence in this latter group was close to that observed in animals immunized with chondroitinase ABC-digested fetal human proteoglycan. The cellular immune reactions to mouse cartilage proteoglycans measured by lymphocyte stimulation were significantly higher in arthritic (SI = 6.27 ± 1.98 SD; $n = 49$) than in nonarthritic mice (SI = 1.56 ± 0.42 SD; $n = 186$), suggesting that these reactions to mouse proteoglycan were not the result of cross-reactions with human proteoglycan. Serum antibody titers, however, were very variable in different groups. Table 2 summarizes the results in selected groups immunized with chondroitinase ABC-digested cartilage proteoglycans (55,71).

D. Immunopathologic Effect of Antibodies of Cartilage Proteoglycans

The work of Kresina and his colleagues (49) has demonstrated that mouse monoclonal antibodies reactive with rabbit large aggregating cartilage proteoglycans cause cartilage damage when injected into rabbits. This was also found in antigen-induced arthritis in rabbits or in normal animals after a single intra-articular injection of recombinant interleukin-1 (72).

When monoclonal antibodies reactive with mouse cartilage proteoglycans were isolated from arthritic Balb/c mice, one antibody caused significant depletion of cartilage proteoglycan from articular and growth plate cartilages when injected into irradiated [to prevent anti-idiotypic antibody production (56)] recipients. Injections were performed using hybridomas secreting this antibody to ensure continued delivery over a period of several weeks (56). The mechanism of this release is not known but may involve the induction of the release of cytokines, such as interleukin-1 (IL-1) and tumor necrosis factor β (TNF-$_\beta$), which are capable of activating chondrocytes to excessively degrade extracellular matrix. It is well established that immune complexes and Fc fragments can stimulate IL-1 production from the monocyte-macrophages, and this may also involve synovial cells (56). Polymorphonuclear leukocytes were not observed in affected joints, although there was a significant accumulation of immunoglobulin. This may be because the antibody is an IgG_1 that can bind little or no complement (73).

Our work on proteoglycan-induced arthritis has also revealed that antibodies that are cytotoxic for chondrocytes are produced (18,54). These may play an important role in the irreversible destruction of articular cartilage, particularly since cell destruction prevents the repair of damaged cartilage.

E. Anti-idiotypic Antibodies in Proteoglycan-Induced Arthritis

Individual analysis of animals for antibody production and cellular reactivity showed that animals that expressed significantly higher responses to native mouse cartilage proteoglycan were at increased risk for arthritis. We frequently found animals with high antibody titers, however, and, at the end of the experiment, with a significantly high cellular reaction (SI > 10.0) to both fetal and mouse proteoglycans without arthritis.

On the other hand, some of the animals developed arthritis at a lower level of immune response (55). This was observed in Balb/c mice immunized with canine or chicken proteoglycans. Autoantibody production without arthritis in animals immunized with these proteoglycans (Table 2) suggested a potential role of anti-idiotypic antibodies in nonarthritic animals exhibiting autoantibodies to mouse proteoglycan (55). Autoantibodies to mouse cartilage proteoglycan from the pooled sera of arthritic animals were purified on immobilized mouse proteoglycan and subsequently labeled with ^{125}I. Serial dilution of sera of nonarthritic and arthritic animals were incubated with these affinity-purified and ^{125}I-labeled antiproteoglycan antibodies, and the immune-precipitated radiolabeled immunoglobulins were determined. In another competitive inhibition assay, serial dilution of arthritic and nonarthritic sera (both expressing autoantibodies to mouse proteoglycan) alone or together were incubated with ^{125}I-labeled mouse cartilage proteoglycan and the antibody-bound radioactivity was measured after protein A precipitation. Our data using these two assays (55) indicate that Balb/c mice immunized with some proteoglycans (e.g., chondroitinase ABC-digested newborn canine articular or chicken sternal proteoglycans) are able to produce antibodies directed against idiotypes of antimouse proteoglycan antibodies since the sera of normal (nonimmunized or adjuvant-injected) or arthritic animals failed to precipitate or inhibit the binding of autoantibodies. The titer of anti-idiotypic antibodies showed, however, large individual differences (e.g., 0.27–40.0 μl sera were required to achieve 50% inhibition). These results suggest that an anti-idiotypic network control may regulate or modulate the formation of pathologic autoantibodies and consequently the development of proteoglycan arthritis in Balb/c mice.

F. Arthritogenic Epitope(s) of Cartilage Proteoglycans

Assays for antibody binding to ^{125}I-labeled intact or chondroitinase ABC-digested mouse proteoglycans inhibited by intact syngeneic (Balb/c) or xenogeneic (e.g., human, bovine, and canine) proteoglycans or proteoglycans treated with proteolytic and/or glycolytic enzymes, affinity-purified antibodies from sera of arthritic animals, and autoantibodies eluted from arthritic joint tissues have been used to study the specificity of autoreactive antibodies in this animal model. These experiments demonstrated (1) cross-reactive antibodies between human and mouse cartilage proteoglycans but not between fetal calf and mouse proteoglycans (56,71), (2) autoantibodies eluted from arthritic tissues with higher affinity and/or reactivity to mouse proteoglycan than to fetal human proteoglycan (71), (3) cytotoxicity of antibodies affinity purified on either mouse or fetal human proteoglycan to both mouse or human chondroycytes (54), and (4) anti-type II collagen and anti-DNA antibodies in some arthritic animals (53).

The possible involvement of immunity of cartilage proteoglycans in arthritic processes has received increasing attention in recent years. Although only a limited number of epitopes on cartilage proteoglycan may be critical in the pathogenesis of arthritis, the association of such immunity or autoimmunity with this animal model has raised many questions about whether the immunity is causal, is a consequence of cartilage destruction, or is a reflection of a molecular mimicry of proteoglycans with bacterial peptidoglycans. It is important to note that inflamed joint tissues were not infected with bacteria or mycoplasma and the electron micrographs showed no evidence of virus particles.

Progressive polyarthritis develops in Balb/c mice immunized with chondroitinase ABC-digested human fetal cartilage proteoglycan. Autoantibodies from arthritic animals and autoreactive monoclonal antibodies raised to mouse proteoglycan cross-react with these arthritogenic proteoglycans. However, the nature of the immunodominant or arthritogenic (auto)epitope(s) is not known. Epitopes on syngeneic mouse cartilage proteoglycan are sensitive to both protease and alkaline treatment, suggesting that the immunodominant (and perhaps the arthritogenic) region(s) of the proteoglycans are related to the core protein. Since chondroitinase ABC digestion is important to expose this immunodominant region and since isolated glycosaminoglycans and their fragments do not react with autoreactive monoclonal antibodies or autoantibodies from arthritic animals, we postulate that these particular epitopes are located on, or near, the chondroitin sulfate attachment region of core protein. However, it is not clear whether these epitopes on arthritogenic proteoglycans are sterically masked from the immune system by chondroitin sulfate chains or are expressed as "new" determinants after modifying the tertiary structure of the core protein by removal of the highly charged chondroitin sulfate side chains.

III. CONCLUSION AND PERSPECTIVES

Proteoglycan-induced arthritis is one of the most promising animal models for studying inflammatory arthritis. In genetically susceptible mice immunized with certain cartilage proteoglycans, the incidence of this inflammatory arthritis is close to 100%. In addition it is progressive, with remissions and exacerbations leading to complete resorption of articular cartilage and intervertebral disks as well as ankylosis of peripheral joints and spine. The pathologic mechanisms involved in this animal model are associated with autoimmune reactions against the mouse's own cartilage proteoglycan. This model advances our understanding of possible mechanisms for human diseases and is useful in the development and testing of therapeutic agents in the treatment of human diseases. However, many questions remain to be answered including the molecular structure of the autoepitope(s), the immunologic aspects of anti-idiotype defense mechanisms detected in animals immunized with certain proteoglycans, the factors involved in the inflammatory process, and the lymphocyte subpopulations that are critical to the development of arthritis.

REFERENCES

1. Hascall, V.C., and Hascall, G.K. (1980). Proteoglycans. In: Cell Biology of Extracellular Matrix. Hay, E.D., ed. Plenum Press, New York, p. 39.
2. Poole, A.R. (1986). Proteoglycan in health and disease: Structures and functions. Biochem. J. 236:1.
3. Rosenberg, L.C., and Buckwalter, J.A. (1986). Cartilage proteoglycans. In: Articular Cartilage Biochemistry. Kuettner, K.E., Schleyerbach, R., and Hascall, V.C., eds. Raven Press, New York, p. 39.
4. Hascall, V.C. (1989). Proteoglycans: The chondroitin sulfate/keratan sulfate proteoglycan of cartilage. ISI Atlas Sci. Biochem. 1:189.
5. Glant, T., Hadas, E., and Nagy, M. (1979). Cell-mediated and humoral immune responses to cartilage antigenic components. Scand. J. Immunol. 9:39.
6. Poole, A.R., Reiner, A., Roughley, P.J., and Champion, B. (1985). Rabbit antibodies to degraded and intact glycosaminoglycans which are naturally occurring and present in arthritic rabbits. J. Biol. Chem. 260:6020.
7. Caterson, B., Calabro, T., Donohue, P.J., and Jahnke, M.R. (1986). Monoclonal antibodies against cartilage proteoglycan and link protein. In: Articular Cartilage Biochemistry. Kuettner, K.E., Schleyerback, R., and Hascall, V.C., eds. Raven Press, New York, p. 59.
8. Glant, T.T., Mikecz, K., and Poole, A.R. (1986). Monoclonal antibodies to protein-related epitopes of human articular cartilage proteoglycans. Biochem. J. 234:31.
9. Herman, J.H., Wiltse, D.W., and Dennis, M.V. (1973). Immunopathologic significance of cartilage antigenic components in rheumatoid arthritis. Arthritis Rheum. 16:287.
10. Glant, T., Lévai, G., and Szücs, T. (1979). The role of immune responses to proteoglycans in joint diseases. In: Biochemistry of Normal and Pathological Connective Tissues, Centre National de la Recherche Scientifique, Paris, Vol. 1. p. 323.
11. Glant, T., Csongor, J. and Szücs, T. (1980). Immunopathologic role of proteoglycan antigens in rheumatoid joint diseases. Scand. J. Immunol. 11:247.

12. Herman, J.H., Herzig, E.B., Crissmann, J.D., Dennis, M.V., and Hess, E.V. (1980). Idiopathic chondrolysis. An immunopathologic study. J. Rheumatol. 7:694.

13. Golds, E.E., Stephen, I.B.M., Esdaile, J.M., Strawczynski, H., and Poole, A.R. (1983). Lymphocyte transformation to connective tissue antigens in adult and juvenile rheumatoid arthritis, osteoarthritis, ankylosing spondylitis, systemic lupus erythematosus and a nonarthritic control population. Cell. Immunol. 82:196.

14. Golds, E.E., and Poole, A.R. (1984). Connective tissue antigens stimulate collagenase production in arthritic diseases. Cell. Immunol. 86:190.

15. Kouri, T. (1985). Etiology of rheumatoid arthritis. Experientia 41:434.

16. Thonar, E.J.-M.A., and Sweet, M.B.E. (1976). Cellular hypersensitivity in rheumatoid arthritis, ankylosing spondylitis and anterior nongranulomatous uveitis. Arthritis Rheum. 19:539.

17. Mikecz, K., Glant, T.T., Baron, M., and Poole, A.R. (1988). Isolation of proteoglycan specific T cells from patients with ankylosing spondylitis. Cell Immunol. 112:55.

18. Mikecz, K., Glant, T.T., Buzas, E., and Poole, A.R. (1988). Cartilage proteoglycans as potential autoantigens in humans and in experimental animals. Agents Actions 23:63.

19. Cole, B.C., Washburn, L.R., Samuelson, C.O., and Ward, J.R. (1982) Experimental models of rheumatoid arthritis systemic lupus erythematosus and scleroderma. In: Scientific Basis of Rheumatology. Panayi, G.S., ed. Churchill Livingstone, Edinburgh, p 22.

20. Goldings, E.A., and Jasin, H.E. (1989). Arthritis and autoimmunity in animals. In: Arthritis and Allied Conditions. McCarty, D.J., ed. Lea & Febiger, Philadelphia, p. 465.

21. Iizuka, Y., and Chang, Y.-H. (1982). Adjuvant polyarthritis. VII. The role of type II collagen in pathogenesis. Arthritis Rheum 25:1325.

22. Griffiths, M.M., Eichwald, E.J., Martin, J.H., Smith, C.B., and DeWitt, C.W. (1981). Immunogenetic control of experimental type II collagen-induced arthritis. I. Susceptibility and resistance among inbred strains of rats. Arthritis Rheum. 24:781.

23. Wooley, P.H., Luthra, H.S., Stuart, J.M., and David, C.S. (1981). Type II collagen-induced arthritis in mice. I. Major histocompatibility complex (I region) linkage and antibody corelates. J. Exp. Med. 154:688.

24. Wooley, P.H., Dillon, A.M., Luthra, H.S., Stuart, J.M., and David, C.S. (1983). Genetic Control of type II collagen-induced arthritis in mice: Factors influencing disease susceptibility and evidence for multiple MHC-associated gene control. Transplant Proc 15:180.

25. Wooley, P.H., Luthra, H.S., Huse, A., and David, C.S. (1985). Regulation of susceptibility to type II collagen-induced arthritis (CIA) by genes mapping exterior to the major histocompatibility complex (H-2) in mice. Arthritis Rheum 28:S42.

26. Battisto, J.R., Smith, R.N., Beckman, K., Sternlicht, M., and Welles, W.L. (1982). Susceptibility to adjuvant arthritis in DA and F_{344} rats. A dominant trait controlled by an autosomal gene locus linked to the major histocompatibility complex. Arthritis Rheum. 25:1194.

27. Trentham, D.E., Townes, A.S., and Kang, A.H. (1977). Autoimmunity to type II collagen: An experimental model of arthritis. J. Exp. Med. 146:857.

28. Trentham, D.E., McCune, W.J., and Susman, P. (1980). Autoimmunity to collagen in adjuvant arthritis of rats. J. Clin. Invest. 66:1109.

29. Courtenay, J.S., Dallman, M.J., Dayan, A.D., Martin, A., and Mosedale, B. (1980). Immunization against heterologous type II collagen induces arthritis in mice. Nature 283:666.

30. Cathcart, E.S., Hayes, K.C., Gonnerman, W. Lazzari, A.A., and Franzblau C. (1984). Experimental arthritis in a nonhuman primate. Clin. Res. 32:462a.

31. VanVollenhoven, R.F., Soriano, A., McCarthy, P.E., Schwartz, R.L., Garbrecht, F.C., Thorbecke, G.J., and Siskind, G.W. (1988). The role of immunity to cartilage proteoglycan in adjuvant arthritis. Intravenous injection of bovine proteoglycan enhances adjuvant arthritis. J. Immunol. 141:1168.

32. Van Eden, W., Holoshitz, J., Nevo, Z., Frenkel, A., Klajman, A., and Cohen, I.R. (1985). Arthritis induced by a T-lymphocyte clone that responds to *Mycobacterium tuberculosis* and to cartilage proteoglycans. Proc. Natl. Acad. Sci. USA 82:5117.

33. Schwab, J.H., Cromartie, W.J., Ohanian, S.H., and Craddock, J.G. (1967). Association of experimental chronic arthritis with the persistence of group A streptococcal cell walls in the articular tissue. J. Bacteriol. 94:1728.

34. Sandson, J., Hamerman, D., Janis, R., and Rojind, M. (1968). Immunologic and chemical similarities between the *Streptococcus* and human connective tissue. Trans. Assoc. Am. Physicians 81:249.

35. Van den Broek, M.F., Van den Berg, W.B., Arntz, O.J., and Van de Putte, L.B.A. (1988). Reaction of bacterium-primed murine T cells to cartilage components: A clue for the pathogenesis of arthritis? Clin. Exp. Immunol. 72:9.

36. Dumonde, D.C., and Glynn, L.E. (1962). The production of arthritis in rabbits by an immunological reaction to fibrin. Br. J. Exp. Pathol. 43:373.

37. Cooke, T.D., and Jasin, H.E.(1972). The pathogenesis of chronic inflammation in experimental antigen-induced arthritis. Arthritis Rheum. 15:327.

38. Graham, R.C., and Shannon, S.L. (1972). Peroxidase arthritis. Am. J. Pathol. 67:69.

39. Tateishi, H., Jasin, H.E., and Ziff, M. (1973). Electron microscopic study of synovial membrane and cartilage in a ferritin-induced arthritis. Arthritis Rheum. 16:133.

40. Brackertz, D., Mitchell, G.F., and Mackay, I.R. (1977). Antigen-induced arthritis in mice. I. Induction of arthritis in various strains of mice. Arthritis Rheum. 20:841.

41. Glant, T., and Olah, I. (1980). Experimental arthritis produced by proteoglycan antigens in rabbits. Scand. J. Rheumatol. 9:271.

42. Glant, T. (1981). Immunology in the pathogenesis of cartilage degradation in experimental arthritis. Semin. Arthritis Rheum. 11:107.

43. Pettipher, E.R., and Henderson, B. (1988). The relationship between cell-mediated immunity and cartilage degradation in antigen-induced arthritis in the rabbit. Br. J. Exp. Pathol. 69:113.

44. Morgan, K., Clague, R.B., Collins, I., Ayad, S., Phinn, S.D., and Holt, P.J.L. (1989). A longitudinal study of anti-collagen antibodies in patients with rheumatoid arthritis. Arthritis Rheum. 32:139.

45. Poole, A.R., Glant, T.T., and Mikecz, K. (1988). Autoimmunity to cartilage collagen and proteoglycan and the development of chronic inflammatory arthritis. In: The Control of Tissue Damage. Glauer, A.M., ed. Elsevier, Amsterdam, p. 55.

46. Champion, B.R., and Poole, A.R. (1981). Immunity to homologous cartilage proteoglycans in rabbits with chronic inflammatory arthritis. Collagen Relat. Res. 1:453.

47. Glant, T. (1982). Induction of cartilage degradation in experimental arthritis produced by allogeneic and xenogeneic proteoglycan antigens. Connect. Tissue Res. 9:137.

48. Kresina, T.F., Rosner, I.A., Goldberg, V.M., and Moskowitz, R.W. (1985). Fine specificity of serum anti-collagen molecules in experimental immune synovitis. Ann. Rheum. Dis. 44:328.

49. Kresina, T.F., Yoo, J.U., and Goldberg, V.M. (1988). Evidence that a humoral immune response to autologous cartilage proteoglycan can participate in the induction of cartilage pathology. Arthritis Rheum. 31:248.

50. Boniface, R.J., Cain, P.R., and Evans, C.H. (1988). Articular responses to purified cartilage proteoglycans. Arthritis Rheum. 31:258.

51. Champion, B.R., Sell, S., and Poole, A.R. (1983). Immunity to homologous collagens and cartilage proteoglycans in rabbits. Immunology 48:605.

52. Glant, T.T., Mikecz, K., Arzomanian, A., and Poole, A.R. (1987). Proteoglycan-induced arthritis in BALB/c mice: Clinical features and histopathology. Arthritis Rheum. 30:201.

53. Mikecz, K., Glant, T.T., and Poole, A.R. (1987). Human cartilage proteoglycan induces progressive polyarthritis and ankylosing spondylitis in BALB/c mice. Orthop. Trans. 11:342.

54. Mikecz, K., Glant, T.T., and Poole, A.R. (1987). Immunity to cartilage proteoglycans in BALB/c mice with progressive polyarthritis and ankylosing spondylitis induced by injection of human cartilage proteoglycan. Arthritis Rheum. 30:306.

55. Glant, T.T., Fülöp, C., Mikecz, K., Buzás, E., Gy.Molnár and Erharhardt, P.(1990) Proteoglycan-specific autoreactive antibodies and T-lymphocytes in experimental arthritis and human rheumatoid joint diseases. Biochem. Soc. Trans. 18:796.

56. Dayer, E., Mathai, L., Glant, T.T., Mikecz, K., and Poole, A.R. (1990). Studies of cartilage proteoglycan-induced arthritis in Balb/c mice: Characterization of polyclonal and monoclonal antibodies that recognize human and mouse cartilage proteoglycan. One monoclonal antibody causes depletion of cartilage proteoglycan in vivo but no synovitis. 33: Sept.

57. Mikecz, K., Glant, T.T., Buzás, E., and Poole, A.R. (1990). Proteoglycan induced polyarthritis can be adoptively transferred to naive (non-immunized) Balb/c mice. Arthritis Rheum. 33:866.

58. Andrews, B.S., Eisenberg, R.A., Theofilopoulos, A.N., Izui, S., Wilson, C.B., McConahey, P.J., Murphy, E.D., Roths, J.B., and Dixon, F.J. (1978). Spontaneous murine lupus-like syndrome. Clinical and immunological manifestations in several strains. J. Exp. Med. 148:1198.

59. O'Sullivan, F.X., Fassbender, H.-G., Gay, S., and Koopman, W.J. (1985). Etiopathogenesis of the rheumatoid arthritis-like disease in MRL/1 mice. The histopathologic basis of joint destruction. Arthritis Rheum. 28:529.

60. Pataki, A., and Rordorf-Adam, C. (1985). Polyarthritis in MRL 1pr/1pr mice. Rheumatol. Int. 5:113.

61. Paul, W.E. (1984). Immune response genes In: Immunogenetics. Paul, W.E., ed. Raven Press, New York, p. 151.

62. Glant, T.T., Mikecz, K., Roughley, P.J., Buzás, E., and Poole, A.R. (1986). Age-related changes in protein-related epitopes of human articular cartilage proteoglycans. Biochem. J. 236:71.

63. Bayliss, M.T., and Ali, S.Y. (1978). Age-related changes in the composition and structure of human articular-cartilage proteoglycans. Biochem. J. 176::683.

64. Sweet, M.B.E., Thonar, E.J.-M.A., and Marsh, J. (1979). Age-related changes in proteoglycan structure. Arch. Biochem. Biophys. 198:439.

65. Roughley, P.J., and White, R.J. (1980). Age-related changes in the structure of the proteoglycan subunits from human articular cartilage. J. Biol. Chem. 255:217.

66. Pal. S., Tang, L.-H., Choi, H., Habermann, E., Rosenberg, L., Roughley, P., and Poole, A.R. (1981). Structural changes during development in bovine fetal epiphyseal cartilage. Collagen Relat. Res. 1:151.

67. Thonar, E.J.-M.A., and Sweet, B.E.(1981). Maturation-related changes in proteoglycans of fetal articular cartilage. Arch. Biochem. Biophys. 208:535.

68. Champion, B.R., Reiner, A., Roughley, P.J., and Poole, A.R. (1982). Age-related changes in the antigenicity of human articular cartilage proteoglycans. Collagen Relat. Res. 2:45.

69. Thonar, E.J.-M.A., Bjornsson, S., and Kuettner, K.E. (1986). Age-related changes in cartilage proteoglycans. In: Articular Cartilage Biochemistry. Kuettner, K.E., Schleyerbach, R., and Hascall, V.C., eds. Raven Press, New York, p. 273.

70. Roughley, P.J., White, R.J., and Glant, T.T. (1987). The structure and abundance of cartilage proteoglycans during early development of the human fetus. Pediatr. Res. 22:409.

71. Glant, T.T., Bayliss, M.T., Hascall, V.C., Mikecz, K., and Gitelis, S. (1990). Proteoglycans from human ostophytes as potential targets of autoimmune reactions. (Manuscript prepared for publication)

72. Pettipher, E.R., Henderson, B., Hardingham, T., and Ratcliffe, A. (1989). Cartilage proteoglycan depletion in acute and chronic antigen-induced arthritis. Arthritis Rheum 32:601.

73. Hardy, R.R. (1986). Complement fixation by monoclonal antibody-antigen complexes. In: Handbook of Experimental Immunology, Vol. 1. (Weir, D.M., Herzenberg, L.A., Blackwell, C., and Herzenberg, L.A., eds.) Blackwell Scientific, London, p. 40.1.

17

Reproduction and Regulation of the Autoimmunity That Induces Cartilage Pathology in Experimental Immune Synovitis

Thomas F. Kresina

Miriam Hospital and Brown University International Health Institute, Providence, Rhode Island

I. EXPERIMENTAL IMMUNE SYNOVITIS: A MODEL OF INFLAMMATORY SYNOVITIS

The use of antigen-induced immune synovitis as an animal model of inflammatory synovitis is based on the postulate that rheumatoid arthritis can be a product of local or systemic immune reactions to an as yet undefined immunogen and that cellular and humoral immune mechanisms mediate inflammation and tissue injury. Therefore, it is suggested that a complex series of immunologically mediated events result in the clinical characteristics of classically defined rheumatoid arthritis, symmetrical chronic synovitis of diarthrodial joints, and synovial lined tendons. Antigen-induced immune synovitis has been widely used as a model for studying the pathophysiology of human rheumatoid arthritis. Similarities between the experimental model of synovitis and human disease include deposition of immune complexes and complement in joint cartilage (1,2), hyperplasia of the synovium (3,4) antibody deposition in the affected synovia (5,6), cell-mediated and humoral immune responses to the genetically distinct interstitial collagens (7), pannus formation, cartilage erosion, and ligament destruction (3,4,7,8). Experimental antigen-induced arthritis has been described in rabbits immunized to homologous or heterologous fibrin (3) and in immunized rabbits receiving articular injections of egg albumin (9), bovine serum albumin (9), cartilage proteoglycan subunits (10), and immunoglobulin (8). Studies characterizing antibody synthesis in these models have noted localization of the antibody specific in the arthritis immunogen in the synovium (1,5). Therefore, chronic monoarthritis of varying intensity can be generated through the use of various antigens with the generation of the characteristic inflammatory synovitis, a function of route of antigen administration, the frequency of challenge, and the specific antigen utilized (11).

Experimental immune synovitis has been utilized as an animal model for the study of the pathophysiology of rheumatoid arthritis. This form of antigen-induced synovitis utilizes homologous rabbit immunoglobulin G (IgG) for the induction of immune synovitis (8). The synovitic pathologic processes developed in this model are similar to those described in rheumatoid arthritis. They include circulating anti-IgG antibodies, marked synovial inflammation characterized by an infiltration of the synovium by immunocompetent cells, pannus formation, and ultimately cartilage erosion and ligament destruction. Although localized inflammation is apparent, the synovitis is manifested as a systemic disease, with the animals observed to have a weight loss or lack of weight gain over the course of chronic synovitis as well as leukocytosis (12). Therefore, experimental immune synovitis induced with homologous IgG represents an animal model of rheumatoid arthritis that exhibits pathologic lesions similar to those of the human disease, and this appears to be well suited to address the issue of the role of autoimmunity to extracellular matrix molecules in the generation and maintenance of synovial inflammation induced by immune-mediated responses.

A pathophysiologic role for cartialge proteoglycan molecules and the interstitial collagens in synovial inflammation and erosion of cartilage matrix that is observed in chronic synovitis has been suggested (13–21). The host response to the interstitial collagens and cartilage proteoglycans is observed in this animal model of human rheumatoid arthritis. Autoimmunity to both cartilage proteoglycan and the interstitial collagens is generated on immunization with IgG molecules. The present review summarizes data that show that a family of monoclonal antibodies specific for diverse epitopes of the proteoglycan molecules induce cartilage pathology similar to that generated in experimental immune synovitis. Data are also presented that indicate that immunotherapy using either hormones (estrogen antagonists) or the induction of antigen-specific tolerance to connective tissue macromolecules can produce a beneficial modulation in the gross pathology and modulate the autoimmune response to connective tissue macromolecules. These studies infer a connectivity between autoimmunity to connective tissue macromolecules and the generation of immune synovitis while also showing that monoclonal antibodies can be generated that mimic autoimmunity and induce cartilage pathology.

II. ARTHRITIS PATHOLOGY IN EXPERIMENTAL IMMUNE SYNOVITIS

In experimental immune synovitis, the synovial inflammation generated ultimately progresses to articular cartilage erosion and ligament destruction. Assessment of the pathologic lesions is performed by grossly assigning equal weight to each of three parameters: cartilage, synovial fluid, and synovium. Patellar, femoral, and tibial cartilage are assessed with pathology scores based on the amount of surface pitting, marginal erosions, ulcerations, and joint disorganization noted. Synovial fluid is scored based on the amount and turbidity of the fluid. For synovium, the level of proliferation and pannus formation are noted. The generation of cartilage and synovial pathology of immune rabbits after the intra-articular injection of homologous IgG is presented in Fig. 1. As can be seen in Fig. 1,

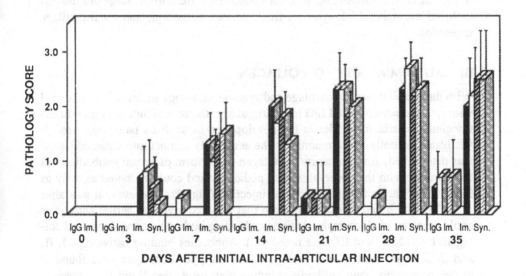

Figure 1 Time course of the expression of gross pathology in IgG-immune (IgG Im) or immune synovitis (Im Syn) rabbits. IgG-immune rabbits were administered 4.0 mg IgG/CFA followed by 2.0 mg IgG/CFA and intra-articular injections of saline twice weekly (days 0–35). Immune synovitis rabbits were administered 4.0 mg IgG/CFA, 2.0 mg IgG/CFA, and intra-articular injections of 1.0 mg IgG in 0.5 ml saline twice weekly, between days 0 and 35. The parameters displayed are for synovial fluid (▰); synovium (▱); femoral cartilage (▨); and tibial cartilage (▨). Pathology scores for these parameters ranged as previously described from 0 to 4 and are expressed as the mean ± SD for individual scores of animals of the group.

gross pathology could be noted as early as 3 days after the initial intra-articular injection of IgG (Im Syn group, Fig. 1). Minimal but consistent values for synovial and cartilage pathology are noted at this early time point, indicative of the initiation of immune synovitis. In this group, fine diffuse cartilaginous surface pitting is noted, as well as synovial proliferation. However, animals receiving intra-articular injection of saline were not observed to portray any gross pathology indicative of immune synovitis (IgG immune group, Fig. 1). Statistically significant gross pathology was noted at 1 week after the initial intra-articular injection in the categories of synovial fluid and femoral and tibial cartilage. In these animals, turbid synovial fluid was noted as well as tibial femoral marginal erosions. All four categories, including synovium, were noted to have statistically significantly elevated gross pathology compared to the saline-injected group 2 weeks after the initial intra-articular injection. This statistically significant elevated gross pathology was observed throughout the time course of the intra-articular injections. The classic rheumatologic lesions observed in the chronic stage of synovitis included excessive thick synovial fluid, pannus formation, and focal cartilage ulcerations.

III. AUTOIMMUNITY TO COLLAGEN

With the establishment of cartilage and synovia pathology in animals immunized with IgG and administered IgG intra-articularly, the role of autoimmunity to extracellular matrix molecules in the development of arthritis pathology was investigated. Initially, autoimmunity to the genetically distinct interstitial collagens was determined. Autoimmunity to collagen in the form of serum antibodies was concomitant with the observable joint pathology and could be noted as early as 3 days after the initial intra-articular injection (Fig. 2). However, it was after 1 week of the initial articular injection that elevated levels of serum antibodies could be noted in all animals. Antibodies binding both native and denatured collagens types I, II, and III were noted (22). Antibodies binding native type I, II, and III collagen molecules as well as denatured type II collagen were found in higher prevalence than antibodies binding denatured type I and III collagens. Statistically significantly elevated levels of these antibodies were apparent at 2 weeks after the initial intra-articular injection. During the time course of an intra-articular injection, elevated levels of antibodies appeared sustained and remained in the range of values determined for the second week of injections. Inhibition studies with preparations of native and denatured interstitial collagens, as well as the cyanogen bromide peptides of type I, II, and III collagens, were performed to determine the binding specificities of the anticollagen antibodies observed in the serum of chronic immune synovitis rabbits. The inhibition data indicated that three populations of antibodies directed to collagenous epitopes were present in the serum of immune synovitis rabbits. They were (1) antibodies directed to the

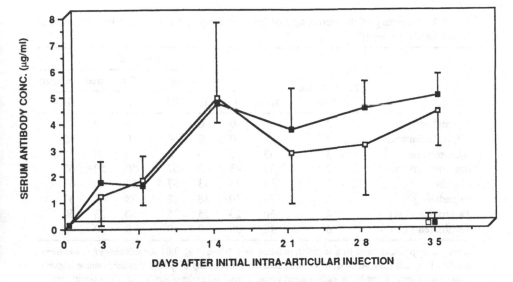

Figure 2   Time course of the antibody response to rabbit type II collagen and cartilage proteoglycan monomer for immune synovitis rabbits (days 3–35). Day 0 and 35 values, approximating no significant measurable antibody levels for collagen or proteoglycan, are presented for IgG-immune rabbits.

helical epitopes of native collagen molecules (however, a small percentage of these antibodies may bind the nonhelical terminal regions of the collagen molecule); (2) antibodies directed to only denatured collagen polypeptide chains; and (3) antibodies recognizing denatured collagen polypeptides and their cyanogen bromide peptide preparations.

In addition, cell-mediated immune responses to rabbit IgG, the native and denatured interstitial collagens, were analyzed in rabbits with chronic immune synovitis (23). As summarized in Table 1, only animals with immune synovitis (Table 1, row 4) were noted to have an incidence of cell-mediated immune responses to both homologous IgG and the native interstitial collagens and their constituent α chains. The relatively high incidence of cell-mediated immune responses to both native and denatured collagens suggests that immunity to structural components of the synovial membrane and the adjacent surface of articular cartilage may play a role in the inflammation observed in immune synovitis. Factors that likely influence the incidence of the autoimmunity noted in immune synovitis animals are the quantitative nature of in vitro cell-mediated immune responses, the outbred nature of the animals, and the lymphatic nature of the cells utilized. This last point reflects the use of peripheral blood lymphocytes is synovial cell lymphocytes infiltrates versus splenic or thymic cells. Nevertheless, these

Table 1 Summary of the Percentage of Immune Response to In Vitro Incubation with Homologous Antigens[a]

Group[b]	Total animal number	IgG	Native collagen			Denatured collagen		
			I	II	III	I	II	III
Normal rabbits	2	0	0	0	0	0	0	0
Adjuvant immune	3	0	0	0	0	0	0	0
IgG immune	3	33	0	0	0	0	0	0
Immune synovitis[d]	7	33	43	43	57	50	50	67
Placebo	7	33	43	43	57	50	50	67
Estradiol	8	71	50	38	38	28	43	57
Tamoxifen (TH)	4	50	25	25	25	50	25	50
Tamoxifen (TL)	6	20	33	0	0	0	0	0

[a]Immune response defined as a stimulation index > 2.0 and $P < 0.01$ for diluent- versus antigen-incubated cultures (23). Analysis of variance indicate a probability of 0.9831 that the immune response to antigens varies among hormonally treated groups compared to the placebo immune synovitis group.
[b]Spleen cells of animals treated with antigens. Adjuvant immune rabbits were rabbits immunized twice with CFA-saline. TH, high-dose tamoxifen treatment group; TL, low-dose tamoxifen treatment group. Immune synovitis rabbits that were administered hormones were given IM injections during the course of intra-articular injections.
[c]Antigens isolated, purified, and utilized at concentrations as described (7).
[d]Seven rabbits analyzed for responses to collagen, six analyzed for responses to IgG.

data show that both a humoral and a cell-mediated autoimmunity to collagen are noted in chronic immune synovitis.

IV. AUTOIMMUNITY TO CARTILAGE PROTEOGLYCAN

Animals exhibiting arthritis pathology associated with experimentally induced chronic immune synovitis were also analyzed for autoimmunity to cartilage proteoglycan. Antibodies recognizing cartilage proteoglycan were observed in the serum of animals with immune synovitis. As shown in Fig. 2, substantial levels of antibodies were noted as early as 3 days after the initial inta-articular injection. Elevated and statistically significant levels of antiproteoglycan antibody were noted as early as 7 days after the initial intra-articular injection, and peak antibody values occurred 2 weeks after the initial intra-articular injection. These antibody levels continued throughout the time course of chronic immune synovitis. Studies were performed to detail the fine antigenic specificity of rabbit antiproteoglycan antibodies and were performed with murine monoclonal antibodies that recognized various regions of the proteoglycan molecule as well as with tryptic peptides of proteoglycan monomer (24). Using a panel of murine monoclonal antibodies, it was observed that antibodies to the chondroitin sulfate-rich region of the proteoglycan molecule, those that recognized native proteoglycan monomer and those that recognized peptides containing the hyaluronic binding region or denatured peptides, showed a limited capacity to inhibit the antiproteoglycan antibody binding to proteoglycan monomer substrate. However, monoclonal antibodies that recognized the keratin sulfate peptides showed inhibitory capacity in all nine rabbit sera tested and significant >40% inhibition in six of the nine rabbits. These data were confirmed using tryptic fragments of the rabbit proteoglycan monomer. As shown in Table 2, tryptic fragments rich in chondroitin sulfate peptides (DEAE I-02-4), were poor inhibitors of binding of the antibody to the proteoglycan substrate (inhibition ranged between 3 and 31%). However, keratin sulfate-rich peptides, that is DEAE II-D1-D4 peptides, inhibited at a much higher level on a per weight basis, in the range of 59–71% inhibition of binding. These data, taken together, indicate that the antibodies, which bind cartilage proteoglycan, that are observed in chronic immune synovitis are heterogeneous in nature but a predominant proportion recognized the proteoglycan molecule containing core protein and associated keratin sulfate (24). These data are particularly relevant in light of the report of antiproteoglycan antibody detection in rheumatoid arthritis (25). In addition, an increasing number of studies (26–28) have shown proteoglycan fragments are released into the serum and or synovial fluids of patients with inflammatory joint disease. Therefore, it is clear that degradation products of proteoglycan, as well as intact monomer, are released from the extracellular matrix into the synovial fluid and serum. The loss of cartilage proteoglycan from the extracellular matrix may be a marker for activating various immune-mediated events, interleukin-1 such as (IL-1) production from activated monocytes (29,30) or production of antiprogeoglycan antibody (31).

V. IMMUNOTHERAPY OF EXPERIMENTALLY INDUCED SYNOVITIS

Autoimmunity to both cartilage proteoglycan and the genetically distinct interstitial collagens is temporally similar to the appearance of gross pathology indicative

Table 2 Summary of Proteoglycan Tryptic Peptide Inhibition of the Binding of Rabbit Antiproteoglycan Antibody Observed in Experimental Immune Synovitis to Rabbit Proteoglycan Monomer[a]

Chondroitin sulfate-rich peptides (%)	Keratin sulfate-rich peptides (%)
3–31	59–71

[a]Percentage inhibition of binding of antibody to substrate in a solid-phase radioimmunoassay as described (29).

of synovitis. To further establish connectivity between joint pathology and autoimmunity, studies were performed to determine if modulation of autoimmunity could be reflected in a reduction of joint arthritis gross pathology.

Initial studies used steroid sex hormones for the modulation of the immune response in arthritis. These reagents were utilized since clinical observations have firmly established that autoimmune diseases occur at a strikingly higher frequency in women compared with men (32,33). In addition, experimental studies suggest a role for estrogens in the modulation of inflammation and pathogenesis of autoimmunity (34,35). In experimental immune synovitis, estradiol has been suggested to influence the severity of inflammation (36) and prostaglandin synthesis by articular chondrocytes (37), the latter being directly correlated to the presence of synovitis (38). The administration of placebo or estradiol to immune rabbits (Table 1, rows 5 and 6) during intra-articular injection of IgG resulted in a high incidence of cell-mediated immunity to homologous IgG as well as the native interstitial collagens and their constituent polypeptide chains. A significant reduction in cell-mediated immune responses to homologous IgG as well as the native interstitial collagens and their constituent α chains was noted particularly with the administration of low-dose tamoxifen during the time course of intra-articular administration of homologous rabbit IgG (Table 1, row 8). As shown in Table 3, the gross pathology in the low-dose tamoxifen group was particularly reduced with regard to the amount of synovial fluid. These data indicate that steroid sex hormones can modulate the autoimmune response to connective tissue macromolecules observed in experimental arthritis and that this immunomodulation can be exhibited in the appearance of gross pathology observed in the animals with immune synovitis (Table 3). Steroid sex hormones likely influence autoimmune

Table 3 Summary of Gross Pathology of Immune Synovitis Rabbits Administered Steroid Sex Hormones

Group	No. animals	Gross pathology[a]		
		Synovitis	Synovial Fluid	Cartilage
Estradiol	8	2.6 ± 0.5	2.0 ± 1.4	2.6 ± 0.4
Tamoxifen (TL)	6	1.8 ± 1.0	0.9 ± 1.4	2.0 ± 1.0
Tamoxifen (TH)	4	2.1 ± 0.9	0.8 ± 1.5	1.9 ± 0.9

[a]Pathologic scores presented as mean $\pm$ SD of the scores for the inidividual animals based on a 0–4 scale as follows. Cartilage: 0, normal; 1, fine diffuse surface pitting; 2, soft modulation of the surface and marginal erosion; 3, focal ulceration of the articular surface; 4, diffuse degrading of the articular surface and joint disorganization. Synovium: 0, normal; 1, hyperemia and minimal proliferation; 2, pannus at joint margin; 3, pannus covering intra-articular structures; 4, replacement of joint structure with pannus. Synovial fluid: 0, normal; 1, minimal but excessive clear fluid; 2, turbid fluid; 3, thick yellow pus; 4, hemorrhagic pus.

responses at the T cell level (32). Estrogens diffuse into cells and bind appropriate cytosolic receptors, and this complex translocates into the nucleus. In the nucleus, the hormone-receptor complex binds to gene response elements adjacent to gene promoter sequences, resulting in the selective stimulation of the rate of transcription of specific genes. The regulatory roles of these specific gene products remain to be determined.

Subsequent studies have used methodologies to induce antigen-specific tolerance to connective tissue macromolecules in experimental immune synovitis. Table 4 shows the suppression of cell-mediated immune responses to both type I and type II collagens in animals that were administered type II collagen intravenously to induce tolerance to interstitial collagens before the induction of immune synovitis. Suppression of cell-mediated immune responses to collagen were not noted in animals given either type IV collagen intravenously for the induction of tolerance to basement membrane collagen or the immune synovitis control group (Table 4, rows 2 and 3). However, rabbits administered type II collagen intravenously were rendered immunologically anergic to type II collagen but not to the arthrogenic molecule, IgG (Table 4, row 1). This observation of reduced cell-mediated immune responses to collagen is once again coupled to a reduction in gross pathology, particularly as observed in the tibial and femoral cartilage (Table 5). These data indicate that immunotherapeutic approaches that involve the suppression of autoimmunity to collagen may be beneficial with regard to the level of cartilage damage observed in animals with experimental immune synovitis.

Table 4 Summary of Cell-Mediated Immune Responses to Native Type I and II Collagen from Splenic Cells Derived from Immune Synovitis Rabbits Preinoculated with Native Collagen

| Collagen type injected[a] | Cell-mediated immune response[b] (stimulation index ± SEM) | | |
| | | Collagen | |
	Rabbit IgG	I	II
II	2.6 ± 0.6	1.7 ± 0.3	1.6 ± 0.2
IV	4.5 ± 0.3	2.5 ± 1.1	3.0 ± 1.3
None	2.1 ± 0.3	2.0 ± 0.2	2.0 ± 0.2

[a]Native type II or type IV collagen administered (20 mg IV) 1 day before the induction of experimental immune synovitis.

[b][^{3}H]Thymidine uptake in vitro of 2×10^5 splenic cells of each rabbit in the group performed in triplicate. Diluent values 1986 ± 262 cpm ($n = 7$). A stimulation index > 2.0 was taken to represent a positive response to incubation with antigen (7).

Table 5 Summary of Gross Pathology of Rabbits Administered Native Collagen Before the Induction of Experimental Immune Synovitis

Collagen type injected[a]	Gross pathology[b]			
		Synovial fluid	Cartilage	
	Synovium		Tibia	Femur
II	2.0 ± 0.1	2.0 ± 1.4	1.0 ± 1.4	0.4 ± 0.5
IV	1.8 ± 0.4	1.6 ± 1.3	2.2 ± 1.3	1.2 ± 1.0
None	2.0 ± 1.0	1.8 ± 1.3	1.8 ± 0.8	1.2 ± 1.0

[a]Native type II or type IV collagen administered (20 mg IV) 1 day before the induction of immune synovitis.
[b]Scoring system 0–4 as described in Table 1: five rabbits per group.

IV. MONOCLONAL ANTIBODIES THAT INDUCE CARTILAGE PATHOLOGY

However, since synovial pathology and synovial fluid levels were not reduced in the antigen-specific tolerized rabbits, these data also indicate that the immunoregulation of autoimmunity to collagen may require coupling to additional immunoregulatory modalities involving autoimmunity to proteoglycan to induce additional beneficial effects on the total gross pathology of immune synovitis. To this point, antibodies that reflect the humoral immune response observed in experimental immune synovitis can cause cartilage pathology (31). In this regard, antiproteoglycan antibodies that recognize the keratin sulfate-rich region of the antibody molecule, when given intravenously to normal animals, induce a series of events that include the deposition of the antiproteoglycan antibody to the surface of the articular cartilage, localization to the articular cartilage of an autologous immune response, and the loss of proteoglycan from cartilage. The loss of proteoglycan from the cartilage can be particularly significant in the femoral cartilage. Therefore, immunotherapy that involves the regulation of autoimmunity to both the interstitial collagens and proteoglycans may be required to totally downregulate chronic immune synovitis.

The present study summarizes the data detailing the observations of autoimmunity to the interstitial collagens and cartilage proteoglycans in an animal model of rheumatoid arthritis. Autoimmunity to collagen in experimental immune synovitis is observed and is heterogeneous with regard to the polymorphic interstitial collagens. In this regard, both cell-mediated and humoral responses are noted to native and denatured type I, II, and III collagens as well as the cyanogen bromide peptides of these collagens. These data are consistent with the large body of information that shows that both cell-mediated and humoral immune responses are observed in patients with rheumatoid arthritis (39–44). Although these studies reveal different immune reactivity to the polymorphism of collagen in patients with rheumatoid arthritis, they suggest that an immune response to collagen may be part of the pathogenesis of rheumatoid arthritis.

The development of autoimmunity to proteoglycan in experimental immune synovitis correlates with reported antiproteoglycan antibody detected in rheumatoid arthritis (25). A number of possible reasons exist why anti-proteoglycan antibody is formed. The production of antiproteoglycan antibody may be due to overcoming tolerance, being secondary to the release of proteoglycan monomer-rich degradation products. Interaction of IgG with proteoglycan could render the proteoglycan cross-reactive to the host response to antigen. Proteoglycan monomers may not be generally encountered by the immune system during development. In addition, the use of adjuvant may be important in the induction of autoimmunity to proteoglycans. The recent data of Oppliger et al. (45), showing that rheumatoid factors bear the conformation internal image of staphylococcal protein A, indicate cross-reactivity between an anti-IgG rheumatoid factor response. The RF antibody noted in this animal model of arthritis may bind to straphylococcal protein A. This observation is noteworthy in light of the recent data of van Eden et al. (15), who have recently shown that in the induction of adjuvant arthritis in rats, a T lymphocyte clone recognizes cartilage proteoglycan as well as *Mycobacterium tuberculosis*. Therefore, the exposure of the immune system to bacterial immunogens during bacterial infection may result in molecules that have cross-reactivity with rheumatoid factor as well as cartilage proteoglycans, thereby inducing autologous autoimmunity, such as that observed in this model of arthritis.

It is also not clear whether proteoglycan can initiate an immune response when molecules are confined to the synovial fluid or whether the macromolecules, or fragments thereof, must be released into the serum first. Boniface et al. (16) has shown that intra-articular injection of purified proteoglycan monomer can cause synovitic changes. Whether proteoglycan monomers are released from the intra-articular space during the course of immune synovitis remains to be determined. Previous physiochemical studies have shown that intact proteoglycan can diffuse from the cartilage (13). As keratin sulfate-containing peptides are released into the serum, it is clear that degradation products of proteoglycan as well as intact monomer are released into the serum as well (26–28). The present studies, detailing autoimmunity to connective tissue macromolecules concomitant with a reduction in specific parameters of arthritis gross pathology, indicate that there is a relationship between autoimmunity to connective tissue macromolecules and the idiopathogenesis of synovitis. This observation is applicable to other models of arthritis, particularly collagen-induced arthritis, in which injection of native type II collagen before the induction of arthritis has been noted to modulate arthritis pathology (46,47). The suppression of synovitis by this methodology in collagen-induced arthritis contrasts with the lack of modulation of synovitis in experimental immune synovitis. The additional observations of autoimmuity to cartilage proteoglycans and high titers of rheumatoid factors noted in experimental immune synovitis may reflect an etiopathogenesis of arthritis that is more complex than that noted in collagen-induced arthritis. In this regard, further studies inducing both immunomodulation of autoimmunity to both collagen and proteoglycans will be required to differentiate the role(s) of reduction of autoimmunity to connective tissue macromolecules and chronic immune synovitis.

VII. SUMMARY

Utilizing an animal model of human rheumatoid arthritis, a series of studies have been performed that detailed the cell-mediated and humoral responses to major cartilage macromolecules, collagen and proteoglycan. In vitro cell-mediated immune responses were observed in experimental immune synovitis using native and denatured interstitial collagens as antigens. In vitro cell-mediated immune responses to these antigens were not noted in control spleen cell cultures derived from normal or antigen-primed nonsynovitis animals. Subpopulation studies noted that the measured immune responses in the synovitis animals were of T cell origin. Suppression of in vitro immune responses to denatured type I, II, and III collagen as well as native type II collagen and type III collagen was noted using low-dose tamoxifen treatment before the induction of immune synovitis. Concomitantly, an effect on the gross pathology was also noted. Administration of low-dose tamoxifen, an estrogen antagonist, was associated with significant improvement in immune synovitis with regard to gross pathology when compared to the placebo or estradiol-treated group. These data suggested that in vivo antiestrogen administration can modulate the in vitro cell-mediated immune responses to connective tissue constituents observed in immune synovitis and concomitantly reduce the observed lesions in the inflammation. Recent studies inducing antigen-specific tolerance to type II collagens have also noted that a reduction in cell-mediated immune responses to the interstitial collagens is observed concomitantly with a reduction in the gross pathology scores of both tibial and femoral cartilage. However, in these studies the amount of synovitis or synovial fluid in animals with experimental immune synovitis was not reduced. These studies suggest that in this animal model of rheumatoid arthritis, synovitis is not induced by the host immune response to an individual connective tissue macromolecule, but likely represents the result of the composite host reponse to both cartilage proteoglycan and the genetically distinct collagens. In this regard, the host response to cartilage proteoglycan noted in this model is heterogeneous with regard to specificity but a relatively large proportion of the antiproteoglycan molecule containing core protein and associated keratin sulfate. Such monoclonal antibodies, on intravenous administration to normal animals, have been shown to home to the surface of the articular cartilage and induce an autologous immune response, as well as promote the loss of proteoglycan from the articular cartilage. These data, taken together, suggest that autoimmunity to both collagen and proteoglycan plays a role in the idiopathogenesis of arthritis and that monoclonal antibodies portraying specifics similar to those of the autologous autoimmune response can mimic humoral immunity and induce arthritis pathology.

REFERENCES

1. Cooke, T.D., Hurd, E.R., Ziff, M., and Jasin, M.E. (1972). The pathogenesis of chronic inflammation in experimental antigen-induced arthritis. II. Preferential localization of antigen-antibody complexes to collagenous tissues. J. Exp. Med. 135:323–338.
2. Cooke, T.D., Hurd, E.R., Jasin, H.E., Bienenstock, J., and Ziff, M. (1975). Identification of immunoglobulin and complement in rheumatoid articular collagenous tissue. Arthritis Rheum. 18:541–551.
3. Dumonde, D.C., and Glynn, L.E. (1962). The production of arthritis in rabbits by an immunological reaction to fibrin. Br. J. Exp. Pathol. 43:373–383.
4. Zvaifler, N.J. (1973). The immunopathology of joint inflammation in rheumatoid arthritis. Adv. Immunol. 161:265–336.
5. Jasin, H.E. and Ziff, M. (1969). Immunoglobulin and specific antibody synthesis in a chronic inflammatory focus: Antigen-induced synovitis. J. Immunol. 102:355–369.
6. Cooke, T.D., and Jasin, H.E. (1972). The pathogenesis of chronic inflammation in experimental antigen-induced arthritis. 1. The role of antigen on the local immune response. Arthritis Rheum. 15:327–337.
7. Kresina, T.F., Rosner, I.A., Goldberg, V.M., and Moskowitz, R.W. (1984). IgG-induced experimental chronic immune synovitis: Cell-mediated immunity to native interstitial collagen molecules and their constitutent polypeptide chains. Cell. Immunol. 87:504–516.
8. Goldberg, V.M., Lance, E.M., and Davis, P. (1974). Experimental immune synovitis in the rabbit. Relative roles of cell mediated and humoral immunity. Arthritis Rheum. 17:993–1005.
9. Glynn, L.E. (1969). Aetiology of rheumatoid arthritis with regard to its chronicity. Ann. Rheum. Dis. 28(Suppl.):3–4.
10. Friedlaender, G.E., Ladenbauer-Bellis, I.M., and Chrisman, O.D. (1983). Immunogenicity of xenogeneic cartilage matrix components in a rabbit model. Yale J. Biol. Med. 56:211–217.
11. Cooke, T.D.V. (1988). Antigen-induced arthritis, polyarthritis and tenosynovitis. In: Handbook of Animal Model for the Rheumatic Diseases, Vol. 1. Greenwald, R.A., and Diamond, H.D., eds. CRC Press, Boca Raton, Florida, pp. 53–81.
12. Rosner, I.A., Boja, B.A., Malemud, C.J., Moskowitz, R.W. and Goldberg, V.M. (1982). Intra-articular hyaluronic acid injection and synovial prostaglandins in experimental immune synovitis. J. Rheumatol. 10:71–78.
13. Evans, C.H., Means, D.C., and Stanitsky, C.L.(1982). Ferrographic analysis of

wear in human joints. Evaluation by comparison with arthroscopic examination of symptomatic knees. J. Bone Joint Surg. 64B:572–578.

14. Saxne, J., Weilham, F.A., Heinegard, D., and Petterson, H. (1985). Difference in cartilage proteoglycan level in synovial fluid in early rheumatoid arthritis and reactive arthritis. Lancet 8447:127–128.

15. van Eden, W., Holshitz, J., Nevo, Z., Frenkel, A., Klajman, A., and Cohen, I.R. (1985). Arthritis induced by a T lymphocyte clone that responds to *Mycobacterium tuberculosis* and to cartilage proteoglycans. Proc. Natl. Acad. Sci. USA 82:5117–5120.

16. Boniface, R.J., Cain, P.R., and Evans, C.H. (1986). Articular responses to purified cartilage proteoglycans (abstract). Trans. Orthop. Res. Soc. 11:147.

17. Poole, A.R. (1986). Connective tissue: Biological and clinical aspects. In: Rheumatology: An Annual Review, Vol. 10. Kuhn, K., and Kries, T., eds. Karger, New York, pp. 316–371.

18. Steffen, C. (1970). Consideration of pathogenesis of rheumatoid arthritis as collagen autoimmunity. Immunobiology 39:219–226.

19. Foidard, J.M., Abe, S., Martin, G.E., et al. (1978). Antibodies to type II collagen in relapsing polychondritis. N. Engl. J. Med. 299:1203–1207.

20. Mesteck, J., and Miller, E.J. (1975). Presence of antibodies specific to cartilage-type collagen in rheumatoid synovial tissue. Clin. Exp. Immunol. 22:453–456.

21. Steffen, C., Ludwig, H., and Knapp, W. (1974). Collagen-anticollagen immune complexes in rheumatoid arthritis synovial fluid cells. Immunobiology 147:229–235.

22. Kresina, T.F., Rosner, I.A., Goldberg, V.M., and Moskowitz, R.W. (1985). Fine specificity of serum anti-collagen molecules in experimental immune synovitis. Ann. Rheum. Dis. 44:328–335.

23. Kresina, T.F., Rosner, I.A., Goldbert, V.M., Boja, B.A., and Moskowitz, R.W. (1984). IgG-induced experimental immune synovitis: Humoral modulation of in vitro splenic immune responses to homologous antigens. Clin. Exp. Immunol. 57:63–72.

24. Yoo, J.U., Kresina, T.F., Malemud, C.J., and Goldberg, V.M.(1987). Epitopes of proteoglycans eliciting an anti-proteoglycan response in chronic immune synovitis. Proc. Natl. Acad. Sci. USA 84:832–836.

25. Glant, T., Csongor, J., and Szucs, T. (1980). Immunopathologic role of proteoglycan antigens in rheumatoid joint disease. Scand. J. Immunol. 11:247–252.

26. Thonar, E.J., Lenz, M.E., Klintworth, G.K., Caterson, B.K., Pachman, L., Glickman, P., Katz, R., Huff, J., and Kuettner, K.E. (1985). Quantification of keratan sulfate in blood as a marker of cartilage catabolism. Arthritis Rheum. 28:1367–1376.

27. Witter, J., Roughley, P.J,. Webber C., Roberts, N., Keystone, E., and Poole, A.R. (1987). The immunologic detection and characterization of cartilage proteoglycan degradation products in synovial fluids of patients with arthritis. Arthritis Rheum. 30:519–529.

28. Saxne, T., Heinegard, D., and Wollheim, F.A. (1987). Cartilage proteoglycans in synovial fluid and serum in patients with inflammatory joint disease. Arthritis Rheum. 30:972–979.

29. Pettipher, E.R., Henderson, B., Hardingham, T., and Ratcliffe, A. (1989). Cartilage proteoglycan depletion in acute and chronic antigen-induced arthritis. Arthritis Rheum. 32:601–607.

30. Dodge, G.R., and Poole, A.R. (1989). Immunohistochemical detection and immunochemical analysis of type II collagen degradation in human normal, rheumatoid, and osteoarthritis articular cartilages and in explants of bovine articular cartilage cultured with interleukin-1. J. Clin. Invest. 83:647–661.

31. Kresina, T.F., Yoo, J.U., and Goldberg, V.M. (1988). Evidence that an antiproteoglycan humoral immune response can induced articular cartilage pathology. Arthritis Rheum. 31:248–257.

32. Ansar, A.S., Penhale, W.J., and Talal, N. (1985). Sex hormones, immune responses and autoimmune diseases. Am. J. Pathol. 121:531–539.

33. Talal, N., and Ansar, A.S. (1987). Sex hormones and autoimmune diseases: A short review. Int. J. Immunother. 3:65–70.

34. Holmdahl, R., Jansson, L., and Andersson, M. (1986). Female sex hormones suppresses development of collagen-induced arthritis in mice. Arthritis Rheum. 29:1501–1509.

35. Holmdahl, R., Jansson, L., Meyersson, B., and Klareskog, L. (1987). Oestrogen-induced suppression of collagen arthritis. I. Long term treatment of DBA/1 mice recudes severity and incidence of arthritis and decreases the anti type II collagen immune response. Clin. Exp. Immunol. 70:372–378.

36. Goldberg, V.M., Moskowitz, R.W., Rosner, I., and Malemud, C. (1981). The role of estrogen and oophorectomy in immune synovitis. Semin. Arthritis. Rheum. 11:134–135.

37. Rosner, I.A., Malemud, C.J., Hassid, A.I., Goldberg, V.M., Boja, B.A., and Moskowitz, R.W. (1983). Estratiol and tamoxifen stimulation of lapine articular chondrocyte prostaglanding synthesis. Prostaglandin 26:123–138.

38. Rosner, I.A., Boja, B.A., Malemud, C.J., Moskowitz, R.W., and Goldberg, V.M. (1983). Intraarticular hyaluronic acid injection and synovial prostaglandin in experimental immune synovitis. J. Rheumatol. 10:71–78.

39. Endler, A.T., Zielinski, C., Meneel, E.J., Smoten, J.S., Schwageri, W., Endler, M., Eberi, R., Frank, O., and Steffen, C.Z. (1978). Leukocyte migration inhibition with collagen type I and collagen type II in rheumatoid arthritis and degenerative joint disease. Rheumatology 37:87–92.

40. Stuart, J.M., Postlethwaite, A.E., Kang, A.H., and Townes, A.S. (1980). Cell mediated immunity to collagen and collagen chains in rheumatoid arthritis and other rheumatic disease. Ann. J. Med. 69:13–18.

41. Smolen, J.S., Menzel, E.J., Scherak, O., Kojer, M., Kolarz, G., Steffen, C., and Mayr, W.R. (1980). Lymphocyte transformation to denatured type I collagens and B lymphocyte alloantigens in rheumatoid arthritis. Arthritis Rheum. 23:424–431.

42. Andriopoulos, N.A., Mesecky, J., Wright, G.P., and Miller, E.J. (1976). Characterization of antibodies to the native human collagens and to their component chains in the sera and the joint fluids of patients with rheumatoid arthritis. Immunochemistry 13:709–712.

43. Michaeli, D., and Fundenberg, H.H. (1974). The incidence and antigenic specificity of antibodies against denatured human collagen in rheumatoid arthritis. Clin. Immunol. Immunopathol. 2:153–159.

44. Stuart, J.M., Huffstutter, E.H., Townes, A.S., and Kang, A.H. (1983). Incidence of specificity of antibodies to types I, II, III, IV and V collagen in rheumatoid

arthritis and their rheumatic diseases as measured by ^{125}I radioimmunoassay. Arthritis Rheum. 26:832–840.

45. Oppliger, I., Nardella, F.A., Stone, G., and Manni, K.M. (1987). Rheumatoid factors bear the conformational internal image of staphylococcal protein A. (abstract). Clin. Res. 35:461A.

46. Cremer, M.A., Hernandez, A.D., Townes, A.S., Stuart, J. M., and Kang, A.H. (1983). Collagen-induced arthritis in rats: Antigen specific suppression of arthritis and immunity by intravenously injected native type II collagen. J. Immunol. 13:2995–3000.

47. Kresina, T.F., and Moskowitz, R.W. (1985). Adoptive transfer of suppression of arthritis in the mouse model of collagen-induced arthritis. Evidence for a type II collagen-specific suppressor T cell. J. Clin. Invest. 75:1990–1998.

18

Serum Keratan Sulfate Concentration as a Measure of the Catabolism of Cartilage Proteoglycans

Eugene J.-M. A. Thonar, James M. Williams, Brian A. Maldonado, Mary Ellen Lenz, Thomas J. Schnitzer, Giles V. Campion, and Klaus E. Kuettner
Rush-Presbyterian–St. Luke's Medical Center, Chicago, Illinois

M. Barry E. Sweet
University of the Witwatersrand, Johannesburg, South Africa

I. INTRODUCTION

Cartilage contains a relatively small number of cells that elaborate an abundant extracellular matrix rich in proteoglycans (PGs) and collagens. The collagens form an insoluble network that gives cartilage its strength and tensile properties (1). This network also entraps the highly deformable PGs that enable the tissue to undergo rapid reversible deformation. A newly synthesized cartilage PG is a very large molecule consisting of a core protein ($M_r = \pm 200,000$ daltons) to which are covalently attached highly negatively charged side chains of chondroitin sulfate (CS) and keratan sulfate (KS), as well as O-glycosidically linked and N-glycosidically linked oligosaccharides (Fig. 1) (2). Several newly synthesized PG monomers interact extracellularly with link protein molecules and a single strand of hyaluronic acid (HA) to form a PG aggregate that is firmly immobilized in the matrix and may reach molecular sizes in excess of 200 million daltons (2).

Proteoglycans and collagens in cartilage are constantly being turned over. Cartilage PGs turn over more rapidly than the collagen network in which they are entrapped. It should be noted that PGs in different cartilages do not necessarily turn over at the same rate (3). The degradation of cartilage PGs during normal turnover is regulated by the chondrocytes, which release proteolytic enzymes in the extracellular milieu. Proteoglycans and HA in cartilage have similar half-lives (4), suggesting the PGs within an aggregate are usually turned over as a unit.

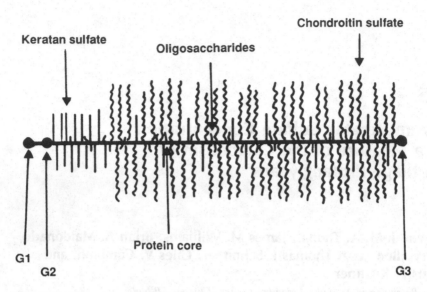

Figure 1 Schematic diagram of the structure of aggregating proteoglycan from cartilage. The protein core contains three globular domains: the binding region (G1), which contains a specific hyaluronic acid binding site involved in aggregation, a second globular domain (G2), and a C-terminal domain (G3). The extended part of the protein core contains a keratan sulfate-rich region and a long chondroitin sullfate attachment region. (Modified after Sheehan et al., Ref. 2.)

Partial degradation of some, but not all, PGs within an aggregate cannot be ruled out at this stage, however. Little is known about the enzymes responsible for the catabolism of cartilage PGs in normal turnover. Recent studies have implied that neutral metalloproteinases may play an important role (5).

Chondrocytes usually synthesize these enzymes in an inactive form. Following activation in the matrix, they are able to cleave the core protein of individual aggregating PG molecules at one or more sites (Fig. 2) but preferentially near the HA binding region. The fragments containing glycosaminoglycans then rapidly diffuse out of the matrix into adjacent body fluids. The fate of the glycosaminoglycan-poor HA binding regions is unclear, but there is increasing evidence that some may remain in the matrix. Indeed, the matrix of adult human cartilage becomes enriched with age in nonfunctional PG fragments, which consist of a HA binding region to which are attached few or no glycosaminoglycan chains (6,7). These glycosaminoglycan-depleted molecules, which almost certainly represent degradation products, represent up to 50% of the PG molecules in the matrix (7).

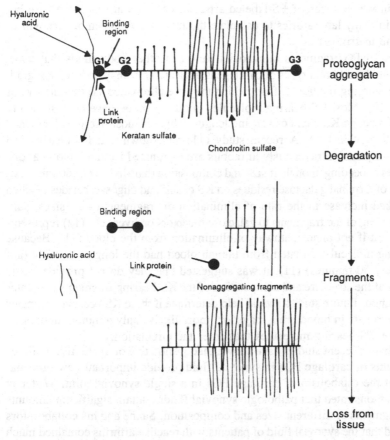

Figure 2 Suggested pathways for proteoglycan degradation in the cartilage matrix. (Modified after Lohmander, Ref. 17.)

The expulsion of large negatively charged PG fragments from the tissue is more than likely facilitated by repulsive forces exerted by the negative charges on PGs present at extremely high concentrations in the matrix. The contention that the diffusion of glycosaminoglycan-bearing fragments from the matrix occurs soon after cleavage of the core protein is supported by the observation that glycosaminoglycan-rich PG fragments are not detected in significant amounts in the matrix (8). Because intact aggregating PGs are not found in significant amounts in the body fluids in contact with the cartilage surfaces, measurements of peptidoglycans in body fluids provide a good measure of the rate of catabolism of cartilage PGs. Researchers have taken advantage of this concept for years. For example, measurements of ^{35}S-labeled fragments appearing in the daily spent

medium in which slices of ^{35}S-labeled articular cartilage are incubated are being used in many laboratories to calculate the rate of catabolism or turnover of
PGs in the matrix (9).

The fate of PG fragments in synovial fluid and other body fluids that make
contact with the different types of cartilage is unclear. They may be further degraded before entering the blood, from which they are eliminated via the kidneys or
the liver (10). Most KS-bearing molecules in human blood have been shown to
consist of a single KS chain of varying length, which is most likely still attached
to a small peptide (10). A recent study (11) has shown that KS-bearing PG
fragments injected intravenously in rabbits are eliminated from the blood at different rates depending upon their size and composition (half-lives = 6–50 minutes).
Exposure of terminal galactose residues on KS chains and oligosaccharides resulted
in a marked increase in the rate of elimination of fragments of all sizes, suggesting binding of the fragments to galactose receptors on liver cells (12) represents
an important if not major pathway of elimination from the blood (11). Because
KS-bearing molecules isolated from human blood had the longest half-life (approximately 50 minutes) (11), it was suggested that they do not provide a true
reflection of the structure and composition of the KS-bearing fragments that enter
the circulation. Future studies should help determine if these KS-bearing fragments
that predominate in blood are a major or, more likely, only a minor subpopulation of the KS-bearing molecules that enter the circulation.

A number of recent studies have shown that quantitative or qualitative analyses
of fragments of cartilage PGs in synovial fluid provide important new information about the catabolism of cartilage PGs in a single synovial joint. Witter et
al. (13) demonstrated that pathologic synovial fluids contain significant amounts
of PG fragments of different sizes and composition. Saxne and his collaborators
(14) found that the synovial fluid of patients with reactive arthritis contained much
higher levels of PG epitope than the synovial fluid of patients with rheumatoid
arthritis (RA) and suggested measurement of the level of the epitope in synovial
fluid could be used as a diagnostic tool. The same group showed levels of PG
epitope decreased significantly following intra-articular injection of glucocorticoid,
suggesting the assay could also be used to monitor disease processes over time
(15). Importantly, some of their subsequent findings suggest that measurement
of the level of PG epitope in synovial fluid could help predict how severe the
destruction in that joint would be in later years (16). Using the same assay,
Lohmander (17) demonstrated that joint trauma causes the release of cartilage
PG fragments into the synovial fluid and suggested that in the acute phase after
injury the synovial fluid levels of PG epitope may be related to the severity of
the trauma but at later stages they may reflect the degree of chronic joint instability.

Whereas measurements of levels of cartilage PG epitopes in synovial fluid provide information about the catabolism of PGs in the cartilages in that joint,
measurements of levels of cartilage PG-related epitopes in blood reflect the

average of what is happening in all the cartilage in the body. However, several studies have shown that this approach can also be used to monitor the rapid and extensive degradation of cartilage PGs in a single joint (18–20). The rationale for measuring KS-bearing fragments in blood is based on the concept that most of the KS–containing PGs in the mammalian body are found in cartilage (hyaline, elastic, and fibrous) (10). Although KS is found in all cartilage in the human body, its concentration varies not only from cartilage to cartilage but also from region to region within a cartilage. For example, it is present at a much higher concentration in the deeper layer than in the most superficial layer of human articular cartilage from the femoral head (21–23). Small amounts of KS are present in body fluids and some noncartilaginous tissues, that is, the compressed regions of tendon (24), aorta (25), cornea (26), but this probably represents a very small percentage of the total KS present in the body. The contention that most of the KS-bearing molecules in blood represent products of the degradation of cartilage PGs is supported by a number of recent studies. In this review we summarize these recent findings that have demonstrated that quantification of KS in serum provides an excellent measure of the rate of catabolism of cartilage PGs.

II. MEASUREMENT OF SERUM KS BY AN ELISA

The development of immunoassays to quantify the different constituents of cartilage PGs has led to a number of important advances by enabling researchers to address questions that would otherwise have remained unanswered. The advantages of using a highly sensitive and specific immunoassay for quantitative analysis are immediately obvious, but the dangers associated with equating measure of epitope recognized by an antibody with amount of protein or glycosaminoglycan present have often been ignored. Accurate quantification of CS- or KS-related epitopes is usually less difficult to achieve than that of some protein constituents. The HA binding region, for example, must first be denatured to prevent it from binding to HA, link protein, or other HA binding region molecules; such interactions have been shown to result in the masking of epitopes (27). Denaturation is easy to achieve, but the need to remove the denaturing agent, which can denature the antibody or suppress antigen-antibody interaction, is a complicating factor.

The enzyme-linked immunosorbent assay (ELISA) we have developed to quantify KS uses a mouse monoclonal antibody specific for a highly sulfated moiety on the KS chain (28,29). The ELISA is represented in diagramatic form in Fig. 3. Important technical aspects of this assay have been described elsewhere in more detail (10,19,30). Although the well-characterized 1/20/5-D-4 antibody (generously donated by Dr. Bruce Caterson, University of North Carolina, Chapel Hill, NC) was used in most studies performed thus far, we have shown that another monoclonal antibody (ET-4-A-4) with apparently identical specificity and similar high affinity yields identical results (29). Importantly, some anti-KS monoclonal

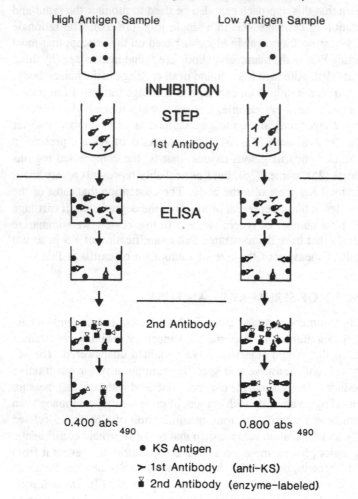

KS ELISA Assay with Inhibition Step

High Antigen Sample   Low Antigen Sample

INHIBITION
STEP
1st Antibody

ELISA

2nd Antibody

0.400 abs$_{490}$ 0.800 abs$_{490}$

● KS Antigen
➤ 1st Antibody   (anti-KS)
▯ 2nd Antibody (enzyme-labeled)

Figure 3 Competitive indirect ELISA for the quantification of keratan sulfate (KS). The KS antigen to be quantified competes with coated KS antigen for binding to the anti-KS antibody. The concentration of KS present in unknowns is calculated by comparing the absorbance value in each case to values generated from known concentrations of costal cartilage KS antigen treated in an identical fashion and run in parallel.

antibodies with similar specificity behave quite differently when used in the ELISA. Thus, the MZ15 anti-KS monoclonal antibody (21) (kindly donated by Dr. Tim Hardingham, Kennedy Institute of Rheumatology, London, England) shows a marked preference for binding to KS insolubilized on the coated plastic and recognizes only poorly the small KS-bearing peptidoglycans present in blood (30). In more recent studies the ELISA was used in a modified form after discovering that lowering the pH of the solutions containing the anti-KS and peroxidase-coupled antimouse antibodies from 7.0 to 5.3 greatly facilitated quantification of KS in rabbit serum (19). ELISAs performed at the lower pH yield steeper inhibition curves for both standards and unknowns, therefore increasing the ability to discriminate between concentrations of antigens that are not markedly different. The lower pH also helps to reduce the background noise. For these reasons, we now use phosphate-buffered saline at pH 5.3 in all our analyses of serum KS.

Mehmet et al. (28) showed that the 1/20/5-D-4 anti-KS antibody recognizes only segments that contain at least three repeating units of (sulfated galactose-sulfated acetylglucosamine). Such highly sulfated sequences have recently been

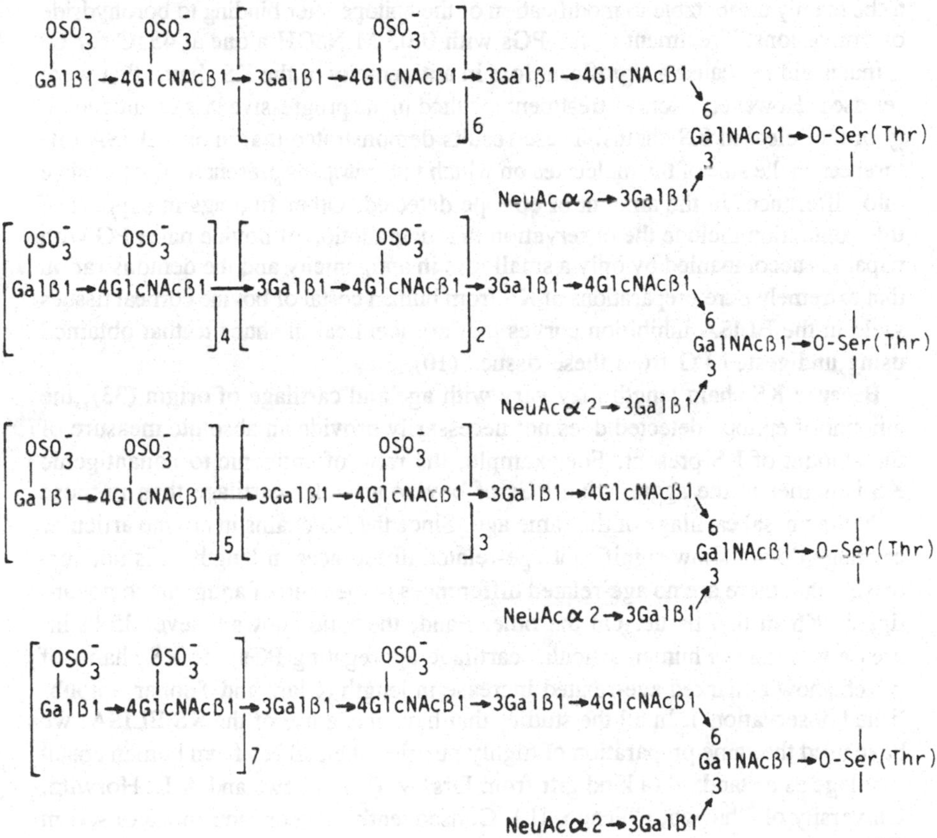

Figure 4 Structure of four keratan sulfate peptidoglycans isolated from nasal cartilage. (After Stuhlsatz et al., Ref. 31, reproduced with the permission of the Biochemical Society.)

shown to be located at the distal, nonreducing, end of the KS chains (Fig. 4) (31). Importantly, the epitope detected by the 1/20/5-D-4 and ET-4-A-4 antibodies is only present in the longest KS chains. These represent less than 15% of all the KS chains present in bovine nasal cartilage aggregating PGs. The ratio of antigenic to nonantigenic chains is identical in the CS-rich and KS-rich regions (32), suggesting the antigenic KS chains are distributed over the whole length of the polysaccharide-attachment region. Previous reports have pointed out that a decrease in the size of the KS-bearing molecule was accompanied by a decrease in the amount of epitope detected in most immunoassays using a variety of anti-KS antibodies, but this does not appear to be the case in our ELISA. Although decreases in antigenicity occur following the release of single KS chains by treatment of bovine nasal PGs with 0.05 M NaOH and 1 M sodium borohydride at 45 °C for 48 h, this was shown to be unrelated to the decrease in the size of the molecule on which the epitope was present. The loss of antigenicity was shown to be mainly attributable to modification of the epitope after binding to borohydride or borate ions. Treatment of the PGs with 0.05 M NaOH alone at 45 °C for 60 minutes did not cause a significant loss in antigenicity of the KS chains that were released. However, a longer treatment resulted in the progressive loss of antigenicity of the released KS chains. These results demonstrated that in our ELISA differences in the size of the molecules on which the epitope is present do not translate into differences in the amount of epitope detected. Other findings in support of this contention include the observation that degradation of bovine nasal PG with papain is accompanied by only a small loss in antigenicity and the demonstration that extremely pure preparations of KS from human costal or bovine corneal tissues yield in the ELISA inhibition curves that are identical in shape to that obtained using undigested PG from these tissues (10).

Because KS chain length may vary with age and cartilage of origin (33), the amount of epitope detected does not necessarily provide an absolute measure of the amount of KS present. For example, the ratio of antigenic to nonantigenic KS is higher in the aggregating PGs of bovine articular cartilage than in those of bovine nasal cartilage of the same age. Since the KS chains in bovine articular cartilage do not show significant age-related differences in length, it is not surprising that there are no age-related differences in the ratio of antigenic to nonantigenic KS in this tissue. On the other hand, the ratio shows a severalfold increase with age in human articular cartilage aggregating PGs, the KS chains of which show a marked age-related increase in length (Glant and Thonar, unpublished observations). In all the studies that have made use of the KS ELISA, we have used the same preparation of highly purified skeletal KS from human costal cartilage as a standard (a kind gift from Drs. M.B. Mathews and A.L. Horwitz, University of Chicago, Chicago, IL). Consequently, all concentrations of serum KS reported in these studies and in this review reflect equivalents of this international standard of KS.

Half-inhibition of binding of the antibody to the coated antigen occurs when the antibody is preincubated with 5 ng human costal cartilage KS per ml. This is equivalent to approximately 150 ng bovine steer nasal cartilage aggregating PG per ml or 35 ng bovine articular cartilage aggregating PG per ml (Fig. 5). Quantification in duplicate requires less than 100 μl human serum or plasma. Importantly, repeated freezing and thawing and long-term storage (up to 4 years) at −50 °C does not cause loss of antigenicity of serum KS.

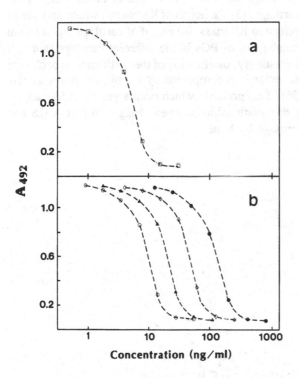

Figure 5 Inhibition curves generated using the keratan sulfate (KS) ELISA. The 1/20/5-D-4 monoclonal antibody specific for KS was incubated overnight in a test tube with an equal volume of a solution containing antigen. Subsequent incubations in the ELISA plate were performed as shown in Fig. 3. Concentration (ng/ml) refers to dry weight of KS or proteoglycan (PG) per ml. (a) international standard of purified KS from human costal cartilage. (b) purified KS from cornea (O), human articular cartilage D1 PG (▲), dogfish cartilage D1 PG (◊), and bovine nasal D1 PG (●). (Reproduced from Thonar et al., Ref. 10, with the permission of the American Rheumatism Association Education Foundation, Atlanta, Georgia.)

III. MEASURE OF THE RATE OF CATABOLISM OF CARTILAGE PROTEOGLYCANS IN NORMAL TURNOVER

Levels of serum KS vary predictably with age (34). They rise progressively during the first 4 years of life and then remain high until 12 years of age (Fig. 6). At this time, concentrations drop markedly and continue to decrease toward the concentrations found in adults. Similar age-related changes in levels of serum KS are found in most species (35). The marked age-related changes in growing children are the result of a multiplicity of changes, all of which contribute to a greater or lesser extent to the pattern of changes. These include progressive changes in (1) the ratio of cartilage mass to body weight or blood volume, (2) the concentration of KS in cartilage, (3) the length of KS chains, which may result in changes in the ratio of epitope to KS mass, (4) extent of cartilage replacement by bone, and (5) rates of catabolism of PGs in the different cartilage that will not be replaced by bone. Interestingly, ossification of the cartilaginous backbone of the rapidly growing deer antler is accompanied by a rapid but transient rise in the level of serum KS (36). This process, which occurs yearly, offers an excellent model for studying the relationship between changes in serum KS and replacement of growing cartilage by bone.

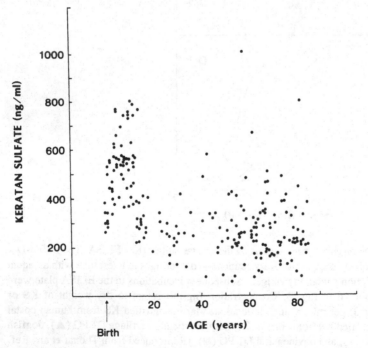

Figure 6 Age-related changes in the concentration of serum keratan sulfate (KS). The concentrations of KS were calculated using purified KS from human costal cartilage as the standard. The values thus represent equivalents of this international standard of KS.

In normal adults, the ratio of cartilage mass to blood volume, the concentration of KS in cartilage, and the size of the KS chains show only moderate changes with increasing age. The amount of cartilage PG catabolized during turnover is replaced via the synthesis and incorporation in the matrix of an equivalent amount of PG. It is worth nothing that the mass of KS present in normal human blood at any one time has been calculated to be about 0.75 mg. This corresponds to about 38 mg cartilage, that is, less than 0.05% of the total mass of cartilage in the body. Because the level of serum KS in normal adults does not fluctuate diurnally or from day to day (18), a single test result can be used as a measure of the metabolic activity of chondrocytes. It should also be noted that moderate (18) or even strenuous exercise, that is, running a marathon (Sweet and Thonar, unpublished observations), does not result in a significant change in levels of serum KS.

The level of serum KS varies, sometimes markedly, from individual to individual. The serum level of cartilage PG core protein epitope shows a similar variation and in children shows a strong correlation with the level of serum KS. This adds strength to the view that the level of serum KS can be used to obtain a good measure of the rate of cartilage PG catabolism. Because PG content remains relatively constant in normal cartilage, measurement of the level of serum KS can be used to obtain a measure of the basal rate of PG turnover in individuals without cartilage disease. This rate can be influenced by systemic factors acting either directly on the chondrocytes or indirectly via the production of other factors able to diffuse into the matrix. For example, we have recently observed that levels of serum KS of asthma patients dropped significantly after a 4 day burst of oral prednisolone (40–60 mg/day; KS levels = 275 ± 58 versus 214 ± 51 ng/ml) (37). The decrease was found to be progressive and to be maintained for at least 30 days after treatment had been stopped. In the same study, these researchers showed treatment of osteoarthritic patients for several weeks with piroxicam did not result in a significant change in the level of serum KS. These exciting findings suggest that measurement of the concentration of KS in blood can be used to study the effect of drugs and other agents on the metabolism of cartilage PGs in vivo.

IV. MEASURE OF CHANGES IN THE RATE OF CARTILAGE PROTEOGLYCAN CATABOLISM IN DISEASE

A. Macular Corneal Dystrophy

The corneal stromal matrix contains two distinct populations of PGs containing either KS or dermatan (chondroitin) sulfate. These PGs play important functional roles: they are located in the interfibrillar spaces and are thought to interact with the collagen fibrils and with each other to maintain the highly ordered matrix structure that provides optical transparency. Macular corneal dystrophy (MCD) is an inherited blinding disease characterized, in part, by the accumulation of opaque deposits containing an abnormal KS PG in the corneal stroma (38). The core protein of this PG is thought to be normal and was shown to be synthesized in normal amounts (39). Although the keratan chains in this PG are normally elongated, they are totally unsulfated (39). The most likely explanation for the lack of sulfation of the keratan chains is a deficiency in a sulfotransferase specific for keratan, a contention supported by the finding that the CS chains are normally sulfated or oversulfated (39).

A major breakthrough in the study of MCD came with the observation that individuals with this condition do not have normally sulfated KS in blood (10). Because the great majority of KS molecules in the circulation represent degradation products of cartilage PGs, this strongly suggested that all O-linked (skeletal) as well as N-linked (corneal) keratan chains in individuals with MCD are unsulfated. This contention is supported by a recent demonstration that the PGs in nasal cartilage and cornea from a patient with MCD are not recognized by an antibody specific for a sulfated moiety on KS chains (40). The findings are of great significance to our understanding of the metabolism of KS. First, they suggest a common sulfotransferase is involved in the sulfation of keratan chains in cartilage and cornea. Second, MCD is not associated with an increased incidence of cartilage disease and consequently it is likely that the presence of sulfate groups on the keratan chains is not essential for the functional properties of cartilage PGs.

Although, as described, most individuals with MCD have no detectable KS in serum, cartilage, and cornea, the observation that normally sulfated KS is present in some patients with the clinical diagnosis of MCD strongly suggests that the disease takes different forms. The type 1 variety, which is the most prevalent, is used to refer to individuals with no detectable sulfated KS in serum, cartilage, and cornea (38). It is clearly diagnosed by an absence of sulfated KS in blood and can thus most likely be diagnosed at birth before clinical symptoms develop. A smaller percentage of individuals have type 2 MCD: they cannot be distinguished clinically from patients with type 1 but have sulfated KS in serum and therefore probably normally sulfated KS in their cartilaginous tissues (38,41). It is worth noting that some of the individuals belonging to this group have normal KS levels but others have levels that are unusually low. It is thus possible that additional groupings may be necessary. Indeed, Edward et al. (41) have reported that an MCD patient with no sulfated KS in serum had detectable amounts of sulfated KS in cornea, although how much was not ascertained.

B. Glycosidase Deficiencies

Because KS and some polylactosamines contain identical long linear segments of the repeat disaccharide (galactose acetylglucosamine), a deficiency in a glycosidase used in the synthesis of a polylactosamine chain can result in an abnormality in KS synthesis. A patient with decreased amounts of membrane-bound forms of galactosyltransferase in microsomal membranes from mononuclear cells was recently found to have an abnormally low level of serum KS (42). Further, the shape of the inhibition curve produced by the serum KS was different from that obtained with normal sera. These results strongly suggest that the connective tissue cells in this patient are also affected by the galactosyltransferase defect and that the deficiency in synthesis of polylactosamines is generalized. As measurement of serum KS is relatively easy to perform, it could prove useful in diagnosing abnormalities in polylactosamine metabolism and in learning more, in each case, about the nature of the deficiency.

C. Abnormalities of Growth

The observation that growing children have elevated levels of serum KS is not unexpected since rapidly growing cartilage containing KS is constantly being eroded and replaced by bone. It is interesting that levels in growing children correlate positively with percentile height (34). Although the significance of this finding is unclear, it is consistent with the contention that the rate of growth is a function of the metabolic activities of chondrocytes. Recent findings have helped support an earlier contention (34) that children with short stature have serum KS levels lower than normal. Children with constitutional delay of maturity (below the 5th percentile for height but not growth hormone deficient) and children who arc growth hormone deficient appear to have abnormally low levels of serum KS (Table 1) (43). Importantly, administration of growth hormone to growth hormone-deficient children resulted in a significant rise in serum KS levels together with

Table 1 Concentrations of Serum Keratan Sulfate (KS) in a General Hospital Pediatric Population (GENPEDS) and in Children with Constitutional Delay of Maturity (CDM) or Growth Hormone Deficiency (GHD)

Group	ng KS per ml (mean $\pm$ SD)
GENPEDS (n = 33, age 8–11)	505 $\pm$ 126[a]
CDM (n = 14, age 8–11)	414 $\pm$ 118[a]
GHD (n = 9, age 8–15)	
Before GH	382 $\pm$ 137[b]
After GH	466 $\pm$ 116[b]

[a]The difference in the means of GENPEDS and children with CDM was statistically significant ($p < 0.05$, two-tailed unpaired t-test) (43).
[b]The difference in the means of the GHD children before and after treatment with growth hormone (GH) was also statistically significant ($p < 0.025$, paired one-tailed t-test) (43).

expected increases in annualized growth rate velocity and plasma levels of insulin-like growth factor 1 (IGF-1) (Table 1) (43). Although this study did not demonstrate that the rise in serum KS occurred relatively soon after the administration of growth hormone, it is possible that measurement of serum KS will prove useful in determining how much growth hormone is necessary in individual cases to induce a response by the chondrocytes in the growing cartilages.

D. Chemonucleolysis

The injection of chymopapain in a single rabbit knee joint causes a three to eightfold transient rise in the level of serum KS (Fig. 7A) (19). Levels rise within 30 minutes

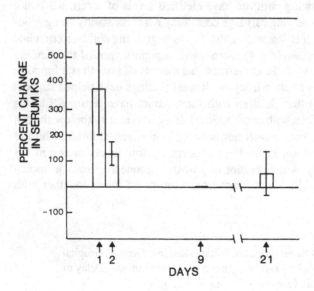

(A)

Figure 7 Changes in levels of serum keratan sulfate (KS) and in articular cartilage PG content following intra-articular injection of chymopapain in a rabbit knee joint. Serum keratan sulfate is expressed as percentage change at various times after the injection (A). The results represent the mean ± SD change in six rabbits (days 1 and 2), four rabbits (day 9), and two rabbits (day 21), respectively. The articular cartilage was taken from the central weight-bearing region of the medial femoral condyle of an injected knee 48 h (B) and 9 days (C) after injection and of a contralateral, noninjected knee (D) 48 h after injection. Single arrows show the articular surface; double arrows show the tidemark. S, subchondral bone. Safranin O-fast green was used as the strain. (Modified from Williams et al., Ref. 19, and reproduced with the permission of the American Rheumatism Association Educational Foundation, Atlanta, GA.)

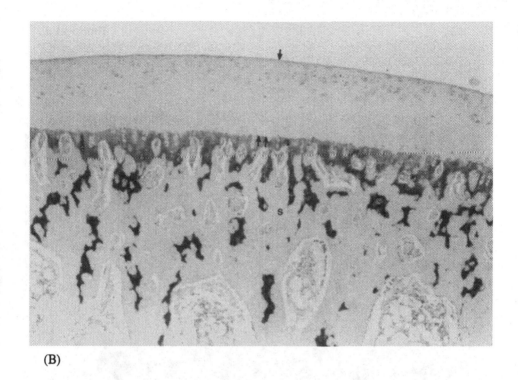

(B)

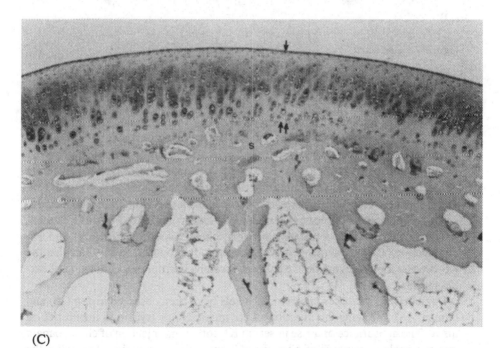

(C)

Figure 7 *Continued*

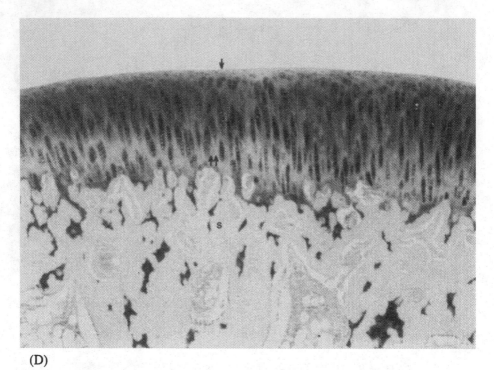

(D)

Figure 7 *Continued*

and remain at a plateau for 24–48 h before returning to preinjection values. In contrast, levels did not change in animals injected intra-articularly with saline or intramuscularly with the enzyme. The articular cartilage in the knee injected with chymopapain shows a marked loss in PG content 48 h after the injection (Fig. 7B). Replenishment of the PGs begins soon thereafter and is evident by day 9 when serum levels have returned to baseline levels (Fig. 7C). Importantly, articular cartilage in the contralateral knee is totally unaffected by this treatment (Fig. 7D). The direct correlation between change in serum KS level and PG degradation but not resynthesis is worth noting. It supports the postulate that the KS-bearing molecules are derived almost exclusively from the degradation of cartilage PGs.

Similar large increases in serum KS levels have been observed in dog (20) and human (18) following the injection of chymopapain or trypsin in intervertebral disks. The appearance of a rise in serum KS following injection of chymopapain into the nucleus pulposus of a herniated human intervertebral disk provides the clinician with direct evidence that the enzyme was active and injected in the correct place and that the PGs in the tissue have been degraded.

E. Cartilage Tumors

The serum KS levels of 24 adult patients bearing cartilage tumors were higher than in age- and sex-matched controls (44). This suggested some of the KS-bearing fragments were derived from the degradation of PGs in the tumors. This is supported by the observation that in 9 of 10 patients levels exhibited a significant decrease following removal of the tumor. As expected, this decrease was highest in patients with benign tumors containing relatively large amounts of KS and a well-differentiated cartilage matrix and lowest in patients with least differentiated tumors containing little KS. Individual differences in the rates of metabolism of PGs in normal cartilage may make it difficult to use serum KS measurements to diagnose the presence of a tumor or ascertain tumor grade, but sequential measurements in such patients may be very useful in monitoring secondary growth of cartilage tumors following primary excision. Alternatively, new monoclonal antibodies directed against other epitopes on the KS chains may allow more specific quantification of tumor-derived KS as opposed to normal cartilage-derived KS.

F. Osteoarthritis

We have obtained evidence that measurements of serum KS provide important new information in the evaluation of patients with osteoarthritis (OA). Sweet et al. (45) elected to study patients with hypertrophic OA, a definite subset of OA characterized by joint narrowing, subchondral sclerosis, and marginal osteophyte formation. Serum levels of KS were considerably higher in 31 patients with this form of OA than in 41 adults without joint disease (OA: mean $\pm$ SD = 475 $\pm$ 178 ng KS per ml; normals: mean $\pm$ SD = 261 $\pm$ 51 ng KS per ml; Fig. 8). Of the patients with OA, 77%, but only 12% of control subjects, had serum levels that were more than 1 SD above the mean of the control group. There were no differences with respect to sex, but levels were slightly although not significantly higher in patients who had received nonsteroidal anti-inflammatory drugs or aspirin than in patients who had received no antirheumatic medication at all. There was a significant linear relationship between serum levels and joint score ($r = 0.370$, $p = 0.041$). However, this relationship was not very strong since only 13.7% of the variation in KS is explained by variation in joint score. These findings strongly suggest that patients with well-characterized hypertrophic OA have considerably higher rates of cartilage PG catabolism than control subjects.

It is important to note that the mean levels of circulating KS in the group of patients studied by Sweet and his collaborators (45) were considerably higher (475 ng KS per ml) than those previously reported for two other groups of randomly selected individuals with OA who were attending an outpatient clinic

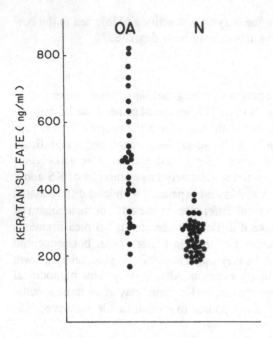

Figure 8 Concentration of keratan sulfate (KS) in the serum of patients with hypertrophic osteoarthritis (OA) and of normal controls (N). (Reproduced from Sweet et al., Ref. 45, with the permission of the American Rheumatism Association Educational Foundation, Atlanta, GA.)

[357 ng KS per ml (10) and 381 ng KS per ml (46)]. Because OA is heterogeneous in regard to etiology, severity of degenerative change, and number of joints involved (47), patients with hypertrophic OA can be considered to represent a definite subset of OA (48). Most of the patients studied by Sweet and his collaborators had multiple joint involvement and Heberden's nodes; the incidence of polyarticular OA was thus very high in this selected group (45).

A recent study of levels of serum KS in 125 patients with knee OA (49,50) is worth noting. Levels were significantly higher in males ($n = 35$, KS = 456 $\pm$ 135 ng/ml) than in females ($n = 90$, KS = 368 $\pm$ 74 ng/ml). Because of the marked sex-related differences, the relationship between KS levels and clinical parameters of OA were evaluated separately in males and females. In females, levels correlated positively with the number of symptomatic joints ($p = 0.04$), Heberden's nodes ($p = 0.04$), and hip symptoms ($p = 0.03$), all features of generalized arthritis. The relationship between serum KS levels and clinical signs of polyarticular disease was less evident in the smaller group of males. This is an exciting finding for it supports the contention that OA of the knee follows a different course in males and females.

The results of all studies performed thus far (10,45,46,50,51) suggest that a single measurement of the concentration of serum KS is not very useful in assessing cartilage destruction in the joints of patients with OA. This is not surprising since KS present in serum was not only derived from cartilaginous structures in the small number of affected joints from all the other cartilage in the body as well. A recent study has shown that cartilage in joints (including intervertebral disk and menisci) constitutes only about 25% of the total mass of cartilage in the immature dog (52). Because this percentage was obtained after exclusion of growth cartilage, it is probably a close approximation of the contribution of joint cartilage in the adult. Consequently, it is likely that increased levels of serum KS in patients with polyarticular OA reflect higher catabolic or metabolic activities in the majority of the cartilaginous tissues rather than in the one or few joints involved. The contention that a generalized disorder of cartilage PG metabolism is present in these individuals is also supported by the observation that 6 months following removal of a large degenerate hip joint serum levels in patients with hypertrophic OA remained markedly elevated (mean $\pm$ SD = 446 $\pm$ 165 ng KS per ml).

Additional support for the concept of a systemic or generalized increase in the rate of metabolism of cartilage PGs in OA comes from recent studies of experimentally-induced OA in the dog (53,54). Transection of the anterior cruciate ligament induced a rapid increase in the concentration of serum KS. This reached a maximum within 2–4 weeks (mean = 186% of presurgery level), decreased slightly thereafter, but remained elevated until 12 weeks postsurgery (mean = 128% of presurgery levels) (54). In contrast, sham operation was not accompanied by any change in the level of serum KS at any time after surgery. Similar increases in serum KS after transection of the anterior cruciate ligament were observed in a separate study (53). Since the PG content of the articular cartilage in the operated knee did not change during this time, the increase in the rate of degradation of PGs was probably accompanied by a corresponding increase in the rate of PG synthesis (54). Although this increase in metabolic activities of chondrocytes could have been restricted to the cartilage in the operated knee, the magnitude of the rise in serum KS suggests it was more systemic or generalized in nature (53). Although the mechanisms involved in this stimulation of PG turnover are unclear, it is possible that factors that stimulate cartilage PG turnover systemically are released into the body fluids from articular cartilage, bone, or synovium of the unstable knee in this canine model of OA.

Abnormally high rates of cartilage PG metabolism would, if sustained for a long time, cause an accelerated accumulation of PG fragments in the extracellular matrix. Fragments containing an intact HA-binding region but few glycosaminoglycan chains have been found to accumulate with age in the articular cartilage of human adults who do not exhibit OA changes. It is tempting to postulate that high concentrations of these nonfunctional PG fragments, which are poor in glycosaminoglycans, adversely affect the functional properties of maximally loaded cartilages. Because OA, a common disorder of human adults, may remain asymptomatic for a long time, measurements of serum KS may help identify individuals at risk or those with early degenerative changes. There appear to be no significant age-related changes in serum levels in adult life, but individual variations clearly exist at any one age (10). Of normal adults aged 23–40 years, 6% have been shown to have serum KS levels greater than 350 ng/ml (46) and it is possible that these individuals with increased PG catabolism or turnover are at an increased risk of developing osteoarthritic changes in several joints. Prospective, long-term follow-up of individuals with high and low serum levels will help test this exciting hypothesis.

G. Rheumatoid Arthritis

Seibel and his collaborators (51) reported that adults with RA have lower serum KS levels than patients with OA or healthy control individuals and concluded that levels of serum KS in patients with RA are abnormally low. Recent findings from our laboratory support the contention that levels are higher in patients with OA than RA but find little evidence to suggest that they are not at least as high as serum KS levels of normal controls (RA: $n = 40$, 308 ± 86 ng KS per ml; OA: $n = 40$, 374 ± 107 ng KS per ml; controls: $n = 45$, 251 ± 78 ng KS per ml). The reasons for the differences between those two studies are unclear. They may have originated from slight differences in the ELISAs that were used but more likely reflect differences in the selection of patients and apparently healthy individuals.

Growing children (aged 5–12) with juvenile rheumatoid arthritis (JRA) have significantly lower levels of serum KS than age-matched children without rheumatic disease (419 ± 100 versus 556 ± 129 ng KS per ml) (55). Although the mean serum KS value was even lower in JRA children on prednisone (399 ± 83 ng KS per ml), treatment with this drug, which has been shown to cause a significant decrease in the levels of serum KS in adults without joint disease (37), did not by itself explain the lower levels in the JRA group as a whole (56). The observation that serum KS levels in children with JRA are as low as in children with constitutional growth delay (43) is worth noting for children in both groups are of shorter stature than normal. This finding thus reinforces the view that the level of serum KS in children provides a measure of rate of growth.

The absence of a significant rise in serum KS in children or adults with inflammatory joint disease and accompanying cartilage degradation suggests that a single measurement of the level of serum KS is not very useful in assessing PG degradation in inflamed joints. The results shown in Fig. 9 indicate that serum

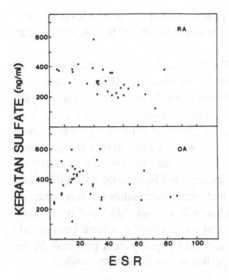

Figure 9 Relationship between serum levels of keratan sulfate (KS) and erythrocyte sedimentation rates (ESR) in patients with rheumatoid arthritis (RA) and osteoarthritis (OA). ESR values represent mm/h.

KS levels in RA appear to be inversely related to the height of the inflammatory response. Interestingly, this relationship was not as evident in OA patients, most of whom had erythrocyte sedimentation rates below 30 mm/h. The association between severe inflammation and decreased level of serum KS is not restricted to inflammatory joint diseases since abnormally low levels of serum KS are also found in patients with acute, nonarthritic infections (51). It is possible products of the inflammatory cascade may be able to induce directly or indirectly, that is via the synthesis of other messengers, a systemic decrease in the rate of catabolism or metabolism of cartilage PGs. At this stage, however, one cannot rule out the possibility that the apparent decrease in serum KS level is caused by an increase in the rate of elimination of KS-bearing fragments from the body fluids (51,57), that is, increase in synovial permeability, increase in rate of clearance by lymphatic drainage, and increase in the uptake of KS-bearing fragments by the reticuloendothelial system.

V. CONCLUSION

Measurements of the concentration of fragments of PGs in body fluids provide important information about the catabolism of PGs in cartilage. Whereas the concentration of cartilage PG-related epitopes in fluids in contact with the tissue can be used to assess the degradation of PGs in a single joint, the level of such epitopes in blood provides a measure of the average rate of turnover of all the cartilage PGs in the body.

Measurement of the concentration of KS in blood has already been shown to be extremely useful in diagnosing some conditions, such as MCD, and in assessing underlying metabolic abnormalities of cartilage PG catabolism or metabolism in disease, such as polyarticular OA. Preliminary findings have shown that it also holds great promise as a tool to monitor the effect of drugs or growth factors on the rate of catabolism of cartilage PGs. It is already evident that this approach can provide important information about many questions that would otherwise have remained unanswered. Insightful questions will have to be posed if we are to achieve success in using blood markers to detect abnormalities or assess changes in cartilage PG metabolism. Future studies will undoubtedly lead to a better understanding of the significance of some of the findings that have proved difficult to interpret. It is hoped they will also build upon recent progress in the field by testing some of the exciting hypotheses that have been made.

ACKNOWLEDGMENTS

This work was supported in part by the William Noble Lane Foundation, grants AG-04736 and 1-P50-AR-39239 from the NIH, and grants from the Rush University Committee on Research, the Illinois Chapter of the Arthritis Foundation, and the South African Medical Research Council.

REFERENCES

1. Mayne, R., and Irwin, M.H. (1986). Collagen types in cartilage. In: Articular Cartilage Biochemistry. Kuettner, K.E., Schleyerbach, R., and Hascall, V.C., eds. Raven Press, New York, pp. 23–35.
2. Sheehan, J.K., Ratcliffe, A., Oates, K., and Hardingham, T.E. (1987). The detection of substructures within proteoglycan molecules. Electron-microscopic immuno-localization with the use of protein A-gold. Biochem. J. 247:267–276.
3. Lohmander, S. (1976). Proteoglycans of hyaline cartilage. Structure, turnover and role in cartilage mineralization. Ph.D. thesis, Karolinska Institute, Stockholm, Sweden.
4. Morales, T.I., and Hascall, V.C. (1988). Correlated metabolism of proteoglycans and hyaluronic acid in bovine cartilage organ cultures. J. Biol. Chem. 263:3632–3638.
5. Woessner, J.F., Jr., and Selzer, M.G. (1984). Two latent metalloproteinases of human articular cartilage that digest proteoglycan. J. Biol. Chem. 259:3633–3638.
6. Roughley, P.J., Poole, A.R., Campbell, I.K., and Mort, J.S. (1986). The proteolytic generation of hyaluronic acid-binding regions derived from the proteoglycans of human articular cartilage as a consequence of aging. Orthop. Res. Soc. Trans. 11:209.
7. Bayliss, M.T., Holmes, M.W.A., and Muir, H. (1989). Age-related changes in the stoichiometry of binding region, link protein and hyaluronic acid in human articular cartilage. Orthop. Res. Soc. Trans. 14:32.

8. Kimura, J.H., Osdoby, P., Caplan, A.I., and Hascall,V.C. (1978). Electron microscopic and biochemical studies of proteoglycan polydispersity in chick limb bud chondrocyte cultures. J. Biol.Chem. 253:4721–4729.

9. Barone-Varelas, J., Schnitzer, T.J., Meng, Q., and Thonar, E.J.-M.A. (1989). Effect of IGF-I on the metabolism of proteoglycans in immature calf and adult steer articular cartilage. Orthop. Res. Soc. Trans. 14:257.

10. Thonar, E.J.-M.A., Lenz, M.E., Klintworth, G.K., Caterson, B., Pachman, L.M., Glickman, P., Katz, R., Huff, J., and Kuettner, K.E. (1985). Quantification of keratan sulfate in blood as a marker of cartilage catabolism. Arthritis Rheum. 28:1367–1376.

11. Maldonado, B.A., Williams, J.M., Otten, L.M., Flannery, M., Kuettner, K.E., and Thonar, E.J.-M.A. (1989). Differences in the rate of clearance of different KS-bearing molecules injected intravenously in rabbits. Orthop. Res. Soc. Trans. 14:161.

12. Schlepper-Schafer, J., Hulsmann, D., Djovkar, A., Meyer, H.E., Herbertz, L., Kolb, H., and Kolb-Bachofen, V. (1986). Endocytosis via galactose receptors in vivo. Ligand size directs uptake by hepatocytes and/or liver macrophages. Exp. Cell Res. 165:494–506.

13. Witter, J., Roughley, P.J., Webber, C., Roberts, N., Keystone, E., and Poole, A.R. (1987). The immunologic detection and characterization of cartilage proteoglycan degradation products in synvoial fluids of patients with arthritis. Arthritis Rheum. 30:519–529.

14. Saxne, T., Heinegard, D., and Wollheim, F.A. (1987). Cartilage proteoglycans in synovial fluid and blood in inflammatory joint disease. Relation to systemic treatment. Arthritis Rheum. 30:972–979.

15. Saxne, T., Heinegard, D., and Wollheim, F.A. (1986). Therapeutic effects on cartilage metabolism in arthritis as measured by release of proteoglycan structures into the synovial fluid. Ann. Rheum. Dis. 45:491–497.

16. Saxne, T. (1989). Molecular markers for joint disease. In: Clinical Impact of Bone and Connective Tissue Markers. Lindh, E., and Thorell, J.I., eds. Academic Press, London, pp. 323–326.

17. Lohmander, L.S. (1988). Proteoglycans of joint cartilage. Structure, function, turnover and role as markers of joint disease. Bailliere's Clin. Rheumatol. 2:37–62.

18. Block, J.A., Schnitzer, T.J., Andersson, G.B.J., Lenz, M.E., Jefferey, R., McNeill, T.W., and Thonar, E.J.-M.A. (1989). The effect of chemonucleolysis on serum keratan sulfate levels in humans. Arthritis Rheum. 32:100–105.

19. Williams, J.M., Downey, C., and Thonar, E.J.-M.A. (1988). Increase in levels of serum keratan sulfate following cartilage proteoglycan degradation in the rabbit knee joint. Arthritis Rheum. 31:557–560. (1988).

20. Oegema, T.R., Swedenburg, S.M., Bradford, D.S., and Thonar, E.J.-M.A. (1988). Levels of keratan sulfate-bearing fragments rise predictably following chemonucleolysis of dog intervertebral discs with chymopapain. Spine 13:707–711.

21. Zanetti, M., Ratcliffe, A., and Watt, F.M.J. (1985). Two subpopulations of differentiated chondrocytes identified with a monoclonal antibody to keratan sulfate. Cell Biol. 101:53–59.

22. Williams, J.M., Katz, R.J., Childs, D., Lenz, M.E., and Thonar, E.J.-M.A. (1988). Keratan sulfate content in the superficial and deep layers of osteophytic and non-fibrillated human articular cartilage in osteoarthritis.Calcif. Tissue Int. 42:162–166.

23. Aydelotte, M.B., Thonar, E.J.-M.A., Lenz, M.E., Schumacher, B.L., and Kuettner, K.E. (1989). Differences in synthesis of keratan sulfate by subpopulations of cultured bovine articular chondrocytes. Orthop. Res. Soc. Trans.14:83.

24. Vogel, K.G., and Thonar, E.J.-M.A. (1988). Keratan sulfate is a component of proteoglycans in the compressed region of bovine flexor tendon, J. Orthop. Res. 6:434–442.

25. Baker, J.R. (1989). Studies of keratan sulphates of aorta and cartilage utilizing MAb 6D2. In: Keratan Sulphate. Chemistry, Biology, Chemical Pathology. Greiling, H., and Scott, J.E., eds. Biochemical Society, London, pp. 30–38.

26. Meek, K.M., Quantock, A.J., Elliott, G.F., Ridgway, A.A.E., Tullo, A., Bron, A.J., and Thonar, E.J.-M.A. (1989). Macular corneal dystrophy: The macromolecular structure of the stroma observed using electron microscopy and synchroton x-ray diffraction. Exp. Eye Res. 49:941–958.

27. Thonar, E.J.-M.A., Kimura, J.H., Hascall, V.C., and Poole, A.R. (1982). Enzyme-linked immunosorbent assay analyses of the hyaluronate binding region and the link protein of proteoglycan aggregate. J. Biol. Chem. 257:14173–14180.

28. Mehmet, H., Scudder, P., Tang, P.W., Hounsell, E.F., Caterson, B., and Feizi, T. (1986). The antigenic determinants recognized by three monoclonal antibodies to keratan sulfate involve sulfate hepta- or larger oligosaccharides of the poly (N-acetyllactosamine) series. Eur. J. Biochem. 157:385–391.

29. Thonar, E.J.-M.A., Meyer, R.F., Dennis, R.F., Lenz, M.E., Maldonado, B., Hassell, J.R., Hewitt, A.T., Stark, W.J., Stock, E.L., Kuettner, K.E., and Klintworth, G.K. (1986). Absence of normal keratan sulfate in the blood of patients with macular corneal dystrophy. Am. J. Ophthal. 102:561–569.

30. Thonar, E.J.-M.A., Lenz, M.E., Maldonado, B., Otten, L., Glant, T., and Kuettner, K.E. Measurement of antigenic keratan sulfate by an enzyme-linked immunosorbent assay (ELISA). In: Methods Used in Research on Cartilaginous Tissues. Maroudas, A., and Kuettner, K.E., eds. Academic Press, New York, in press.

31. Stuhlsatz, H.W., Keller, R., Becker, G., Oeben, M., Lennartz, L., Fischer, D.C., and Greiling, H. (1989). Structure of keratan sulphate proteoglycans: Core proteins, linkage regions, carbohydrate chains. In: Keratan Sulphate. Chemistry, Biology, Chemical Pathology. Greiling, H., and Scott, J.E., eds. Biochemical Society, London, pp. 1–15.

32. Maldonado, B., Kuettner, K.E., and Thonar, E.J.-M.A. (1988). Characterization of antigenic keratan sulfate in the KS-rich and CS-rich regions of cartilage proteoglycans. Orthop. Res. Soc. Trans. 13:44.

33. Thonar, E.J.-M.A., and Kuettner, K.E. (1987). Biochemical basis of age-related changes in proteoglycans. In: The Biology of the Extracellular Matrix: Biology of Proteoglycans. Wight, T.N., and Mecham, R.P. eds. Academic Press, New York, pp. 211–246.

34. Thonar, E.J.-M.A., Pachman, L.M., Lenz, M.E., Hayford, J., Lynch, P., and Kuettner, K.E. (1988). Age related changes in the concentration of serum keratan sulphate in children. J. Clin. Chem. Clin. Biochem. 26:57–63.

35. Thonar, E.J.-M.A., Klintworth, G.K., Meyer, R.F., Lenz, M.E., and Kuettner, K.E. (1986). Absence of normal skeletal keratan sulfate in some articular cartilages. Orthop. Res. Soc. Trans. 11:151.

36. Dinsmore, C.E., Goss, R.J., Lenz, M.E., and Thonar, E.J.-M.A. (1986). Correlations between phases of deer antler regeneration and levels of serum keratan sulfate. Calcif. Tissue Int. 39:244–247.

37. Campion, G., Schnitzer, T., Zeitz, H., and Thonar, E. (1989). The effect of oral administration of prednisolone and of the non-steroidal anti-inflammatory drug (NSAID) piroxicam on serum keratan sulfate (KS). Arthritis Rheum. 32(4):S105.

38. Yang, C.J., SundarRaj, N., Thonar, E.J.-M.A., and Klintworth, G.K. (1988). Immunohistochemical evidence of heterogeneity in macular corneal dystrophy. Am. J. Ophthalmol. 106:65–71.

39. Hassell, J.R., SundarRaj, N., Cintron, C., Midura, R., and Hascall, V.C. (1989). Alterations in the synthesis of keratan sulphate proteoglycan in corneal wound healing and in macular corneal dystrophy. In: Keratan Sulphate. Chemistry, Biology, Chemical Pathology. Greiling, H., and Scott, J.E., eds. Biochemical Society, London, pp. 215–225.

40. Thonar, E.J.-M.A., Edward. D.P., Srinivasan, M., Lenz, M.E., and Tso, O.M. (1990). Absence of keratan sulfate in the serum, cartilage and corneal proteoglycans of a patient with type 1 macular corneal dystrophy. Orthop. Res. Soc. Trans. 15:333.

41. Edward, D.P., Yue, B.Y.J.T., Sugar, J., Thonar, E.J.-M.A., SundarRaj, N., Stock, E.L., and Tso, M.O.M. (1988). Heterogeneity in macular corneal dystrophy. Arch. Ophthalmol. 106:1579–1583.

42. Fukuda, M.N., Masri, K.A., Dell, A., Thonar, E.J.-M.A., Klier, G., and Lowenthal, R.M. (1989). Defective glycosylation of erythrocyte membrane glycoconjugates in a variant of congenital dyserythropoietic anemia type II: Association of low level of membrane-bound form of galactosyl transferase. Blood 73:1331–1339.

43. Pachman, L.M., Green, O.C., Lenz, M.E., Hayford, J., and Thonar, E.J.-M.A. (1990). Increase in serum concentration of keratan sulfate following treatment of growth hormone deficiency with growth hormone. J. Ped. 116:400–403.

44. Kliner, D.J., Gorski, J.P., and Thonar, E.J.-M.A. (1987). Keratan sulfate levels in sera of patients bearing cartilage tumors. Cancer 59:1931–1935.

45. Sweet, M.B.E., Coelho, A., Schnitzler, C.M., Schnitzer, T.J., Lenz, M.E., Jakim, I., Kuettner, K.E., and Thonar, E.J.-M.A. (1988). Serum keratan sulfate levels in osteoarthritis patients. Arthritis Rheum. 31:648–652.

46. Thonar, E.J.-M.A., Schnitzer, T.J., and Kuettner, E.K. (1987). Quantification of keratan sulfate in blood as a marker of cartilage catabolism. J. Rheumatol 14 (Suppl. 14):23–24.

47. Sokoloff, L., and Hough, A.J. (1985). Pathology of osteoarthritis. In: Arthritis and Related Conditions. McCarty, D.J., ed. Lea & Febiger, Philadelphia, pp. 1377–1399.

48. Peyron, J.G. (1986). Osteoarthritis: The epidemiologic viewpoint. Clin. Orthop. 213:13–19.

49. Campion, G.V., McCrae, F., Schnitzer, T.J., Watt, I., Dieppe, P.A., and Thonar, E.J. (1989). Do serum levels of keratan sulfate help us with the heterogeneity of osteoarthritis? Orthop. Res. Soc. Trans. 14:162.

50. Campion, G., McCrae, F., Schnitzer, T., Lenz, M., Dieppe, P., and Thonar, E. (1989). Serum and synovial fluid (SF) keratan sulfate (KS) levels in osteoarthritis (OA) of the knee. Arthritis Rheum. 32(4):S105.

51. Seibel, M.J., Towbin, H., Braun, D.G., Kiefer, B., Muller, W., and Paulsson, M. (1989). Serum keratan sulphate in rheumatoid arthritis and different clinical subsets of osteoarthritis. In: Keratan Sulphate: Chemistry, Biology, Chemical Pathology. Greiling, H., and Scott, J.E., eds. Biochemical Society, London, pp. 191–198.

52. Attencia, L.J., McDevitt, C.A., Nile, W.B., and Sokoloff, L. (1989). Cartilage content of an immature dog. Connect. Tissue Res. 18:235–242.

53. Brandt, K.D., and Thonar, E.J.-M.A. (1989). Lack of association between serum keratan sulfate concentrations and cartilage changes of osteoarthritis after transection of the anterior cruciate ligament in the dog. Arthritis Rheum. 32:647–651.

54. Manicourt, D.H., Pita, J.C., Thonar, E.J.-M.A., and Howell, D.S. (1989). A decrease in the size of proteoglycan aggregates is an early event in experimental canine osteoarthritis. Orthop. Res. Soc. Trans. 14:503.

55. Pachman, L.M., Lenz, M.E., Caterson, B., Jacobitz, J., Kuettner, K.E., and Thonar, E.J.-M.A. (1985). Serum keratan sulfate (KS) concentrations are lower in children with juvenile rheumatoid arthritis (JRA) than in children without rheumatic disease. Arthritis Rheum. 28(4):S99.

56. Pachman, L.M., Hayford, J., Lynch, P.A., Jacobitz, J., Lenz, M.E., Kuettner, K.E., and Thonar, E.J.-M.A. (1987). Comparisons of serum levels of keratan sulfate (KS) with height in the general outpatients pediatric hospital population (GENPEDS), constitutional growth delay (GD) and in juvenile rheumatoid arthritis (JRA). Arthritis Rheum. 30:S20.

57. Wallis, W.J., Simkin, P.A., and Nelp, W.B. (1987). Protein traffic in human synovial effusions. Arthritis Rheum. 30:57–63.

19

Cross-Reactive Idiotypes of Rheumatoid Factors in Arthritis and Related Diseases

Pojen P. Chen* and Dennis A. Carson*
Scripps Clinic and Research Foundation, La Jolla, California

I. INTRODUCTION

Rheumatoid factors (RF) are antibodies against IgG. High titers of such autoantibodies are found in most patients with rheumatoid arthritis (RA). Since RFs are reviewed extensively in the preceding chapter, we restrict ourself mainly to the most current studies on the cross-reactive idiotypes (CRI) of RFs. Interested readers are referred to our two recent reviews for details (1,2).

Idiotypes are the uniquee antigenic determinants of antibody molecules. They are defined serologically by anti-idiotypic antibodies or anti-idiotypes. The study of idiotypes has greatly advanced our understanding of antibody structures and immunoglobulin (Ig) genetics. Particularly, it has been established that hypervariable regions or complementarity-determining regions (CDR) are the structural correlates of many idiotypic determinants (3,4). Moreover, although an idiotype was originally defined as the unique antigen of an antibody molecule, it was soon demonstrated that some idiotypes were shared by antibodies with the same and/or different antigen specificities and were termed cross-reactive idiotypes (CRIs). Importantly, analyses of CRIs have revealed that some CRIs are phenotypic markers of Ig variable region (V) genes, and individual or private idiotypes are markers for Ig genes that have diversified somatically (4). Thus,

---

*Present affiliation: University of California, San Diego, La Jolla, California.

anti-CRI antibodies have been very useful tools for delineating the genetic basis for antibody responses.

In addition, recognizing the idiotypes could represent potential targets for internal immune regulatory mechanisms, Lindemann and Jerne independently proposed the concept of an immunologic network (5,6). This elegant theory has guided immunologists and research clinicians in their thinking and experimentation. Elements of the immune network have been shown to function in vivo, and anti-idiotypes have been used successfully in treating some B cell malignancies.

II. CROSS-REACTIVE IDIOTYPES OF MONOCLONAL RHEUMATOID FACTORS

Although RFs were originally discovered in patients with RA, they have also been associated with some IgM paraproteins from patients with cryoglobulinemia and chronic lymphocytic leukemia (CLL) of B cell type (7–10). The cryoglobulins have been classified into three groups (9). Type I cryoglobulins consist of only monolconal Ig molecules and are found mainly in patients with lymphoproliferative diseases, such as multiple myeloma and Waldenström's macroglobulinemia. Type II cryoglobulins are made of a monoclonal antibody together with polyclonal IgG. Type III cryoglobulins are composed of polyclonal antibodies and polyclonal Ig (or non-Ig) molecules. Based on their composition, type II and III cryoglobulins are often called "mixed cryoglobulins." Most type II cryoglobulins contain monoclonal IgM RFs and polyclonal IgG and occur frequently in patients with Waldenström's macroglobulinemia, chronic active hepatitis, or Sjögren's syndrome (SS). In contrast, type III cryoglobulins are often associated with autoimmune conditions. Because of the common occurrence of monoclonal RFs from patients with the type II cryoglobulinemia, they have been used extensively in delineating the idiotypes and molecular genetics of human RFs.

A. The Wa, PSL2, PSL3,, an 17.109 CRIs and Humkv325 Germline Gene

In 1973, Kunkel et al. used classic rabbit polyclonal anti-idiotypes to describe two major CRIs, termed Wa and Po (11). They were expressed on 60 and 20% of monoclonal IgM RFs, respectively. Interestingly, the same authors noted that all Wa-positive RFs contained light chains of the kIIIb sub-subgroup, which constitutes only about 13% of total Ig x chains (12). Subsequently, Capra and coworkers showed that two Wa-positive RFs shared similar amino acid sequences in their light-chain variable regions, and two Po-positive RFs were similar in their heavy-chain variable regions (13,14). These data implied that the Wa CRI was associated mainly with the RF light chains and the Po CRI was dependent on the RF heavy chains.

To define the structural and genetic basis of the Wa CRI, we synthesized a peptide (PSL2) corresponding to the second hypervariable (region/CDR) of the

RF Sie light chain and used this peptide to immunize rabbits. The resulting anti-PSL2 antiserum bound specifically to the RF Sie light chains and to the light chains of all Wa-positive RFs tested (15,16). Similarly, antibodies were generated against the third hypervariable (region/CDR) of the Sie light chain (PSL3), and the resulting anti-PSL3 antiserum reacted with most of the Wa-positive RF light chains examined (17). Combined, these data showed that most, if not all, Wa-positive light chains were very similar and indicated that these light chains might derive from a single x light chain V (Vk) gene.

In addition to these two rabbit polyclonal peptide-induced anti-CRI antibodies, we generated a murine monoclonal anti-CRI (17.109) from a mouse immunized with the same Wa-positive RF, Sie (18). The 17.109 antibody reacted efficiently with both intact RF molecules and their separated light chains and inhibited the binding of RFs to human IgG Fc fragments, indicating that the 17.109 CRI depends on the light chains in the region of the antigen binding site. It reacted with about 30–50% of monoclonal IgM RFs, including 11/14 Wa-positive monoclonal RFs, but not with any of two Po-positive monoclonal RFs. All 17.109-positive RFs were positive for the PSL2-CRI (2,19,20).

Subsequently we compared the reported light-chain amino acid sequences of RFs that were reactive with both anti-peptide antibodies and found these sequences were indeed very similar, suggesting strongly that such RF light chains were encoded by a single Vk gene, designated Vk(RF) (16). To isolate this putative gene, we screened two human DNA libraries three times with three different probes, namely NG9/3, Humkv301, and Humkv305. Eventually, the putative Vk(RF) gene was isolated from a human placenta and was designated Humkv325 (2,21–23). The deduced amino acid sequence of Humkv325 is identical to four RF light-chain sequences and differs from the other eight sequences by one to seven amino acid residues only (2,24,25). These data thus clearly demonstrated that RF light chains from many unrelated individuals are encoded by a single Vk gene with no or limited somatic mutations and implied that Humkv325 exists widely in humans.

Is Humkv325 the genetic basis for the Wa CRI? Among nine Wa-positive RFs that have been characterized by amino acid sequencing, all light chains utilize Humkv325 together with three different Jk gene segments, including Jk1 (for Bor, Cur, Glo, Gol, Sie, and Wol), Jk2 (for Gar, Got),and Jk4 (for Kas) gene segments (2). The VJ rearrangement results in different junctional amino acid residues, including Arg (for Cur, Gol, Got, and Wol), Gln (for Bor and Sie), Leu (for Glo), Phe (for Kas), and Tyr (for Gar). Regarding the heavy chains of these RFs, serologic analysis showed that Cur and Got utilize the Vh2 heavy chains, Glo uses the Vh3 heavy chain, and the remaining six RF employ the Vh1 heavy chains (2,26). Of four RFs whose heavy chains have been sequenced, all have Jh4 gene segments but they differ extensively from each other in the second and the third hypervariable (regions/CDRs). The latter CDR is generated by the VDJ joining.

Thus, the accumulated data indicate that all Wa-positive RF share two common elements, Jh4 and Humkv325. Since no CRI has ever been assigned to the Jh region, it is likely that Humkv325 is the structural and genetic basis for the Wa CRI.

B. The 6B6.6 CRI and Humkv328 Germline Gene

Recently, a murine monoclonal anti-CRI (designated 6B6.6) was generated from a mouse immunized sequentially with the human monoclonal RFs Cor and Lew (27). Significantly, the anti-CRI reacted with 7 of 26 IgM RFs, but with only 3 of 137 IgM without RF acivity (28). In addition, the anti-idiotype bound to the separated light chains of the CRI-positive RFs, and a sequence comparison of 6B6.6-positive RF light chains revealed that they shared similar amino acid sequences, suggesting that the 6B6.6 CRI may be the phenotypic marker of another Vk gene (13,29).

To isolate the second RF-associated Vk gene, we used the rearranged Vk gene for the CRI-positive RF Les (ka31es) to screen a genomic library and isolated a new Vk gene, Humkv328 (29,30). It shared with ka31es 1315 of 1331 nucleotides at the DNA level and 109 of 112 amino acid residues at the protein level (including the leader peptide) (29,31). Together, these data indicated that kv328 or its allelic form(s) is the corresponding germline gene for the rearranged Les light-chain gene, as well as other RF light chains bearing the 6B6.6 CRI.

C. The G6 CRI and Humha1LR Rearranged Gene

In addition to the two aforementioned RF light chain-associated CRIs, a RF heavy chain-associated CRI (designated G6) has also been analyzed in detail (32). This CRI was displayed by about 30% of monoclonal RFs and by 80–90% of monoclonal RFs that bore the phenotypic markers of Humkv325 (i.e., PSL2, PSL3, and 17.109) (2). The heavy chains of two G6-positive RFs (i.e., Bor and Kas) were shown to share a 86% homology (25). Subsequently, we found that these two Vh sequences were 91–93% homologous to the Humha1LR-rearranged Vh gene (renamed from the 783 gene) from the LR CLL, a CD5/Leu-1-positive B cell tumor frequently expressing surface Ig with self reactivities (33–35). In contrast, they were quite different from all other reported Vh1 germline genes (33). Importantly, the DNA sequence of ha1LR is almost identical to 51P1 cDNA isolated from a fetal liver, except one base near the VD junction that probably reflects the imprecise joining of the Vh gene segment and the D gene segment (36). Taken together, these data led us to suggest that, except one base near the VD junction, ha1LR is the unmutated form of a germline Vh gene that encodes most, if not all, G6-positive RF heavy chains as well as 51P1 cDNA of the fetal antibody repertoire.

Very recently, Kipps et al. sequences the G6-positive heavy chains from two CLL and found they were 99% homologous to ha1LR (37). Furthermore, in collaboration with Dr. Katherine A. Siminovitch (Toronto, Canada), we found the heavy chain from a RF-secreting hybridoma (designated Humha113) was 99% homologous to ha1LR (unpublished data). Thus, it is clearly established that, except one base near the VD junction, halLR is the unmutated form of a germline Vh gene that encodes most, if not all, G6-positive heavy chains.

It should be noted that the G6 CRI is very similar to the Cc1 CRI (2,38). Among monoclonal RFs, the Ccl antibody reacted with 18 of 19 17.109-positive RFs, and the 17.109 antibody reacted with 18 of 26 Ccl-positive RFs. Thus, in addition to G6, halLR is very likely to be the genetic basis of the Ccl CRI.

III. CROSS-REACTIVE IDIOTYPES OF POLYCLONAL RHEUMATOID FACTORS

In contrast to the monoclonal RFs from patients with cryoglobulinemia, RFs from patients with RA and SS are polyclonal, as indicated by their heterogeneous binding properties, their light-chain constituents of both x and λ types, and their idiotypic profiles (1).

By hemagglutination inhibition assay with polyclonal anti-idiotypes, the Wa, Po, and other RF-associated CRIs were detected in some polyclonal IgM RFs in RA patients (39). Similarly, using the polyclonal anti-Wa antibodies in cytoplasmic staining of the pokeweed mitogen (PWM)-stimulated blood lymphocytes, the CRI was found in about 10% of plasma cells in most seropositive and some seronegative RA patients, as well as in about 50% of seronegative juvenile RA (JRA) patients (40–42). In contrast, Wa CRI was detected in about 2% of mitogen-stimulated plasma cells in the age-matched normals (40,41). In addition, some low-molecular-weight (7S) IgM monomers without RF activity from seropositive RA patients were found to inhibit the cytoplasmic staining with the rabbit anti-Wa antiserum, indicating that such IgM molecules expressed the Wa CRI (43).

In a separate study using an anti-idiotypic antiserum against the polyclonal RF from an RA patient, CRI was detected on RF in four of the patient's first-degree relatives, but not in five unrelated RA patients (44). The results suggested that the expression of RF-associated CRI was allotypically restricted and might be influenced by the polymorphisms in immunoglobulin loci,

In addition to polyclonal anti-idiotypes, one monoclonal anti-idiotype (H5) was shown to identify a CRI in about 50% of polyclonal IgM RFs and IgG RFs from unrelated RA patients (45). However, H5 reacted with both the Wa-positive RF Sie and the Po-positive RF Pom. Since Sie and Pom differ greatly from each other in their light- and heavy-chain variable regions, it is likely that H5 may represent the internal image of IgG, similar to the "internal image" type of anti-CRI antibodies that bind to most RFs regardless of their variable region structures (46,47). Accordingly, CRIs defined by such anti-CRI do not have any genetic implications.

On the other hand, CRIs that depend mainly on the primary structure of the RF variable regions have been found in polyclonal RFs from RA and SS patients, thus suggesting that some polyclonal RFs in RA patients may utilize the same V genes as do the monoclonal RFs in patients with cryoglobulinemia. For example, G6 CRI was detected in the sera from 8 of 14 RA patients, but not from 6 normal individuals (32); the Ccl and Fcl anti-idiotypes each bound to RFs from 4 of 5 RA patients, and the Lcl anti-idiotype reacted with RFs from 5 of 5 RA patients (38). In addition to monoclonal anti-idiotypes, the peptide-induced anti-PSL2 antiserum was shown to react with the affinity-enriched RFs from 5 of 5 RA and 4 of 4 SS patients, indicating that Humkv325 is employed to generate polyclonal RFs (19). Compared to the PSL-2-CRI, the PSL3 and 17.109 markers were expressed less frequently. Only 1 of 5 RA patients carried the PSL3-positive RF, compared to 3 of 4 SS patients (19). Similarly, 17.109 CRI was detected in sera from most patients with SS, but not from RA patients (19). By cytoplasmic staining, 17.109-CRI was found on 2–4% of lymphocytes in the salivary tissue of SS patients but was not detected in rheumatoid synovial membranes (19,48). Very recently, in an extensive study of sera from 87 RA patients and 53 normal controls, 17.109 CRI was detected in 33% of RA patients but in none of the normal subjects (49). Similarly, 6B6.6 was detected in 44% of RA patients, but in only 4% of normal subjects. When detected, the CRI-positive RFs constituted only a very small fraction of the IgM RFs, 0.7% ± 0.9% for 17.109 and 0.9% ± 2.2% for 6B6.6. These observations were consistent with the failure to detect CRI in polyclonal RFs from different RA patients by polyclonal anti-idiotypes generated against polyclonal RFs (50). It is obvious that such reagents consist of many antibodies specific for mainly private idiotypes and few CRIs; each is shared by only a very small fraction of RFs from other individuals.

IV. DISCUSSION

As reviewed here, idiotypic analyses of human monoclonal RFs derived mainly from individuals with cryoglobulinemia, who rarely had RA, showed that there were some major RF-associated CRIs. Subsequent molecular studies of these CRIs revealed that they all represent the phenotypic markers of some human Ig V genes. In addition to monoclonal RFs, some of these RF-associated CRIs were expressed by various portions of polyclonal RFs in 10–50% patients with RA and primary SS.

It is noteworthy that Humkv325 is identical to the light chains of four RFs derived from four unrelated individuals (2). Similarly, we found the heavy chain of an anti-DNA antibody is identical to the VH26 germline gene and to the 30P1 cDNA derived from two unrelated individuals (51). Together, these data demonstrate that some RFs and other autoantibodies can be encoded by the unmutated germline Ig V genes and that such V genes are conserved in outbred human populations, indicating that these RF and autoantibody-associated V genes have been preserved through evolution and may serve some important biologic functions.

Recent studies of RFs and other autoantibodies have revealed not only that autoantibodies are found regularly in the preimmune repertoire of normal individuals (thus, they are termed natural autoantibodies) but also that a high frequency of proliferating autoreactive B cells are detected in neonates (35,52–54). In humans, Humkv328 gene (for the 6B6.6-positive RF light chains) and Humha1LR-corresponding Vh gene (for the G6-positive RF heavy chains) belong to a restricted set of V genes expresed in a day 130 fetal liver (36,55). The early antibody repertoire also contained the products of VH26 (for 16/6-positive anti-DNA heavy chain) and 20P1-corresponding Vh gene (for 4B4 anti-Sm heavy chain) (56). These findings are very provocative and speak strongly that RFs and other natural autoantibodies may be very important during the early development stages.

By sequence comparison, Humkv325 sequence is identical to the light-chain variable region of an autoantibody (Pie) against intermediate filament (IF) and differs by only one amino acid residue from the light-chain variable region of an autoantibody (Son) against low-density lipoprotein (LDL) (57). As expected, both Son and Pie are positive for the PSL2 and PSL3 CRIs (2). These data demonstrate that a single human Vk gene encodes various CRI-positive autoantibodies with different binding specificities. Similarly, the light chain of the C6B2 anti-DNA antibody is 99% homologous to the Humkv328 gene that encodes the 6B6.6-positive RF light chains (58), and the heavy chain of the Ab25 anti-thyroglobulin antibody is 98% similar to the VH26 gene that encodes the 16/6 CRI-positive heavy chains of anti-DNA antibodies (59). Taken together, these results provide the molecular basis for the idiotypic connectivity of autoantibodies and suggest that, to some extent, human autoantibodies might be encoded by a restricted set of Ig V genes.

It has been shown in humans and mice that autoreactive B cell precursors are often in a proliferative state (60–62). Accordingly, it is conceivable that B cells expressing the kv325 gene are likely to react with self components and thus may be stimulated by autoantigens to proliferate constantly. The continual cell cylcing would render the kv325-bearing cells exceptionally susceptible to abnormal clonal expansion and malignant transformation (23). If substantiated, this hypothesis may explain why the kv325 gene is expressed by a large proportion of CLL and is overly represented among Ig paraproteins and/or Bence-Jones light chains.

In addition to autoantibodies, Humkv325 is likely to encode the light chain of a human monoclonal IgG anticytomegalovirus (CMV) antibody (Evl-15) (63). It has been reported that A/J mice use an unmutated Vh gene to generate DNA binding antibodies and employ the same Vh gene with some somatic diversifications to produce antiarsonate antibodies (64). Combined, these findings indicate that in certain instances autoantibodies may be directly encoded by germline V genes that serve as the precursor genes for antibodies against exogenous antigens.

To explain these astounding and provocative observations, Coutinho and his colleagues recently proposed a "network" model (65). They contend that, in the sterile fetal environment, the neonatal B cell repertoire is comprised largely of cells expressing the idiotypically connected and self reactive V genes and such B cells react with each other and/or are stimulated by autoantigens to proliferate and eventually form a functional network providing the framework for distinguishing self from nonself. With maturation, the self reactive B cell repertoire diminishes in size, representing only about 20% of the preimmune B cell repertoire and interacting with the 80% of nonautoreactive resting B cells that are not connected to the network. Upon exposure to conventional antigens, the latter B cells respond and, through somatic mutation and other diversification mechanisms, produce high-affinity classic antibodies. If this hypothesis is proven, it is probably the abnormal expression and diversification of RFs and other autoantibodies, rather than their mere presence, that is responsible for the pathogenesis of systemic autoimmune diseases.

ACKNOWLEDGMENTS

This is publication number 5961-BCR from the Research Institute of Scripps Clinic, La Jolla, California. Funding for this research supported in part by grants AR39039, AR33489, and AR25443 from the National Institutes of Health.

We thank Drs. J.D. Capra, S. Fong, B. Frangione, F. Goni, T.J. Kipps, W.J. Koopman, R. Jefferies, M.F. Liu, R.A. Mageed, R.E. Schrohenloher, and K.A. Siminovitich for their significant contributions toward collaborative studies of human rheumatoid factors. We acknowledge the excellent technical assistance of S. Singha and the secretarial assistance of Ms. Jane Uhle and Mrs. Nancy Noon in the preparation of this manuscript.

REFERENCES

1. Chen, P.P., Fong, S., and Carson, D.A.(1987). Rheumatoid factor. Rheum. Dis. North Am. 13:545.
2. Chen, P.P., Fong, S., Goni, F., Silverman, G.J., Fox, R.I., Liu, M.-F., Frangione, B., and Carson, D.A. (1988). Cross-reacting idiotypes on cryoprecipitating rheumatoid factor. Springer Semin. Immunopathol. 10:35.

3. Rudikoff, S.(1983). Immunoglobulin structure-function correlates: Antigen binding and idiotypes. Contemp. Top. Mol. Immunol. 9:169.

4. Rajewsky, K., and Takemori, T. (1983). Genetics, expression, and function of idiotypes. Annu. Rev. Immunol. 1:569.

5. Lindemann, J. (1973). Speculation on idiotypes and homobodies. (Journal title misplaced) 124C:171.

6. Jerne, N.K. (1984). Idiotypic networks and other preconceived ideas. Immunol. Rev. 79:5.

7. Metzger, H. (1969). Myeloma proteins and antibodies (editorial). Am. J. Med. 47:837.

8. Preud'homme, J.L., and Seligmann, M. (1972). Anti-human immunoglobulin G activity of membrane-bound monoclonal immunoglobulin M in lymphoproliferative disorders. Proc. Natl. Acad. Sci. USA 69:2132.

9. Winfield, J.B.(1983). Cryoglobulinemia. Hum. Pathol. 14:350.

10. Merlini, G., Farhangi, M., and Osserman, E.F. (1986). Monoclonal immunoglobulins with antibody activity in myeloma, macroglobulinemia and related plasma cell dyscrasias. Semin. Oncol. 13:350.

11. Kunkel, H.G., Agnello, V., Joslin, F.G., Winchester, R.J., and Capra, J.D. (1973). Cross-idiotypic specificity among monoclonal IgM proteins with anti-gammaglobulin activity. J. Exp. Med. 137:331.

12. Kunkel, H.G., Winchester, R.J., Joslin, F.G., and Capra, J.D. (1974). Similarities in the light chains of anti-gamma globulins showing cross-idiotypic specificities. J. Exp. Med. 139:128.

13. Capra, J.D., and Klapper, D.G. (1976). Complete amino acid sequence of the variable domains of two human IgM anti-gamma globulins (Lay/Pom) with shared idiotypic specificities. Scand. J. Immunol 5:677.

14. Andrews, D.W., and Capra, J.D. (1981). Complete amino acid sequence of variable domains from two monoclonal human anti-gamma globulins of the Wa cross-idiotypic group: Suggestion that the J segments are involved in the structural correlate of the idiotype. Proc. Natl. Acad Sci. USA 78:3799.

15. Chen, P.P., Fong, S., Normansell, D., Houghten, R.A., Karras, J.G., Vaughan, J.H., and Carson, D.A. (1984). Delineation of a cross-reactive idiotype on human autoantibodies with antibody against a synthetic peptide. J. Exp. Med. 159:1502.

16. Chen, P.P., Goni, F., Fong, S., Jirik, F., Vaughan, J.H., Frangione, B., and Carson, D.A. (1985). The majority of human monoclonal IgM rheumatoid factors express a "primary structure-dependent" cross-reactive idiotype. J. Immunol. 134:3281.

17. Chen, P.P., Goni, F., Houghten, R.A., Fong, S., Goldfien, R., Vaughan, J.H., Frangione, B., and Carson, D.A. (1985). Characterization of human rheumatoid factors with seven antiidiotypes induced by synthetic hypervariable region peptides. J. Exp. Med. 162:487.

18. Carson, D.A., and Fong, S.(1983). A common idiotype on human rheumatoid factors identified by a hybridoma antibody. Mol. Immunol. 20:1081.

19. Fong, S., Chen, P.P., Gilbertson, T.A., Weber, J.R., Fox, R.I., and Carson, D.A. (1986). Expression of three cross reactive idiotypes on rheumatoid factor autoantibodies from patients with autoimmune diseases and seropositive adults. J. Immunol. 137:122.

20. Chen, P.P., Fong, S., Goni, F., Houghten, R.A., Frangione, B., Liu, F., and Carson, D.A. (1987). Analyses of human rheumatoid factors with antiidiotypes induced by synthetic peptides. Monogr. Allergy 22:12.

21. Chen, P.P., Albrandt, K., Orida, N.K., Radoux, V., Chen, E.Y., Schrantz, R., Liu, F.-T., and Carson, D.A.(1986). Genetic basis for the cross-reactive idiotypes on the light chains of human IgM anti-IgG autoantibodies. Proc. Natl. Acad. Sci. USA 83:8318.

22. Radoux, V., Chen, P.P., Sorge, J.A., and Carson, D.A.(1986). A conserved human germline Vk gene directly encodes rheumatoid factor light chains. J. Exp.Med. 164:2119.

23. Chen, P.P., Albrandt, K., Kipps, T.J., Radoux, V., Liu, F.-T., and Carson, D.A. (1987). Isolation and characterization of human VkIII germline genes: Implications for the molecular basis of human VkIII light chain diversity. J. Immunol. 139:1727.

24. Goni, F., Chen, P.P., Pons-Estel, B., Carson, D.A., and Frangione, B. (1985). Sequence similarities and cross-idiotypic specificity of L chains among human monoclonal IgM-K with anti-gammaglobulin activity. J. Immunol. 135:4073.

25. Newkirk, M.M., Mageed, R.A., Jefferis, R., Chen, P.P., and Capra, J.D.(1987). Complete amino acid sequences of variable regions of two human IgM rheumatoid factors, BOR and KAS of the Wa idiotypic family, reveal restricted use of heavy and light chain variable and joining region gene segments. J. Exp. Med. 166:550.

26. Silverman, G.J., Goldfien, R.D., Chen, P., Mageed, R.A., Jefferis, R., Goni, F., Frangione, B., Fong, S., and Carson, D.A. (1988). Idiotypic and subgroup analysis of human monoclonal rheumatoid factors: Implications for structural and genetic basis of autoantibodies in humans. J. Clin. Invest. 82:469.

27. Schrohenloher, R.E., and Koopman, W.J. (1986). An idiotype common to rheumatoid factors from patients with rheumatoid arthritis identified by a monoclonal antibody. Arthritis Rheum. 29:S28.

28. Crowley, J.J., Goldfien, R.D., Schrohenloher, R.E., Spiegelberg, H.L., Silverman, G.J., Mageed, R.A., Jefferis, R., Koopman, W.J., Carson, D.A.,and Fong, S. (1988). Incidence of three cross-reactive idiotypes on human rheumatoid factor paraproteins. J. Immunol 140:3411.

29. Chen, P.P., Robbins, D.L., Jirik, F.R., Kipps, T.J., and Carson, D.A. (1987). Isolation and characterization of a light chain variable region gene for human rheumatoid factors. J. Exp. Med. 166:1900.

30. Jirik, F.R., Sorge, J., Fong, S., Heitzmann, J.G., Curd, J.G., Chen, P.P., Goldfien, R., and Carson, D.A. (1986). Cloning and sequence determination of a human rheumatoid factor light-chain gene. Proc. Natl. Acad. Sci. USA 83:2195.

31. Liu, M.F., Robbins, D.L., Crowley, J.J., Sinha, S., Kozin, F., Kipps, T.J., Carson, D.A., and Chen, P.P. (1989). Characterization of four homologous light chain variable region genes which are related to 6B6.6 idiotype positive human rheumatoid factor light chains. J. Immunol. 142:688.

32. Mageed, R.A., Dearlove, M., Goodall, D.M., and Jefferis, R. (1986). Immunogenic and antigenic epitopes and immunoglobulins. XVII. Monoclonal anti-idiotypes to the heavy chain of human rheumatoid factors. Rheumatol. Int. 6:179.

33. Chen, P.P., Liu, M.-F., Glass, C.A., Sinha, S., Kipps, T.J., and Carson, D.A.

(1989). Characterization of two Ig Vh genes which are homologous to human rheumatoid factors. Arthritis Rheum. 32:72.

34. Casali, P., and Notkins, A.L.(1989). Probing the human B-cell repertoire with EBV: Polyreactive antibodies and CD5+ B lymphocytes. Annu. Rev. Immunol. 7:513.

35. Sthoeger, Z.M., Wakai, M., Tse, D.B., Vinciguerra, V.P., Allen, S.L., Budman, D.R., Lichtman, S.M., Schulman, P., Weiselberg, L.R., and Chiorazzi, N. (1989). Production of autoantibodies by CD-5-expressing B lymphocytes from patients with chronic lymphocytic leukemia. J. Exp. Med. 169:255.

36. Schroeder, H.W., Jr., Hillson, J.L., and Perlmutter, R.M. (1987). Early restriction of the human antibody repertoire. Science 288:791.

37. Kipps, T.J., Tomhave, E., Pratt, L.F., Duffy, S., Chen, P.P., and Carson, D.A. (1989). Developmentally restricted VH gene is expressed at high frequently in CD5 B cell malignancies. Proc. Natl. Acad. Sci. USA 86:5913.

38. Ono, M., Winearls, C.G., Amos, N., Grennan, D., Gharavi, A., Peters, D.K., and Sissons, J.G.P. (1987). Monoclonal autobodies to restricted and cross-reactive idiotopes on monoclonal rheumatoid factors and their recognition of idiotope-positive cells. Eur. J. Immunol. 17:343.

39. Forre, O., Dobloug, J.H., Michaelsen, T.E., and Natvig, J.B. (1979). Evidence of similar idiotypic determinants on different rheumatoid factor populations. Scand. J. Immunol. 9:281.

40. Bonagura, V.R., Kunkel, H.G., and Pernis, B. (1982). Cellular localization of rheumatoid factor idiotypes. J. Clin. Invest. 69:1356.

41. Kunkel, H., Posnett, D., and Pernis, B. (1983). Anti-immunoglobulins and their idiotypes: Are they part of the immune network? Ann. N.Y. Acad. Sci. 418:324.

42. Ilowite, N.T., Wedgwood, J.F., and Bonagura, V.R. (1989). Expression of the major rheumatoid factor cross-reactive idiotype in juvenile rheumatoid arthritis. Arthritis Rheum 32:265.

43. Bonagura, V.R., Mendez, L., Agostino, N., and Pernis, B. (1987). Monomeric (7S) IgM found in the serum of rheumatoid arthritis patients share idiotypes with pentameric (19S) monoclonal rheumatoid factors. J. Clin. Invest. 79:813.

44. Pasquali, J.-L., Fong, S., Tsoukas, C.D., Vaughan, J.H., and Carson, D.A.(1980). Inheritance of immunoglobulin M rheumtoid factor idiotypes. J. Clin. Invest. 66:863.

45. Pasquali, J.-L., Urlacher, A., and Storck, D.(1983). A highly conserved determinant on human rheumatoid factor idiotypes defined by a mouse monoclonal antibody. Eur. J. Immunol. 13:197.

46. Fong, S., Gilbertson, T.A., Chen, P.P., Karras, J.G., Vaughan, J.H., and Carson, D.A. (1986). The common occurrence of internal image type anti-idiotypic antibodies in rabbits immunized with monoclonal and polyclonal human IgM rheumatoid factors. Clin. Exp. Immunol. 64:570.

47. Oppliger, Z.R., Nardelli, F.A., Stone, G.C., and Mannik, M. (1987). Human rheumatoid factors bear the internal image of the Fc binding region of staphylococcal protein A. J. Exp. Med. 166:702.

48. Fox, R.I., Chen, P.P., Carson, D.A., and Fong, S. (1986). Expression of a cross reactive idiotype on rheumatoid factor in patients with Sjogren's syndrome. J. Immunol. 136:477.

49. Koopman, W.J., Schrohenloher, R.E., and Carson, D.A. (1989). Dissociation of expression of two cross-reactive idiotopes (CRI) on rheumatoid factors (RF) in rheumatoid arthritis (RA) sera. Arthritis Rheum. 32:S126.

50. Nelson, J.L., Nardella, F.A., Oppliger, I.R., and Mannik, M. (1987). Rheumatoid factors from patients with rheumatoid arthritis posses private repertoires of idiotypes. J. Immunol. 138:1391.

51. Chen, P.P., Liu, M., Sinha,S., and Carson, D.A. (1988). A 16/6 idiotype positive anti-DNA antibody is encoded by a conserved Vh gene with no somatic mutation. Arthritis Rheum. 31:1429.

52. Fong, S., Chen, P.P., Vaughan, J.H., and Carson, D.A. (1985). Origin and age-associated changes in the expression of a physiologic autoantibody. Gerontology 31:236.

53. Avrameas, S., Guilbert, B., Mahana, W., Matsiota, P., and Ternynck, T. (1988). Recognition of self and non-self constituents by polyspecific autoreceptors. Int. Rev. Immunol. 3:1.

54. Zouali, M., Stollar, B.D., and Schwartz, R.S.(1988). Origin and diversification of anti-DNA antibodies. Immunol. Rev. 105:137.

55. Hillson, J.L., Schroeder, H.W., and Pelmutter, R.M. (1989). Expression of antibody genes associated with self-specificities by human fetal B lymphocytes. (Arthritis Rheum. 32:S135.

56. Sanz, I., Dang, H., Takei, M., Talal, N., and Capra, J.D. (1989). V-H sequence of a human anti-Sm autoantibody. J. Immunol. 142:883.

57. Pons-Estel, B., Goni, F., Solomon, A., and Frangione, B. (1984). Sequence similarities among kIIIb chains of monoclonal human IgMk autoantibodies. J. Exp. Med. 160:893.

58. Hoch, S. (1989). A polyreactive anti-DNA antibody uses a RL light chain. Arthritis Rheum. 32:S41.

59. Sanz, I., Casali, P., Thomas, J.W., Notkins, A.L., and Capra, J.D. (1989). Nucleotide sequences of eight human natural autoantibody V-H regions reveals apparent restricted use of V-H families. J. Immunol. 142:4054.

60. Fong, S., Gilbertson, T.A., Huenkien, R.J., Singhal, S.K., Vaughan, J.H., and Carson, D.A.(1985). IgM rheumatoid factor autoantibody and immunoglobulin producing precursor cells in the bone marrow of humans. Cell. Immunol. 95:157.

61. Portnoi, D., Freitas, A., Holmberg, D., Bandeira, A., and Coutinho, A. (1986). Immunocompetent autoreactive B lymphocytes are activated cycling cells in normal mice. J. Exp. Med. 164:25.

62. Holmberg, D., Freitas, A.A., Portnoi, D., Jacquemart, F., Avrameas, S., and Coutinho, A. (1986). Antibody repertoires of normal BABL/c mice: B lymphocyte populations defined by state of activation. Immunol. Rev. 93:147.

63. Newkirk, M.M., Gram, H., Heinrich, G.F., Ostberg, L., Capra, J.D., and Wasserman, R.L. (1988). The complete protein sequences of the variable regions of the cloned heavy and light chains of a human anti-cytomegalovirus antibody reveal a striking similarity to human rheumatoid factors of the Wa idiotypic family. J. Clin. Invest. 81:1511.

64. Naparstek, Y., Andre-Schwartz, J., Manser, T., Wysocki, L.J., Breitman, L., Stollar, B.D., Gefter, M., and Schwartz, R.S. (1986). A single germline VH gene segment

of normal A/J mice encodes autoantibodies characteristic of systemic lupus erythematosus. J. Exp. Med. 164:614.

65. Coutinho, A., Grandien, A., Faro-Rivas, J., and Mota-Santos, T.A. (1988). Idiotypes, tailors and networks. Ann. Inst. Pasteur Immunol. 139:599.

20

Characterization of Rheumatoid Factors Using Monoclonal Anti-idiotypic Reagents

Mary Ann Accavitti and Ralph E. Schrohenloher
University of Alabama at Birmingham, Birmingham, Alabama

William J. Koopman
University of Alabama at Birmingham, Birmingham Veterans' Administration Hospital, Birmingham, Alabama

I. INTRODUCTION

Rheumatoid factors (RF) are defined as autoantibodies that bind to IgG molecules. A large portion of RF are of the IgM isotype, but the existence of IgA-RF and IgG-RF is now well established (1,2). Classically, the term RF has been used to describe autoantibodies that react with determinants in the constant or Fc portion of the IgG heavy chain. More recent experiments, however, indicate that there is a distinct group of RF that have specificity for both the Fab and Fc fragments of IgG (3,4). This unique group of RF, called epibodies, is discussed in greater detail here. Transient synthesis of RF is routinely observed in mice (5,6) and humans (7,8) during secondary immune responses. In addition, RF are readily produced upon in vitro stimulation of peripheral blood B cells from healthy adults (9–11), and low levels of circulating RF can occasionally be detected in normal adults (12). In view of the conservation of RF in the B cell repertoire and the regularity with which these autoantibodies appear in normal individuals, it is likely that RF perform some beneficial functions. For example, RF are capable of accelerating the clearance of immune complexes and enhancing complement binding by relatively small complexes of IgG and antigen (13) and may therefore play an important role in facilitating clearance of antigen.

A. RF Production in Disease

Although transient production of RF appears to be a normal physiologic function, the persistent synthesis of these autoantibodies occurs in a number of pathologic conditions. Elevated levels of RF are detected in patients with rheumatoid arthritis (RA), Sjögren's syndrome, mixed cryoglobulinemia, and a variety of other pathologic states, listed in Table 1. In patients with RA, RF are present not only in the serum but in synovial fluid as well (14). The notion that there is local production of RF in rheumatoid joints is supported by the detection of RF-secreting plasma cells in synovial tissue (15,16). Similarly, in Sjögren's syndrome, plasma cells producing RF of the IgA class are found in salivary gland infiltrates (17).

B. Specificity of RF

The initial discovery of circulating RF was based on the ability of sera from patients with RA and other diseases to agglutinate sheep red blood cells coated with subagglutinating amounts of rabbit antibody or bacteria similarly coated with human antibody (18,19). Subsequent experiments demonstrated that RF present in RA sera also cross-reacted with other mammalian immunoglobulins (Igs), including bovine, equine, porcine, and guinea pig IgG (20). The broad spectrum of cross-reactivity observed with RF in the sera of RA patients reflects the conservation of Ig heavy chains throughout evolution. Early analysis of IgG-binding

---

Table 1 Selected Diseases Associated with Elevated Serum RF

Chronic Bacterial Diseases
  Subacute bacterial endocarditis
  Tuberculosis
  Syphilis
  Leprosy
Viral Diseases
  Rubella
  Infectious mononucleosis
  Cytomegalovirus
  Influenza
Parasitic Diseases
Chronic Inflammatory Diseases
  Sarcoidosis
  Periodontal disease
  Pulmonary interstitial disease
  Liver disease
Hypergammaglobulinimic Purpura

---

autoantibodies indicated that rheumatoid sera contained a subpopulation of RF that exhibited preferential reactivity toward rabbit IgG (21). The selectivity of these antibodies for rabbit IgG, however, was less obvious in the presence of heat-aggregated human IgG, suggesting that the epitope(s) recognized by these RF is merely more accessible in rabbit IgG populations (21).

In addition to cross-reacting with heterologous immunoglobulins, a subpopulation of human RF in RA sera appears to recognize epitopes on nuclear antigens. For example, Hannestad demonstrated that all the RF activity and antinuclear antibody (ANA) in two distinct autoimmune sera could be removed by affinity chromatography on an IgG-Sepharose column (22). A subsequent study indicated that the RF were cross-reacting with nucleosomes, the repeating histone-DNA subunit of chromatin (23).

In vitro analysis of RF indicates that these antibodies readily form precipitates with soluble aggregates of human IgG formed by heating or chemical cross-linkage (24). Precipitation is not readily inhibited by the addition of native monomeric human IgG. Similarly, RF-mediated agglutination of IgG-coated RBCs, although strongly inhibited by the addition of aggregated human IgG, is minimally affected by the presence of 7S IgG (24). Such findings imply that IgM-RF selectively bind to complexed forms of IgG. Nonethless, the frequent detection of 22S immunoglobulin complexes in rheumatoid sera provide ample evidence for the in vivo interaction of 19S IgM-RF with monomeric 7S IgG (24). The preferential binding of RF to aggregated IgG likely indicates that aggregated IgG acts as a multivalent antigen, allowing a single IgM molecule to bind to multiple sites on the same complex. Under these circumstances, the effective energy of interaction is higher with aggregated IgG than with native IgG or antigen-bound IgG (25).

The Fc region of the IgG molecule contains the second and third homology regions (domains) of two identical γ chains joined by disulfide bonds (Fig. 1). Much experimental effort has been directed toward identifying those portions of the Fc fragment recognized by RF. To date, a minimum of five RF-reactive regions on the Fc fragment have been identified (2). Some of these regions consist of genetically determined Gm markers; others correspond to isotypic determinants distributed among the four subclasses of IgG (Table 2). Since patients with RA typically produce a heterogenous population of RF, several different specificities may be present in an individual serum.

A significant proportion of the RF activity in RA sera is directed toward the isotypic marker, Ga, found on IgG_1, IgG_2, and IgG_4 molecules. The location of the Ga marker has been tentatively assigned to the $C\gamma2$ domain (26). An epitope corresponding to Ga is found on rabbit IgG, which accounts in part for the strong cross-reactivity of RF in RA sera with rabbit immunoglobulin. The integrity of the Ga-like structure on rabbit γ chains requires the presence of both $C\gamma2$ and $C\gamma3$ domains (26). Other γ chain determinants recognized by RF include a number of genetically determined allotypic structures called Gm antigens. Gm markers

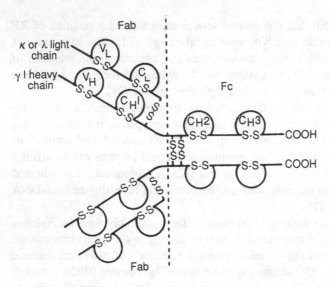

Figure 1 Polypeptide chain structure of human IgG₁ (62). The Fc region of the IgG molecule contains the second and third homology regions (domains) of two identical γ chains joined by disulfide bonds.

Table 2 Localization of IgG Antigens Interacting with RF

	Heavy Chain Constant Region	
Subclass	CH2	CH3
IgG₁	Ga	Gm(a)
	Non-b1	Gm(x)
IgG₂	Ga	Non-a
	Non-b1	
IgG₃	Gm(g)	Non-a
	Gm(b1)	
	Non-b1	
IgG₄	Ga	γ4 Non-a

Source: Data from Natvig, J.B., Gaardner, P.I., and Turner, M.W. IgG antigens of the Cγ2 and Cγ3 homology regions interacting with rheumatoid factors. Clin. Exp. Immunol. 12:177, 1972.

targeted by RF activity include the Gm(a) and Gm(x) groups present in the Cγ3 region of IgG$_1$ and the Gm(b1) and Gm(g) groups located in the Cγ3 region of IgG$_3$ (27). In addition to the Gm structures, a number of RF appear to recognize isoallotypic or antithetical groups (28,29). These two terms are used to describe determinants that occur as genetic variants in one immunoglobulin subclass, but they are present on all molecules of at least one other subclass (2). For example, the non-a determinant, an isotypic determinant present on all IgG$_2$ and IgG$_3$ molecules, occurs as an allotypic marker antithetical to Gm(a) on IgG$_1$ antibodies. Another non-a marker, called γ4, is found on antibodies of the IgG$_4$ subclass. Similarly, non-b1 is antithetical to Gm(b1) in IgG$_3$ but isotypic in IgG1 and IgG2. The location of the various epitopes recognized by RF is illustrated in Fig. 2.

C. Epibodies

The variable regions of immunoglobulin molecules contain antigenic determinants capable of evoking an antibody response (30). The term "idiotope" has been coined

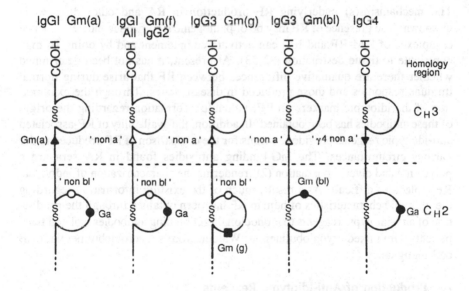

Figure 2 Location of sites reactive with RF in several human IgG molecules. The Gm(a), non-a, and γ4 non-a sites are shown in the approximate positions established for these structures; however, the location of the reactive sites in the CH2 homology region is speculative. (Redrawn from Natvig, J.B., Gaardner, P.I., and Turner, M.W. IgG antigens of the Gγ2 and Cγ3 homology regions interacting with rheumatoid factors. Clin. Exp. Immunol. 12:177, 1972.)

to describe individual antigenic determinants of the variable region. Antisera directed against these epitopes are referred to as anti-idiotypic reagents. While producing mouse antisera to variable region determinants of human IgM paraproteins, Bona and colleagues noted that a portion of these anti-idiotypic antibodies also reacted with the Fc portion of γ heavy chains (4). Antibodies demonstrating this type of dual specificity were called epibodies. The occurrence of epibodies in humans is evidenced by the identification of monoclonal rheumatoid factors that react with both the Fab and Fc region of autologous IgG (31). A possible explanation for the epibody phenomenon is the presence of homologous amino acid sequences in the Fc and Fab portions of some immunoglobulins (1). It has also been proposed that in vivo production of epibodies results from immune responses to Fc binding proteins on bacteria and viruses (1,13). Under these circumstances, the complementary determining region (CDR) of antibodies against Fc binding proteins may mimic structures found in the Fc fragment, resulting in recognition by RF.

II. IDIOTYPIC MARKERS ON RF

The mechanisms(s) underlying RF production in RA and other diseases is unknown. The presence of RF may be of pathogenic significance, however, since complexes of IgM-RF and IgG can activate complement and by doing so may contribute to tissue destruction (32,33). At present, it has not been determined whether there are qualitative differences between RF that arise during normal immune responses and those produced in disease states. Through the examination of the idiotypic markers on RF, valuable information regarding the origin of these antibodies has been obtained. In addition, the availability of RF-associated anti-idiotypic reagents provides a means for the comparison of RF produced under various circumstances. The IgG-binding antibodies found in RA sera are a polyclonal and diverse population (2), rendering the characterization of individual RF molecules difficult. As a result, much of the existing information regarding the idiotypic characteristics of human RF has been obtained through the production of anti-idiotypic reagents to monoclonal IgG-binding antibodies isolated from patients with mixed cryoglobulinemia, Waldenström's macroglobulinemia, or B cell malignancy (1).

A. Production of Anti-Idiotypic Reagents

Early studies examining the idiotypic markers on human RF were carried out with polyclonal anti-idiotypic antisera raised in rabbits (34,35). These reagents are typically produced by immunizing rabbits with the relevant Ig molecule in combination with Freund's complete adjuvant. In some cases, F(ab')$_2$ fragments are used as the immunizing antigen. The resultant antisera are then extensively absorbed with irrelevant immunoglobulin from the homologous species to remove antibodies directed against constant region determinants. Polyclonal anti-idiotypic reagents contain antibodies to a variety of antigenic determinants, including light- and heavy-chain idiotopes, as well as combinatorial determinants contributed to by both heavy- and light-chain regions. The advent of hybridoma technology (36) has greatly facilitated the production of anti-idiotypic reagents. Since monoclonal antibodies (MAb) react with a single antigenic determinant they are potentially ideal reagents for the localization and characterization of individual idiotopes. In addition, the use of monoclonal anti-idiotypic reagents eliminates the laborious absorption process required for the production of polyclonal anti-idiotypic antisera.

B. Cross-Reactive Idiotypes of RF

The availability of a significant number of human paraproteins with RF activity has facilitated the identification of idiotypic markers on this type of autoantibody. In pioneering experiments, Kunkel and colleagues demonstrated that 60% of a panel of monoclonal RF from unrelated individuals reacted with a rabbit antiserum produced against the monoclonal IgM-RF WA (34). Subsequently, it was demonstrated that all antibodies bearing the WA cross-reactive idiotype (CRI) had light chains belonging to the minor VKIIIb sub-subgroup (37). Additional RF-associated CRI that have been identified with rabbit antisera include the PO and BLA markers (34,35). The prevalence of these CRI on monoclonal RF is not as great as that observed for the WA epitope. Amino acid sequence analysis of heavy chains of monoclonal RF expressing the PO CRI indicate restricted use of VHIII heavy chains; however, the structural basis for the serologically defined PO CRI remains uncertain (38,39,40). The BLA CRI appears to be a conformational determinant requiring the integrity of both heavy and light chains (41). RF bearing the BLA idiotype are notable for their cross-reactivity with nuclear antigens (35,41).

More recent studies have utilized MAbs to identify CRI on RF. Carson and coworkers generated a MAb, designated 17.109, that reacts with RF paraproteins expressing light chains within the KIIIb sub-subgroup (42,43). Subsequent experiments indicate that the 17.109 CRI is a marker for the VK325 germline gene (44). This point is discussed in greater detail in the next chapter.

III. THE 6B6.6 CROSS-REACTIVE IDIOTYPE

In an effort to produce additional RF-specific anti-idiotypic reagents, our laboratory used a panel of seven monoclonal RF paraproteins: LAY (IgM,$\varkappa$), SLO(IgM,$\varkappa$), MIL(IgM,$\varkappa$), POM(IgM,$\varkappa$), COR(IgM,$\varkappa$), LEW(IgM,$\varkappa$), and SCH (IgA,$\varkappa$). In initial experiments, rabbit (Fab')$_2$ anti-idiotypic antisera were prepared against each of the paraproteins and tested for reactivity with all other members of the panel (Table 3). Our analysis indicated that two of the antibodies, *COR* and *LEW*, had at least one idiotope in common. Subsequent experiments with isolated heavy and light chains of these two RF determined that these antibodies shared a minimum of two CRI: one on the light chain and one on the heavy chain. In view of the problems inherent in using polyclonal antiserum to characterize individual idiotopes, we initiated production of MAbs specific for the major CRIs of COR and LEW RF.

The first fusion experiment was designed to generate MAbs to the CRI on the x light chains of COR and LEW. DBA $\times$ Balb/c F_1 mice were immunized with 100 μg of COR light chain in complete Freund's adjuvant injected subcutaneously as described by Lieberman et al. (45). The mice were boosted with 100 μg LEW light chain in 0.15 M sodium chloride 3 weeks after the primary injection. Lymphocytes from the popliteal and inguinal lymph nodes were subsequently fused with the P3X63-Ag8.653 myeloma cell line (46). Approximately 14 days after fusion, culture supernatants were screened for reactivity with COR, LEW, and DAU light chains by enzyme-linked immunosorbent assay (ELISA). Hybridomas producing antibody that reacted with the light chains from COR and LEW, but not with light chains from DAU (a human monoclonal paraprotein without RF activity), were subcloned, expanded, and grown in ascites by standard procedures.

A. Specificity of MAb 6B6.6

Our initial fusion generated MAb 6B6.6, an IgG_1x molecule that strongly bound to microtiter wells coated with COR and LEW IgM RF (Fig. 3). In addition, the MAb exhibited weak activity for IgM RFs POM and MIL and essentially no activity for the IgM RF LAY or IgA RF SCH. MAb 6B6.6 did not bind to

Table 3 Relative Activity of Anti-Id Panel for Various Monoclonal RF by the Inhibition Assay[a]

F(ab')$_2$ Anti-Id	Monoclonal RF						
	LAY	SLO	MIL	POM	COR	LEW	SCH
Anti-LAY	100	—	—	—	—	—	—
Anti-SLO	—	100	—	—	—	—	—
Anti-MIL	—	29	100	—	—	—	—
Anti-POM	—	—	5	100	0.6	—	—
Anti-COR	—	—	3	6	100	68	0.2
Anti-LEW	—	—	—	—	66	100	—
Anti-SCH	—	—	—	0.4	6	5	100

[a]SCH is an IgAx protein; all others are IgMx.

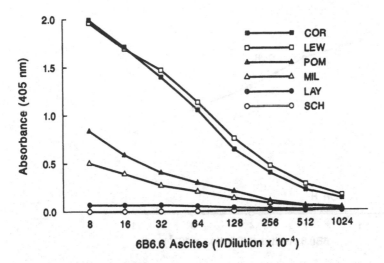

Figure 3 ELISA binding curves of MAb 6B6.6 with human monoclonal rheumatoid factors Microtiter wells coated with (■——■) COR IgM, (□——□) LEW IgM, (▲——▲) POM IgM, (△——△) MIL IgM, (●——●) LAY IgM, and (○——○) SCH IgA (0.01 mg/ml) were reacted with 6B6.6 ascites diluted in BSA-PBS diluent as indicated on the abscissa and developed with alkaline phosphatase-labeled F(ab')$_2$ fragments of goat antimouse IgG antibody followed by substrate.

wells coated with heavy chains isolated from the COR and LEW proteins, thus localizing the relevant idiotype to the light chain (Fig. 4). By the Western blot technique, the specificity of MAb 6B6.6 for the L chains of COR, LEW, MIL, and POM IgM RF was confirmed.

Anti-idiotypic reagents specific for the antigen-binding site or paratope of an antibody molecule would be expected to block antigen binding. As is illustrated in Fig. 5, the reaction of both COR and LEW RF with 6B6.6 in solution inhibited their binding to IgG-coated microtiter wells. This finding suggests that MAb 6B6.6 recognizes an epitope in or near the IgG binding site of these proteins. The failure of 6B6.6 to inhibit the IgG binding of POM and MIL may simply reflect the weaker affinity of the MAb for these two proteins. It is also possible that POM and MIL express only a portion of the CRI.

As illustrated in Table 4, the four 6B6.6-reactive IgM-RF all contained light chains belonging to the xIIIa sub-subgroup. Assignment of light chains to the xIIIa sub-subgroup was based on amino acid sequence analysis of amino-terminal portions of selected RF light chains. x chains from COR, LEW, MIL, and DAU contained an alanine residue at position 9 rather than the glycyl residue characteristic of the xIIIb sub-subgroup (47). The close association between the 6B6.6 marker and xIIIa light chains clearly distinguishes this idiotope from 17.109

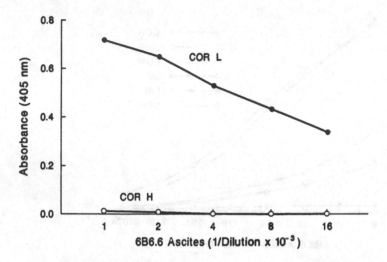

Figure 4 Reaction of MAb 6B6.6 with the heavy (H) and light (L) polypeptide chains of COR IgM by ELISA. Microtiter wells were coated with isolated COR heavy (O——O) and light (●——●) chains (0.01 mg/ml) and reacted with 6B6.6 ascites diluted in BSA-PBS diluent as indicated on the abscissa. The wells were then developed with alkaline phosphatase-labeled F(ab')$_2$ fragments of goat antimouse IgG followed by substrate.

since the latter is present only on light chains in the xIIIb sub-subgroup. In addition, the 6B6.6 CRI was not detected on RFs SCH and GLO, two 17.109 CRI-positive proteins included in the panel. Although the 6B6.6 idiotope was present on all IgM-RF paraproteins in our panel with xIIIa light chains, it was not detected on DAU, an IgM molecule having xIIIa light chains but lacking RF activity. In view of this finding, it is likely that MAb 6B6.6 identifies a subgroup of xIIIa light chains that is frequently associated with RF activity.

To determine if the 6B6.6 CRI was related to the PO CRI, two paraproteins bearing this marker (POM and LAY) were included in our panel. The reaction of MAb 6B6.6 with only one of the two proteins indicates that the 6B6.6 idiotype is distinct from the PO idiotype. This is not surprising in view of previous amino acid sequencing studies indicating that LAY uses VxI light chains in contrast to the VxIII light chains of POM (47a). To distinguish 6B6.6 CRI-positive RF from the BLA group described by Agnello et al. (35,41), immunofluorescence studies were performed using mouse kidney substrate. Since these experiments indicated that the 6B6.6-positive RF did not cross-react with nuclear antigens, it is highly unlikely that these antibodies are related to those in the BLA idiotypic group.

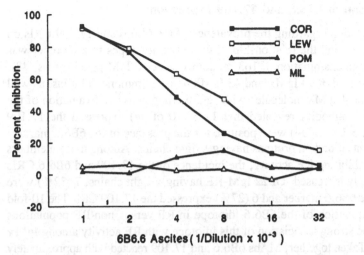

Figure 5 Inhibition of RF binding to IgG-coated microtiter wells by MAb 6B6.6. Microtiter wells coated with human IgG (0.05 mg/ml) were reacted with preincubated mixtures containing equal volumes of RF (50 ng/ml) and 6B6.6 ascites diluted in BSA-PBS diluent as indicated on the abscissa and developed with alkaline phosphatase-labeled $F(ab')_2$ fragments of rabbit anti-human IgM antibody followed by substrate: (■——■) COR IgM; (□——□) LEW IgM; (▲——▲) POM IgM; (△——△) MIL IgM.

Table 4 Reaction of Human Monoclonal Immunoglobulins with MAb 6B6.6 Anti-COR Idiotype and a Control MAb (6A6.7) of the Same Isotype but Specific for an Unrelated Antigen by ELISA[a]

Protein	Specificity	Light chain (reference)	Absorbance (×1000)	
			MAb 6B6.6	MAb 6A6.7
COR IgM	RF	κIIIa	1475	0
LEW IgM	RF	κIIIa	1333	0
POM IgM	RF	κIIIa	281	12
MIL IgM	RF	κIIIa	162	9
LAY IgM	RF	κI	16	0
GLO IgM	RF	κIIIb	12	15
SCH IgA	RF	κIIIb	0	0
DAU IgM	Unknown	κIIIa	0	0

[a]Microtiter wells coated with the IgM or IgA proteins were reacted with 100 ng/ml dilutions of the respective MAb for 3 h at room temperature, and bound antibody was subsequently detected by reaction with alkaline phosphatase-labeled goat $F(ab')_2$ antimouse antibody.

B. Comparison of 6B6.6 and 17.109 Expression

Further information regarding the prevalence of the 6B6.6 and 17.109 CRIs on immunoglobulins and the relationship of these two idiotopes to each other was acquired through examination of 163 randomly selected IgM paraproteins (48). The panel consisted of 94 IgMϰ and 43 IgMλ non-RF immunoglobulins, as well as 22 IgMϰ and 4 IgMλ molecules with IgG-binding activity. Evaluation of the non-RF IgMϰ antibodies revealed that 11% (10 of 94) expressed the 17.109 idiotope while 3% (3 of 94) were positive for the presence of the 6B6.6 marker. Neither CRI was found on proteins having λ light chains. Among those members of the panel exhibiting RF activity, the incidence of the 17.109 and 6B6.6 CRIs was significantly increased. Of 22 IgM-RF having ϰ light chains, 7 (32%) were positive for the 6B6.6 marker and 6 (27%) expressed the 17.109 CRI. The 10-fold increase in expression of the 6B6.6 idiotope in RF versus non-RF populations emphasizes the strong association of this idiotope with RF activity among IgMϰ paraproteins. Taken together, MAbs 6B6.6 and 17.109 reacted with approximately two-thirds of IgMϰ RFs included in the panel. However, in no instance were the two CRI present on the same molecule, emphasizing that expression of these two idiotopes is mutually exclusive.

C. Germline Origin of 6B6.6

The detection of a particular idiotope on denatured light (or heavy) chains of antibodies from unrelated individuals raises the possibility that the idiotope is encoded by a germline immunoglobulin gene. In view of the significant number of monoclonal paraproteins bearing the 6B6.6 CRI, it appeared probable that this idiotope, like 17.109, was the product of a germline V ϰ gene. Evidence for this supposition was provided when Chen and collagues isolated germline gene Humkv328, which encodes an amino acid sequence highly homologous to those found in light chains bearing the 6B6.6 CRI (49–51).

IV. CRI OF RF HEAVY CHAINS

Several laboratories have generated MAbs specific for CRIs located on the heavy chains of IgM RFs. MAb G6, for example, was produced by fusing lymphocytes from mice immunized with the RF paraprotein KOK, a member of the WA group (52). It was subsequently determined that the epitope recognized by this antibody was present not only on the immunizing protein but also on other RFs expressing the WA CRI. More recent experiments have determined that the G6 idiotype is present on VHI heavy chains likely encoded by germline gene ha1LR (53). In examining the prevalence of the G6 idiotype among 163 IgM paraproteins (described earlier), Crowley et al. (48) found that 14 members of the panel (9%) were positive for this idiotope. Especially noteworthy was the high prevalence of RF activity among IgM molecules bearing the G6 idiotype. Of 14 paraproteins expressing this marker, 9 (64%) exhibited IgG binding, indicating that the G6 idiotype is frequently, although not exclusively, found on RF molecules. Another interesting observation was the frequent pairing of G6-bearing heavy chains with 17.109-positive light chains. This heavy and light chain combination was observed with eight paraproteins, five of which possessed RF activity. Since three of the proteins displaying the G6-17.109 CRI combination were not RF, it is clear that the coexpression of these two idiotypes does not guarantee IgG-binding capability. Pairing of a 6B6.6-positive light chain with a G6-positive heavy chain was not observed.

Another CRI found on the heavy chains of IgM RF is defined by MAb Lc1 (54). The mice used to produce this MAb were immunized with a monoclonal IgM RF isolated from a patient with mixed cryoglobulinemia. Subsequent experiments determined that MAb Lc1 not only reacted with the immunizing antibody but also bound weakly to several other monoclonal RF. Moreover, the Lc1 CRI was detected on polyclonal RF in all five of the RA sera tested for the presence of this idiotype. Although MAb Lc1 does not react with isolated heavy or light chains, the results of recent experiments suggest that the Lc1 CRI requires heavy chains derived from the VH4 gene family (55).

A. Production of MAbs 5-14, 6-8, and 6-10

Our own efforts to identify CRIs on RF heavy chains have focused on two 6B6.6-positive IgM paraproteins, COR and LEW, which also have at least one heavy chain epitope in common (56). MAbs to the shared heavy chain idiotope(s) of COR and LEW were produced in a manner similar to that used to generate the MAb 6B6.6 (see Sec. III). Mice were initially immunized with 100 μg COR heavy chain in CFA, followed 3 weeks later by 50 μg of LEW heavy chain in saline. Lymphocytes from the popliteal and inguinal lymph nodes were fused with X63-Ag8.653 myeloma cells 3 days after challenge. Approximately 14 days after fusion, supernatants were tested for reactivity with heavy chains from proteins COR, LEW, and DAU. Hybridomas producing antibody that reacted with the heavy chains from COR and LEW, but not from DAU, were cloned, expanded, and grown in ascites.

B. Characterization of MAbs 5-14, 6-8, and 6-10

The fusion produced three MAbs, 5-14 (IgG$_{2b}$$\varkappa$), 6-8 (IgG$_3$$\varkappa$), and 6-10 (IgG$_{2b}$$\varkappa$), which reacted with IgM RFs COR and LEW but not with other paraproteins in a panel that included members of the WA and PO groups. Antibodies 6-8 and 6-10 were similar in that by a direct binding assay they exhibited strong binding to the COR paraprotein and somewhat weaker binding to the LEW paraprotein; however, MAb 5-14 was distinguished from the other two antibodies by its substantially lower level of reactivity with LEW IgM compared to COR IgM. To localize the determinant(s) recognized by the three MAbs, ELISA wells were coated with isolated heavy and light chains from the COR and LEW proteins. As illustrated in Table 5, all three MAbs reacted exclusively with heavy chain-coated wells, verifying the specificity of each antibody for a μ chain determinant. In agreement with previous ELISA data using intact molecules, MAbs 6-10 and 5-14 were more reactive with COR heavy chains than with those isolated from LEW. Despite their strong binding to COR IgM; however, none of the MAbs inhibited the RF activity of this protein in solution.

Although the epitope specificities of the three MAbs have not yet been determined, the similarity of their patterns of cross-reactivity suggests that they recognize the same idiotypic structure. However, the differences among the MAbs in the extent of cross-reactivity with LEW IgM RF or its heavy chains suggest that the epitope detected by MAb 5-14 differs somewhat from that detected by MAbs 6-8 and 6-10. Taken together, the results indicate that each of the monoclonal antibodies detects a μ chain idiotope expressed on COR IgM that is also either partially or completely present on LEW IgM. In view of the failure of the MAbs to inhibit IgG binding by the COR RF, it is likely that the CRI defined by the three antibodies does not reside in the active site but represents instead a framework antigen related to the heavy-chain variable region used in this molecule. This hypothesis is corroborated by the results of recent experiments, performed in collaboration with Drs. Greg Silverman and Dennis Carson, which indicate that MAbs 6-8 and 5-14 identify a determinant(s) present on a subset of heavy chains derived from the VH4 gene family which also express the Lc1 idiotope (55).

V. ASSOCIATION OF 6B6.6⁺ LIGHT CHAINS WITH VH4 HEAVY CHAINS

Previously described studies have demonstated that RFs with light chains bearing the 17.109 CRI frequently have G6-positive heavy chains derived from the VH1 gene family. This finding did not hold true for RF expressing the 6B6.6

Table 5 Reaction of MAbs with Heavy and Light Chains of COR and LEW by ELISA

	Absorbance ($\times$1000)		
Chain	MAb 5-14	MAb 6-8	MAb 6-10
COR heavy	1164	1119	1229
COR light	5	3	14
LEW heavy	360	1109	721
LEW light	3	5	8

CRI. Experiments performed in collaboration with Silverman and Carson have provided information concerning the type of heavy chains found in association with 6B6.6-positive light chains (5). As illustrated in Table 6, of nine monoclonal RFs bearing the 6B6.6 CRI, seven (or approximately 80%) utilized heavy chains originating from the VH4 gene family. The other two 6B6.6-positive RF (MIL and POM) had heavy chains associated with VH3 genes. It was of further interest that six of seven RF with VH4 heavy chains were reactive with MAb 6-10. The data in Table 6 also demonstrate the close relationship between the 6-10 and Lc1 CRIs. In all the cases examined, RFs expressing the Lc1 CRI also reacted with MAb 6-10. Despite the frequent coexpression of these two CRIs, there is evidence to indicate that these two idiotypic markers are distinct. First, MAb Lc1 inhibits IgG binding by RFs bearing this idiotope, whereas MAb 6-10 does not. Furthermore, a large number of IgM cold agglutinins exhibit weak reactivity with MAb 6-10 but fail to express the Lc1 CRI (55). Another distinguishing characteristic between MAbs 6-10 and Lc1 is that the former binds to isolated heavy chains whereas the latter does not. Such findings suggest that MAbs 6-10 and Lc1 identify different epitopes; indeed, the available data indicate that the Lc1 marker defines a subpopulation of VH4-derived, 6-10-positive heavy chains that are strongly associated with IgG binding.

VI. PREVALENCE OF CRIs ON POLYCLONAL RF

Several studies have examined the prevalence of various CRIs on polyclonal RFs in RA sera. In 107 IgM RF-containing RA sera, we detected 6B6.6-reactive RF in approximately 60% of the samples, at concentrations ranging from 0.02 to 6 μg/ml. More than 50% of the panel of RA sera, however, contained less than 0.5 μg of 6B6.6-positive RF per ml (56A). We observed no correlation between the amount of IgM RF present in the sera and the level of 6B6.6-positive RF.

Table 6 Characterization of VH Use in 6B6.6-positive Monoclonal RF

RF	MAb 6B6.6	VH	MAb 6-10	MAb Lc1
COR	+	VH4	+ +	+
LEW	+	VH4	+ +	+
ORI	+	VH4	+ +	+
7	+	VH4	+ +	+
51	+	VH4	+ +	+
108	+	VH4	+ +	+
LES	+	VH4	−	−
MIL	+	VH3	−	−
POM	+	VH3	−	−

Our study also quantitated the amount of 6B6.6 CRI$^+$ RF in 50 RA synovial fluids with known titers of IgM RF. The idiotope was detected on IgM RFs in 24 (48%) of the fluids at concentrations ranging from 0.3 to 13 μg/ml. As with RA sera, the level of 6B6.6-reactive RF detected in the synovial fluids did not correlate with the amount of IgM RF present. It is clear from these studies that RFs expressing the 6B6.6 CRI are present in a significant number of RA patients but account for only a small proportion of the total RF.

Using an ELISA inhibition assay, Carson and coworkers probed RA sera for the presence of RF expressing the 17.109 idiotope (57). The assay was based on the ability of MAb 17.109 to block IgG binding by RF. Under the conditions of this assay, marginal inhibition was observed in 4 of 8 samples, indicating that a small proportion of the RF in RA sera bear the 17.109 CRI. In contrast, RF activity in all 6 sera from patients with Sjögren's syndrome (SS) was significantly inhibited by MAb 17.109. In another study, utilizing an immunoblot assay, substantial levels of 17.109 CRI$^+$ RFs were detected in 12 of 15 sera from patients with SS (58). Direct-binding studies indicated that RFs bearing the CRI were mainly of the IgA class and to a much lesser extent, the IgM class. Moreover, B cells containing 17.109$^+$ Ig in their cytoplasm were prevalent in the salivary glands of 11 of 12 SS patients. In view of these data, it is apparent that a large proportion of the IgA RFs found in this disease express the 17.109 CRI.

More recent studies performed in this laboratory employed a sensitive direct-binding ELISA to determine the relationship between 6B6.6-positive and 17.109-positive RF in sera from 86 RA patients and 49 normal controls (58a). Although detectable levels of CRI$^+$ RF were seldom present in control sera, they frequently occurred in sera from RA patients. Of the sera tested 48% were positive for 6B6.6$^+$ RF, 35% for 17.109$^+$ RF, and 21% of the samples were positive for both CRI. When detected, CRI$^+$ RF were present in low concentrations (6B6.6: 1.12 $\pm$ 1.57 μg/ml; 17.109: 1.20 $\pm$ 1.15 μg/ml) and constituted a small fraction (less than 1%) of the total IgM RF in these sera. As in previous studies, there was no correlation between the levels of CRIs detected and the amount of IgM RF present in the sera.

VII. DISCUSSION

Experiments performed in this and other laboratories have generated polyclonal and monoclonal reagents specific for RF-associated CRIs. Although RFs expressing these structurally defined CRIs are found in a significant number of RA sera, represent only a small fraction of the total RF. The failure to detect a predominant CRI on these autoantibodies implies that the RFs produced in this disease express a variety of different idiotypes and argues for the involvement of a multitude of germline V genes. Alternatively, it is possible that relatively few germline genes encode RFs but that these genes undergo extensive somatic mutation in diseases like RA.

One obstacle in the identification of RF-associated CRI in RA has been the sparcity of cloned RF obtained from patients with this disease. To date, most of the monoclonal RFs used to probe for the presence of RF-associated CRIs have been obtained from patients with cryoglobulinemia or B cell malignancy. It is possible that these RF do not accurately reflect the population of RF produced during such autoimmune phenomena as RA (13).

Although there have been many attempts to produce RF-secreting hybridomas by fusion of lymphocytes from RA patients, the problems inherent in human hybridoma technology have made this a difficult undertaking. For example, peripheral blood lymphocytes (PBL) contain relatively few activated B cells and as a result must be stimulated with mitogen before fusion. Under these circumstances, even if RF-secreting hybridomas are obtained, they may result from the fusion of mitogen-activated B cells rather than B cells activated in vivo during autoimmune phenomena.

A number of laboratories, including our own, have attempted to isolate and fuse B cells from rheumatoid synovium and synovial fluids. Recently, Robbins et al. (59) produced two stable IgM RF-secreting hybridomas by fusing rheumatoid synovial cells isolated from two different patients. Idiotypic analysis of these and other RF should provide interesting information regarding the characteristics of RF present at the site of tissue destruction in RA.

Experience with MAbs directed against RF-associated CRIs has indicated that some monoclonal anti-idiotypic reagents are not useful for probing the genetic origin of these autoantibodies. For example, some anti-idiotypic MAbs recognize private idiotypes that arise upon somatic mutation of germline V genes or result from unique V and D segment joining events (60). MAbs specific for private idiotypes are highly reactive with the particular autoantibody used for immunization but would not be likely to recognize comparable autoantibodies produced by unrelated individuals. Monoclonal anti-idiotypic antibodies, which are the internal image of the RFs used for immunization, have CDRs that resemble the Fc portion of IgG. Such anti-idiotypic reagents bind to a variety of RF regardless of their genetic origin and thus do not provide information regarding the expression of a particular germline V gene (61). Among the anti-idiotypic reagents produced to date, those that have proven most useful for probing the structural diversity of RF have been those that recognize epitopes that appear to be encoded by germline genes. Examples of this type of anti-idiotypic reagent include MAbs 6B6.6 and 17.109.

A novel approach to the preparation of anti-idiotypic reagents to RF-associated CRI was recently introduced by Carson and colleagues (13). Their strategy was to produce rabbit antisera to synthetic peptides corresponding to two light-chain hypervariable region sequences found in the IgM RF paraprotein SIE. The resulting antisera, referred to as PSL2 and PSL3, reacted with epitopes located in the second and third hypervariable regions of SIE light chains, respectively. This technique has been used effectively to determine the structure of light chains associated with RF.

As additional germline V genes sequences are identified, the use of peptide immunogens will greatly facilitate the production of anti-idiotypic reagents to structurally defined epitopes. The availability of these antibodies, coupled with the acquisition of RF-secreting hybridomas from RA patients, will undoubtedly provide further insight into the genetic origin of RF and the mechanism by which they are produced in RA.

ACKNOWLEDGMENTS

Funding for this research supported in part by NIH grants AR-20614, AR-03555, and AI-18745 and the Veteran's Administration Research Program.

REFERENCES

1. Carson, D.A. (1985). In: *Textbook of Rheumatology*. Kelley, W.N., Harris, E.D., Ruddy, S., and Sledge, C.B., eds. W.B. Saunders, Philadelphia, pp. 664–679.
2. Koopman, W.J., and Schrohenloher, R.E. (1985). Rheumatoid factor. In: Rheumatoid Arthritis. Etiology, Diagnosis, Management. ner Utsig, P.D. Zvaifler, N.J., and Ehrlich, E.E., eds J.B. Lippincott, Philadelphia, pp. 217–241.
3. Chen, P.O., Fong, S., Houghten, R.A., and Carson, D.A. (1985). Characterization of an epibody: An antiidiotype which reacts with both the idiotype of rheumatoid factors (RF) and the antigen recognized by RF. J. Exp. Med. 161:323–331.
4. Bona, C.A., Finley, S., Waters, S., and Kunkel, H.G. (1982). Anti-immunoglobulin antibodies. III. Properties of sequential anti-idiotypic antibodies to heterologous anti-gamma globulins. Detection of reactivity of anti-idiotype antibodies with epitopes of Fc fragments. J. Exp. Med. 156:986–999.
5. Coulie, P., and Van Snick, J. (1983). Rheumatoid factors and secondary immune responses in the mouse. II. Incidence, kinetics and induction mechanisms. Eur. J. Immunol. 13:895–899.
6. Nemazee, D.A., and Sato, V.L. (1983). Induction of rheumatoid antibodies in the mouse: Regulated production of autoantibody in the secondary humoral response. J. Exp. Med. 158:529–545.
7. Welch, M.J., Fong, S., Vaughan, J.H., and Carson, D.A. (1983). Increased frequency of rheumatoid factor precursor B lymphocytes after immunization of normal adults with tetanus toxoid. Clin. Exp. Immunol. 51:299–305.
8. Aho, K., Konttinen, A., Rajasalmi, M., and Wager, O. (1962). Transient appearance of the rheumatoid factor in connection with prophylactic vaccination. Acta Pathol. Microbiol. Immunol. 56:478–479.
9. Slaughter, L., Carson, D.A., Jensen, F.C., Holbrook, T.L., and Vaughan, J.H. (1978). In vitro effects of Epstein-Barr virus on the peripheral blood mononuclear

cells from patients with rheumatoid arthritis and normal subjects. J. Exp. Med. 148:1429–1434.

10. Rodriguez, M.A., Ceuppens, J.L., and Goodwin, J.S. (1982). Regulation of IgM rheumatoid factor production in lymphocyte cultures from young and old subjects. J. Immunol. 128:2422.

11. Koopman, W.J., and Schrohenloher, R. (1980). In vitro synthesis of IgM rheumatoid factor by lymphocytes from healthy adults. J. Immunol. 125:934.

12. Wernick, R., LoSpalluto, J.J., Fink, C.W., and Ziff, M. (1981). Serum IgG and IgM rheumatoid factors by solid phase radioimmunonassay: A comparison between adult and juvenile rheumatoid arthritis. Arthritis Rheum. 24:1501.

13. Carson, D.A., Chen, P.P., Fox, R.I., Kipps, T.J., Jirik, F., Goldfien, R.D., Silverman, G., Radoux, V., and Fong, S. (1987). Rheumatoid factors and immune networks. Annu. Rev. Immunol. 109.

14. Winchester, R.J., Agnello, V., and Kunkel, H.G. (1970). Gamma globulin complexes in synovial fluids of patients with rheumatoid arthritis: Partial characterization and relationship to lowered complement levels. Clin. Exp. Immunol. 6:689.

15. McCormick, J.N. (1963). An immunofluorecsence study of rheumatoid factor. Ann. Rheum. Dis. 22:1.

16. Munthe, E., and Natvig, J.B. (1972). Immunoglobulin classes, subclasses and complexes of IgG rheumatoid factor in rheumatoid plasma cells. Clin. Exp. Immunol. 12:55.

17. Anderson, I.G., Cummings, N.A., Asofsky, R., Hylton, M.B., et al. (1972). Salivary gland immunoglobulin and rheumatoid factor synthesis in Sjögren's syndrome. Am. J. Med. 53:456.

18. Lamont-Havers, R.W. (1955). Nature of serum factors causing agglutination of sensitized sheep cells and group A hemolytic streptococci. Proc. Soc. Exp. Biol. Med. 88:35.

19. Waller, M.V., and Vaughan, J.H. (1956). Use of anti-Rh sera for demonstrating agglutination activating factor in rheumatoid arthritis. Proc. Soc. Exp. Med. 92:198.

20. Butler, V.P., Jr., and Vaughan, J.H. (1965). The reaction of rheumatoid factor with animal gamma-globulins: Quantitative considerations. Immunology 8:144.

21. Williams, R.C., Jr., and Kunkel, H.G. (1963). Separation of rheumatoid factors of different specificities using columns conjugated with gamma-globulin. Arthritis Rheum. 6:665.

22. Hannestad, K. (1978). Certain rheumatoid factors with both IgG and an antigen associated with cell nucleii. Scand. J. Immunol. 7:127.

23. Hannestad, K., and Stollar, B.D. (1978). Certain rheumatoid factors react with nucleosomes. Nature 275:671.

24. Franklin, E.C., Holman, H.R., Müller-Eberhard, H.J., and Kunkel, H.G. (1957). An unusual protein component of high molecular weight in the serum of certain patients with rheumatoid arthritis. J. Exp. Med. 105:425.

25. Gaarder, P.I., and Natvig, J.B. (1974). The reaction of rheumatoid anti-Gm antibodies with native and aggrevated Gm-negative IgG. Scand. J. Immunol 3:559.

26. Natvig, J.G., Gaarder, P.I., and Turner, M.W. (1972). IgG antigens of the $C\gamma2$ and $C\gamma3$ homology regions interacting with rheumatoid factors. Clin. Exp. Immunol 12:177.

27. Natvig, J.B., Gaarder, P.I., and Turner, M.W. (1972). IgG antigens of the $\gamma2$ and $C\gamma3$ homology regions interacting with rheumatoid factors. Clin. Exp. Immunol. 12:177.

28. Gaarder, P.I., and Natvig, J.B. (1970). Hidden rheumatoid factors reacting with "non a" and other antigens of native autologous IgG. J. Immunol. 105:928.

29. Gaarder, P.I., and Natvig, J.B. (1972). Two new antigens of human IgG, "non b⁰" and "non-b¹" related to the Gm system. J. Immunol. 108:617.

30. Bona, C., and Hiernaux, J. (1981). Immune response: Idiotype anti-idiotype network, Crit. Rev. Immunol. 2:33-81.

31. Goldman, M., Renversez, J.C., and Lambert, P.H. (1983). Pathological expression of idiotypic interactions: Immune complexes and cryoglobulins. Springer Semin. Immunopathol. 6:33-47.

32. Schmid, F.R., Roitt, I.M., and Rocha, M.J.(1970). Complement fixation by a two-component antibody system: Immunoglobulin G and immunoglobulin M anti-globulin (rheumatoid factor). Paradoxical effect related to immunoglobulin G concentration. J. Exp. Med. 132:673.

33. Tanimoto, K., Cooper, N.R., Johnson, J.S., and Vaughan, J.H. (1975). Complement fixation by rheumatoid factor. J. Clin. Invest. 55:437.

34. Kunkel, H.G. Agnello, V., Joslin, F.G., Winchester, R.J., and Capra, J.D. (1973). Cross-idiotypic specificity among monoclonal IgM proteins with anti-γ-globulin activity. J. Exp. Med. 137:331-342.

35. Agnello, V., Arbetter, A., de Kasep, G.I., Powell, R. Tan, E.M., and Joslin, F. (1980). Evidence for a subset of rheumatoid factors that cross-react with DNA-histone and have a distinct cross-idiotype. J. Exp. Med. 151:1514-1527.

36. Kohler, G., and Milstein, C. (1975). Continuous cultures of fused cells secreting antibody of predefined specificity. Nature 256:495.

37. Kunkel, H.G., Winchester, R.J., Joslin, F.G., and Capra, J.D. (1974). Similarities in the light chains of anti-gamma-globulins sharing cross-idiotypic specificities. J. Exp. Med. 139:128-136.

38. Capra, J.D., and Klapper, D.G. (1976). Complete amino acid sequence of the variable domains of two human IgM anti-gamma globulins (Lay/Pom) with shared idiotypic specificities. Scand. J. Immunol. 5:677.

39. Capra, J.D., and Kehoe, J.M. (1974). Structure of antibodies with shared idiotype: The complete sequence of the heavy chain variable regions of two immunoglobulin M anti-gamma globulins. Proc. Natl. Acad. Sci. USA 71:4032-4036.

40. Newkirk, M.M., and Capra, J.D.(1987). Restricted usage of immunoglobulin variable genes in human antibodies. In: The Immunoglobulin Gene. Honjo, T., Rabbits, T., and Alt, F.W., eds. Academic Press, New York.

41. Agnello, V., and Barnes, J.L. (1986), Human rheumatoid factor crossidiotypes I. WA and BLA are heat-labile conformational antigens requiring both heavy and light chains. J. Exp. Med. 164:1809.

42. Carson, D.A., and Fong, S. (1983). A common idiotype on human rheumatoid factors identified by a hybridoma antibody. Mol. Immunol. 20:1081-1087.

43. Fong, S., Chen, P.P., Gilbertson, T.A., Fox, R.I., Vaughan, J.H., and Carson, D.A. (1985). Structural similarities in the kappa light chains of human rheumatoid

factor paraproteins and serum immunoglobulins bearing a cross-reactive idiotype. J. Immunol. 135:1955–1960.

44. Radoux, V., Chen, P.P., Sorge, J.A., and Carson,D.A. (1986). A conserved human germline Vx gene directly encodes rheumatoid factor light chains. J. Exp. Med. 164:2119.

45. Lieberman, R., Potter, M., Humphrey, Jr., W., Mushinski, E.B., and Vrana, M. (1975). Multiple individual and cross-specific idiotypes on 13 levan-binding myeloma proteins of BALB/c mice. J. Exp. Med. 142:106–119.

46. Kearney, J.F., Radbruch, A., Liesegang, B., and Rajewsky, K. (1979). A new mouse myeloma cell line that has lost immunoglobulin expression but permits the construction of antibody-secreting hybrid cell lines. J. Immunol. 123:1548–1550.

47. Ledford, D.K., Goñi, F., Pizzolato, M., Franklin, E.C., Solomon, A., and Frangione, B. (1983). Preferential association of xIIIb light chains with monoclonal human IgMx autoantibodies. J. Immunol. 131:1322–1325.

47a. Kunkel, H.G., Winchester, R.J., Joslin, F.G., and Capra, J.D. (1974). Similarities in the light chains of anti-gamma-globulins showing cross-idiotypic specificities. J. Exp. Med. 139:128.

48. Crowley, J.J., Goldfien, R.D. Schrohenloher, R.E., Spiegelberg, H.L., Silverman, G.J., Mageed, R.A., Jefferis, R., Koopman, W.J., Carson, D.A., and Fong, S. (1988). Incidence of three cross-reactive idiotypes on human rheumatoid factor paraproteins. J. Immunol. 140:3411–3418.

49. Chen, P.P., Robbins, D.L., Jirik, F.R., Kipps, T.J, and Carson, D.A. (1987). Isolation and characterization of a light chain variable region gene for human rheumatoid factors. J. Exp. Med. 166:1900.

50. Jirik, F.R., Sorge, J., Fong, S., Heitzmann, J.G., Curd, J.G., Chen, P.P., Goldfien, R., and Carson, D.A. (1986). Cloning and sequence determination of a human rheumatoid factor light-chain gene. Proc. Natl. Acad. Sci. USA 83:2195.

51. Liu, M.-F., Robbins, D.L., Crowley, J.J., Sinha, S., Kozin, F., Kipps, T.J., Carson, D.A., and Chen, P.P. (1989). Characterization of four homologous light chain variable region genes which are related to 6B6.6 idiotype positive human rheumatoid factor light chains. J. Immunol. 142:688.

52. Mageed, R.A., Dearlove, M., Goodall, D.M., and Jefferis, R. (1986). Immunogenic and antigenic epitopes of immunoglobulins. XVIII. Monoclonal anti-idiotypes to the heavy chain of human rheumatoid factors. Rheumatol. Int. 6:179.

53. Kipps, T.J., Tomhave, E., Pratt, L.F., Duffy, S., Chen, P.P., and Carson, D.A. (1989). Developmentally restricted V$_H$ gene is expressed at high frequency in CD5 B cell malignancies. Proc. Natl. Acad. Sci. 86:5913.

54. Ono, M., Winearls, C.G., Amos, N., Grennan, D., Gharavi, A., Peters, D.K., and Sissons, J.G.P. (1987). Monoclonal antibodies to restricted and cross-reactive idiotopes on monoclonal rheumatoid factors and their recognition of idiotope-positive cells. Eur. J. Immunol. 17:343.

55. Silverman, G.J., Schrohenloher, R.E., Accavitti, M.A., Koopman, W.J., and Carson, D.A. VH4 gene expression in human monoclonal cold agglutinins and rheumatoid factors. Arthritis and Rheumatism. In press.

56. Schrohenloher, R.E., Accavitti, M.A., and Koopman, W.J. (1988). Occurrence of a μ-chain idiotope in two human monoclonal RF which also share a x-chain idiotope. Scand. J. Rheumatol. (Suppl.) 75:102.

56a. Schrohenloher, R.E., Accavitti, M.A., Bhown, A.S., and Koopman, W.J. (1990). Monoclonal antibody 6B6.6 defines a cross-reactive kappa light chain idiotope on human monoclonal and polyclonal rheumatoid factors. Arthritis Rheum. 33:187.

57. Fong, S., Chen, P.P., Gilbertson, T.A., Weber, J.R., Fox, R.I., and Carson, D.A. (1986). Expression of three cross-reactive idiotypes on rheumatoid factor autoantibodies from patients with autoimmune diseases and seropositive adults. J. Immunol. 137:122.

58. Fox, R.I., Chen, P., Carson, D.A., and Fong, S. (1986). Expression of a cross-reactive idiotype on rheumatoid factor in patients in Sjögren's syndrome. J. Immunol. 136:477.

58a. Koopman, W.J., Schrohenloher, R.E., and Carson, D.A. (1990). Dissociation of expression of two rheumatoid factor cross-reactive kappa light chain idiotypes in rheumatoid arthritis. J. Immunol. 144:3468.

59. Robbins, D.L., Kenny, T.P., Larrick, J.W., and Wistar, R. (1989). Two unique human monoclonal IgM rheumatoid factors derived from rheumatoid synovial cell secreting hybridomas. Arthritis Rheum. 32:S102.

60. Rajewsky, K., and Takemori, T. (1983). Genetics, expression, and function of idiotypes. Annu. Rev. Immunol. 1:569.

61. Fong, S., Gilbertson, T.A., Chen, P.P., Karras, J.G., Vaughan, J.H. and Carson, D.A. (1986). The common occurrence of internal image type anti-idiotypic antibodies in rabbits immunized with monoclonal and polyclonal human IgM rheumatoid factors. Clin. Exp. Immunol. 64:570.

62. Edelman, G.M. (1970). The covalent structure of a human γG-immunoglobulin. XI. Functional implications. Biochemistry 9:3197.

21

The Human Anti-DNA Idiotype (16/6 Idiotype)

Howard Amital-Teplizki and Yehuda Shoenfeld
Sheba Medical Center and Tel-Aviv University Medical School, Tel-Hashomer, Israel

I. INTRODUCTION

Antibodies are often associated with autoimmune diseases and are characterized in several ways. Most frequently they are defined according to their antigen-binding specificities, as anti-acetylcholine receptor, antistreptolysin, or anti-DNA. An additional way of classifying antibodies is by the antigenic determinants, which are usually located in the variable regions of the antibodies, in other words, by their idiotypes. These markers distinguish antibody molecules, even if they share a common class or subclass, or antigen binding properties.

A major transition in the field of idiotypic research was brought about during the last decade with the generation of hybridoma technology by Köhler and Milstein (1). Utilization of this method for production and analysis of autoantibody idiotypes in systemic lupus erythematosus (SLE) is of major importance for several reasons. It contributes to the classification of immunoglobulins into idiotypically related families, which aids tracing autoantibody origins. Idiotypes also link antibodies in the context of idiotypic networks, as postulated by Jerne (2). Detection of idiotypes and their corresponding anti-idiotypes that emerge in autoimmune diseases may assist in a better comprehension of their pathogenetic role. Furthermore, their identification may help to determine the immunoregulatory deficit from which they stem. And last but not least, there may be therapeutic potential in the utilization of idiotypes and anti-idiotypes to restore immunoregulatory equilibrium in autoimmunity.

In this chapter we review the characteristics of monoclonal anti-DNA idiotypes and we focus on their pathogenic role in autoimmune diseases.

II. ANTI-DNA IDIOTYPES IN THE MRL 1pr/1pr LUPUS-PRONE MURINE STRAIN

Several studies have focused on the production of hybridoma-derived monoclonal antibodies in animal models, prone to develop a SLE-like disease (3–6). In these animals circulating autoantibodies appear in the sera along with the development of clinical autoimmune disorders. Mice belonging to the MRL lpr/lpr murine strain develop lupuslike serology with an associated lymphorproliferative disease. Of their serum anti-DNA antibodies, 50% bear idiotypes that cross-react with a monoclonal anti-DNA antibody generated from lymphocytes of mice from the same strain and designated H130 (3). In this strain, the concentration of H130 idiotype increases in parallel to the progress of the SLE-like syndrome. Yet levels of the H130 idiotype are not fully correlated with titers of anti-DNA antibodies detected in sera since only 50% of serum anti-DNA antibodies carry this idiotype, whereas 40% of the antibodies possessing this idiotype bind to DNA (3). This idiotype is not confined to a single strain. On the contrary, its existence has been established in other autoimmune strains. Morever, lymphocytes taken from normal mice after being stimulated in vitro with mitogens can secret antibodies carrying the H130.

III. HUMAN ANTI-DNA ANTIBODIES AND THEIR RELATED IDIOTYPES

An extension of these observations has been completed in humans as well Table 1. Utilizing the human-human hybridoma technique, human anti-DNA monoclonal antibodies were generated and thoroughly scrutinized (7). Fusions were performed with either peripheral blood lymphocytes or splenocytes derived from seven unrelated lupus patients with the human lymphoblastoid cell line termed GM 4672 (derived from a patient with multiple myeloma). Exogenous antigenic stimulation was not committed before fusion, thus favoring spontaneous production of autoantibodies by the "naturally" aroused B cells. Although the yield of successful fusions was significantly lower among human hybridomas in contrast to mice fusions, the ratio of human-SLE autoantibody-secreting hybridoma (25%) compared favorably with the ratio reported on MRL lpr/lpr autoantibody-producing hybridoma (9–58%) (8). Among 30 human SLE monoclonal autoantibodies selected for their binding capacity to denatured DNA, 18 reacted with three or more additional polynucleotides, including native DNA, left-handed double-helical DNA (Z-DNA), poly(I), and poly(dT); 10 reacted with both nucleic acids and

Table 1 Representative Idiotypes of Anti-DNA Antibodies (Summared in Ref. 151)

Autoantibody	Ag specificity	Idiotype	Anti-idiotype	Cross-reactive/private	% Frequency in SLE patients
Human					
Anti-DNA	DNA	16/6	p. rabbit	CRI	50
		134	Antisera	CRI	40
		32/15	p. rabbit and m. monoclonal	CRI	28
Anti-DNA	DNA	3I	m. anti-3 I	CRI	90
		8.12	m. anti-8.12	CRI	50
		TOF	p. rabbit antisera	CRI	70
		AM	p. rabbit antisera	CRI	88
Murine anti-DNA					
MRL/1pr	DNA	H-130	p. rabbit antisera	CRI	—
(B/W)F$_1$	DNA	F-227	p. rabbit antisera	CRI	—

the phospholipid cardiolipin (9). Interestingly, all anti-DNA antibodies derived from human-human hybridomas belonged to the IgM isotype.

The polyspecific nature of the monoclonal human anti-DNA antibodies parallels observations concering MRL lpr/1pr monoclonal anti-DNA antibodies (10). These cross-reactions share similar binding patterns exhibited by serum antibodies of SLE patients (11).

The polyspecificity demonstrated by the human SLE monoclonal antibodies imply that the common epitope is probably an antigen carried by all the polynucleotides mentioned. Since the three-dimensional conformation of the different polynucleotides may vary considerably, the most likely target of the monoclonal antibodies is a structure comprising the backbone of these molecules, the phosphodiester bond. Similar to polynucleotides, cardiolipin is composed of phosphodiester bonds, thus clarifying the observed-cross-reactivity of the anti-DNA monoclonal antibodies with this phospholipid, as well as the biologically false-positive serologic test for syphilis among patients with SLE. Yet the specificity of these monoclonal antibodies differs strikingly from that found in sera of animals following deliberate immunization by Z-DNA (a right-handed helical synthetic double-stranded DNA molecule). In contrast to the broad spectrum of the monoclonal anti-DNA affinity, the induced anti-Z-DNA are highly specific for the Z-DNA molecule (12). These distinctions between binding characteristics of serum DNA binding antibodies and hybridoma-generated monoclonal antibodies may reflect different immunoregulatory processes that modulate autoantibody production. One of the outstanding traits engaging anti-DNA antibodies is their ability to react with cytoskeletal proteins (13). This aspect of lupus autoantibodies not only enlarges the spectrum of their binding properties but also offers several pathogenetic routes eliciting tissue injury as well.

The cytoskeletal structure we studied belonged to the intermediate filament subclasses, which probably anchor the nucleus to the cytoplasm, yet their precise role has not been completely elucidated. Several types of intermediate filaments have been described according to their cellular origin: vimentin in mesenchymal cells, desmin in muscular cells, neurofilaments in neurons, and others (14). All types bear a certain resemblance when compared by electron microscopy, X-ray diffraction, and amino acid sequencing (15).

Antibodies reacting with cytoskeletal proteins were reported to occur in both healthy and diseased states (16–19), for instance, in sera taken from mice of the MRL/++ autoimmune strain, antiintermediate filament antibodies were detected in contrast to antibodies directed against tubulin [a cytoskeletal protein with a role in cellular mitosis, adherence, and intercellular recognition (20,21)], which appear more frequently in hamsters (22). In humans, autoantibodies against tubulin or intermediate filaments have been found among patients with infectious mononucleosis (23). An affinity to cytoskeletal proteins was observed among 29 human hybridoma-derived monoclonal anti-DNA antibodies. Of these, 17 were found to bind to the cytoskeleton of mink lung cells, tested by the indirect immunofluorescence assay (13). The specificity of this binding was substantiated by prior application of DNAse to the cellular specimen. No abatement of the anti-DNA antibody reactivity with cytoskeletal components could be observed following this procedure.

However, similar treatment abolished the antinuclear activity of these monoclonal antibodies with epithelial cells, anticytoskeletal activity could not therefore be related to adherent DNA. Incubation with either DNA or vimentin completely blocked this binding.

An absolute ratification of the cross-reactivity between anti-DNA and antivimentin antibodies was achieved by showing that a previous application of an antivimentin monoclonal antibody eliminated any further cytoskeletal protein staining of anti-DNA antibodies, and vice versa. These data were established by the immunoblot technique, showing reactivity of the monoclonal anti-DNA antibodies to a 54 kD polypeptide consistent with vimentin.

The capacity of antinucleic antibodies to bind with cytoskeletal structures broadens the spectrum of cross-reacting epitopes recognized by the anti-DNA monoclonal antibodies. Although a shared phosphodiester-containing structure was clarified with affinities to monoclonal anti-DNA antibodies resembling those of anti-DNA and antiphospholipid, it is not evident whether this finding applies to the antivimentin potential of these antibodies. An alternative to a shared epitope on vimentin and nucleic acids is the possibility that the anti-DNA antibodies may have multiple independent specificities. Beyond their ability to bind to cytoskeletal components, the monoclonal lupus autoantibodies can react with diverse classes of cells as well.

Hannestad and Johannessen (24) found that 5 of 24 sera with antinuclear activity titers of 1:250 or more contained antinuclear antibodies that bound to a normal viable human mononuclear cells and granulocytes, but not to erythrocytes. The antibodies eluted from cell membranes were shown to possess antinuclear activity, in particular at 37 °C. Later it was ascertained that the antilymphocyte antibodies were absorbed following incubation with nuceli (25). These findings support the notion that lymphopenia, which is so often encountered in SLE, may be partially mediated by humoral mechanisms. Later we reported on lymphocytotoxicity mediated by 2 of 25 monoclonal hybridoma-derived anti-DNA autoantibodies (26). The antibodies reacted with normal B and T cells at 4 °C as well as at 37 °C. The lymphocytotoxic activity of the monoclonal anti-DNA antibodies could be inhibited by prior incubation of the monoclonal antibodies with polynucleotides or anti-idiotypes raised against their common anti-DNA idiotype, whereas prior incubation of the cells with DNAse did not substract the lymphocytotoxic effect.

Several possibilities can account for the binding of anti-DNA antibodies to lymphocyte membrane. Double-stranded DNA has been identified in the plasma membrane fraction of a long-term human blastoid cell culture line (27). In another work, nuclear materials could be detected within 6–9 h after commencement of culture (28). Yet in this study both the use of DNAse and the treatment of fresh lymphocytes with antibodies exclude this possibility. On these grounds an antigenic determinant that resides within lymphocytes membranes and nucleic materials (as phosphodiester bonds that comprise these two elements) may be attributed to this cross-reactivity. However, one cannot exclude the propositions of Lane and Kaprowski (29) and Richards et al. (30) regarding binding of monoclonal antibodies to diverse molecules via polyfunctional combining sites. Lymphocytotoxic antibodies may be ascribed to some of the immunoregulatory perturbations occurring in SLE. Some investigators reported that lysis occurs preferentialy, with T lymphocytes killing T suppressors in particular (31,32), perhaps mediating the B cell hyperactivity observed in SLE (26).

The binding of anti-DNA monoclonal autoantibodies is not confined solely to the normal population of lyphocytes. It was obseved that 7 anti-DNA antibodies of 60 human monoclonal lupus autoantibodies derived from three patients with SLE reacted with Raji cells by the indirect immunofluorescence technique and by radioimmunoassay (33). The binding of hybridoma-derived anti-DNA autoantibodies to Raji cells could be significantly abrogated by antecedent incubation of the autoantibodies with polynucleotides and cardiolipin.

The Raji lymphoblastoid cell lines are used to determine and purify immune complexes in many clinical conditions, particularly in SLE (34,35). Previous studies indicated that anti-DNA antibodies by themselves can react with Raji cell membrane, thus overestimating the quantity of immune complexes in conditions associated with the presence of anti-DNA antibodies (36). Although adherence of nuclear material to cell membrane is well known in cells growing for long periods in culture (29), the lack of effect of prior treatment of Raji cells with DNAse precluded this mechanism.

Experiments done with control IgM and IgG that did not bind to Raji cells excluded the involvement of Fc receptors presence on Raji cells. This notion is supplemented by the study of Tron and associates (37) showing that there is no binding of immunoglobulin to the putative Fc receptor on the Raji cell membrane. The identification of polypeptides on various mammalian cell membranes to which mouse monoclonal anti–double-stranded DNA antibodies and antibodies originating from SLE patients reacted (38,39) might account for the described phenomenon. This is consistent with the anti-DNA antibody recognition of membranous epitopes on nonlymphoid cells by anti-DNA antibodies (7,9,38–41). We have recently shown that anti-DNA monoclonal antibodies attached to human cortical brain tissue utilizing the indirect immunofluorescent assay (40).

Similar binding was exhibited by incubation of a rabbit monoclonal antiasialo GM_1 antibody, a ganglioside that is a constituent of the human brain (42). Furthermore, we showed that these two monoclonal antibodies competed on binding to a common site located on the neuronal membrane (40). Furthermore, the binding of the lupus autoantibodies could be blocked by prior absorption on nuclear and bovine brain extracts (40), and their specificity was ascertained by the negligible inhibition following absorption with mammalian splenic and hepatic extracts. Similarly, ssDNA, poly(I), poly(G), Ro(SSA), La(SSB), and RNP abrogated the autoantibody attachment to brain tissue.

These results are in line with those published by Hanley and associates (43), who found by Western immunoblots that antineuronal antibodies react with RNP, Sm, Ro, and La. The immunostaining of human cortical brain cells by these monoclonal antibodies perfectly resembled that observed by immuofluorescent studies utilizing sera of SLE patients, in particular those with neuropsychiatric involvement (44,45).

It is important to mention that cross-reactivity between neuroreactive and lymphocytotoxic antibodies has been similarly shown in sera of SLE patients (46). Last probably not least of the great scope of affinities by the lupus anti-DNA monoclonal antibodies is the reactivity to platelets (7,9). Undoubtedly, the mechanisms providing this large range of specificities remain to be revealed (47,48).

IV. CLINICAL CORRELATIONS OF ANTI-DNA ANTIBODIES

Anti-ds-DNA serum autoantibodies have been known for the last three decades as one of the hallmarks of SLE (49). They are detectable in up to 75% of lupus patients, depending on disease activity and selection of assay method (50). Virtually 90% of SLE patients produce anti ds-DNA antibodies when repeated tests are done (51), yet the prompt measurement of anti-DNA antibody titers has only minor accordance to the level of disease activity.

To compensate for this drawback we analyzed serologic results of 56 lupus patients (mostly outpatients) using a graded index of disease activity (50). Antibodies to ssDNA, dsDNA, RNA, poly(dT), poly(I), and cardiolipin were compared in cohorts of patients sharing similar clinical activity but different disease symptomatology (50).

No correlation between multiple antigen binding of lupus sera and clinical activity could be established. For instance, of 11 patients judged to be clinically inactive, 6 had four or more raised levels of IgG autoantibodies in their sera (50). In other studies different classifications were used on the number of systems involved (51,52). Partial degrees of correlation were found. However, the validity of these findings are equivocal since minor symptoms in three systems may be graded "severely active" whereas a life-threatening neurologic involvement may be referred to as mildly active.

To overcome these obstacles we assessed the concordance between serum anti-DNA idiotype concentrations and disease activity. All the idiotypes evaluated in the study were thoroughly scrutinized following their generation by the human hybridoma technique (7,9). High levels of 16/6 Id (one of the most investigated anti-DNA idiotypes) were revealed in 46 of the 98 SLE patients in the study, in contrast to 4 slightly elevated titers among 96 healthy controls (53).

After division into two subsets on grounds of clinical activity, 40 of 74 patients (54%) with active disease were found to have augmented levels of the 16/6 idiotype compared to 6 of 24 patients (25%) whose disease was in remission. Similar results were obtained following analysis of the patient sera by levels of another lupus anti-DNA idiotype, 32/15 Id: 28% among those with active disease had high concentrations of this idiotype versus 4% among those with quiescent disease (53).

Studying serially collected sera presented a notable correlation of the 16/6 Id concentration with disease activity among 8 of 12 patients (53). Such sequential idiotype measurements in SLE patients may be beneficial, determining or predicting disease activity. In one of the reported cases, the level of 16/6 Id declined earlier than that of anti ds-DNA antibodies just before the onset of clinical remission. In another patient a rise of 16/6 Id concentration took place during disease exacerbation without a concomitant increase in anti-dsDNA antibodies (53).

Solomon and associates (54) described a case of an active SLE patient in whom anti-dsDNA antibodies were undetectable but level of the idiotype they studied was raised. We also showed that 16/6 Id measurement may offer a more accurate tool to estimate disease activity (55).

Although the lupus anti-DNA idiotypes were first associated with their binding to DNA, it was acknowledged that they are not confined solely to anti-DNA antibodies (56). This observation is, in part, based on experiments showing that after immunoabsorption of serum anti-DNA antibodies the 16/6 Id could still be detected.

A remarkable occurrence is a case of an SLE patient whose lymphocytes spontaneously secreted large quantities of 16/6 Id DNA-reactive antibodies during an active phase of the disease but during clinical remission his lymphocytes mainly generated in vitro 16/6 Id DNA nonreactive antibodies, provided they were first stimulated by lectins (57). The results described are in concordance with those of Diamond and Solomon (58), who reported an 80% prevalance of an idiotype designated 3I among lupus patients with serum anti-DNA activity. This idiotype has no linkage to the DNA binding site. Concurrently, Zouali and Eyquem (59) identified an additional anti-DNA antibody idiotype, temed TOF, which was preset among 31 of 34 patients tested. These converging observations imply that, owing to the wide distribution of the lupus idiotypes among SLE patients with no common genetic origin, these idiotypes emerge from a restricted number of germline genes that exist among the patients.

V. IDIOTYPE NETWORK AND ANTI-DNA IDIOTYPES

Jerne (2) postulated that any given individual possesses thousands of idiotypes reflecting the infinite conformational possibilities of foreign antigen structures. As lympohocytes identify a broad range of antigenic determinants, they may also be able to recognize other idiotypes carried on antibodies secreted by other lymphocytes. Therefore, similar to the manner in which an autobody removes an antigen circulating in the blood stream, an anti-idiotype may be triggered and exert the termination of another idiotype production.

One of the benefits provided by the hybridoma technique is a better comprehension of idiotypic networks in disease and health. This is exemplified by the idiotypic cross-reactivity detected among seven hybridoma-derived IgM anti-DNA antibodies originating from seven unrelated SLE patients (60).

The anti-idiotype antibodies that disclosed this cross-reactivity were generated by immunization of animals with IgM monoclonal antibodies derived from two unrelated lupus patients. Anti-idiotypic binding to the Fc portion of the autoantibodies could be excluded, since no binding was observed following incubation with pooled immunoglobulins obtained from normal persons, nor did they bind to monoclonal immunoglobulins obtained from patients with monoclonal gammaopathies.

The anti-idiotypic antibodies seemed to react with components near the antigen binding site of the monoclonal antibodies. This was elucidated by abrogration of monoclonal idiotypes binding to their homologous anti-idiotypes by prior incubation with their antigens. The reaction of the lupus idiotype 32/15 to its corresponding murine anti-idiotype was inhibited almost entirely by poly(dT) and poly(I) and partially by dsDNA (60). Binding of rabbit-derived anti-32/15 was inhibited by the three nucleic acid polymers, yet in a different order of affinities from which they attached to the 32/15 Id (60). herefore it could be concluded that each monoclonal anti-idiotype reacted with a selective small structure localized within the variable region of the homologous idiotype. A similar phenomenon was observed regarding the idiotype designated 16/6 Id. The autoantibody 16/6 attached to poly (I), poly(dT), and ssDNA, but its binding to rabbit anti-16/6 could be inhibited only by poly(I). Interestingly, rabbit anti-16/6 could block 16/6 binding to ssDNA.

Of the 60 human hybridoma-derived lupus monoclonal antibodies, 20 showed no avidity to the two anti-idiotypic reagents that were mentioned. These 20 monoclonal antibodies had no binding properties to poynucleotides or cardiolipin that could distinguish them for other anti-DNA autoantibodies (60). Of the remaining 40 autoantibodies, 15 cross-reacted with one antiidiotype, 10 with two anti-idiotypes, and 15 with three antiidiotypes.

Of the monoclonal autoantibodies derived from five patients, nine reacted exclusively with mouse anti-32/15 and the mouse anti-idiotype (anti-32/15) reacted with hybridoma anti-DNA antibodies derived from six of the seven patients comprising the study. On the grounds of these assays, we believe that rabbit anti-16/6 Id, rabbit anti-32/15 Id, and mouse anti-32/15 identified different structures localized within the variable regions of the anti-DNA antibodies. This is noteworthy since it indicates that a particular family of epitopes is distributed among lupus autoantibody idiotypes. Solomon and associates (54) reported parallel findings with a monoclonal anti-idiotype antibody produced following immunization of a mouse with partially purified anti-DNA antibodies. The antibodies originated from an SLE patient. The reagent detected cross-reactivity among serum idiotypes of eight of nine patients with SLE, as well as with monoclonal anti-dsDNA antibodies of all IgG subclasses. However, the anti-idiotype did not react with the binding site of the anti-DNA antibodies since it did not inhibit their binding to ds-DNA. Similarly, DNA did not affect the reactivity of the anti-idiotype reagent with anti-DNA antibodies.

It is well known that idiotypic cross-reactivity appears among monoclonal antibodies derived from strains of lupus-prone mice as NZB $\times$ NZWF$_1$ (4,5) or MRL lpr/lpr (3). This phenomenon should not be attributed solely to the inbred strain origin since Datta et al. (61) found that NZB mice can generate autoantibodies that share idiotypes with monoclonal anti-DNA antibody derived from a genetically unrelated MRL 1pr/lpr mice.

VI. LUPUS IDIOTYPE ANTIBODY IN OTHER AUTOIMMUNE STATES

Overlapping clinical and laboratory features are often encountered in autoimmune rheumatic states. Even when distinct in clinical presentations and prognostic outcomes, different autoimmune conditions may share various properties, such as:

1. Similar defects in suppressor T cell functions (62)
2. Increased incidence of complement component deficiencies (63)
3. Association with the same or related major histocompatibility complexes (64)
4. Existence of families with a concurrent occurrence of several autoimmune disorders (65)
5. Preferential presence of specific phenotypes on the Fc portion of immunoglobulins in different diseases, such as myasthenia gravis, Graves' disease, and type 1 diabetes mellitus (66)

A rather interesting element that embraces various autoimmune diseases is the occurrence of autoantibodies (67,68). Anti-DNA antibodies have been described in a variety of autoimmune conditions, in particular anti-ssDNA, yet the significance of these finding and any pathologic role they fulfill remains obscure.

We determined the presence of the common lupus idiotype 16/6 in sera of 170 patients with different autoimmune disorders excluding SLE (68).

The results clearly reflected that the anti-DNA idiotype is detected in high concentration, particularly among patients with Graves' disease (37.5%), polymyositis (40%), Sjögren's syndrome (17%), and multiple sclerosis (16%) (68). These incidence rates were compared to 0% found in 77 normal healthy controls. Patients with scleroderma were notably found to lack 16/6 Id in their sera. The high prevalence of the 16/6 Id in sera of patients with rheumatic condition was not confined to one type of anti-DNA idiotype. A high concentration of another anti-DNA idiotype termed 134 Id was demonstrated as well. This idiotype appears in sera of approximately 60% of SLE patients. Among 70 serum samples representing various autoimmune conditions, the 134 Id was detected in 17 of 27 samples (63%) in which the 16/6 Id was found, versus merely 8 of 43 (19%) serum samples in which the 16/6 Id was absent (69). This occurrence was not owing to an outstanding nonspecific hyperreactivity of the engaged serum samples, since no detection of an unrelated antihepatitis B surface antigen could be shown (69). Further analysis of lupus idiotypes was carried out among patients with chronic liver diseases (70); the 16/6 Id was detected among 58 of 88 (66%) patients with chronic liver disorders, and the 134 Id was encountered among 43 of the patients (49%) and the 32/15 Id in 13 (15%). Distinct diagnostic groups displayed different lupus anti-DNA idiotypic profiles. Patients with primary biliary cirrhosis and chronic active hepatitis had mainly the 16/6 Id, whereas among patients with either alcoholic or cryptogenic cirrhosis both the 16/6 Id and the 134 Id were the main idiotypes recorded.

Although a considerable correlation among the different idiotypes was disclosed, no concordance was revealed between the lupus idiotypes and the unrelated antihepatitis B surface antigen idiotype. In addition, no association between immunoglobulin concentrations and appearance of lupus idiotypes could be found. These results substantiate early reports indicating the appearance of antinuclear antibodies in sera of patients with chronic liver disease (71,72). These findings extend the scope of those already recognized linking rheumatic diseases and chronic liver diseases. Several examples of such linkage are arthritis, skin lesions, and Sjögren's syndrome, as well as laboratory evidence, such as hypergammaglobulinemia, immune complexes, and common autoantibodies (73).

Another rheumatic condition associated with the appearance of antinuclear autoantibodies is drug-induced lupus. Drug-induced lupus bears many clinical and serologic characteristics of SLE; however, involvement of the central nervous system and the kidneys is very rare, as is the appearance of anti-dsDNA antibodies (74). Nevertheless, high titers of antibodies against other nuclear components were identified, such as antihistone (75–77) and anti-ssDNA antibodies (78). Several theories have been raised to explain the development of autoimmune phenomena that accompany long-term drug treatment. Binding of drugs to nucleic acids may elicit their denaturation and ultimately the formation of immunogenic DNA, which promotes the appearance of anti-DNA antibodies (75). Other explanations propose that antibodies produced against the drug cross-react with nuclear components.

Rabbits immunized with a hydralazine-human serum albumin conjugate generated antibodies to hydralazine, ssDNA, and dsDNA (78). Furthermore, anti-DNA antibodies were absorbed by the hydralazine-albumin conjugate, implying the possible existence of shared epitopes. Other findings implicated in the direct impact of drugs on the immune system that brings about the emergence of autoantibodies were demonstrated with procainamide (77–80). These observations are based on the augmentation of B cell responses to procainamide mediated by inhibition of suppressor T cells; N-acetylprocainamide fails to produce similar results (79). In another study it was suggested that procainamide activates the helper T cell population (80). We have examined the presence of two common idiotypes 16/6 Id and 32/15 Id among 67 patients on treatment with procainamide (81). Raised concentrations of 16/6 Id and 32/15 were detected among 37 and 24% of the patients, respectively.

Furthermore, five of eight patients who developed drug-induced lupus had both idiotype levels raised (81). In some the idiotype levels reached those recorded in sera of patients with active SLE. A correlation could be found between the 16/6 Id titer and ssDNA and antihistone antibody titers in the group as a whole. These serologic similarities may point to the relatedness of drug-induced lupus and SLE. However, other immunologic markers contradict these findings, such as the observed higher frequency of HLA-B8, DR2, and DR3 among SLE patients versus the prevalent finding of HLA-DR4 among patients with drug-induced lupus due to antecedent therapy with hydralazine (82).

Anti-DNA idiotypes are associated with other rheumatic diseases. Recently we produced a monoclonal antibody following fusion of peripheral blood lymphocytes of a patient with manifestations of polymyositis with a lymphoblastoid cell line (83). Interestingly, this patient did not carry the 16/6 Id in her serum antibodies, nor did she have any detectable serum anti-DNA activity. Yet the monoclonal antibody we developed was 16/6 Id positive, which had anti-DNA binding capacity. Furthermore, a second monoclonal antibody generated following the establishment of remission did not carry the 16/6 Id nor it did bind to DNA (83).

The association between high levels of 16/6 Id and autoimmune phenomena is obviously dependent on an appropriate environmental, hormonal, and genetic background (64). This concept is clearly demonstrated by patients with monoclonal gammopathies in whom monoclonal antibody concentration may reach striking levels. We reported on an 8.7% prevalence of the 16/6 Id in serum samples obtained from 265 patients. Of the 23 16/6 Id-positive detected, 7 had benign monoclonal gammopathy, 3 multiple myeloma, 3 Waldenström's macroglobulinemia, five mixed essential cryoglobulinemia, and 5 monoclonal cryoglobulinemia (84). In 11 of the 16/6 Id-positive serum samples, antinucleic acid activity was found as well. However, only 1 patient (with essential mixed cryoglobulinemia) had symptomatology resembling rheumatic disease.

These data should not come as a surprise, since other studies revealed the autoantibody activity of monoclonal antibodies in patients with plasma cell dyscrasias, such as rheumatoid factor activity, anti-red blood cells, cardiolipin, albumin, thyroglobulin, DNA, and histone activities (85–89).

Although the autoantibody activity may be interpreted as an epiphenomenon, it has been shown that they may take part in the pathogenesis of disease as well. This was noted by IgM monoclonal antibody from a patient with chronic lymphocytic leukemia that cross-reacted with DNA and phosphorylated neuronal constituents. It suggested that this antibody may have mediated the pathogenesis of a neuropathy that appeared in this patient (89).

VII. ANTI-DNA IDIOTYPES IN NORMAL INDIVIDUALS

Serum from normal humans and mice contains low levels of antibodies that react with dsDNA (90–92). Moreover, precursor B cells committed to the production of anti-DNA antibodies have been identified (67). In culture, anti-DNA antibodies were induced following a polyclonal stimulus of B cells by lipopolysaccharide (93) and Epstein-Barr virus (94) or after induction of a graft-versus-host reaction in normal mice (95). Similarly, hybridomas derived from lymphocytes of normal individuals (57,96) and healthy animals (97) were shown to generate monoclonal anti-DNA antibodies, thereby establishing the concept that common anti-DNA idiotypes are an integral part of the normal repertoire of the immune system. Datta and associates (57) reported the in vitro production of 16/6 Id by lymphocytes of normal subjects and lupus patients.

Using biosynthetic labeling, immunoprecipitation, and sodium dodecyl sulfate (SDS)-polyacrylamide gel electrophoresis, their findings indicated that the 16/6 Id exists on two distinct populations of antibodies. The first, conserved in normal subjects, is of uncertain antigenic specificity and is represented dominantly by the 16/6 Id set that appears after pokeweed mitogen stimulation of normal individuals. The second is observed on antibodies binding to nucleic acids and becomes prominent during clinical relapse of SLE (57).

VIII. INFECTION AND LUPUS IDIOTYPES

One of the most important factors associated with induction of autoimmunity, with ominous impact on the natural history of this group of diseases, are infectious agents. Viruses, bacteria, and parasites may participate as ubiquitous triggers in the breakdown of immune tolerance by several mechanisms. Mimicry between host tissue components and microbial agents have been reported in many communications. Several examples of these occurrences are blood group substances and bacterial polysaccharides, cardiac tissue and streptococcal polysaccharides, kidney tissue and *Escherichia coli* lipopolysaccharides, and brain components and the capsular polysaccharides of *Nesseria meningitidis* group B and *E. coli* K1 (98–102). Other evidence proposes that this association is elicited by polyclonal activation stimulated by infections. The temporal relationship between a specific infection and the appearance of a disease is classically demonstrated by the development of rheumatic fever following a streptococcal infection (97) or the presentation of diabetes mellitus type I after coxsackie virus or mumps epidemics (100,101).

Other mechanisms involved are the induction of class II major histocompatibility complex (MHC) antigens in target tissues leading to their elimination by host T lymphocytes and the cross-reactivity between microbial and host antigens via anti-idiotypic networks (102). Infectious diseases lead to the occurrence of anti-DNA antibodies as in tuerculosis (103), and trypanosomiasis (104,105). In one study a rabbit injected with *Schistosoma japonicum* developed anti-ssDNA antibodies and severe nephropathy (106).

Atkinson and associates demonstrated a marked similarity between four monoclonal anti-DNA idiotypes and the amino acid sequence of Waldenström's IgM antibody that binds to the 3,4-pyruvylated galactose in the *Klebsiella* polysaccharide K30, designated WEA. Complete identity of the NH_2-terminal sequences of the four 16/6 idiotype-positive IgM autoantibody light chains and the WEA IgM light chain could be noted, with a single exception of the amino acid threonine substituting for glycine 34 in the WEA protein (107). In contrast, another anti-DNA monoclonal antibody not carrying the 16/6 Id showed no homology to the WEA antibody (108). It was noted that the WEA antibody not only had a striking similarity to the 16/6 Id monoclonal anti-DNA antibodies but carried the idiotype itself (107). It seems unlikely that the V genes of 16/6 were conserved through the ages to specify anti-DNA antibodies. It is more plausible that the original specificity of this idiotype was of bacterial origin. These results were further endorsed by interesting data carried out in recent studies. In the first, polyclonal stimulation of peripheral blood mononuclear cells obtained from six normal subjecs were carried out by incubation with polyclonal activators (Epstein-Barr virus, pokeweed mitogen, group A streptococcus, straphylococcus, and klebsiella). After 7 days of incubation, significantly increased levels of the 16/6 Id were secreted only by klebsiella-stimulated cells (109), whereas secretion of total immunoglobulins was enhanced by all mitogens (110).

These results are complemented by the second observation that an increased incidence of high titers of 16/6 Id (and antipolynucleotide activity) was detected in the sera of patients with *Klebsiella* infection, compared to patients with other gram-negative infections and normal controls (111).

Further cues implicate that mycobacterial infections are engaged with the development of autoimmune processes (40,44,103,112–117). A variety of autoantibodies, including antinuclear antibodies (112), anticardiolipin antibodies (113), and rheumatoid factor (113), were detected in sera of patients infected with *Mycobacterium leprae*.

In a recent study (114), monoclonal antituberculosis antibodies, which are known to react with different species of mycobacteria, were found to bind to ssDNA as well as to other polynucleotides. The binding of the anti-TB antibodies to ssDNA could be inhibited by prior incubation of these antibodies with ssDNA and with the different polynucleotides. Human and mouse monoclonal anti-DNA antibodies derived from patients and mice with SLE (among them antibodies carrying the 16/6 Id) reacted with three mycobacterial cell wall glycolipids shared by all mycobacteria.

This binding could also be inhibited by DNA and other polynucleotides. These anti-DNA antibodies and the anti-TB antibodies competed with each other on their binding to ssDNA, and finally, a murine anti-TB antibody was shown to carry the dominant 16/6 Id and to have antinuclear reactivity (114).

This association was substantiated by further analysis of serum samples obtained from patients with active untreated pulmonary tuberculosis. Among 57 tuberculosis patients, 34 (60%) had increased levels of the 16/6 Id, compared to only 1 of 28 matched controls; increased autoantibody activity to polynucleic acids and cardiolipin were found as well (103).

In parallel to these results, antibodies to mycobacterial glycolipids appear in two different patterns among patients with SLE. The first subset of patients possesses an elevated anti-glycolipid antibody titer as high as that detected among tuberculosis patient, whereas the second subset has extremely low levels, even below those recorded in a group of normal healthy controls. This second group could be delineated by their central nervous system symptomatology, which was absent in the first high antiglycolipid titer group (115).

These data paralleled those reported by Hirano and associates (118), who detected autoantibodies against a cerebral ganglioside, "asialo CM_1," which is a component of white and gray matter in the central nervous system. Among patients with SLE-associated neurologic disorders, the titer of these antibodies was high for long periods before and after acute neurologic exacerbation, yet their level diminished during the appearance of neurologic symptoms. All these findings lead to a suggestive antigenic mimicry existing between mycobacterial and cerebral glycolipids.

As reported, cross-reactivity was ascertained between cerebral gangliosides and DNA by a monoclonal antibody derived from a patient with chronic lymphocytic leukemia complicated by a neuropathy (89). Therefore, we decided to assess the binding properties of monoclonal antiasialo GM_1, murine monoclonal antimycobacterial glycolipids, and human lupus anti-DNA antibodies carrying the 16/6 Id. IgG antimycobacterial glycolipids and three IgM anti-DNA, 16/6 Id-positive antibodies reacted with tissue sections from the frontal cortex of a man who expired from a nonneurologic unrelated disease, using the indirect immunofluorescence assay. Polynucleic acids [ss-DNA, poly(I), and poly(G)] abrogated the attachment of the monoclonal antibodies to the brain tissue sections as well as purified mycobacterial glycolipids and bovine brain extracts. The antineuronal affinity of these antibodies was further validated by the rather negligible inhibition presented by either liver or spleen extracts (40).

A similar trend was detected by analyzing binding the properties of antineuronal antibodies in sera of SLE patients. Of SLE patients with neuropsychiatric symptoms, 81% had these antineuronal antibodies in their sera compared to 17% among other SLE patients. However, regardless of the existence of neurologic disease, these antibodies' avidity to brain tissue was blocked by either bovine brain extract or mycobacterial glycolipids (44).

These studies emphasize the pertinent pathogenic role of cross-reactive antimycobacterial antibodies and antineuronal antibodies in SLE, especially among patients with an associated neuropsychiatric disease. These antibodies may penetrate the central nervous system via a "leaky" blood-brain barrier damaged by a vasculitic process, entailing a cytopathic effect to brain tissue. More of the facts typing mycobacterial infections with autoimmunity are reviewed thoroughly elsewhere (44).

Tabe 2 summarizes the various binding characteristics of anti-DNA anti-bodies carrying the 16/6 Id. In Table 3 we have listed the clinical conditions in which increased titers of the 16/6 Id were recorded.

Table 2 Binding Characteristics of Anti-DNA Antibody Carrying the 16/6 Id

1. ssDNA, synthetic polynucleotides (poly [dT], poly[I], and poly[G]) (9).
2. dsDNA (83)
3. Cardiolipin (55)
4. Platelet membrane (7)
5. Lymphocytes membrane (e.g., Raji cell (33)
6. Lymphocytotoxic (26)
7. Tuberculous glycolipids (102,114,115)
8. *Klebsiella* polysaccharides (102,107,109)
9. Brain glycolipids (40)
10. Cytoskeletal proteins (e.g., vimentin) (13)

Source: From Ref. 148.

Table 3 Clinical Conditions Associated with Increased Titers of 16/6 Id

1. Active SLE, correlation with clinical activity (53,55)
2. Sera of first-degree relatives of patients with SLE (69,113)
3. C_4 complement component deficiency (135)
4. Healthy subjects with IgA deficiency (140)
5. Other autoimmune diseases, e.g., chronic liver diseases (70) and autoimmune thyroid diseases (68)
6. Drug-induced lupus (81)
7. Monoclonal gammapathies, e.g., multiple myeloma and Waldenström's macroglobulinemia (84)
8. Sera of patients with active infection with mycobacteria (102,103,116) and *Klebsiella* (109,111)
9. Deposition in afflicted kidney (141) and skin (142) of SLE patients and brain (40)
10. In naive mice in which SLE was induced by immunization with 16/6 Id (increased 16/6 Id in mice sera of murine origin [146,147])
11. Normal subjects (57,109)
12. Offspring of mothers with SLE (131)

Source: From Ref. 143.

IX. GENETIC ASPECTS OF LUPUS IDIOTYPES

Evidence of a genetic basis for SLE has been accumulated in different communications. Population studies indicated a marked ethnic variance disclosed by a Hawaiian study that found prevalence rates per 100,000 people to range from 5.8 among among whites to 24.1 in the Chinese (119).

Support for genetic grounds was gained after positive association between HLA-DR antigens and SLE was established. It is generally accepted that among whites the presence of DR2 and DR3 is associated with increased risks of developing SLE. Among the Japanese, only DR2 was correlated with the manifestation of SLE, whereas among black Americans preliminary result suggest that DR3 showed a slight concordance with lupus (120).

Other HLA studies have consistently shown associations with A1 and B8 as well (121). The frequency of the Gm allotypes 1, 17, 5, 6, and 13 were found to be higher among black American SLE patients (122).

Inherited complement deficiency states, notably those of the classic pathway, have also been noted (123). In a recent study more than 80% of white SLE patients were found to have a silent or null allele of C4a or C4b (and in one patient, C2) equated with 40% of a matched normal control group (124). In approximately 4% of SLE patients a positive family history is revealed (125), yet in many asymptomatic relatives of lupus patients hypergammaglobulemia (126), raised circulating immune complex levels (127), serum autoantibodies (128), and decreased suppressor T cell function (129) are reported as well. We extended these observations by showing a high incidence of the lupus anti-DNA idiotypes 16/6 Id and 32/15 Id among first-degree relatives of SLE patients, 24 and 7%, respectively (130). These data imply that 16/6 Id is a genetically associated marker and is not necessarily pathogenetic.

No distinction could be made between male and female relatives regarding the presence of the DNA idiotypes (130). These data differ from previous communications showing that female relatives are primarily involved with T suppressor abnormal function or with the augmented frequency of anti-nuclear factor (127,129). More evidence on the familial characteristics of the lupus idiotypes comes from a report on the vertical transmission of autoantibody expression through generations (131). Sera from six mothers and their paired offspring were screened for the presence of the common anti-DNA idiotype 16/6 Id. Of three active SLE mothers, two, as well as their matched offspring, had increased levels of 16/6 Id. In a third clinically active pair a high concentration of anti-DNA idiotypes were recorded in cord serum only, but maternal serum was negative for the 16/6 Id, favoring the de novo production of this idiotype by the fetus (131). This finding may be explained by the immunogenic environment in which the fetus resides, similar to reports of affected newborns of myasthenic mothers (132).

Additionally, elevated titers of autoantibodies, mostly of the IgG isotype, were observed among the clinically active mothers. Similarly, all offspring of clinically active SLE mothers showed increased IgG autoantibodies to a variety of antigens, but IgM antibodies were detected in only one fetus (131). Parallel results corroborated these data by the detection of a 30% prevalence of the lupus idiotype 134 among first-degree relatives of SLE patients. This idiotype is highly common among SLE patients (45%) yet is not confined to anti-dsDNA antibodies (69). These data reflect the concept that germline genes encode these relatively public (common) idiotypes. Another alternative may stress that the frequent idiotype presence represents a dominant immunoglobulin rearrangement in both the patients and their first-degree relatives (70).

The genetic aspects of rheumatic diseases have been partly better understood since the mapping of chromosome 6, revealing the approximate location of the complement component's genes (C2 and C4) and the major histocompatability complex genes (133). C2 deficiency is the most common congenital complement component deficiency. Among patients with C2 deficiency, connective tissue diseases emerge more often, SLE in particular (134). Up to a third of these patients suffer from a lupus skin involvement (134).

We analyzed a family of a female SLE patient who had raised levels of the 16/6 Id in her serum (135). Among family members, elevated concentration of this idiotype could be detected as well. This family was notable since many of its members were C4 deficient. A sister of the propositus subsequently developed SLE. Of eight members examined, seven had C4 deficinecy and all except one of these seven had a raised 16/6 Id level. The one member without a deficiency had normal 16/6 Id levels. In addition we analyzed the autoantibody characteristics of another immunodeficiency state, selective IgA deficiency. This disease is generally regarded as a permanent, genetically inherited state with multifactorial etiologies (136). Despite seeing the most common immunodeficiency disorder, the majority of IgA-deficient people are asymptomatic. However, there is an association with various allergic disorders, frequent upper respiratory tract infections, gastrointestinal diseases, malignancies, and autoimmune phenomena. Numerous autoimmune features turn out to coexist with IgA deficiency, such as SLE, rheumatoid arthritis, dermatomyositis, and polymyositis, (136–139). To determine whether serologic markers of autoimmune diseases similarly coexist with IgA deficiency as clinical manifestations, we analyzed autoantibody patterns in samples of IgA-deficient patients (140). Of the tested sera, 37% proved to harbor autoantibody activity directed against cardiolipin, 29% against ssDNA, and 22% against dsDNA; however, only a minority of 12% of the patients carried detectable titers of the 16/6 Id (140). The utilization of autoantibody screening among IgA-deficient patients may aid in identifying those who are prone to develop a more harsh course of the disease, yet a prospective study is warranted to establish this hypothesis.

X. THE PATHOGENETIC ROLE OF LUPUS IDIOTYPES

One of the major questions that arises concerning the lupus anti-DNA idiotypes is whether these idiotypes are a reflected epiphenomenon of the pathogenic process taking place in the organism or are directly involved in the development of the autoimmune disorder.

This enigma was partly resolved by the detection of immunoglobulins carrying the 16/6 Id in the glomerular basement membrane and mesangium of 11 of 26 kidney biopsies of lupus patients (141). Similar results were obtained screening skin biopsies of 24 lupus patients. Up to 45% of the immunoglobulins at the dermal-epidermal junction were found to share idiotyes compared to 30% of 23 patients with diskoid lupus (142).

The demonstration of these common idiotypes at the site of the lupus renal lesion strongly suggests that they may be engaged in the immunopathogenesis of the disease. In the skin, however, idiotypes were detected within lesional and nonlesional areas; therefore, elicitation of the cutaneous involvement cannot be clearly defined on grounds of anti-DNA idiotypes. Moreover, anti-DNA antibodies were never unequivocally demonstrated in the dermal-epidermal junction.

The vigorous pathogenetic potency of th 16/6 Id is best illustrated by a recently reported breakthrough concerning the development of autoimmunity in general and SLE in particular. Until lately, it was accepted that it was not possible to induce SLE in animal models by either DNA immunization or challenge with anti-DNA antibodies. Yet, by serial injections of the common anti-DNA idiotype 16/6 Id in murine strains that are not susceptible to spontaneous autoimmune diseases, we were able to induce an SLE-like syndrome. Accepted hallmarks of SLE appeared amaong the injected mice, such as high erythrocyte sedimentation rate, leukopenia, and proteinuria (143). Serologic features of SLE were detectable as well, exhibited by antinuclear antibodies, anti-ssDNA, and anti-dsDNA antibodies, anti-SSA, anti-SSB, antiribonucleoprotein, and anti-Sm antibodies. The mice had sustained high titers of both anti-16/6 idiotype antibodies as well as detectable 16/6 idiotype. By immunohistochemistry, antibodies bearing the 16/6 idiotype of mouse origin were shown to be deposited in the kidney, and this was further elucidated by electron microscopy to be deposits of immune complexes. Several previous studies failed to induce a lupuslike syndrome following injections of DNA owing to the nonimmunogenicity of DNA (144). A similar outcome was achieved following the injection of naive mice with several monoclonal anti-DNA antibodies (145). Interestingly, injection of NZB/WF mice with monoclonal anti-DNA antibodies was followed by a transient clinical amelioration (144).

Immunization of the former strain with the 16/6 Id brought on the disease earlier, and after 3 months all five of immunized mice were struck by the disease in comparison to one of five of the nonimmunized mice. After 9 months all five immunized mice expired, as opposed to one of five of the control mice (143).

Further studies have confirmed the pathogenetic importance of the 16/6 idiotype. A similar lupuslike syndrome was induced in mice following immunization with SA-1 (146). This IgM monoclonal antibody was derived from a patient with active polymyositis, and it was shown to react with DNA and bear the 16/6 idiotype (83). A later IgM monoclonal antibody (lacking anti-DNA affinity and not bearing the 16/6 Id) was generated from the same patient yet during clinical remission failed to induce such a disorder (146)].

As mentioned previously, a mouse monoclonal antimycobacterial glycolipid, designated TB-68, was found to carry the 16/6 idiotype and bind to DNA (114). The injection of this disease produced a similar syndrome, whereas another antimycobacterial glycolipid, termed T-72, which had anti-DNA affinity but lacked the 16/6 Id, did not induce such a disease (147). Several variables influenced the nature of the inductive lupuslike syndrome. The disorder was found to be strain dependent (147). Thus the disease was most easily induced in Balb/c mice (H-2^a), C3H/SW (H-2^b), AKR (H-2^k), and SJL (H-2^m) strains but C57BL/6 (H-2^b) and CH/He(H-2^k) were relatively resistant to such an induction. The development of an overt syndrome was concordant with the ability of the mice to respond to the injected 16/6 idiotype. The variables leading to the development of autoimmune features are open to debate, yet it seems that some important pathogenetic mechanisms have been elucidated.

How does the 16/6 lupus idiotype induce an autoimmune process? One of the theories is based on the idiotypic network. In other words, if anti-idiotypic antibodies are directed against the internal image of the antibody's antigen binding site, a conformational mimicry of the original antibody can be produced (148). Thus immunization of mice with monoclonal anti-idiotypic antibody against the 16/6 Id may result in the production of anti-anti-16/6 Id antibodies that possess the 16/6 Id and have anti-ssDNA activity (148). This stimulus may alter the threshold of immunotolerance to various autoantigens. Such an inclination comes from the fact that mice injected with a monoclonal anti-16/6 Id (anti-anti-DNA) antibody constantly produced anti-DNA antibodies even after clearance of the immunizing agent (148). On the cellular level we observed that DNA-specific T cells could be detected during the induction of the lupus syndrome in mice. These autoreactive T cells were found only following the formation of anti-16/6 Id determinants (either on antibodies or on T cells).

Another factor determining the course of the disease was external manipulation of the sex hormone balance. Castration of Balb/c males enhanced the development of autoimmune serologic markers; testosterone administration to female mice postponed their emergence (149).

These studies took place with only one anti-DNA idiotype; however it is conceivable that other pathogenic idiotypes coexist as well. Suenaga and associates (150) described a shift in anti-DNA idiotypes in SLE. They followed a patient with SLE for several years; at the beginning of follow-up he had lupus nephritis, and later he developed central nervous system involvement. With this clinical alternative a parallel disappearance of the first idiotype and a generation of a new idiotype could be observed.

Taken together it is tempting to assume that via the appearance of autoantibodies following an external stimulus, anti-idiotypic that mimic autoantigens may be generated. These anti-idiotypes can consequently perturb the existing immunotolerance of an individual to various auto-antigens. If a proper hormonal, genetic, and environmental setting coexists with this shift, autoimmune disorders may evolve.

ACKNOWLEDGMENTS

Supported in part by a grant given by the Chief Ministry of Health in Israel, and Mifal Hapais.

REFERENCES

1. Kohler, G., and Milstein, C. (1975). Continuous cultures of fused cells secreting antibody of predefined specificity. Nature 256:495.
2. Jerne, N.K. (1974). Towards a network theory of the immune system. Ann. Immunol. (Paris) 125c:373.

3. Rauch, J., Murphy, E., Roths, J.B., Stollar, B.D., and Schwartz, R.S. (1982). A high frequency idiotypic marker of anti-DNA autoantibodies in MRL-1pr/lpr mice. J. Immunol. 129:236-241.

4. Tron, F., Guern, C., Cazenane, P.A., and Bach, J. F. (1982). Intrastrain recurrent idiotypes among anti-DNA antibodies of (NZB × NZW) F_1 hybrid mice. Eur. J. Immunol. 12:761-766.

5. Marin, T.N., Lawton, A.R., III, Kearney, J.F.T., and Briles, D.E. (1982). Anti-DNA autoantibodies in (NZB × NZW) F_1 mice are clonally heterogeneous, but the majority share a common idiotype. J. Immunol. 128:668-674.

6. Hahn, B.H., and Ebling, F.M. (1984). A public idiotype is present on spontaneous cationic IgG antibodies to DNA from mice of unrelated lupus-prone strains. J. Immunol. 133:3015-3019.

7. Shoenfeld, Y., Hsu Lin, S.C., Gabriels, J.E., Silberstein, J.C., Furie, B.C., Furie, B., Stollar, B.D., and Schwartz, R.S. (1982). Production of human human hybridomas. J. Clin. Invest. 70:205-208.

8. Andrezejewski, C., Jr., Stollar, B.D., Lalor, T.N., and Schwartz, R.S. (1980). Hybridoma autoantibodies to DNA. Immunology 124:1499-1502.

9. Shoenfeld, Y., Rauch, J., Massicotte, H., Datta, S.K., André-Schartz, J., Stollar, B.D., and Schwartz, R.S. (1983). Polyspecificity of monoclonal lupus autoantibodies produced by human human hybridomas. N. Engl. J. Med. 308:414-420.

10. Hahn, B.H., Ebling, F., Freeman, S., Cleringer, G., and Davie, J. (1983). Production of monoclonal murine antibodies to DNA by somatic cell hybrids. Arthritis Rheum. 23:942-945.

11. Stollar, B.D., and Papalian, M. (1980). Secondary structure in denatured DNA is responsible for its reactions with antinative DNA antibodies of systemic lupus erythematosus sera. J. Clin. Invest. 66:210-219 (1980).

12. Lafer, E.M., Moller, A., Nordheim, A., Stollar, B.D., and Rich, A. (1981). Antibodies specific to left-handed Z-DNA Proc. Natl. Acad. Sci. USA 78:3546-3550.

13. Andre-Schwartz, J., Datta, S.K., Shoenfeld, Y., Isenberg, D.A., Stollar, B.D., and Schwartz, R.S. (1984). Binding of cytoskeleton proteins by monoclonal anti-DNA lupus autoantibodies. Clin. Immunol. Immunopathol. 31:261-271.

14. Lazarides, E. (1982). Intermediate filaments: A chemically heterogeneous, developmentally regulated class of proteins. Annu. Rev. Biochem. 51:219-250.

15. Steinert, P.M., Steven, A.C., and Roop, D.R. (1985). The molecular biology of intermediate filaments. Cell 42:411-420.

16. Osorn, M., Franke, W.W., and Weber, K. (1977). The visualization of a system of filaments 7-10 nm thick in cultured cells of an epitheloid line (PtK2) by immunofluorescence microscopy. Proc. Natl. Acad. Sci. USA 74:2490-2494.

17. Karsenti, E., Guilbert, B., Bornens, M., and Avrameas, S. (1977). Antibodies to tubulin in nonimmunized animals. Proc. Natl. Acad. Sci.USA 74:3997-4001.

18 Dighiero, G., Lymperi, P., Mazie, J.C., Roarye, S., Butler-Brown, G.S., Whalen, R.G., and Avrameas, S. (1983). Murine hybridomas secreting natural monoclonal antibodies reacting with self antigens. J. Immunol. 131:2267-2272.

19. Gordon, W.E., Bushnell, A., and Burridge, K. (1978). Characterizaton of the intermediate (10 nm) filaments of cultured cells using an autoimmune rabbit anti-serum. Cell 13:249-261.

20. Brinkley, B.R. (1982). Organization of the cytoplasm. Cold Spring Harbor Symp. Quant. Biol. 46:1029–1040.

21. Geiger, B. (1983). Membrane-cytoskeleton interaction. Biochim. Biophys. Acta 737:305–341.

22. Wide, K.S., Lucaites, V., and Watson, P.K. (1983). Murine monoclonal autoantibodies to cytoskeletal elements derived from autoimmune mice. Fed. Proc. 42:5392.

23. Mead, G.M., Cowin, P., and Whitehouse, J.M. (1980). Antitubulin antibody in healthy adults and patients with infectious mononucleosis and its relationship to smooth muscle antibody (SMA). Clin. Exp. Immunol. 39:328–336.

24. Hannestad, D., and Johannessen, A. (1976). Polyclonal human antibodies to IgG (rheumatoid factors) which cross-react with cell nuclei. Scand. J. Immunol. 5:541–547.

25. Searles, R.P., Messner, R., and Bankhurst, A.D. (1979). Cross reactivity of antilymphocyte and antinuclear antibodies in systemic lupus erythematosus. Clin. Immunol. Immunopathol. 14:292–299.

26. Shoenfeld, Y., Zamir, R., Joshua, H., Lavie, G., and Pinkhas, J. (1985). Human monoclonal anti-DNA antibodies react as lymphocytotoxic antibodies. Eur. J. Immunol. 15:1024–1028.

27. Lerner, R.A., Meinke, W., and Goldstein, D.A. (1971). Membrane associated DNA in the cytoplasm of diploid human lyphocytes. Proc. Natl. Acad. Sci. USA 68:1212–1216.

28. Holers, V.M., and Kotzin, B.L. (1984). Anti-DNA antibodies (abstract). Clin. Res. 32:40a.

29. Lane, D., and Koprowski, H. (1982). Molecular recognition and the future of monoclonal antibodies. Nature 296:200–202.

30. Richards, F.F., Konigsberg, W.H., and Rosenstein, R.W. (1975). On specificity of antibodies. Science 187:130–134.

31. Rivero, S.J., Diaz-Jovanen, E., and Alarcon-Segovia, D. (1978). Lymphopenia in systemic lupus erythematosus clinical, diagnostic and prognostic significance. Arthritis Rheum. 21:295–305.

32. Sakane, T., Steinberg, A.D., Reeves, J.O., and Green, I. (1979). Studies of immune functions of patients with systemic lupus erythematosus. J. Clin. Invest. 63:954–965.

33. Shoenfeld, Y., Smordinsky, N.I., Lavie, G., Hazaz, B., Joshua, H., and Pinkhas, J. (1985). Human lupus monoclonal autoantibodies bind to Raji cells. Immunol. Lett. 11:121–126.

34. Theofilopoulos, A.N., Wilson, C.B., Bokisch, V.A., and Dixon, F.J. (1974). Binding of soluble immune complexes to human lymphomablastoid cells. J. Exp. Med. 140:1230–1244.

35. Theofilopoulos, A.N. Wilson, C.B., and Bixon, F.J. (1976). The Raji cell radioimmunoassay for detecting complexes in human sera. J. Clin. Invest. 57:169–182.

36. Anderson, C.L., and Stillman, W.S. (1980). Raji cell assay for immune complexes. Evidence for detection of Raji-directed immunoglobulin G. antibody in sera from patients with systemic lupus erythematosus. J. Clin. Invest. 66:353–360.

37. Tron, F., Jacob, L., and Bach, J.F. (1980). Binding of a murine monoclonal anti-DNA antibody to Raj cells. Implications for the interpretation of the Raj cell assay for immune complexes. Eur. J. Immunol. 14:283–286.
38. Jacob, L., Lety, M.A., Monterio, R.C., Jacob, F., Bach, J.F., and Louvard, D. (1987). Altered cell-surface protein(s), cross-reactive with DNA, on spleen cells of autoimmune lapic mice. Proc. Natl. Acad. Sci.USA 84:1362–1363.
39. Jacob, L., Lety, M.A., Choquette, D., Viard, J.P., Jacob, F., Louvard, D., and Bach, J.F. (1987). Presence of antibodies against a cell-surface protein, cross-reactive with DNA, in systemic lupus erythematosus: A marker of the disease. Proc. Natl. Acad. Sci. USA 84:2956–2959.
40. Amital-Teplizki, H., Avinoach, I., Kooperman, O., Blank, M., and Shoenfeld, Y. (1989). Binding of monoclonal anti-DNA and anti-TB glycolipids to brain tissue. Autoimmunity 1:87–94.
41. Pischel, K.D., and Bluestein, H.G. (1986). Neuron reactive antibodies in systemic lupus erythematosus. In: Immunology of Rheumatic Diseases. Gupta, S., and Talal, N., eds. Plenum Medical Book Company, New York, p. 237.
42. Ando, S. (1983). Gangliosides in the nervous system. Neurochem. Int. 5:507–537.
43. Hanley, J.G., Behmann, S., and Denburg, J.A. (1987). Neural antibody specificities in systemic lupus erythematosus (SLE) (abstract). Arthritis Rheum. 30:554.
44. Avinoach, I., Teplizki, H., Kuperman, O., Caotes, A.R.M., Sukenik, S., and Shoenfeld, Y. (1990). Characteristics of antineuronal antibodies in SLE patients with and without central nervous system involvement: The role of mycobacterial cross-reacting antigens. Isr J Med Sci 26:367–373.
45. Bluestein, H.G. (1979). Heterogeneous neurocytotoxic antibodies in systemic lupus erythematosus. Clin. Exp. Immunol. 35:210.
46. Bluestein, HG., and Zvaifler, N.J. (1976). Brain-reactive lymphocytotoxic antibodies in the serum of patients with systemic lupus erythematosus J. Clin. Invest. 57:509–516.
47. Holborow, E.J., Weir, D.M., and Johnson, G.D. (1957). A serum factor in lupus erythomatosus with affinity for tissue nuclei. Br. Med. J. 2:732–733.
48. Stollar, B.D. (1981). Anti-DNA antibodies. Clin. Immunol. Allergy 1:243–260.
49. Weinstein, A., Bordwell, B., Stone, B., Tibetts, C., and Rothfield, N.F. (1983). Antibodies to native DNA and serum complement (C3) levels. Am. J. Med. 74:206–216.
50. Isenberg, D.A., Shoenfeld, Y., and Schwartz (1984). Multiple serologic reactions and their relationship to clinical activity in systemic lupus erythematosus. Arthritis Rheum. 27:132–128.
51. Schur, P.H., Monroe, M., and Rothfield, N. (1972). The jn G subclass of antinuclear and antinucleic acid antibodies. Arthritis Rheum. 15:174–182.
52. Pennebaker, J.B., Gilliam, J.N., and Ziff, M. (1977). Immunoglobulin classes of DNA-binding activity in serum and skin in systemic lupus erythematosus. J. Clin. Invest.60:1331–1338.
53. Isenberg, D.A., Shoenfeld, Y., Madaio, M.P., Rauch, J., Reichlin, M., Stolar, B.D., and Schwartz (1984). Anti-DNA antibody idiotypes in systemic lupus erythematosus. Lancet 2:417–421.
54. Solomon,G., Schiffenbauer, J., Keiser, H.D., and Diamond, B. (1983). The use of monoclonal antibodies to identify shared idiotypes on human antibodies to native

DNA from patients with systemic lupus erythematosus. Proc. Natl. Acad. Sci. USA 80:850–854.

55. Isenberg, D.A., Colaco, C.B., Dudeney, C., Todd-Pokropek, A., and Snaith, M.L. (1986). A study of the relationship between anti-DNA antibody idiotypes and anti-cardiolipin antibodies with disease activity in systemic lupus erythematosus. Medicine (Baltimore) 65:46–55.

56. Madaio, M.P., Schattner, A., Schattner, M., and Schwartz, R.S. (1986). Lupus serum and normal human serum containing anti-DNA antibodies with the same idiotypic marker. J. Immunol. 137:2535–2540.

57. Datta, S.K., Naparstek, Y., and Schwartz, R.S. (1983). In vitro production of an anti-DNA idiotype by lymphocytes of normal subjects and patients with systemic lupus erythematosus. Clin. Immunol. Immunopathol. 38:302–308.

58. Diamond, B., and Solomon, G. (1981). A monoclonal antibody that recognizes anti-DNA antibodies in patients with systemic lupus erythematosus. Ann. N.Y. Acad. Sci. 418:379–385.

59. Zouali, M., and Eyquem, A. (1984). Idiotypic restriction in human autoantibodies to DNA in systemic lupus erythematosus. Immunol. Lett. 7:187–193.

60. Shoenfeld, Y., Isenberg, D.A., Rauch, J., Madaio, M.B., Stollar, B.D., and Schwartz, R.S. (1983). Idiotypic cross-reactions of monoclonal human lupus autoantibodies. J. Exp. Med. 158:718–730.

61. Datta, S.K., Stollar, D., and Schwartz, R.S. (1983). Normal mice express idiotypes related to the autoantibody idiotypes inherited by lupus mice. Proc. Natl. Acad. Sci. USA 80:2723–2727.

62. Miller, K.B., and Schwartz, R.S. (1982). Genetic factors predisposing to autoimmune diseases: Autoimmunity and suppressor T lymphocytes. Adv. Intern. Med. 27:281–313.

63. Kelly, W.N., et al., eds. (1985). Textbook of Rheumatology, 2nd ed. W.B. Saunders, Philadelphia.

64. Shoenfeld, Y., and Schwartz, R.S. (1984). Immunologic and genetic factors in autoimmune diseases. N. Engl. J. Med. 311:1019–1029.

65. Lippman, S.M., Arnett, F.C., Conley, C.L., Ness, P.M., Meyers, D.A., and Bias, W.B. (1982). Autoimmune hemolytic uremia, chronic thrombocytopenic purpura and systemic lupus erythematosus. Am. J. Med. 73:827–840.

66. Nakao, Y., Matsumoto, H., Tsuji, Myazaki, T., Massoka, T., Nakayama, S., Kinoshita, K., Shingaui, T., Matsui, T., and Fujita, T. (1984). IgG heavy chain allotypes (Gm) a genetic marker for human chromosome 14q32 and G28-36, haematopoietic malignancies. Clin. Exp. Immunol. 56:628–636.

67. Schattner, A. (1987). The origin of autoantibodies. Immunol. Lett. 14:143–153.

68. Shoenfeld, Y., Ben-Yehuda, O., Messinger, Y., Bentwitch, Z., Rauch, J., and Isenberg, D.A. (1988). Autoimmune diseases other than lupus share common anti-DNA idiotypes. Immunol. Lett. 17:445–450.

69. Dudeney, C., Shoenfeld, Y., Rauch, J., Jones, M., MacWorthy, Y., Tavassoli, M., Shall, S., and Isenberg, D.A. (1986). A study of anti-poly(ADP-ribose) antibodies and an anti-DNA antibody idiotype and other immunological abnormalities in lupus family members. Ann. Rheum. Dis. 45:502–507.

70. Konikoff, F., Isenberg, D.A., Kooperman, O., Kennedy, R.C., Rauch, J. Theodor, E., and Shoenfeld, Y. (1987). Common lupus anti-DNA idiotypes in chronic liver diseases. Clin. Immunol. Immunopathol. 43:265–272.

71. Kurki, P., Gripenberg, M., Teppo, A.M., and Salaspuro, M. (1984). Profiles of antinuclear antibodies in chronic active hepatitis, primary biliary cirrhosis and alcoholic liver disease. Liver 4:134–138.

72. Gurian, L.E., Rogoff, T.M., Ware, A.J., Jordon, R.E., Combes, B., and Gillian, J.W. (1985). The immunologic diagnosis of chronic active autoimmune hepatitis: Distinction from systemic lupus erythematosus. Hepatology 5:397–402.

73. Meyer Zum Buschenfelde, K.H., Manns, M., and Trautmann, F. (1984). Autoimmunity in chronic active liver diseases' relationship to SLE. In: Recent Advances in Systemic Lupus Erythematosus. Lambert, P.H., Perrin, L., and Isui, S., eds., Academic Press, London, pp. 259–269.

74. Shoenfeld, Y., Andre-Schwartz, J., Stollar, B.D., and Schwartz, R.S. (1987). Anti-DNA antibodies. In: Systemic Lupus Erythematosus. Lahita, R.G., ed. p. 237.

75. Lee, S.L., and Chase, P.H., (1975). Drug induced lupus erythematosus: A critical review. Arthritis Rheum. 5:83–103.

76. Bluestein, H.G., Redelamn, O., and Zvaifler, N.J. (1981). Procainamide-lymphocyte reaction. A possible explanation for drug-induced autoimmunity. Arthritis. Rheum. 24:1019–1023.

77. Totoritis, M.C., Tan, E.M., MaNally, E.M., and Rubin,R.I. (1988) Association of antibody to histone complex H2A-H2B with symptomatic procainamide-induced lupus. N. Engl. Med. 318:1431–1436.

78. Yamauchi, Y., Litwin, A., and Adams, B. (1975). Induction of antibodies to nuclear antigens in rabbits by immunization with hydralazine human serum albumin conjugates. J. Clin. Invest. 56:958–969.

79. Ochi, T., Goldings, E.A., Lipsky, P.E., and Ziff, M. (1983). Immunomodulatory effect of procainamide in man: Inhibition of human suppressor T-cell activity in vitro. J. Clin. Invest. 71:36–45.

80. Miller, K.B., and Salem, D. (1982). Immune regulatory abnormalities produced by procainamide. Am. J. Med. 73:487–492.

81. Shoenfeld, Y., Vilner, Y., Reshef, T., Klajman, A., Skibin, A., Kooperman, D., and Kennedy, R.C. (1987). Increased presence of common systemic lupus erythematosus (SLE), anti-DNA idiotypes (16/6 Id, 32/15 Id) is induced by procainamide. J. Clin. Immunol. 74:410–419.

82. Batchelor, J.R., Welsh, K.I., Tinoco, R.M., Dollery, C.I., and Huges, G.R.V., (1980). Hydralazine-induced SLE: Influence of HLA-DR and sex on susceptibility. Lancet 1:1107–1109.

83. Shoenfeld, Y., Livne, A., Argov, S., Krupp, M., Fleishmakher, Sukenik, S., and Teplizki, H. (1988). A human monoclonal anti-DNA antibody derived from a patient with polymyositis having the common lupus 16/6 idiotype. Immunol. Lett. 19:77–84.

84. Shoenfeld, Y., Ben-Yehuda, O., Naparstek, Y., Wilner, Y., Frolichman, R., Schattn, A., Lavie, G., Joshua, H., Pinkhas, J., Kennedy, R.C., Schwartz, R.S., and Pick, A.I. (1986). The detection of a common idiotype of anti-DNA antibodies in the sera of patients with monoclonal gammopathies. J. Clin. Immunol. 6:194–204.

85. Seligmann, M., and Brouet, J.C. (1973). Antibody activity of human myeloma globulins. Semin. Hematol. 10:163–177.

86. Intrator, L., Andre, C., Chenal, C., and Sulton, C. (1979). A monoclonal macroglobulin with antinuclear activity. J. Clin. Pathol. 32:450–454.

87. Zouali, M., Fine, J.M., and Eyquen, A. (1984). Anti-DNA autoantibody activity and idiotypic relationships of human monoclonal proteins. Eur. J. Immunol. 14:1085–1090.

88. Shoenfeld, Y., El-Roeiy, A., Ben-Yehuda, O., and Pick, A.I. (1987). Detection of anti-histone activity in sera of patients with monoclonal gammopathies. Clin. Immunol. Immunopathol. 42:2508.

89. Freddo, L., Hays, A.P., Nickerson, K.G., Spatz, L., McGinnis, S., Liberson, R.A., Vadeler, C.A., Shy, M.E., Autilio-Gambetti, L., Grauss, F.C., Patito, F., Chess, I., and Latov, N. (1986). Monoclonal anti-DNA IgMk in neuropathy binds to myelin and to a conformational epitope bound by phospatidic acid and gangliosides. J. Immunol. 137:3821–3825.

90. Rubin, R.L., and Carr, R.I. (1979). Anti-DNA activity of IgG (ab1)2 from normal human serum. J. Immunol. 122:1604–1607.

91. Hasselbacher, P., and LeRoy, E.C. (1974). Serum DNA binding activity in healthy subjects and in rheumatic disease. Arthritis Rheum. 17:63–71.

92. Smith, H.R., Green, D.B., Raveche, E.S., Smathers, P.A., Gershon, P.K., and Steinberg, A.B. (1982). Studies of the induction of anti-DNA antibodies in normal mice. J. Immunol. 129:2332–2334.

93. Izui, S., Zaldivar, N.M., Scher, I., and Lambert, P.H. (1977). Mechanism for induction of anti-DNA antibodies by bacterial LPS in mice. Anti-DNA induction by LPS without significant release of DNA in circulating blood. J. Immunol. 119:2151–2156.

94. Hoch, S., Schur, P.H., and Schwaber, J. (1983). Frequency of anti-DNA antibody producing cells from normal and patients with SLE. Clin. Immunol. Immunopathol. 27:28–37.

95. Lewis, R.M., Armstrong, M.Y.K., and Andre-Schwartz, J. (1968). Chronic allogenic disease. I. Development of glomerulonephritis. J. Exp.Med. 128:653–663.

96. Cairns, E.J., Block, J., and Bell, D.A. (1984). Anti-DNA autoantibody producing hybridomas of normal human lymphoid cell origin. J. Clin. Invest. 74:880–887.

97. Monier, J.C., Brochier, J., Moreira, A., Salt, C., and Roux, B. (1984). Generation of hybridoma antibodies to double-stranded DNA from non-autoimmune BALB/c strain: Studies on anti-idiotype. Immunol. Lett. 8:61–68.

98. Throns, C.J., and Morris, J.A. (1985). Common epitopes between mycobacterial and certain host tissue antigens. Clin. Exp. Immunol. 61:323–328.

99. Zabriskie, J.B. (1982). Rheumatic fever; a streptococcal-induced autoimmune disease? Pediatr. Annu. 11:383–396.

100. Christiansen, M.L., Pachman, L.M., Maryjowski, M.C., and Freidman, J.C. (1983). Antibody to Coxsackie-B virus increased incidence in sera from children with recently diagnosed juvenile dermatomyositis. Arthrit. Rheum. 26:S24.

101. King, M.L., Shaikah, A., Bidwell, D., Voller, A., and Banatvak, J.E. (1983). Coxsackie-B-virus-specific IgM responses in children with insulin-dependent (juvenile onset; type 1) diabetes mellitus. Lancet 1:1397–1399.

102. Shoenfeld, Y., and Cohen, I.R. Infection and autoimmunity. In: The Antigens, Vol. VIII. Sela, M., ed. Academic Press, New York, pp.307-325.

103. Sela, O., El-Roeiy, A., Isenberg, D.A., Kennedy, R.C., Colaco, C.B., Pinkhas, J., and Shoenfeld, Y. (1987). A common anti-DNA idiotype in sera of patients with active pulmonary tuberculosis. Arthritis Rheum. 30:50-56.

104. Greenwood, B.M. (1974). Possible role of B-cell mitogen in hypergammaglobulinaemia in malaria and trypanasomiasis. Lancet 1:435-436.

105. Lindsley, H.B., Kysela, S., and Steinberg, A.D. (1976). Nucleic acid antibodies in African trypanosomiasis. Studies in Rhesus monkeys and man. J. Immunol. 113:1921-1927.

106. Jones, C.E. (1977). Schistosomajaponicum: Anti-DNA responses, serum cryogelatification and cryoprecipitation phenomena in infected rabbits. Exp. Parasitol. 42:261-273.

107. Atkinson, P.M., Lampan, G.W., Furie, B.C., Naparstek, Y., Schwartz, R.S., Stollar, B.D., and Furie, B. (1985). Homology of the NH_2-terminal amino acid sequences of the heavy and light chains of human monoclonal lupus autoantibodies containing the dominant 16/6 idiotype. J. Clin. Invest. 75:1138-1143.

108. Naparstek, Y., Duggan, D., Schattner, A., Madio, M.P., Goni, F. Frangione, B., Stollar, D.B., Kabat, E.A., and Schwartz, R.S. (1985). Immunochemical similarities between monoclonal antibacterial Waldentrom's macroglobulins and monoclonal anti-DNA lupus autoantibodies. J. Exp.Med. 161:1525-1538.

109. El-Roiey, A., Gross, W.L., Leudemann, J., Isenberg, D.A., and Shoenfeld, Y. (1986). Preferential secretion of a common anti-DNA idiotype (16/6 Idx) and anti-polysaccharide antibodies by normal mononuclear cells following stimulation with Klebsiella pneumoniae. Immunol. Lett. 12:313-319.

110. Shoenfeld, Y., Teplizki, Buskila, D., Leudeman, J., and Gross, W. Immunoglobulin secretion of mononuclear cells induced by various mitogens. Int. J. Immunopharmacol. 4:347-352.

111. El-Roiey, A., Sela, O., Isenberg, D.A., Feldman, R., Colaco, B.C., Kennedy, R.C., and Shoenfeld, Y. (1987). The sera of patients with Klebsiella infections contain a common anti-DNA idiotype (16/6 Id) and polynucleotide activity. Clin. Exp. Immunol. 67:507-515.

112. Ruge, H.G.S., Fromm, G., Fohner, F., and Guinto, R.B.S. (1960). Serological findings in leprosy: An investigation into the specificity of various serological tests for syphilis. Bull. WHO 23:793-802.

113. Mathews, L.J., and Trautman, J.R. (1965). Clinical and serological profiles in leprosy. Lanet 2:915-917.

114. Shoenfeld, Y., Vilner, Y., Coates, A.R.M., Joyce, R., Lavie, G., Shaul, D., and Pinkhas, J. (1986). Monoclonal anti-tuberculosis antibodies react with DNA, and monoclonal anti-DNA autoantibodies react with Mycobacterium tuberculosis. Clin. Exp. Immunol. 66:255-261.

115. Teplizki, H., Buskila, D., Argov, S., Isenberg, D.A., Coates, A.R.M., Sukenik, S., Horowitz, Y., and Shoenfeld, Y. (1987). Low serum antimycobacterial glycolipid antibody titers in the sera of patients with systemic lupus erythematosus associated with central nervous system involvement. J. Rheumatol. 14:507-511.

116. Shoenfeld, Y., and Isenberg, D.A. (1988). Mycobacteria and autoimmunity. Immunol. Today 9:178–181.
117. Hughes, G.R.V. (1979). Connective Tissue Disease, 2nd ed. Blackwell Scientific, Oxford, pp. 4–5.
118. Hirano, T., Hashimoto, H., and Shiokawa, Y. (1980). Antiglycolipid autoantibody detected in the sera from systemic lupus erythematosus patients. J. Clin. Invest. 66:1437–1440.
119. Serdula, M.K., and Rhoades, G.G. (1979). Frequency of systemic lupus erythematosus in different ethnic groups in Hawaii. Arthritis Rheum. 22:339–350.
120. Woodrow, J.C. (1988). Immunogenetics of systemic lupus erythematosus. J. Rheumatol. 15:197–199.
121. Walport, M.J., Black, C.M., and Batchelor, J.R. (1982). The immunogenetic of systemic lupus erythematosus. Clin. Rheum. Dis. 8:3–21.
122. Frederick, J.A., Pandey, J.P., Chen, Z., Fudenberg, H.H., Ainsworth, S.K., and Dobson, R.L. (1983). Gm allotypes in blacks with systemic lupus erythematosus. Hum. Immunol., 8:177–181.
123. Rynes, R.I. (1982). Inherited complement deficiency states and SLE. Clin. Rheum. Dis. 8:28–47.
124. Fielder, A.H.L., Walport, M.J., Batchelor, J.R., Rynes, R.I., Black, C.M., Dodi, I.A., and Hughes, G.R.V. (1983). Family study of the major histocompatibility complex in patients with systemic lupus erythematosus: Importance of null alleles of C4A and C4B in determining disease susceptibiility. Br. Med. J. 286:425–428.
125. Estes, D., and Christian, C.L. (1971). The natural history of systemic lupus erythematosus by prospective analysis. Medicine (Baltimore) 50:85–95.
126. Morteo, O.G., Franklin, E.C., McEwen, C., Rythyon, J., and Tanner, M. (1961). Studies of relatives of patients with systemic lupus erythematosus. Arthritis Rheum. 4:356–363.
127. Elkon, K.B., Walport, M.J., Rynes, R.I., Black, C.M., Batchelor, J.R., and Hughes, C.R. (1983). Circulating CIg binding complexes in relatives of patients with systemic lupus erythematosus. Arthritis Rheum. 26:921–924.
128. Lehman, T.J.A., Curd, J.G., Zvaifler, N.J., and Hanson, V. (1982). The association of antinuclear antibodies, antilymphocyte antibodies and C4 activation among the relatives of children with systemic lupus erythematosus. Arthritis Rheum. 25:556–561.
129. Miller, K.B., and Schwartz, R.S. (1979). Familial abnormalities of suppressor cell function in systemic lupus erythematosus. N. Engl. J. Med. 301:803–809.
130. Isenberg, D.A., Shoenfeld, Y., Walport, M., MacWorth-Young, C., Dudeney, C., Todd-Pokropek, A., Brill, S., Weinberger, A., and Pinkhas, J. (1985). Detection of cross reactive anti-DNA antibody idiotypes in the serum of systemic lupus erythematosus patients and their relatives.Arthritis Rheum. 28:999–1007.
131. El-Roiey, A., Gleicher, N., Isenberg, D.A., Kennedy, R.C., and Shoenfeld, Y. (1987). A common anti-DNA idiotype and other autoantibodies in sera of offspring of mothers with systemic lupus erythematosus. Clin. Exp. Immunol. 68:528–534.
132. Lefvert, A.K., and Osterman, P.O. (1983). Newborn infants to myasthenic mothers. A clinical study and an investigation of acetylcholine receptors antibodies in 17 children. Neurology 33:133–138.
133. Weitkamp, L.R., and Lamm, L.U. (1982). Report of the committee on the genetic

constitution of chromosome 6 Cytogenet. Cell. Ent. 32:130–143.

134. Angello, V. (1978). Complement deficiency states. Medicine (Baltimore) 57:1–24.

135. Shoenfeld, Y., Brill, S., Weinberger, A., Pinkahs, J., and Isenberg, D.A. (1986). High levels of a common anti-DNA idiotype (16/6) a genetic marker of SLE. Acta Haematol. (Basel) 76:107–109.

136. Oen, K., Petty, R.E., and Schroeder, M.L. (1982). Immunoglobulin A deficiency: Genetic studies. Tissue Antigens 19:174–182.

137. Koistinen, J. (1975). Selective IgA deficiency in blood donors. Vox Sang.29:192–202.

138. Ammann, A.J., and Hong, R. (1971). Selective IgA deficiency: presentation of 30 cases and a review of the literature. Medicine (Baltimore) 60:223–236.

139. Ammann, A.J., and Hong, R. (1971). Selective IgA deficiency and autoimmunity. N. Engl. J. Med. 284:985–986.

140. Goshen, E., Livne, A., Krupp, M., Hammarstrome, L., Digheiro, G., Slor, H., and Shoenfeld, Y. (1989). Antinuclear and related autoantibodies in sera of healthy subjects with IgA deficiency. J. Autoimmun. 2:51–60.

141. Isenberg, D.A., and Collin, C. (1985). Detection of cross reactive anti-DNA antibody idiotype on renal tissue bound immunoglobulins from lupus patients. J. Clin. Invest. 76:287–294.

142. Isenberg, D.A., Dudeney, C., Wojharenska, F., Bhogal, B.S., Rauch, J. Schattner, A., Napparstek, Y., and Duggan, D. (1985). Detection of cross reactive anti-DNA idiotypes on tissue bound immunoglobulins from skin biopsies of lupus patients. J. Immunol. 135:261–264.

143. Mendlovic, S., Brocke, S., Shoenfeld, Y., Ben-Bassat, M., Meshorer, A., Bakimer, R., and Mozes, E. (1988). Induction of a systemic lupus erythematosus-like syndrome in mice by a common human anti-DNA idiotype. Proc. Natl. Acad. Sci. USA 85:2260–2264.

144. Hahn, B.H., and Ebling, F.M. (1982). Suppression of NZB/NZW murine nephritis by administration of a syngeneic monoclonal antibody to DNA. J. Clin. Invest. 71:1726–1736.

145. Cukier, R., and Tron, F. (1985). Monoclonal anti-DNA antibodies; an approach to studying SLE nephritis. Clin. Exp. Immunol. 62:143–149.

146. Blank, M., Mendlovic, S., Mozes, E., and Shoenfeld, Y. (1988). Induction of SLE like disease in naive mice with a monoclonal anti-DNA antibody derived from a patient with polymyositis carrying the 16/6 Id. J. Autoimmun. 1:683–691.

147. Mendelovic, S., Brocke, S., Shoenfeld, Y., et al. The genetic regulation of the inductin of experimental SLE in mice Semin. J. Immunol. (in press).

148. Shoenfeld, Y., Amital-Teplizki, H., Mendlovic, S., Blank, M., Mozes, E., and Isenberg, D.A. (1989). The role of the human anti-DNA idiotype 16/6 in autoimmunity. Clin. Immunol. Immunopathol. 51:313–325.

149. Blank, M., Mendelovic, S., Fleishmakher, Mozes, E., and Shoenfeld, Y. The effect of hormones on induction of experimental systemic lupus erythematosus in mice J. Rheumatology (in press).

150. Suengaga, R., Munoz, P.A., Bright, S.W., and Abdou, N.I. (1988). Spontaneous shift of anti-DNA antibody idiotypes in systemic lupus erythematosus. J. Immunol. 140:3508–3514.

151. Horsfall, A.C., and Isenberg, D.A. (1988). Idiotypes and autoimmunity: A review of their role in human disease. J. Autoimmun. 1:7–30.

22

Immunoregulation in Systemic Lupus Erythematosus by Idiotypic Network: Possible Future Therapeutic Implications

Nabih I. Abdou and Ronsuke Suenaga
St. Luke's Hospital of Kansas City, Kansas City, Missouri

I. INTRODUCTION

Idiotypes (Ids) and their anti-idiotypes (anti-Ids) constitute a complex network of interactions at the serum and lymphocyte receptor levels (1). Each Id within the repertoire could be considered a self antigen for which complimentary anti-Id is formed. The anti-Id could therefore be essential for the induction of self tolerance and the prevention of autoimmunity. Abnormalities of the Id-anti-Id network could lead to the expression or expansion of autoreactive cell clones (2–4).

In this brief review we focus on our work, which deals with the regulation of anti-DNA antibodies by anti-Id in patients with systemic lupus erythematosus (SLE), their families, and laboratory personnel who handle lupus sera. Several issues are discussed:

1. Do autoanti-Ids against anti-DNA Id exist in sera of lupus patients, and if so, do they inversely correlate with SLE disease activity?
2. Can autoanti-Ids against anti-DNA modulate the cellular network of anti-DNA Ids?
3. Do autoanti-Ids exist in sera of healthy family members of lupus patients? If so, is the production of autoanti-Id in family members dependent on genetic background?

465

4. Do autoanti-Ids exist in sera of normal personnel who are healthy but handle lupus sera or nucleic acids?
5. Do anti-DNA Ids spontaneously shift to other Ids over time?
6. Do anti-DNA Ids have target organ specificity?
7. Can IgG anti-DNA be distinguished by its isotype-restricted Id from IgM anti-DNA?

II. IMMUNOREGULATION OF ANTI-DNA IDIOTYPES BY AUTOANTIIDIOTYPES IN HUMAN SLE

Our earlier work demonstrated the presence of autoanti-Ids in sera of inactive SLE patients (5). Characterization of the anti-Ids has shown this activity to be localized in the F(ab')$_2$ portion of IgG, not due to a rheumatoid factor. The anti-Id could bind to anti-DNA Id and form immune complexes that could be detected in sera of lupus patients by the C1q binding assay. Anti-Ids were specific for anti-DNA antibodies but not specific for anti-tetanus toxoid antibodies isolated from the same patient.

Our work has also demonstrated an inverse correlation between the serum levels of anti-Ids and those of anti-DNA Ids or disease activity of the same lupus patient (5). This has been confirmed by performing a long-term 6 year follow-up study of a large number of lupus patients followed by us (6). In this study, anti-Ids could be detected only in sera of patients with inactive disease.

At the cellular level, anti-Ids were shown by us to suppress the binding of DNA to DNA-binding mononuclear cells from active lupus patients (7). Furthermore, anti-Ids inhibited the in vitro secretion of anti-DNA from B cells of active lupus patients without inhibiting polyclonal IgG secretion from the same cells. This study strongly suggests, therefore, that anti-Ids could also regulate the cellular network in human SLE. We have not, however, been able to conclude from this earlier work whether anti-Ids directly downregulate the B cell clones or whether their effect is mediated via a suppressor cellular mechanism.

These observations of ours (5–7) and the findings by others (8–11) indicate that in human SLE anti-Ids play a role in the modulation of Id expression and secretion and are probably involved in the induction and maintenance of disease remission.

III. IMMUNOREGULATION BY ANTI-IDIOTYPES IN FAMILIES OF LUPUS PATIENTS: LACK OF GENETIC INFLUENCE

In a large study of 64 first-degree relatives of 24 lupus patients, we have shown that family members' sera compared to healthy controls without a family history of lupus, had higher binding activity to F(ab')$_2$ fragments of IgG anti-DNA than to those of IgG non-anti-DNA (12). Inhibition experiments have shown that the anti-Id is directed against the framework determinants, not against the antigen binding sites of the Id. The anti-Ids present in the sera of the family members were directed against cross-reactive anti-DNA Ids and were not restricted to the Ids of the lupus proband. Age, sex, and blood relationship to the lupus patient did not influence the presence of anti-Ids in the family members. The presence of anti-F(ab')$_2$ antibodies directed against anti-DNA antibodies of thc lupus proband in family members has also been reported by others (13).

It is still unclear if environmental factors or close contact with lupus probands is responsible for the induction of the anti-Id in the family members. The lack of genetic influence on the production of anti-Ids in families of lupus patients has recently been shown by us (14). In a detailed study of one large family of 17 members of a lupus patient, we could not detect correlation between HLA types or null alleles of the lupus family members and the presence of spontaneous auto anti-Ids. In family studies of myasthenia gravis patients, however, a positive correlation has been reported between HLA haplotypes, the levels of antiacetylcholine receptor antibodies, and anti-Id in siblings and children of patients with myasthenia gravis (15).

IV. IMMUNOREGULATION BY ANTI-IDIOTYPES IN LABORATORY PERSONNEL EXPOSED TO LUPUS SERA OR TO NUCLEIC ACIDS

Individuals exposed to lupus sera or to nucleic acids had significantly higher binding to F(ab')$_2$ fragments of IgG anti-DNA compared to unexposed controls (16). Binding to the anti-DNA F(ab')$_2$ fragments was significantly higher than to the non-anti-DNA or the normal F(ab')$_2$ fragments.

The presence of anti-Id in the laboratory personnel indicates that these individuals have been sensitized to the anti-DNA. We could not, however, detect anti-DNA in the sera of these individuals, probably due to the regulatory role of anti-Id or to the binding of anti-DNA to the anti-Id in vivo. Therefore, these observations suggest the role of environmental factors in the induction of anti-Id. Exposure to the Id or to the antigen induces the production of a specific anti-Id that maintains the balance of the Id–anti-Id network and prevents the expression of the autoimmune state.

V. SPONTANEOUS SHIFT OF ANTI-DNA IDIOTYPES

If the production of anti-DNA antibodies is downregulated by autoanti-Ids, as we reviewed in the preceding sections, then treatment with exogenous anti-Id can be theoretically effective. In fact, preliminary experiments by Hahn and Ebling (17) have shown that the treatment of lupus mice with the anti-Id raised against murine monoclonal anti-dsDNA antibodies succeeded in the transient decrease in the serum levels of anti-DNA antibodies and prolongation of the life span of the treated mice. However, it eventually led to a rebound that resulted in the production of anti-DNA bearing different Id and caused fatal nephritis. In human B cell lymphoma, a similar escape of cell surface Ids of lymphoma cells following serotherapy or during monitoring by the specific anti-Id has been reported (18,19).

Because suggestions have been made to monitor SLE disease activity by following the levels of anti-DNA Ids (20) or to suppress or eliminate the corresponding Id-secreting clones by anti-Id for treatent for SLE (17,21), it is important to know whether Id expression spontaneously shifts over time in human SLE. We therefore examined Id expression of two anti-DNA antibodies prepared at 5 year intervals from the same lupus patients (22). Polyclonal or monoclonal anti-Id was raised against each of these two anti-DNA antibodies. All anti-Id reagents were specific to Id on or near the antigen binding sites. By direct binding or inhibition studies, all anti-Ids reacted significantly with the homologous anti-DNA used for immunization of animals and reacted poorly with the anti-DNA prepared from a differently dated serum, indicating that these two anti-DNA antibodies expressed distinct Ids. Serial kinetic studies of Id expression of anti-DNA using anti-Ids as probes clearly demonstrated a spontaneous shift of anti-DNA Id.

Although the precise mechanism for the Id shift is unclear, a possible mechanism could be a shift of an Id$^+$ cell population to pre-existing Id$^-$ clones bearing distinct Ids. This could be secondary to regulatory pressure by the Id–anti-Id network. It is likely that autoanti-Id or anti-Id T cells may play a role in regulating the expression of certain Id$^+$ populations of anti-DNA clones. The "Id switch" observed by Hahn and Ebling was shown to be due to expanding pre-existing Id-negative clones (23) or to "Id spreading," involving helper T cells (24).

Although we do not know at the present time whether the observed Id shift is a general phenomenon for all anti-DNA Ids, it should be given special consideration in future strategy for the treatment of SLE by anti-Id.

VI. ORGAN SPECIFICITY OF ANTI-DNA IDIOTYPES

The Id shift observed by us (22) appeared to correlate with changes in the clinical manifestations of the lupus patient whom we studied between 1982 and 1986. This lupus patient had nephritis in 1982 and cerebritis without nephritis in 1986. We therefore characterized these two anti-DNA antibody preparations, BS-82 and BS-86 (25). Direct binding and inhibition studies showed that the BS-82 had more specific antigen binding activity and avidity to dsDNA than the BS-86. Furthermore, the BS-82 showed more cationic quality than the BS-86 upon isoelectric focusing and Western blot analysis. Thus, as has been described in the literature (26–30), the BS-82 had more nephritogenic nature than the BS-86, and these qualities of the BS-82 were consistent with the presence of active nephritis in 1982. The BS-86 anti-DNA Id was associated with cerebritis in our patient and had immunochemical characteristics different from those of the BS-82 anti-DNA Id of the same patient (25).

The organ or tissue specificity of anti-DNA has been reported (26–30). The association of neuropathy and anti-DNA antibody that binds to myelin has been reported (31). Characterization of anti-DNA Ids and their correlation to the predominant clinical organ manifestations in SLE is of current interest to us at the serum and tissue levels.

In future strategies of immunomodulation of the lupus patient disease activity by anti-Ids, attention should be paid not only to the phenomenon of Id shift but also to the possibility that various anti-DNA Ids could have organ or tissue specificity.

VII. ISOTYPE-RESTRICTED Id OF ANTI-DNA

IgG class anti-DNA antibodies have generally been considered pathogenic, whereas certain IgM class anti-DNA may be less pathogenic or even non-pathogenic. The predominance of IgM anti-DNA antibodies have been shown to correlate with milder disease in human SLE (32,33). Moreover, naturally occurring autoantibodies have recently been described that are mainly of IgM class and cross-react with a variety of autoantigens, including DNA (34). This type of autoantibody has even been proposed to play a physiologic (35) or protective (36) role for the normal equilibrium of the immune system.

Therefore, there may be an Id difference between IgG and IgM anti-DNA antibodies due to qualitative differences of both classes of anti-DNA. To test this possibility, we investigated Id sharing between IgG and IgM anti-dsDNA antibodies that coexisted in serum of an active lupus patient (37). Partially purified IgM anti-dsDNA antibodies by affinity chromatography were tested for the ability to react with the rabbit anti-Id recognizing private Id on coexisting IgG anti-dsDNA antibodies. Only negligible idiotypic cross-reactions were observed between the two classes of anti-DNA (37).

Although certain cross-reactive Ids of human anti-DNA antibodies have been shown to be expressed on IgG and IgM anti-DNA (38,39), our study suggests that it is feasible to develop anti-Id detecting specific Ids on pathogenic IgG anti-DNA and distinguishing them from IgM nonpathogenic anti-DNA. Studies of murine anti-DNA Ids have recently shown that pathogenic anti-DNA antibodies are idiotypically distinct from nonpathogenic anti-DNA (23,30). Anti-Id reagents directed against the pathogenic Ids would therefore be an ideal tool to use in the immunomodulation of the pathogenic anti-DNA antibodies in SLE.

VIII. CONCLUSION

Clinicians and researchers have been struggling to elucidate the mechanisms by which autoimmune diseases occur and to apply such knowledge to the specific therapy of SLE. Here we demonstrated that one of the major immunoregulatory mechanisms in SLE is the Id–anti-Id network of anti-DNA antibody. Autoanti-Ids against anti-DNA exist and appear to down regulate anti-DNA production in lupus patients and probably prevent family members of lupus patients or normal laboratory personnel—who are sensitized with Id or antigen—from the expression of the autoimmune state. The idea of using exogenous anti-Id as a therapeutic reagent becomes attractive, but we must consider the spontaneous shifts of anti-DNA Id that we have clearly demonstrated. We also demonstrated the possibility of target organ specificity of anti-DNA Id and the existence of isotype-restricted anti-DNA Id. All this information will in the future lead to the development of more specific anti-Id reagents targeted only against the pathogenic or the organ-specific anti-DNA Ids.

ACKNOWLEDGMENTS

The work presented in the paper was supported by NIH Grant AM29674, by a generous grant by the Evans family to St. Luke's Hospital, the Lupus Foundation, Kansas City Chapter of the Lupus Foundation, and by the Sheryl N. Hirsh Award of the Philadelphia Lupus Chapter. We are also grateful to M. Evans, M. Hatfield, K. Smith, and H. Wall for technical assistance and to G. Schroder and A. Knight for secretarial assistance. The understanding and cooperation of the lupus patients and their families made these studies feasible.

REFERENCES

1. Jerne, N.K. (1974). Towards a network theory of the immune system. Ann. Immunol. (Paris) 125C:373–389.
2. Urbain, J., Collignon, C., Franssen, J.D., Mariame, B., Leo, B., Vansanten, G.U., Walle, P.V., Wickler, M., and Wuilmart, C. (1979). Idiotypic networks and self-recognition in the immune system. Ann. Immunol. 130C:281–291.
3. Talal, N. (1978). Autoimmunity and the immunologic network. Arthritis Rheum. 21:853–861.
4. Roitt, I.M., Male, D.K., Cooke, A., and Lydyard, P.M. (1983). Idiotypes and autoimmunity. Springer Semin. Immunopathol. 6:51–66.
5. Abdou, N.I., Wall, H., Lindsley, H.B., Halsey, J.F., and Suzuki, T. (1981). Network theory in autoimmunity. In vitro suppression of serum anti-DNA antibody binding to DNA by anti-idiotypic antibody in systemic lupus erythematosus. J. Clin. Invest. 67:1297–1304.
6. Abdou, N.I., Smith, K., and Ramsey, M. (1984). Regulation of anti-DNA antibody by antiidiotypic antibody in inactive lupus sera (abstract). Arthritis Rheum. 27:S84.
7. Abdou, N.I., Wall, H., and Clancy, J. (1981). The network theory in autoimmunity. In vitro modulation of DNA-binding cells by anti-idiotype antibody present in inactive lupus sera. J. Clin. Immunol. 1:234–240.

8. Nasu, H., Chia, D.S., Taniguchi, O., and Barnett, E.J. (1982). Characterization of anti-F(ab')$_2$ antibodies in SLE patients. Evidence for cross-reacting autoanti-idiotypic antibodies. Clin. Immunol. Immunopathol. 25:80–85.

9. Zouali, M., and Eyquem, A. (1983). Idiotypic anti-idiotypic interactions in systemic lupus erythematosus. Demonstration of oscillatory levels of anti-DNA autoantibodies and reciprocal anti-idiotypic activity in a single patient. Ann. Immunol. (Inst. Pasteur) 134C:377–391.

10. Silvestris, F., Bankhurst, A.D., Searles, R.P., and Williams, R.C. (1984). Studies of anti-F(ab')$_2$ antibodies and possible immunologic control mechanisms in systemic lupus erythematosus. Arthritis Rheum. 27:1387–1396.

11. Silvestris, F., Williams R.C., Jr., Frassanito, M.A., and Dammcco, F. (1987). In vitro inhibition of anti-DNA producing cells from systemic lupus erythematosus patients by autologous anti-F(ab')$_2$ antibodies. Clin. Immunol. Immunpathol. 42:50–62.

12. Abdou, N.I., Suenaga, R., Hatfield, M., Evans, M., and Hassanein, K.M. (1989). Anti-idiotypic antibodies directed against anti-double stranded DNA antibodies in sera of families of lupus patients. J. Clin. Immunol. 9:16–21.

13. Silvestris, F., Searles, R.P., Bankhurst, A.D., and Williams, R.C. (1985). Family distribution of anti-F(ab')$_2$ antibodies in relatives with systemic lupus erythematosous. Clin. Exp. Immunol. 60:329–338.

14. Suenaga, R., Hatfield, M., Jones, E., Jones, J.V., and Abdou, N.I. (1989). Lack of correlation between HLA types and anti-idiotypic production in family members of a lupus patient. Clin. Immunol. Immunopathol. 52:126–132.

15. Lefvert, A.K., Pirskanen, R., and Svanborg, E. (1985). Anti-idiotypic antibodies, acetylcholine receptor antibodies and disturbed neuromuscular function in healthy relatives to patients with myasthenia gravis. J. Neuroimmunol. 9:41–53.

16. Hatfield, M., Evans,M., Suenaga, R., Hassanein, K.M., and Abdou, N.I. (1987). Anti-idiotypic antibody against anti-DNA in sera of laboratory personnel exposed to lupus sera or nucleic acids. Clin. Exp. Immunol. 70:26–34.

17. Hahn, B.H., and Ebling, E.M. (1984). Suppression of murine lupus nephritis by administration of an anti-idiotypic antibody to anti-DNA. J. Immunol. 132:187–190.

18. Meeker, T., Lowder, J., Cleary, M.L., Stewart, S., Warnke, R., Sklar, J., and Levy, R. (1985). Emergence of idiotype variants during treatment of B-cell lymphoma with anti-idiotype antibodies. N. Engl. J. Med. 312:1658–1665.

19. Raffeld, M., Neckers, L., Lango, D.L., and Cossman, J.(1985). Spontaneous alteration of idiotype in a monoclonal B-cell lymphoma: Escape from detection by anti-idiotype. N. Engl. J. Med. 312:1653–1658.

20. Isenberg, D.A., Shoenfeld, Y., Madaio, M.P., Rauch, J., Reichlin, M., Stollar, B.D., and Schwartz, R.S. (1984). Anti-DNA antibody idiotypes in systemic lupus erythematosus. Lancet 2:417–421.

21. Sasaki, T., Muryoi, T., Tamate, O., Ono, Y., Koide, Y., Ishida, N., and Yoshinaga, K. (1986). Selective elimination of anti-DNA antibody-producing cells by anti-idiotypic antibody conjugated with neocarzinostatin. J. Clin. Invest. 77:1382–1386.

22. Suenaga, R., Munoz, P.A., Bright, S.W., and Abdou, N.I. (1988). Spontaneous shift of anti-DNA antibody idiotypes in systemic lupus erythematosus. J. Immunol. 140:3508–3514.

23. Hahn, B.H., and Ebling, F.M. (1987). Idiotypic restriction in murine lupus; high frequency of three public idiotypes on serum IgG in nephritic NZB/NZW F1 mice. J. Immunol. 138:2110–2118.

24. Ebling, F.M., Ando, D.G., Sahakian, N.P., Kalunian, K.C., and Hahn, B.H. (1988). Idiotypic spreading promotes the production of pathogenic autoantibodies. J. Autoimmun. 1:47–61.

25. Suenaga, R., Munoz, P.A., Hon, S.H. and Abdou, N.I. (1989). Characterization of two anti-DNA antibodies bearing distinct idiotypes. Correlation with clinical manifestations. J. Autoimmun. 2:297–306.

26. Koffler, D., Schur, P.H., and Kunkel, H.G. (1967). Immunologic studies concerning the nephritis of systemic lupus erythematosus. J. Exp. Med. 26:607–623.

27. Winfield, J.B., Faiferman, I., and Koffler, D. (1977). Avidity of anti-DNA antibodies in serum and IgG glomerular eluates from patients with systemic lupus erythematosus. Association of high avidity anti-native DNA antibody with glomerulonephritis. J. Clin. Invest. 59:90–96.

28. Ebling, F.M., and Hahn, B.H. (1980). Restricted subpopulations of DNA antibodies in kidneys of mice with systemic lupus: Comparison of antibodies in serum and renal eluates. Arthritis Rheum. 23:392–403.

29. Dang, H., and Harbeck, R.J. (1984). The in vivo and in vitro glomerular deposition of isolated anti-double stranded DNA antibodies in NZB/W mice. Clin. Immunol. Immunopathol. 30:265–278.

30. Gavalchin, J., and Datta, S.K. (1987). The NZB/SWR model of lupus nephritis. II. Autoantibodies deposited in renal lesions show a distinctive and restricted idiotypic diversity. J. Immunol. 138:138–148.

31. Freddo, L., Hays, A.P., Nickerson, K.G., Spatz, L., McGinnis, S. Lieberson, R., Vedeler, C.A., Shy, M.E., Gambetti, L.A., Grauss, F.C., Petito, F., Chess, L., and Latov, N. (1986). Monoclonal anti-DNA IgM K in neuropathy binds to myelin and to a conformational epitope formed by phosphatidic acid and gangliosides. J. Immunol. 137:3821–3825.

32. Pennebaker, J.B., Gilliam, J.N., and Ziff, M. (1977). Immunoglobulin classes of DNA binding activity in serum and skin in systemic lupus erythematosus. J. Clin. Invest. 60:1331–1338.

33. Abdou, N.I., Lindsley, H.B., Pollock, A., Stechschulte, D.J., and Wood, G. (1981). Plasmapheresis in active lupus erythematosus: Effect on clinical, serum, and cellular abnormalities. Case report. Clin. Immunol. Immunopathol. 19:44–54.

34. Avrameas, S., Dighiero, G., Lymberi, P., and Guilbert, B. (1983). Studies on natural antibodies and autoantibodies. Ann. Immunol. (Inst. Pasteur) 134D:103–113.

35. Graber, P. (1983). Autoantibodies and the physiological role of immunoglobulins. Immunol. Today 4:337–340.

36. Cohen, I.R., and Cooke, A. (1986). Natural autoantibodies might prevent autoimmune disease. Immunol. Today 7:363–364.

37. Suenaga, R., and Abdou, N.I. (1988). Private idiotypes on human polyclonal IgG anti-DNA antibodies are not expressed on coexisting IgM anti-DNA antibodies in systemic lupus erythematosus. Clin. Immunol. Immunopathol. 49:251–260.

38. Madaio, M.P., Schattner, A., Schattner, M., and Schwartz, R.S. (1986). Lupus serum and normal human serum contain anti-DNA antibodies with the same idiotypic markers. J. Immunol. 137:2535–2540.

39. Davidson, A., Preud'homme, J., Solomon, A., Chang, M.Y., Beede, S., and Diamond, B. (1987). Idiotypic analysis of myeloma proteins and anti-DNA activity of monoclonal immunoglobulins bearing an SLE idiotype in man. J. Immunol. 138:1515–1518.

23

Clinical Trial Design and Concepts Specific for Biologic Agents in the Treatment of Rheumatic Diseases

Vibeke Strand

XOMA Corporation, Berkeley, and University of California San Francisco School of Medicine, San Francisco, California

I. INTRODUCTION

It is generally recognized that the current therapeutic armamentarium for treatment of rheumatoid arthritis (RA) falls short of both patients' and physicians' expectations. The limited treatment successes which have been achieved with a variety of immunosuppressive therapies, coupled with our rapidly expanding comprehension of the immune system, make biologically based therapeutic products uniquely attractive as new treatments for RA and other autoimmune diseases.

Several characteristics distinguishing the development process for biologic agents are outlined in this chapter. As illustrative examples, the experience gained in the preliminary analysis of two phase II trials in RA of a new biologic product, CD5 Plus, an immunoconjugate composed of a monoclonal antibody and a toxin moiety, is presented.

The rational and efficient development of a new biologic agent for the treatment of such autoimmune diseases as RA is difficult. Although the design of newer biologic products typically is based on scientific data, it is unclear how relevant a sound scientific rationale may be in a disease where the pathogenesis is uncertain. Animal models of this disease may not predict which agents are clinically useful. Rheumatoid arthritis is a heterogeneous disease with a variable course; it can be difficult to identify a response or a responsive patient population. It is a disease for which no definitive treatment is available. The high placebo response typically observed in clinical studies makes controlled trials a necessity in virtually every phase of development.

These difficulties are compounded by the fact that there are no universally agreed upon clinical outcome measurements to define efficacy. Across a variety of studies, multiple analytic methods have been utilized. Although criteria for response to therapy have been established, such as the "gold standard" criteria for lack of progression of x-ray changes or the American College of Rheumatology (ACR) criteria for clinical remission, neither auranofin nor methotrexate (recently approved as DMARDs, disease modifying antirheumatic drugs) have met these criteria. There is a need for a grading system which can be universally applied to assess clinical response in a disease such as RA (1).

Understandably, there exists a great deal of enthusiasm for studying new biologically based therapies in the treatment of rheumatoid arthritis. Unfortunately, we need to learn much more about this disease before the development process of a biologic agent in RA can be considered rational and efficient. Nonetheless, there are certain characteristics of biologic products which may allow more rapid evaluation of their potential efficacy, and require consideration in the design and analysis of clinical trials.

II. ISSUES SPECIFIC TO BIOLOGIC AGENTS

Several issues specific to biologics distinguish their development process from that of traditional drugs and immunosuppressives. Typically, biologic agents are given parenterally, although the future will bring designer compounds that may be orally active. For most cytokines the axiom has been to use the maximal tolerated dose (MTD), e.g. "industrial strength doses" as opposed to pharmacologic or physiologic doses. Cytokines are administered systemically; targeted delivery at a level that would mirror their physiologic function on a cell to cell basis has yet to be efficiently designed. Although the goal has been to alter very specific functions, systemic effects are usually observed.

In general, the biologic agents we study in autoimmune disease therapy have immunomodulatory functions. The goal is to utilize them as therapeutic agents to acheive either a sustained or maximal augmentation of a relevant immune effector function. To accomplish this without concomitantly diminishing other immune functions, in other words, while maintaining immune surveillance, may be difficult. Intervening in the immune system with its cell circuitry and redundant cytokine cascades remains similar to manipulating a black box. For example, how do we know when we dissect one small part of an immune function and examine it in an in vitro system, that we're relevantly mirroring an in vivo occurrence? Further, the toxicity of some of these biologic agents may exclusively be their effect on other immune effector functions.

Most biologic agents will engender some type of a human immune response; this has been true as well with the newer chimeric antibodies. Do these immune responses pose a problem? Patients take recombinant human insulin, have an immune response, and still gain clinical effect from the administered insulin. This has been noted with cytokines, is observed with monoclonal antibodies, and will be true for other biologic products. The human immune response may alter the pharmacokinetics of the administered agent, but may not change its effect. Perhaps we should consider the human immune response, not as a roadblock, but as one of many considerations in the development process of a biologic product.

III. BIOLOGIC MARKERS

A very important aspect of studying biologic agents is the use of biologic markers to measure the effect of their administration. Since most of these agents are immunomodulatory, it is appropriate to utilize an immune assay marker to indicate that the agent has been successfully administered, internalized, and noted to have had an effect. Such a marker may or may not eventually correlate with a therapeutic endpoint.

A variety of biologic markers have been used in this fashion. Based upon some of the changes in immune assays reported with long-standing methotrexate therapy, we may be close to identifying some disease-specific measures (2). Whether we can develop an efficient panel that includes disease-specific and agent-specific markers remains unclear. Furthermore, these types of immunologic assays are expensive to perform; samples must be specially transported and studied immediately. The comparability of results in a multicenter protocol must be assured. Issues relevant to the dose-response relationship for these biologic markers are critical if we are to depart from clinical doses other than MTD. Moreover, the type of clinical intervention may determine the availability of such samples. As an example, it would be ideal to perform joint aspirations and/or biopsies before and after therapy. Yet, in our studies with CD5 Plus, the rapid onset of clinical effect made it impossible to aspirate joints after therapy because the effusions had resolved.

Finally, it may be difficult to discern meaningful correlations between biologic markers and early clinical observations. By indicating when the agent has its "on" and "off" effect, biologic markers can facilitate more efficient clinical development. They may not be and may never become surrogate markers, but they make it possible to identify that the biologic product has been successfully delivered and has had a biologic effect.

IV. PHASE I STUDIES

Traditionally, Phase I studies are safety studies. They are also designed to examine a variety of characteristics about the agent in question, the one exception being efficacy. Nonetheless, it is hoped that every Phase I study will offer some inkling of potential efficacy. This may be possible with newer biologic agents particularly if they are potent and have a rapid onset of effect.

In Phase I, studies of pharmacodynamics, assays of biologic function, host immune response, and observations of clinical tolerability should be used to define the "window" of potential therapeutic effect—the active dose range. Ideally, a careful titration method will allow identification of the maximal tolerated dose (MTD) and the "no-effect" dose. With certain biologic agents that have high tolerability profiles, MTD may be the maximal amount of protein that can be administered in a given setting, and can be less specific to the product. Whether a no-effect dose can be defined depends on the agent. If it is possible, this may be the control dose utilized in subsequent studies. Although a no-effect dose may lack activity with short-term administration in a Phase I study, there is the possibility of benefit with chronic or repetitive administration in subsequent protocols, and patients may thus be offered potential clinical effect.

It is important to consider using a placebo control in a Phase I study, defining a no-effect dose, and substituting that dose for placebo in subsequent studies. An argument for employing other types of controls in later studies is the necessity for observing patients with autoimmune disease over a long period of time. As with pharmaceutical studies, it is difficult to maintain patients in a placebo arm for a sufficient period of time to then allow open label administration. And with biologic agents, it may be very difficult to perform blinded administration, given the acute effects often observed after administration of recombinant proteins in humans.

An example of such a Phase I protocol is a dose-ranging study where of six patients at a given dose level, four will receive agent and two will receive placebo (Fig. 1). This type of design is extremely useful in defining tolerability issues. Utilizing biologic markers in such a study offers additional information about the agent's activity. Using a placebo control is an early study offers the relative ease of re-enrolling patients at subsequent dose levels for a second opportunity to receive active drug. In a Phase I study, unblinding can occur at the end of a given dose level before progression to the next.

- Consider using a **control** in the first study

- 6 patients / dose level
  - 4 receive agent
  - 2 placebo

- Control for toxicity and activity

Figure 1 Phase I protocol.

In studying biologic agents, if an accurate biologic marker is available, it is possible to look at single administration of the product and after an appropriate washout period, move to repetitive administration, even in the same patient at the same dose level. A typical design consists of one-time administration, washout for 14 days during which time results of the analyses can be studied, followed by administration every day for three days. This protocol can be adhered to provided assays for serum levels and biologic activity are performed and analyzed rapidly. Results of the previous administration course can be used to accurately confirm the appropriate washout periods and readministration schedules. This can be a very efficient phase I design, allowing repetitive administration at each dose level, provided all measurements have returned to baseline prior to the next administration. Similarly, with appropriate careful monitoring, it may be possible with some agents to start with IV dosing and proceed to either IM or SQ administration. Biologic agents are uniquely suited to these types of complicated and labor-intensive Phase I studies.

As most of these agents are immunomodulators, it is important, even in the Phase I study, to enroll patients with active disease. It is unlikely that information gained in normal human subjects will be generalizable to the patient population. Many biologic products have been introduced into malignant disease settings and subsequently studied in autoimmune diseases such as rheumatoid arthritis. Again, it is not readily apparent how much of the information from a study in malignant disease can be generalized into another clinical setting. Often the issues of tolerability are distinctly different among different patient populations, not to mention confounding difficulties with concomitant medications and other organ system involvement. One is reminded of the old clinical "saw" that patients with rheumatoid arthritis are extremely sensitive to the administration of many types of drugs. Our experience with CD5 Plus has shown distinctly different tolerability profiles in patients with graft vs. host disease compared with patients with rheumatoid arthritis. Additionally, in studies of several other autoimmune diseases such as diabetes and aplastic anemia, the tolerability profile varied among the different patient populations.

Given that the agent will be studied in patients with rheumatoid arthritis, which population should be selected? Do you start with the refractory patients to whom you having nothing else to offer? If so, will you learn anything in the Phase I study? Information can be gained about tolerability. If an effect is not seen, does that mean that the agent should be abandoned; or that it should be studied in patients with earlier, presumably more modifiable disease?

There are multiple safety issues to consider in the administration of biologic products. Given the species specificity of many agents, the supraphysiologic doses, redundancy of circuitry, and our limited understanding of an intact human immune system, it may be difficult to predict the tolerability profile for a given agent. Such a profile may change significantly when the product is administered as a bolus intravenously versus as a continuous infusion, underscoring the importance of studying dose and route of administration questions separately. With many of the recombinant human proteins, it is difficult to obtain a meaningful tolerability profile in any of the short-term toxicology studies in nonhuman animals, including primates. Nor may it be possible to predict the human immune response from information in animal studies. Consequently, initial administration of a new agent must start at a very low dose, possibly 10 to 100 times lower than MTD in animal studies. With the goal to escalate to a true MTD, a well-executed Phase I study will require a wide range of doses, since early administration effects may be more difficult to predict than with a pharmaceutical agent.

Finally, what do you do if the well-designated Phase I study fails to demonstrate any effect, yet there are alterations in a biologic marker? This may suggest that a different patient population should be studied once safety data have been collected in patients with refractory disease. It may necessitate studying a different dosing regimen or more closely examining the setting in which the agent is administered. Are patients receiving too many additional agents for their disease which may mask the effect? These questions are of particular concern in a Phase I protocol where the patient will be offered little if any therapeutic benefit.

In summary, there are several important points to consider carefully in Phase I studies of biologic agents. Too often, these questions are asked belatedly in the middle of Phase II of III studies. The efficiency and technical excellence of the Phase I studies will largely determine the pace of the clinical development of product.

V. PHASE II

By definition, Phase II studies are designed to examine the potential efficacy of a product. With some biologic agents, it may be possible to combine Phase I and II type studies, depending upon the experience with the agent in other disease states. Again, it is important to select a responsive patient population. As these are early efficacy studies, it is necessary to utilize adequate washout periods, intent to treat analyses, and blinding to the treatment and dose.

It is critical to select a sensitive instrument to quantitate the "delta," or change, in order to gain information regarding the potential efficacy of the agent. This is especially true in typical Phase II, short-term studies of chronic diseases where little clinical change may be evident. This is analogous to the attempts to define surrogate markers in the recent AIDS clinical trials. In most autoimmune diseases, and certainly in rheumatoid arthritis, there are no surrogate markers or (a more preferable term) leading indicators. At the present time, the most rational procedure may be to select the biologic markers appropriate for the new agent and disease in question, to try to identify potential leading indicators and, ultimately, to validate these against clinical endpoints in subsequent longer term, multicenter controlled Phase III studies.

A potentially useful design for a Phase II study is to examine randomized treatment of a high dose versus a moderate dose, against a no-effect dose defined in the previous Phase I protocol. The moderate and high doses are selected based upon changes in pharmacodynamics or biologic markers in the earlier study; the no-effect dose could have clinical effect with either more prolonged or repetitive administration. Careful attention must be paid to the pharmacodynamics of the agent. Dose comparison studies can be difficult to interpret for efficacy unless there is a steep dose–response curve.

In Phase II studies, it is important to examine dosing and dose schedules that would be practical for treating patients in an outpatient setting. We have learned much about the self-administration of agents such as gamma interferon (IFNγ) at home, yet rheumatoid arthritis therapy is not yet like cancer chemotherapy, where complicated methods of self-administration are commonplace. As rheumatologists gain more experience with the administration of biologic agents, this situation should change very quickly. Rheumatoid arthritis will remain a disease which will be treated in an ambulatory setting. Thus, it is important, if the tolerability profile allows, to consider studying a variety of methods for parenteral administration in a come-and-go ambulatory setting.

Provided the doses are well tolerated, additional information may be gained regarding longer term treatment by continuing open label administration beyond the formal protocol time. To maximize this information patients must be followed until there is either a loss of clinical effect or toxicity intervenes. It is particularly important in rheumatoid arthritis to define specific criteria for patient dropout and subsequent treatment with another agent in order to understand the durability of clinical effect.

In addition to selecting a responsive patient population for Phase II studies, it is also necessary to select a relatively homogeneous disease population. This is true for rheumatoid arthritis, and perhaps even more relevant for multiple organ system diseases such as lupus and scleroderma. Given the relatively short period of time which these studies are conducted and the long duration of the disease process, it may be best to select disease involvement of only one or two organ systems where changes can be measured in a relatively short period of time. This has been well demonstrated in trials of systemic sclerosis. Other than skin scores, it is difficult to document changes in internal organ involvement. In a study protocol, it is equally difficult to stipulate that patients undergo invasive procedures on a regular basis in order to document potential internal changes. Similarly, there is the axiom that patients with earlier rheumatoid arthritis respond better to treatment. That observation may be confounded by the fact that there may be a more pronounced placebo response in this population. Realistically, it may be important

```
• High dose vs. low dose vs. NE dose

• Select a responsive patient population

• Utilize leading indicators
        • Biologic markers
        • MRI
        • MHAQ

• Pilot efficacy trials —> GO/NO GO decision
```

Figure 2 Considerations for Phase II protocols.

to design separate protocols for patients with early, moderate, and refractory rheumatoid arthritis.

Phase II studies are pilot efficacy studies. They should be designed to allow a "GO/NO GO" decision regarding further development of the product for that indication. This requires a careful selection of leading indicators and clinical outcome measures (Fig. 2).

VI. PHASE III STUDIES

At the end of Phase II studies, the clinical product should be well characterized. The timing of onset of therapeutic action should be known. Appropriate protocol design will proceed from a thorough understanding of the expected treatment effect, based on the earlier studies. Again, if the prior studies have not been controlled, this treatment effect can be overestimated by as much as two to three times.

It is critical when progressing to larger multicenter studies, to ensure that the patient populations are well stratified. For example, it is difficult to enroll 600 rheumatoid arthritis patients easily or efficiently, even if one has 60 centers participating. To be more efficient, and accomplish product development with a smaller number of patients, it is important to make the study population as homogeneous as possible. Several multicenter trials in early, moderate, and late disease may be the most appropriate plan.

Again, these trials should be blinded and randomized. An active controlled study with well-defined parameters for dropout and efficacy may best demonstrate the true effect of a new agent in its potential clinical setting. Provided the previous protocols have been well controlled, it may be possible to eliminate a placebo control and instead utilize an active control such as methotrexate. Both in-

```
• Select specific patient populations

• Multicenter

• Blinded; randomized

• Control:
      Active vs. accepted agent?
      Placebo with crossover to active control
      Multiple agent studies
```

Figure 3 Considerations for Phase II/III protocols.

tramuscular gold or oral methotrexate, administered once a week, are easily adapted to blinded administration. Typically, active controlled trials are less sensitive and the statistical analysis can be very problematic, unless the new therapy is clearly superior to the active control (Fig. 3).

The issues regarding placebo for biologic agents are a little different. As the majority of these products cause clinical symptoms such as fever, malaise, and fatigue following administration, careful work in the early Phase I and II trials to blunt that response with premedication (as is commonly used with chemotherapeutic agents) is necessary.

In chronic autoimmune diseases with variable courses, crossover studies remain problematic. Finally, if utilizing a placebo arm, it becomes extremely difficult to maintain patients in that arm for a significant period of time. Although that has been possible in the Cooperative Systematic Studies of the Rheumatic Diseases (CSSRD) studies, there remains the difficulty of defining the true motivation of certain patients remaining in long-term clinical studies.

It is easy to underestimate the importance of utilizing stringent criteria for drop out due to loss of clinical effect. Once patients have experienced a significant benefit from a potential new therapy, it is frustrating for them to continue in a study as the benefit is lost. In our recent trials with CD5 Plus, it was very clear that patients dropped out as their disease reactivated well *before* disease activity reached baseline (pretreatment) levels. Having experienced significant improvement made them (and their treating physicians) intolerant of even mild worsening in their disease status (Fig. 4).

Rheumatologists recognize the polypharmacy of the treatment of rheumatoid arthritis, upon which is frequently superimposed a study of new therapeutic agents.

> • Collect "early" and chronic outcome measures
>   Traditional clinical endpoints
>   Include functional and/or health status measures
>   Validate the "leading indicators" used in Phase II
>
> • Stringent criteria for lack of clinical effect vs. response
>   Paulus criteria: 20% vs. 50%
>   Total joint count vs. tenderness and swelling scores

Figure 4 Outcome measures Phase II/III protocols.

The concurrent administration of multiple DMARDs has become increasingly popular. Realizing this, and understanding certain cytokine cascades which occur in inflammatory processes, suggests that clinical trials utilizing the concurrent or simultaneous administration of multiple biologic agents are probable in the near future. This will pose additional difficulties unless each agent's effect is well characterized before sequential or combination dosing is studied.

An important component of Phase III studies is the collection of both early and later outcome measurements (Fig. 4). In RA one must use the traditional clinical endpoints and, if the study extends more than 12 months, fine detail (industrial grade) hand films should be performed. A functional or health status measurement that reflects changes the patient may perceive as important should be included. This later multicenter trial can collect the information to validate the leading indicator used in the Phase II study against clinical outcome. Ideally, utilizing the perspective gained in the Phase III study, it may be possible to correlate the biologic markers of Phase I to the leading indicators of Phase II to the final clinical outcome measurements demonstrated with long-term administration of the new agent. Although we have not been able to accomplish this with current immunosuppressive therapies, perhaps the study of biologic agents will enable us to do so in the future (Fig. 5).

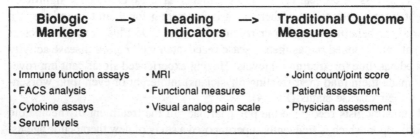

Figure 5 Correlation of biologic markers to clinical outcome measures is an important goal in the development process of biologic agents.

VII. LEADING INDICATORS →OUTCOME MEASUREMENTS

It has been possible to define surrogate markers for certain cardiovascular therapeutic applications. In the last several years, much effort has been expended with clinical trials in AIDS to define a surrogate marker for progression of disease. Peripheral CD4 T-cell counts may be the best such measure, but controversy still surrounds their use. In autoimmune diseases, and especially in rheumatoid arthritis, we have yet to define such a leading indicator. Similar to the AIDS Clinical Trials Group (ACTG) protocols, we shall have to study a variety of measures until a correlation can be validated.

Joint counts, scores, physician assessment, patient assessment, erythrocyte sedimentation rate (ESR), and morning stiffness are universally employed measures. However, significant changes in any of these parameters may not be observable in early clinical trials. Even in long-term studies, controversy exists regarding the utility of ESR, rheumatoid factor, or C-reactive protein (CRP) measurements. The rational study of a new biologic agent in autoimmune disease may require that patients undergo multiple immune function assays on a regular basis. Measuring a variety of biologic markers can be methodologically difficult, and the amount of blood drawn on a regular basis will be carefully monitored by current Investigational Review Board practices. Further, most rheumatologists believe either a health status questionnaire or a functional measurement is important, even if such measures have not been utilized in the approval process of traditional DMARDs (3–7). Pilot studies of new agents may not demonstrate significant change in the traditional clinical outcome measurements. Since no biologic marker has yet been demonstrated to correlate with clinical outcome, it is important to consider a variety of potential leading indicators which could then be standardized for Phase III studies (Fig. 6).

There are several strong candidates for "standard" leading indicators (Fig. 5). A variety of validated functional measurements may be useful, particularly for measuring response in early disease. The Modified Health Assessment

```
• Agent specific biologic markers

• MRI

• Functional measures
     • MHAQ
        • Problem elicitation technique

• Visual analog pain scale
```

Figure 6 Candidates for leading indicators.

Questionaire (MHAQ) may be a leading indicator in patients with chronic disease once significant functional impacts upon lifestyle have already occurred. The visual analog pain scale is a well validated sensitive indicator and is remarkably easy to use unless you are working with a foreign speaking patient population. The newer magnetic resonance imaging techniques (MRI) may be the best candidates for a leading indicator in early trials as they can sensitively define synovial proliferation. However, procedures are extremely expensive and require further validation.

In summary, outcome measurements should define disease modification and be capable of identifying change in the patient population selected. These measurements should be important to the patient, particularly as there are times when joint counts and scores do improve, yet patients don't feel any better. A rational "GO/NO-GO" decision regarding further development of an agent should ideally be based on an objective measurement that does not improve with placebo. We know there is a placebo response in our traditional clinical measurements, in the functional measures, and the health status questionnaires. Given the recognition of the CNS-immune system axis, it is likely a placebo response affects MRI results as well. Thus the importance of blinded controlled trials in the early phases of clinical development cannot be overestimated.

Alternatively, biologic agents may be the exception to the long rheumatologic tradition of partially effective DMARDs. If one has an agent with a very rapid onset (as can be possible with a biologic), and a very profound response, traditional clinical outcome measurements of joint counts, scores, etc. may change very quickly, even in patients with refractory disease. This may obviate the need for a "leading indicator" in the Phase II studies as efficacy may be demonstrated in a shorter period of time. Nonetheless, the utility of identifying a leading indicator would remain; with a very "powerful" new agent, such a measure could show change in a Phase I study.

VIII. COMPOSITE OUTCOME MEASUREMENTS

This brings us to the final discussion: how to select appropriate clinical outcome measurements. Efficacy parameters must be defined prior to the initiation of Phase III studies. To date, only traditional clinical measures have been utilized to support the approval of new DMARD therapies, e.g., auranofin and methotrexate (8,9), although enthusiasm among rheumatologists exists for the use of a variety of functional or health status measures (3–7). The recognition that the development process for biologic agents is sufficiently different from that for pharmaceutical products may allow for greater flexibility in the choice of composite outcome measures. Yet the broad range of agents under study may necessitate selecting such measures on a case by case basis.

The use of functional or health status measures may be more relevant to defining efficacy in earlier Phase II studies than in later multicenter trials. Phase III studies, designed to establish efficacy in a specific therapeutic setting, will require demonstration of change in traditional clinical outcome measures. At the present time efficacy, even measured by traditional parameters, is defined differently, according to the CSSRD, clinical trial consortia, and the Food and Drug Administration, Center for Drugs Evaluation and Research (FDA, CDER) which has reviewed all prior DMARD submissions.

As an example, the CSSRD defines important improvement in either swelling or tenderness joint counts as: the number of joints affected by swelling (or tenderness) at the time of evaluation compared with the number of joints affected by swelling (or tenderness) at baseline. The (number of joints improved minus the number of joints worsened at the time of evaluation) must be ≥ 30–50% of the number of joints involved at baseline. This is scored separately from patient and physician assessment of improvement (10–14).

Similarly, Weinblatt, in his trials of methotrexate, defined significant improvement as a decrease of ≥ 50% in the total joint swelling index and in the total joint pain/tenderness index. Moderate improvement was defined as 30–49% decrease in total joint indices. Again patient and physician assessment of response were scored separately (15,16).

Neither of these scoring methods allow a composite evaluation of "overall improvement." In reviewing the data for the long awaited approval for methotrexate as a DMARD, the reviewer for the FDA, CDER defined a composite improvement score. He used the CSSRD method of evaluation summing the responses as: Greater or equal to three of the four parameters as improved, or two improved with none demonstrating worsening (4).

Paulus attempted to define a "placebo response" across a variety of DMARD studies by evaluating the clinical outcome of the placebo-treated population in four CSSRD protocols (17,18). These studies examined a variety of DMARDS, from relatively "effective" agents such as methotrexate and D-penicillamine, to "mild" agents such as auranofin. He developed a composite method which excluded the response of 94% of the patients receiving placebo. This scoring method utilizes the joint tenderness score, the joint swelling score, duration of morning stiffness, ESR, and patient and physician assessment. A composite change in four of these six parameters of less than or equal to 20% improvement in the scores, length of AM stiffness, or ESR; or less than two grades improvement (out of 5) in patient or physician assessment distinguished response to placebo compared with treatment with active drug.

Such a method requires validation in a variety of other studies of potential DMARD therapy. However, it is reasonable to expect that this placebo response, identified in four different protocols over a total of six years of study, may accurately reflect the magnitude of such effect in placebo-controlled studies. This method of analysis can be (retrospectively) applied and may allow comparison between different studies (18). Paulus successfully applied his criteria to the placebo-treated patients in a fifth CSSRD study. Similarly, Weinblatt has reported the response data in patients receiving hydroxychloroquine and either subcutaneous IFNγ or placebo. The clinical response, as defined by total joint index in both groups, was high: 44% for agent; 45% for placebo (19). However, applying the Paulus criteria for ≤ 20% response identified 9% of the placebo population and 20% of the IFNγ-treated group (20).

Similarly, it may be possible to utilize a composite method, such as the "Paulus criteria" to define efficacy. The same six parameters could be scored for ≥ 40% or ≥ 50% improvement in four of the six criteria. This will require validation in a variety of studies, but can be utilized in conjunction with the application of traditional as well as functional measures of efficacy. Further, the patient and physician assessments could be converted to visual analog scales, rather than discrete graded boxes which must be checked. This would allow easy measurement of 40 or 50% improvement. And such a scale may be more accurate, as it is more difficult for both patient or physician to recall their prior responses on a scale rather than checking the same numbered box.

An example of the utility of such analyses is given in the following discussion of preliminary data from our Phase II studies of CD5 Plus in rheumatoid arthritis.

IX. CD5 PLUS TREATMENT OF RHEUMATOID ARTHRITIS

CD5 Plus is an immunoconjugate composed of a murine IgG_1 monoclonal antibody to the cell surface antigen CD5 linked to the A chain of ricin, a protein synthesis inhibitor. Ricin is a naturally occurring toxin, purified from castor beans. During manufacture the A chain is isolated from the B chain, which attaches to the cell surface and mediates internalization of the ricin molecule. In effect, the monoclonal antibody is substituted for the B chain, and thus confers specificity to the toxin moeity. The CD5 antigen is present on 95–97% of mature peripheral T cells in humans, as well as a small population of B cells which may play a role in autoantibody production. CD5 Plus is selectively cytotoxic in vitro for mature human T cells in the nanogram per milliliter concentration range. Its cytotoxic effect upon $CD5^+$ cells is three to four logs greater than the ricin A chain itself or other immunoconjugates comprised of antibodies to other cell surface antigens (21).

Clinical experience with the use of CD5 Plus was first gained in the treatment of graft vs. host disease following bone marrow transplantation. Doses utilized in these studies have ranged from 0.10 to 0.50 mg/kg/day for 10–14 days of treatment (22).

A Phase I study performed in 16 patients with RA yielded promising results. All patients had active, refractory disease, having failed at least two immunosuppressive therapies. Four patients each received doses of 0.05, 0.10, 0.20, or 0.33 mg/kg/day for 5 days. A dose response was observed in the flow cytometry (FACS) data, showing more significant depletion of $CD5^+$ T cells at doses of 0.20 and 0.33 mg/kg/day. Rapid normalization of peripheral T-cell counts occurred within 15–30 days of administration (Fig. 7), (23).

Clinically, responses were observed in eight patients, at all four doses. Long-term responses, defined as significant decreases in total joint counts and scores, were seen in three patients, lasting more than 14 months. These patients received doses of 0.05, 0.10, and 0.33 mg/kg/day, respectively, and remained off all DMARD therapy for as long as 24 months after treatment. Clinical effect was

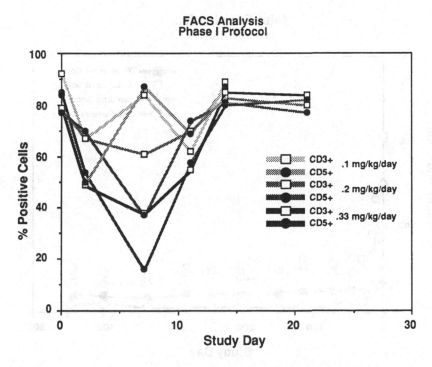

Figure 7 Flow cytometric analysis of representative patients from the Phase I study. At each dose level further depletion of $CD3^+$ and $CD5^+$ peripheral T cells can be noted. Percent positive cells plotted allows for comparison across patients.

noted within the first 30 days of administration of the agent; and continued long after normalization of the peripheral T-cell count (Fig. 8).

Mild to moderate constitutional symptoms, typical following the administration of biologic proteins, were observed during the treatment days. Fever with and without rigor, associated with nausea, fatigue, and malaise were seen. Symptoms decreased when premedication with acetaminophen, diphenhydramine, and metaclopromide was administered. In some patients, myalgias and muscle weakness were noted after later infusions, although muscle tenderness and creatine phosphokinase (CPK) elevations were rarely seen. These symptoms defined the MTD of 0.33 mg/kg/day for the five-day treatment regimen. Increased extravascular volume, manifested by pedal and/or periorbital edema, occurred after

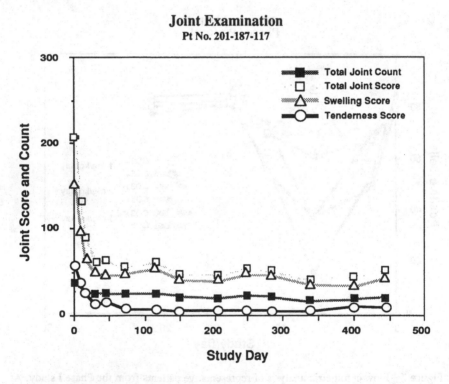

Figure 8 Joint examination scores and counts of one of the three patients with long-term (> 14 months) response in the Phase I protocol.

treatment, not associated with abnormalities of renal or hepatic function. All treatment-related symptoms resolved without sequelae.

Based on this promising information, two Phase II protocols were designed to further examine the effects of this agent in RA. We wished to extend this experience to patients with early, aggressive as well as moderate disease. We also wanted to identify potential biologic markers that would predict efficacy or identify potential responders.

The two protocols, 01 and 02, were multicenter trials, and designed to enroll patients who had failed either methotrexate or azathioprine. At the discretion of the investigator, the patient could continue to receive immunosuppressive therapy at the failed dose. CD5 Plus was administered for 5 day courses at doses of 0.20 or 0.33 mg/kg/day. The distinction between the patient enrollment in the two protocols was disease duration. In protocol 01 disease duration was not specified; in 02 it was required to be less than 3 years (Table 1).

A total of 79 patients entered the two protocols; 54 in study 01, 25 in study 02. This is a preliminary analysis of 60 of the 79 patients; 40 in 01; 20 in 02. Of these patients, a majority continued to receive prednisone in doses of 10 mg or less and a minority remained on concurrent immunosuppressive therapy (Table 2). From our preliminary analysis, the continuing administration of either methotrexate or azathioprine did not appear to confound the effect of CD5 Plus. The average disease duration of patients in study 01 was 10.8 years, in 02 it was 1.9 years. As expected, all patients in protocol 02 were functional class II.

Data from FACS analyses following treatment were similar to the pattern observed in the Phase I protocol and served as a biologic marker of drug administration. A representative example is shown in Figure 9. Again, counts normalized 30–45 days following administration of CD5 Plus. This pattern was typical of the majority of patients, although in some, changes in absolute counts were less striking. A separate study of immune function assays and more detailed FACS

Table 1 Characteristics of Patients Enrolled in the Two Phase II Protocols

01: • Failed MTX or AZA (continued in 19/40)
• Disease duration 10.8 years
• Age 50.8 years
• Functional class II or III

02: • Failed MTX (continued in 3/20)
• Disease duration 1.9 years
• Age 46.5 years
• Functional class II

Table 2 Doses of CD5 Plus and Concomitant Medication Administered to 60 Patients in the Preliminary Analysis: Protocols 01 and 02

	Protocol 01	Protocol 02
Treated	54	25
Re-treated	4	2
Interim analysis	40	20
Medication:		
CD5 Plus		
0.20	17/40	8/20
0.33	23/40	12/20
Prednisone	37/40	9/20
MTX	16/40	3/20
AZA	3/40	0/20

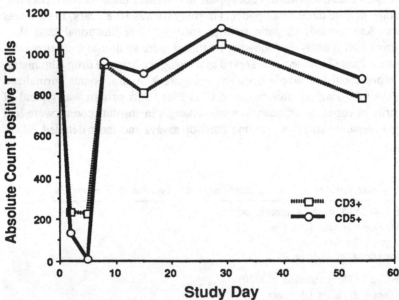

FACS Analysis
Pt No. 210-234-255

Figure 9 Flow cytometric analysis of a representative patient in protocol 02, depicting absolute number of CD3$^+$ and CD5$^+$ T cells. Maximum depletion is demonstrated at day 5 with reconstitution following.

analyses of T-cell subsets was performed on 12 of the 79 patients in both protocols who did not receive concomitant immunosuppressive therapy. Despite detailed analysis, neither the immune assays nor the FACS data were found to predict clinical response (24,25).

Total joint counts as well as scores for swelling and pain/tenderness often decreased by study day 8, three days after a single course of drug administration. In patients who had a sustained clinical response, these counts and scores remained significantly improved as long as six months post study. Joint examination results for four such patients are plotted in Figures 10–13. The total joint count is highlighted, demonstrating a ≥50% improvement in all four patients.

To study this further, we at XOMA elected to analyze the data from our Phase II studies in several different ways. We compared the composite score based on

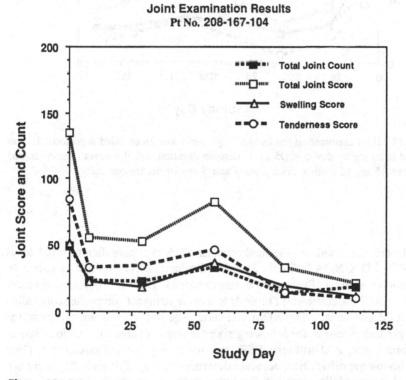

Figure 10 Joint examination results in a 57-year-old male enrolled in protocol 01 who received 0.33 mg/kg/day of CD5 Plus for 5 days. Disease duration was 9.7 years. He continued to receive 10 mg of methotrexate weekly and 10 mg of prednisone daily.

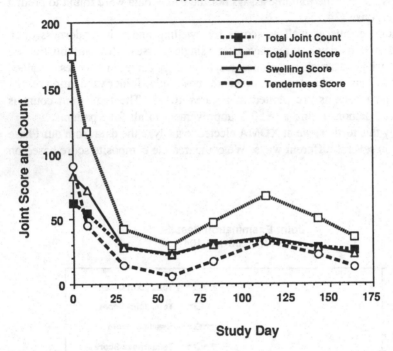

Figure 11 Joint examination results in a 61-year-old woman enrolled in protocol 01 who received 0.20 mg/kg/day of CD5 Plus. Disease duration was 9.4 years. She continued to receive 15 mg of methotrexate weekly and 8 mg of prednisone daily.

CSSRD criteria, used for the methotrexate SBA (9), hereafter referred to as "CSSRD, MTX NDA"; (Table 3) to the Paulus criteria, defined as either ≥ 20% improvement ("Paulus, 20% improvement") or ≥ 50% improvement ("Paulus, 50% improvement) (Table 4) to a more stringent composite score called the "XOMA criteria." The XOMA criteria required ≥50% improvement (or 2 of 5 grades) in four of the following six parameters (Table 5): total joint score, total joint count, AM stiffness, ESR, or patient or physician assessment. (Due to methodologic difficulties, accurate determination of ESR and CRP were not obtained at every follow-up visit. For these studies alone, the Paulus criteria were modified to include improvement in either RF, ESR, or CRP. However, this criterion was not, in effect, evaluable after month one.)

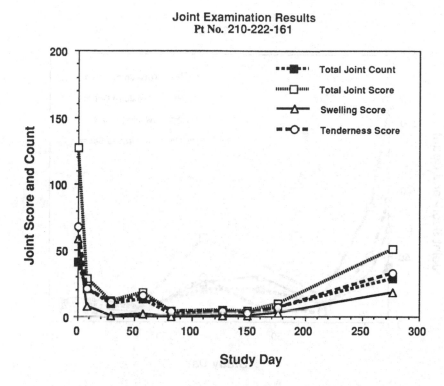

Figure 12 Joint examination results in a 48-year-old male enrolled in protocol 02 who received 0.33 mg/kg/day. Disease duration was less than one year and clinical response is still being measured at day 275. During this period of time, concomitant daily prednisone dosage of 7.5 mg was tapered to 3 mg/4 mg alternate days. He received no concomitant immunosuppressive therapy.

Table 3 Outcome Measurements for DMARDs in Rheumatoid Arthritis According to CSSRD, MTX NDA Criteria: Individual Patient Improvement—Composite Methods

Parameters	Criteria
Joint tenderness count	$\dfrac{\text{\# Improved - \# Worsened}}{\text{\# Involved at baseline}} \geq 50\%$
Joint swelling count	
Investigator assessment	≥ 3 Improved or
Patient assessment	≥ 2 Improved with none worse

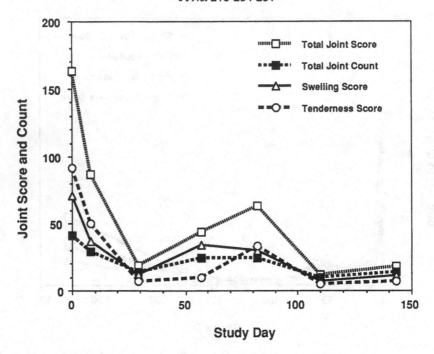

Figure 13   Joint examination results in a 44-year-old woman enrolled in protocol 02 who received .33 mg/kg/day. Concomitant medication was methotrexate 20 mg weekly.

We hoped that this comparison might help to distinguish drug effect from presumed placebo response, recognizing that these were uncontrolled trials, and the data preliminary. We present this as an attempt to quantify the magnitude of response to therapy and agree that it well may be overestimated. We plan to use this data to design the next controlled trial and to select the appropriate outcome measures for subsequent protocols.

We applied these four methods to the patients in protocol 02, patients with early disease (Table 6). Of the 20 patients, 30 days following treatment the CSSRD criteria indicated all patients had responded. The Paulus 50% improvement criteria and the XOMA criteria identified 15 responders. For comparison purposes, the

Table 4 Outcome Measurements for DMARDs in Rheumatoid Arthritis According to Paulus Criteria:
Individual Patient Improvement—Composite Methods

Parameters	Criteria
Joint tenderness score	≥ 4 Improved by 50%
Joint Swelling score	or
AM Stiffness	Improvement by 2 of 5 grades
ESR	≥ 4 Improved by 20%
Investigator assessment	or
Patient Assessment	Improvement by 2 of 5 grades

Excludes 94% of placebo patients in 4 CSSRD studies (range 71–97%) (18).

Table 5 Outcome Measurements for DMARDs in Rheumatoid Arthritis According to XOMA Analysis:
Individual Patient Improvement—Composite Methods

Parameters	Criteria
Total joint score	≥ 4 Improved by ≥ 50%
Total joint count	or
AM stiffness	2 of 5 Grades
ESR	
Investigator assessment	
Patient assessment	

Table 6 Rheumatoid Arthritis Phase II Interim Analysis, Composite Response Criteria: Protocol 02

	Month 1	Month 2	Month 3	Month 4	Month 5
Evaluable Patients	20	17	13	4	3
Patients Improved					
CSSRD, MTX NDA	20	12	6	2	3
Paulus Criteria (≥ 20%)	17	7	6	2	3
Paulus Criteria (≥ 50%)	15	7	5	2	2
XOMA Criteria	15	7	4	2	2
Total Joint Count (≥ 50%)	14	8	2	2	2
Exited	0	3	3	7	1
Follow up pending	0	0	1	2	0

number of patients with $\geq 50\%$ improvement in total joint count was 14. As one follows this analysis out to months two through five of the study several points become evident. In general, the CSSRD, MTX NDA criteria tended to overestimate the number of responders; the XOMA criteria appear more stringent. Beyond month three and later, the number of responders identified by any of the criteria become the same.

If we look at the specific analyses according to each composite method, the reasons for this convergence become clear (Tables 7–10). At the first and second months the patient and physician were both impressed by the drug's effect, consistently more than the changes seen in either joint tenderness or swelling counts. By the time month three responses were analyzed, there was more consistent agreement among the criteria. We interpret this to be related to a placebo effect which is progressively lost from month one to three.

In summary, all of the patients can be classified as responders at month one using the most lenient criteria, and 75% by the most stringent. Using an intent to treat analysis (thereby including all those for whom data are not yet available, or who have exited the study), 10% have sustained responses identified at months five and six.

Table 7 CSSRD, MTX NDA Criteria, Protocol 02

		Month 1	Month 2	Month 3	Month 4	Month 5
# of patients		20	17	13	4	3
Improvement	: Tender joint count	13	10	2	2	2
	: Swollen joint count	13	10	3	2	2
	: Pt. impress of drug	19	9	6	3	3
	: Phys. impress of drug	20	12	6	2	3
No change	: Tender joint count	7	5	8	2	1
	: Swollen joint count	7	5	8	2	1
	: Pt. impress of drug	1	7	4	0	0
	: Phys. impress of drug	0	4	5	1	0
Worsening	: Tender joint	0	2	3	0	0
	: Swollen joint	0	2	2	0	0
	: Pt. impress drug	0	1	3	1	0
	: Phys. impress drug	0	1	2	1	0
Overall Response	: Better	20	12	6	2	3
	: No Change	0	4	4	1	0
	: Worse	0	1	3	1	0
# Not Evaluated	: Exited	3	3	7	1	1
	: Follow up pending	0	1	2	0	1

Table 8 Paulus Criteria, 20% Improvement, Protocol 02

		Month 1	Month 2	Month 3	Month 4	Month 5
# of patients		20	17	13	4	3
Improvement	: Tender joint score	15	13	8	4	3
	: Swollen joint score	16	12	6	2	2
	: Morning stiffness	17	10	7	3	3
	: Either RF, CRP or ESR	5	0	0	0	0
	: Pt. impress of drug	19	9	6	3	3
	: Phys. impress of drug	20	12	6	2	3
Overall Response	: Yes	17	7	6	2	3
	: No	3	10	7	2	0
# Not Evaluated	: Exited	3	3	7	1	1
	: Follow up pending	0	1	2	0	1

Table 9 Paulus Criteria, 50% Improvement, Protocol 02

		Month 1	Month 2	Month 3	Month 4	Month 5
# of patients		20	17	13	4	3
Improvement	: Tender joint score	12	11	4	2	2
	: Swollen joint score	13	11	4	2	2
	: Morning stiffness	16	10	6	3	3
	: Either RF, CRP or ESR	4	0	0	0	0
	: Pt. impress of drug	19	9	6	3	3
	: Phys. impress of drug	20	12	6	2	3
Overall Response	: Yes	15	7	5	2	2
	: No	5	10	8	2	1
# Not Evaluated	: Exited	3	3	7	1	1
	: Follow up pending	0	1	2	0	1

Table 10 XOMA Criteria, Protocol 02

		Month 1	Month 2	Month 3	Month 4	Month 5
# of patients		20	17	13	4	3
Improvement	: Total joint score	15	10	4	2	2
	: Total joint count	14	8	2	2	2
	: Morning stiffness	16	10	6	3	3
	: Either RF, CRP or ESR	4	0	0	0	0
	: Pt. impress of drug	19	9	6	3	3
	: Phys. impress of drug	20	12	6	2	3
Overall Response	: Yes	15	7	4	2	2
	: No	5	10	9	2	1
# Not Evaluated	: Exited	3	3	7	1	1
	: Follow up pending	0	1	2	0	1

Examining protocol 01, in patients with longer duration disease, there is a broader spread in the composite response criteria (Table 11). The most stringent criterion, $\geq 50\%$ decrease in total joint count, identifies a subset of the responding patients at each interval (Tables 12–15). The CSSRD, MTX NDA score overestimates responders, and the other composite criteria come to agreement by month three. Examining the individual scores, again there is an impressive

Table 11 Rheumatoid Arthritis Phase II Interim Analysis, Composite Response Criteria: Protocol 01

	Month 1	Month 2	Month 3	Month 4	Month 5
Evaluable Patients	40	32	18	12	7
Patients Improved					
CSSRD, MTX NDA	25	14	9	7	5
Paulus Criteria ($\geq 20\%$)	27	11	10	7	5
Paulus Criteria ($\geq 50\%$)	**19**	9	5	7	5
XOMA Criteria	**13**	7	6	6	5
Total Joint Count ($\geq 50\%$)	7	5	6	3	3
Exited	0	8	10	3	3
Follow up pending	0	0	4	4	2

Table 12 CSSRD, MTX NDA Criteria, Protocol 01

		Month 1	Month 2	Month 3	Month 4	Month 5
# of patients		40	32	18	12	7
Improvement	: Tender joint count	14	7	7	8	5
	: Swollen joint count	10	11	7	3	4
	: Pt. impress of drug	28	16	8	7	5
	: Phys. impress of drug	24	15	9	8	6
No change	: Tender joint count	22	22	10	3	1
	: Swollen joint count	26	18	11	9	3
	: Pt. impress of drug	8	8	5	3	2
	: Phys. impress of drug	15	13	5	2	1
Worsening	: Tender joint count	4	3	1	1	1
	: Swollen joint count	4	3	0	0	0
	: Pt. impress of drug	4	8	5	2	0
	: Phys. impress of drug	1	4	4	2	0
Overall Response	: Better	25	14	9	7	5
	: No Change	12	15	6	5	2
	: Worse	3	3	3	0	0
# Not Evaluated	: Exited	0	8	10	3	3
	: Follow up pending	0	0	4	4	2

response in patient and physician assessment, which carries the analysis for the CSSRD criteria, but which is less prominent in the other composite methods. Comparing the XOMA criteria with the Paulus 50% improvement indicates total joint scores to be more lenient than total joint count, but this difference diminishes after month two.

Table 13 Paulus Criteria, 20% Improvement, Protocol 01

		Month 1	Month 2	Month 3	Month 4	Month 5
# of patients		40	32	18	12	7
Improvement	: Tender joint score	30	15	13	9	6
	: Swollen joint score	24	18	12	9	6
	: Morning stiffness	22	15	12	10	6
	: Either RF, CRP or ESR	19	0	0	0	0
	: Pt. impress of drug	28	16	8	7	5
	: Phys. impress of drug	24	15	9	8	6
Overall Response	: Yes	27	11	10	7	5
	: No	13	21	8	5	2
# Not Evaluated	: Exited	0	8	10	3	3
	: Follow up pending	0	0	4	4	2

Table 14 Paulus Criteria, 50% Improvement, Protocol 01

		Month 1	Month 2	Month 3	Month 4	Month 5
# of patients		40	32	18	12	7
Improvement	: Tender joint score	19	8	7	8	6
	: Swollen joint score	10	11	7	4	4
	: Morning stiffness	19	13	11	9	6
	: Either RF, CRP or ESR	13	0	0	0	0
	: Pt. impress of drug	28	16	8	7	5
	: Phys. impress of drug	24	15	9	8	6
Overall Response	: Yes	19	9	5	7	5
	: No	21	23	13	5	2
# Not Evaluated	: Exited	0	8	10	3	3
	: Follow up pending	0	0	4	4	2

Table 15 XOMA Criteria, Protocol 01

		Month 1	Month 2	Month 3	Month 4	Month 5
# of patients		40	32	18	12	7
Improvement	: Total joint score	13	8	7	6	6
	: Total joint count	7	5	6	3	3
	: Morning stiffness	19	13	11	9	6
	: Either RF, CRP or ESR	13	0	0	0	0
	: Pt. impress of drug	28	16	8	7	5
	: Phys. impress of drug	24	15	9	8	6
Overall Response	: Yes	13	7	6	6	5
	: No	27	25	12	6	2
# Not Evaluated	: Exited	0	8	10	3	3
	: Follow up pending	0	0	4	4	2

Thirty days following treatment, 33% of the patients with moderate disease can be considered responders. At months five and six, 12.5% continue to show clinical benefit, using all the composite criteria. The magnitude of the acute improvement in both studies appears to be impressive and may be comparable to methotrexate or cyclosporine (26) but will require future controlled trials to be accurately assessed.

Further, in a controlled trial it will be interesting to study the correlation between patient and physician assessment and objective measures of joint pain/tenderness and swelling. From this preliminary analysis it is not clear that these outcome parameters vary in parallel. This may be a phenomenon of treatment with a new biologic agent, not dissimilar to the high placebo response observed with parenteral administration of IFNγ by Weinblatt (19).

Methodologically, this analysis offers several points for consideration. We believe that it is worthwhile to pursue a composite scoring system so that individual patient responses may be more readily compared. We are planning to utilize both the Paulus 50% improvement and the XOMA criteria for efficacy analysis in future controlled trials of CD5 Plus. We hope to correlate functional measures and visual analog pain scores with these composite criteria. Finally we believe the Paulus 20% criteria may be useful in identifying those patients for whom placebo effect is not the cause for their clinical improvement.

This is an exciting time for the development of new therapeutic agents for the treatment of autoimmune diseases. The unique properties of biologically based products may indeed offer us the opportunity to finally correlate scientific data with ultimate clinical outcome. This is a learning process that will require continuing cooperation between academic and clinical investigators, the biotechnology industry, and regulatory agencies.

REFERENCES

1. Williams, J.H. (1990). Methods of clinical measurement. Curr. Opin. Rheumatol. 2:309.
2. Weinblatt, M.E., Trentham, D.E., Fraser, P.A., Holdsworth, D.E., Falchuk, K.R., Weissman, B.N., and Coblyn, J.S. (1988). Long-term prospective trial of low-dose methotrexate in rheumatoid arthritis. Arthr. Rheum. 31:167.
3. Bombardier, C., Ware, J. Russell, I.J., Larson, M., Chalmers, A., Read, J. L., and the Auranofin Cooperating Group. (1986). Auranofin therapy and quality of life in patients with rheumatoid arthritis. Am. J. Med. 81:565.
4. Tugwell, P., Bombardier, C., Watson, B.W., Goldsmith, C., Grace, E., Bennett, K.J., Williams, H.J., Egger, M., Alarcón, G.S., Guttadauria, M., Yarboro, C., Polisson, R.P., Szydlo, L., Luggen, M.E., Billingsley, L.M., Ward, J.R., and Marks, C. (1990). Impact of quality of life assessed by traditional standard-item and individualized patient preference health status questionnaires. Arch. Int. Med. 150:59.

5. Liang, M.H. (1988). Functional and health status or quality of life measures: state of the art. In: Proceedings: Early Decisions in DMARD Development. Arthritis Foundation, Atlanta, Georgia, pp. 97–103.

6. Bellamy, N., Meenan, R., Fries, J., Tugwell, P., and Gerber, L. (1988). Panel discussion. New functional measures: do they overcome problems and how can they be improved? In: Proceedings: Early Decisions in DMARD Development. Arthritis Foundation, Atlanta, Georgia, pp. 121–133.

7. Weisman, M.H. (1988). Discussion VII. In: Proceedings: Early Decisions in DMARD Development. Arthritis Foundation, Atlanta, Georgia, pp. 134–137.

8. Summary Basis of Approval, Auranofin, NFS 18–689, Food and Drug Administration, U.S. Department of Health and Human Services (5/24/85).

9. Summary Basis of Approval, Methotrexate, NDA 8085/S028, Food and Drug Administration, U.S. Department of Health and Human Services (10/31/88).

10. Williams, J.H., Ward, J.R., Reading, J.C., Egger, M.J., Grandone, J.T., Samuelson, C.O., Furst, D.E., Sullivan, J.M., Watson, M.A., Guttadauria, M., Cathcart, E.S., Kaplan, S.B., Halla, J.T., Weinstein, A., and Plotz, P.H. (1983). Low-dose D-penicillamine therapy in rheumatoid arthritis. Arthr. Rheum. 26:581.

11. Ward, J.R., Williams, J.H., Egger, M.J., Reading, J.C., Boyce, E., Altz-Smith, M., Samuelson Jr., C.O., Willkens, R.F., Solsky, M.A., Hayes, S.P., Blocka, K.L, Weinstein, A., Meenan, R.F., Guttadauria, M., Kaplan, S.B., and Klippel, J. (1983). Comparison of auranofin, gold sodium thiomalate, and placebo in the treatment of rheumatoid arthritis. Arthr. Rheum. 26: 1303.

12. Paulus, H.E., Williams, H.J., Ward, J.R., Reading, J.C., Egger, M.J., Coleman, M.L., Samuelson, Jr., C.O., Willkens, R.F., Guttadauria, M., Alarcón, G.S. Kaplan, S.B., MacLaughlin, E.J., Weinstein, A., Wilder, R.L., Solsky, M.A., and Meenan, R.F. (1984). Azathioprine versus D-penicillamine in rheumatoid arthritis patients who have been treated unsuccessfully with gold. Arthr. Rheum. 27: 721.

13. Williams, H.J., Willkens, R.F., Samuelson Jr., C.O., Alarcón, G.S., Guttadauria, M., Yarboro, C., Polisson, R.P., Weiner, S.R., Luggen, M.E., Billingsley, L.M., Dahl, S.L., Egger, M.J., Reading, J.C., and Ward, J.R. (1985). Comparison of low-dose oral pulse methotrexate and placebo in the treatment of rheumatoid arthritis. Arthr. Rheum. 28:721.

14. Williams, H.J., Ward, J.R., Dahl, S.L., Clegg, D.O., Willkens, R.F., Oglesby, T., Weisman, M.H., Schlegel, S., Michaels, R.M., Luggen, M.E., Polisson, R.P., Singer, J.Z., Kantor, S.M., Shiroky, J.B., Small, R.E., Gomez, M.I., Reading, J.C., and Egger, M.J. (1988). A controlled trial comparing sulfasalazine, gold sodium thiomalate, and placebo in rheumatoid arthritis. Arthr. Rheum. 31:702.

15. Weinblatt, M.E., Coblyn, J.S., Fox, D.A., Fraser, P.A., Holdsworth, D.E., Glass, D.N., and Trentham, D.E. (1985). Efficacy of low-dose methotrexate in rheumatoid arthritis. N. Engl. J. Med. 312: 818.

16. Weinblatt, M.E., Kaplan, H., Germain, B.F., Merriman, R.C., Solomon, S.D., Wall, B., Anderson, L., Block, S., Irby, R., Wolfe, F., Gall, E., Torretti, D., Biundo, J., Small, R., Coblyn, J., and Polisson, R. (1990). Low-dose methotrexate compared with auranofin in adult rheumatoid arthritis. Arthr. Rheum. 33:330.

17. Paulus, H.E. (1988). Pilot efficacy studies: Identifying their role in drug development and rationale for their use: Paulus model. In: Proceedings: Early Decisions in DMARD Development. Arthritis Foundation, Atlanta, Georgia, pp. 56–58.
18. Paulus, H.E., Egger, M.J., Ward, J.R., Williams, H.J., and the Cooperative Systematic Studies of Rheumatic Diseases Group. (1990). Analysis of improvement in individual rheumatoid arthritis patients treated with disease-modifying antirheumatic drugs, based on the findings in patients treated with placebo. Arthr. Rheum. 33: 477.
19. Weinblatt, M.E. (1990). Substantial placebo response with parenteral therapy in active rheumatoid arthritis. 33:S152.
20. Weinblatt, M.E. (1990). Personal communication.
21. Investigational Drug Brochure: XomaZyme CD5 Plus, June 14, 1990.
22. Byers, V.S., Henslee, P.J., Kernan, N.A., Blazar, B.R., Gingrich, R., Phillips, G.L., LeMaistre, C.F., Gilliland, G., Antin, J.H., Martin, P., Tutscha, P.J., Trown, P., Ackerman, S.K., O'Reilly, R.J., and Scannon, P.J. (1990). Use of an anti-pan T-lymphocyte ricin A chain immunotoxin in steroid-resistant acute graft-versus-host disease. Blood 75: 1426.
23. Caperton, E., Byers, V., Shepard, J., Ackerman, S., and Scannon, P.J. (1989). Treatment of refractory rheumatoid arthritis (RA) with antilymphocyte immunotoxin. Arthr. Rheum. 24: S130.
24. Byers, V.S., Scannon, P., Fishwild, D. Henkel, C., Hall, M., Drajesk, J., Ackerman, S., and Strand, V. (1990). Patients with rheumatoid arthritis treated with a pan-T-lymphocyte immunotoxin; Phase II studies. FASEB 4: A1855.
25. Strand, V., and Fishwild, D. and the XOMA Rheumatoid Arthritis Investigators Group (1990). Treatment of rheumatoid arthritis with an anti-CD 5 immunoconjugate: clinical and immunologic findings and preliminary results of re-treatment. Arthr. Rheum. 33: S25.
26. Tugwell, P. Bombardier, C., Gent, M., Bennett, K.J., Bensen, W.G., Carette, S., Chalmers, A., Esdaile, J.M., Klinkhoff, A.V., Kraag, G.R., Ludwin, D., and Roberts, R.S. (1990). Low-dose cyclosporin versus placebo in patients with rheumatoid arthritis. Lancet 305:1051.
27. Nordstrom, D.M., West, S.G., Andersen, P.A., and Sharp, J.T. (1987). Pulse methotrexate therapy in rheumatoid arthritis. Ann. Int. Med. 107: 797.
28. Tugwell, P., Bennett, K., and Gent, M. (1987). Methotrexate in rheumatoid arthritis. Ann. Int. Med. 107: 358.
29. Kremer, J.M., and Lee, J.K. (1988). A long-term prospective study of the use of methothrexate in rheumatoid arthritis. Arthr. Rheum 31: 577.
30. Cannon, G.W., Pincus, S.H., Emkey, R.D., Denes, A., Cogen, S.A., Wolfe, F., Saway, P.A., Jaffer, A.M., Weaver, A.L., Cogen L., and Schindler, J.D. (1989). Double-blind trial of recombinant γ-interferon versus placebo in the treatment of rheumatoid arthritis. Arthr. Rheum. 32: 964.
31. Weinblatt, M.E., and Maier, A.E. (1990). Longterm experience with low dose weekly methotrexate in rheumatoid arthritis. J. Rheumatol. 17 (Suppl. 22): 33.
32. Cannon, G.W., Emkey, R.D., Denes, A., Cohen, S.A., Saway, P.A., Wolfe, F., Jaffer, A.M., Weaver, A.L., Cohen, L., Gulinello, J., Kennedy, S.M., and Schindler, J.D. (1990). Prospective two-year followup of recombinant interferon-γ in rheumatoid arthritis. J. Rheumatol. 17: 304.

Index

About the Editor

Thomas F. Kresina is an Associate Professor of Medicine at the Program in Geographic Medicine and in the Division of Rheumatology, the Miriam Hospital, Brown University, as well as Director of Research at the Program in Geographic Medicine, Brown University International Health Institute, Providence, Rhode Island. The author of over 100 papers, articles, abstracts, and book chapters, Dr. Kresina is a member of the American Association of Pathologists, American Association of Immunologists, Orthopedic Research Society, New York Academy of Sciences, American Association for the Advancement of Science, and American Federation for Clinical Research, among others. He received the B.S. degree (1975) in biomedical engineering from the Catholic University of America, Washington, D.C., and Ph.D. degree (1979) in biochemistry from the University of Alabama in Birmingham.

Printed in the United States
by Baker & Taylor Publisher Services

Printed in the United States
by Baker & Taylor Publisher Services